Community Mental Health

Lois A. Ritter, EdD, MA, MS
California State University, East Bay

Shirley Manly Lampkin, RN, MSN, PhD
University of California at San Francisco, School of Nursing

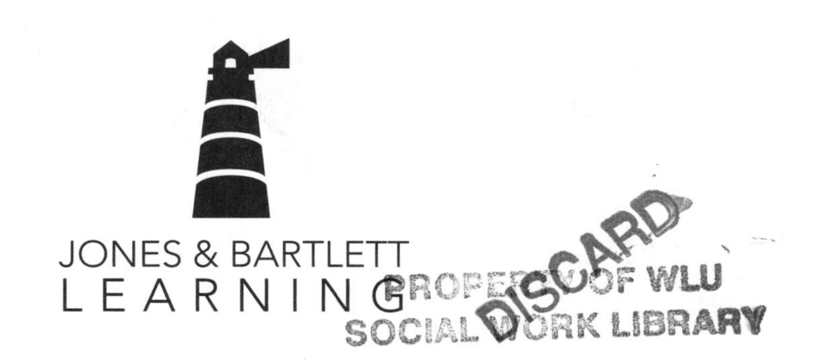

World Headquarters
Jones & Bartlett Learning
40 Tall Pine Drive
Sudbury, MA 01776
978-443-5000
info@jblearning.com
www.jblearning.com

Jones & Bartlett Learning
Canada
6339 Ormindale Way
Mississauga, Ontario L5V 1J2
Canada

Jones & Bartlett Learning
International
Barb House, Barb Mews
London W6 7PA
United Kingdom

Jones & Bartlett Learning books and products are available through most bookstores and online booksellers. To contact Jones & Bartlett Learning directly, call 800-832-0034, fax 978-443-8000, or visit our website, www.jblearning.com.

Substantial discounts on bulk quantities of Jones & Bartlett Learning publications are available to corporations, professional associations, and other qualified organizations. For details and specific discount information, contact the special sales department at Jones & Bartlett Learning via the above contact information or send an email to specialsales@jblearning.com.

Production Credits
Publisher, Higher Education: Cathleen Sether
Senior Acquisitions Editor: Shoshanna Goldberg
Senior Associate Editor: Amy L. Bloom
Editorial Assistant: Prima Bartlett
Production Manager: Julie Champagne Bolduc
Production Assistant: Sean Coombs
Associate Marketing Manager: Jody Sullivan
V.P., Manufacturing and Inventory Control: Therese Connell
Project Management: Thistle Hill Publishing Services, LLC
Composition: Dedicated Business Solutions
Cover Design: Kristin E. Parker
Photo Research and Permissions Supervisor: Christine Myaskovsky
Associate Photo Researcher: Sarah Cebulski
Cover Images: (background) © Wingedsmile/Dreamstime.com; (left to right) © Ron Chapple Studios/Dreamstime.com, © Felix Mizioznikov/ShutterStock, Inc., © Arne9001/Dreamstime.com, © Monkey Business Images/ShutterStock, Inc.
Printing and Binding: Malloy, Inc.
Cover Printing: Malloy, Inc.

Library of Congress Cataloging-in-Publication Data
Ritter, Lois A.
Community mental health / Lois A. Ritter, Shirley Manly Lampkin.
p. ; cm.
Includes bibliographical references and index.
ISBN-13: 978-0-7637-8380-8 (pbk.)
ISBN-10: 0-7637-8380-3 (pbk.)
1. Community mental health services. I. Lampkin, Shirley Manly. II. Title.
[DNLM: 1. Community Mental Health Services. 2. Mental Disorders—prevention & control. 3. Mental Health. WM 30]
RA790.R526 2011
362.196′89–dc22

2010033532

6048

Printed in the United States of America
14 13 12 11 10 10 9 8 7 6 5 4 3 2 1

DEDICATION

To my brother Gary, who taught me about love and life by never saying too much but by showing me the way. The gifts that he has given to me are priceless, and I am eternally grateful. —LR

I am deeply indebted to my parents, Edward and Doris Manly. Most of what is good in me seems to have come from you. I would like to thank my mother in particular for her unwavering support and encouragement. She consistently had more confidence in me than I had in myself. Mother, you were my number-one fan. I miss and love you tremendously. To my sisters Sandra and Mildred, and brothers Robert, David, and Timothy, and to my godparents, Mr. and Mrs. Robert Brewer and Mr. and Mrs. Ray Roundtree and Joyce, thank you all for your love and kindness. —SML

CONTENTS

PREFACE

The past century has brought about remarkable progress in public health through innovation and research in medical and social science. These achievements are extraordinary; however, mental health and illness continue to be neglected and viewed as ancillaries to physical health. Tragic and devastating disorders such as schizophrenia, depression, bipolar disorder, Alzheimer's disease, autism, and other mental disorders affect nearly 1 in 5 Americans in any year, yet these conditions frequently continue to be spoken of in whispers and with shame. In addition, our communities are inundated with conditions such as substance abuse, violence, and child and elder abuse. Mental health advocates as well as researchers, scientists, government officials, and consumers have supported the idea that mental health be integrated into mainstream health. The authors of this book agree with that ideology and approach.

Studies related to psychological, behavioral, and societal events are an exciting and dynamic area of scientific research and human inquiry. The completion of the human genome project as well as other biological and social research endeavors have contributed to contemporary mental health research and deepen the understanding of how mental and physical health are integrated.

We know more today about how to treat mental illness effectively and appropriately than we know with certainty about how to prevent mental illness and promote mental health. For obvious reasons we need to increase our efforts on prevention; this area is in need of immediate attention.

The mental health field is plagued by disparities in the availability of and access to its services. These disparities can easily be seen through racial and ethnic lenses, but these are not the only disparity lines. A key contributor to mental health disparities is financial status. Financial barriers sometimes prevent access to mental health care, whether one has health insurance with inadequate mental health benefits or is one of the 46 million Americans who lack health insurance at all. Over time, we have allowed stigma, lack of mental health services, and other barriers to seeking mental health services to exist. It is time to remove these barriers.

Promoting mental health for all Americans will require scientific knowledge but, even more importantly, a societal commitment to the needed investment. The investment does not call for massive budgets; rather, it calls for the willingness of each of us to educate ourselves and others about mental health and illness and to confront the attitudes, fear, and misunderstanding that remain as barriers before us. It is our intent that *Community Mental Health* will help usher this needed education and commitment.

This book is primarily written for public health professionals working in the area of mental health. The target audience includes community outreach workers, public health program planners and evaluators, social workers, and program administrators. The book does not cover the clinical aspects of mental health care, such as psychopharmacology. The content does include a wide breadth of topics related to community mental health including indicators of illness and problems (e.g., violence), methods of prevention and promotion, evaluation, and research. The overarching goal is to provide the essential skills, tools, and knowledge to enable mental health professionals to identify and help prevent mental health problems and provide effective programs for communities encountering symptoms of mental disorders or illness.

To accomplish this overarching goal, the authors have divided this book into five units. Each unit, with the exception of Unit V, has two or more chapters with common themes.

Unit I, "Understanding Mental Illness," begins with Chapter 1, "Foundations of Community Mental Health and Illness," which defines terminology and key concepts that set the foundation for the remainder of the text. It addresses the history of mental illness and common stigmas and myths. Chapter 2, "Fundamentals of Mental Illness," addresses the etiology, types, symptoms, diagnosis, and treatment methods. Chapter 3 explores how culture and mental health interact. It discusses the ways that mental health and illness are perceived by different cultures and factors that healthcare professionals need to consider when working with diverse communities. Culture-bound syndromes are explained, and the chapter ends with a discussion of the role of discrimination and mental illness in specific racial and ethnic groups.

Unit II, "Governance and the Mental Health Care System," addresses legal issues for mental health professionals working with mentally ill patients on an individual and community level and the mental health care system. Chapter 4, "Legal and Ethical Issues in Mental Health Practice," explains laws and regulations that limit and protect mentally ill patients, communities, and healthcare professionals. Ethical principles and decision-making guidelines are discussed to assist mental health community professionals in making the difficult ethical decisions they encounter. Chapter 5, "The Mental Health Care System," provides information that will help healthcare professionals work within the system and better equip them to help patients, families, and communities understand the complex mental health system and how to maneuver through it. The content in this chapter will be useful to those working in community mental health to comprehend the policies and resources that impact the treatment process.

Unit III, "Mental Health Across the Lifespan," addresses mental health and illness during three broad stages of life. Chapter 6 focuses on children and adolescents, Chapter 7 concentrates on adults, and Chapter 8 spotlights older adults. The common mental health challenges and illnesses that occur at each stage of life are described.

Unit IV, "Community Mental Health," provides an overview of community problems and interventions. Chapters 9 to 12 describe common community mental health problems that our communities are struggling with today, such as violence in schools, gangs, and substance abuse. The section ends with Chapter 13, "Prevention and Health Promotion in Community Mental Health," which focuses on prevention strategies and frameworks, mental health promotion, and research, as well as planning and evaluating community mental health programs.

Unit V contains Chapter 14, "A Vision for the Future." This final chapter explores the agenda for community change to improve the services and care for mentally ill patients and families and to promote and implement prevention programs. It further addresses the general changes that are needed and encourages professionals to assist with moving our nation forward in terms of mental health prevention and treatment and reducing or eliminating stigmas.

Instructor resources, including PowerPoint Presentations, an Instructor's Manual, and TestBank questions, are available as free instructor downloads. Contact your sales representative for access.

We hope that the information contained in the book will introduce you to the causes, diagnosis, treatment, and prevention of mental health and illness at the community level. This book is intended to be the beginning of your journey to helping build and implement prevention programs, improving mental health care treatment and the systems in which they reside, and reducing the stigmas that exist so our nation can advance prevention methods and reduce—and we hope eliminate—barriers to mental health care treatment for all Americans.

ACKNOWLEDGMENTS

Although there are two names on the cover of this book, numerous people contributed, and we would like to express our gratitude to them. We extend a special thanks to those who provided us with permission to reprint their work in this textbook. We also are grateful to the Jones & Bartlett Learning team, who assisted with the writing, editing, design, and marketing of this book. We would like particularly to acknowledge Shoshanna Goldberg and Amy Bloom at Jones & Bartlett Learning for their efforts. We are indebted to the reviewers for their thoughtful and valuable suggestions: Karen Sladyk, PhD, OTR, FAOTA, Bay Path College, and Gerald "Jerry" Thompson, MSN, RN, Samuel Merritt University, San Mateo Learning Center. We also are grateful to Leslie Mueller and Jenny Le, students at California State University, East Bay, who assisted with the development of the ancillary materials that accompany this text. Our families, friends, and colleagues are probably the most deserving of our gratitude. They provided continuous encouragement, support, and recognition throughout the process.

ABOUT THE AUTHORS

Lois A. Ritter, EdD, MA, MS, is an assistant professor in the nursing and health sciences department at California State University, East Bay. She teaches community health, research, and evaluation classes. Dr. Ritter does consulting work in public health and education. She has more than 20 years of experience in the healthcare field and has designed and implemented community programs and conducted evaluations at both the statewide and national levels. She has a doctorate in education and master's degrees in health science and anthropology.

Shirley D. Manly Lampkin, RN, MSN, PhD, has more than 25 years of experience developing and implementing community-based health promotion and prevention programs, working with vulnerable populations and speaking on diversity in health care locally and abroad. She lectures in the departments of community health systems, family health care, and physiological nursing at the University of California at San Francisco, School of Nursing. Dr. Manly Lampkin has won numerous prestigious awards for her accomplishments and contributions to the community and nursing and serves on several boards. She received her bachelor's and master's degrees at Samuel Merritt School of Nursing and her doctorate at the University of California at San Francisco School of Nursing where she currently serves as Dean of Academic Services and Diversity Enhancement.

UNIT I Understanding Mental Illness

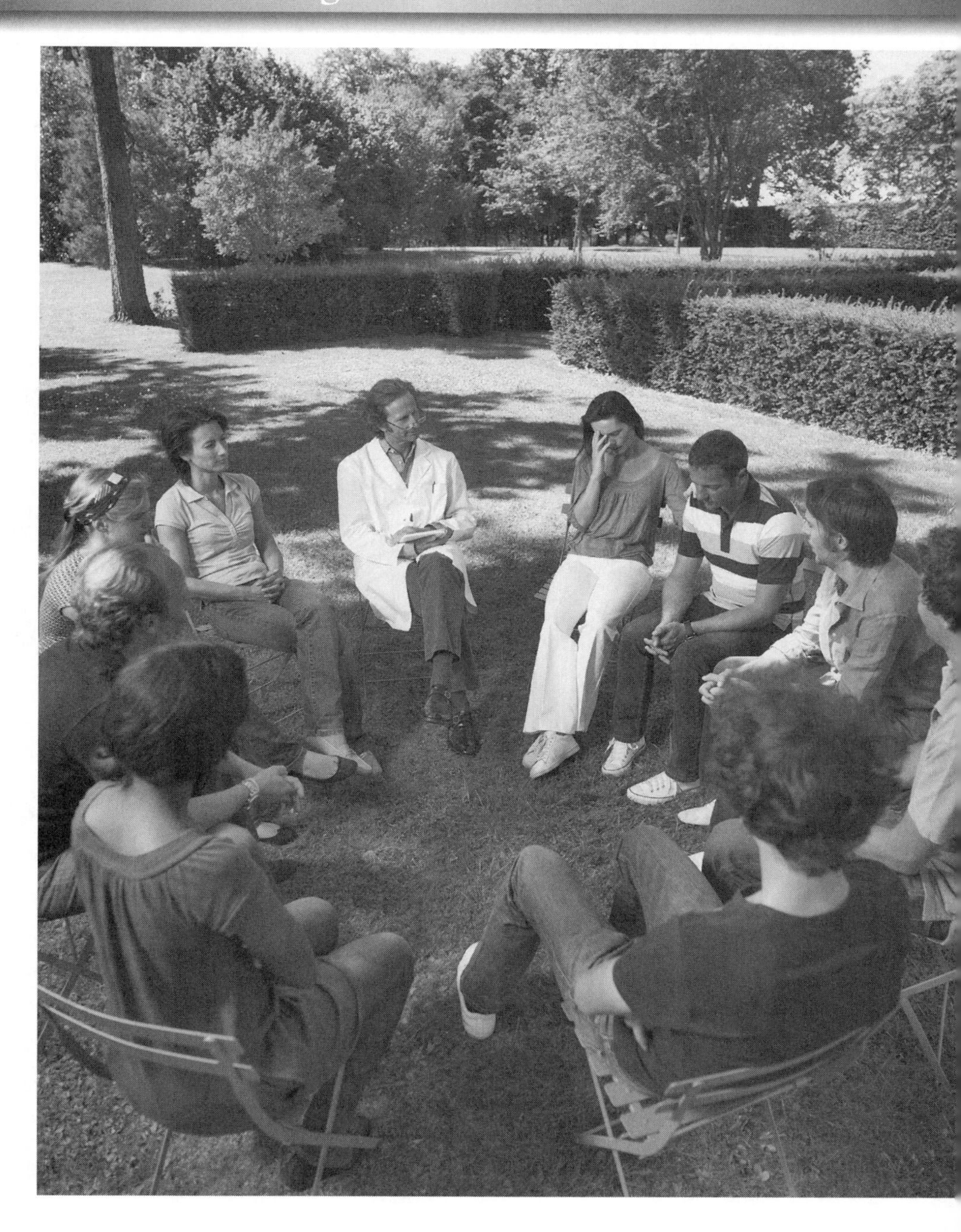

CHAPTER 1

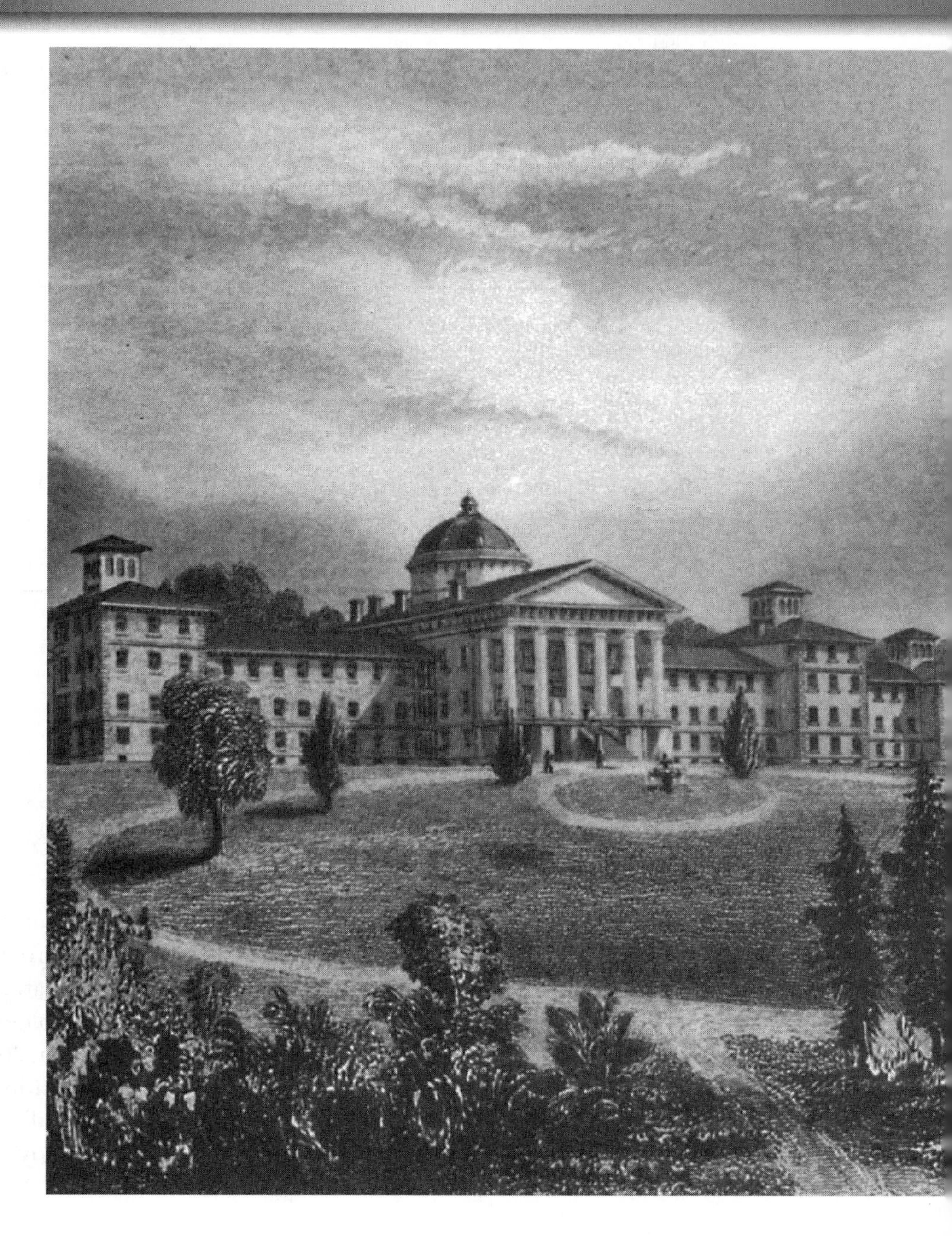

Foundations of Community Mental Health and Illness

CHAPTER OBJECTIVES

1. Define community, community mental health, mental health, and mental illness.
2. Describe the history of mental illness.
3. Explain five reasons for improving community mental health.
4. Explain the stigmas surrounding mental health and the reasons behind them.
5. Explain how community affects mental health.
6. Describe two types of communities.
7. List the five levels of community.
8. List the six elements of a community.

KEY TERMS

- Assertive Community Training (ACT)
- Asylums
- Community
- Community mental health
- Culture
- *Diagnostic and Statistical Manual of Mental Disorders (DSM)*
- Disability-adjusted life years (DALYs)
- Electroconvulsive therapy
- Lobotomy
- Mental disorders
- Mental health
- Mental health problems
- Mental illness
- Psychopathology
- Public health
- Seasonal affective disorder
- Somatic

Mental health and **mental illness** are often not considered part of mainstream health and are afterthoughts in our nation's health system. Mental health problems and illnesses such as dementia, schizophrenia, depression, bipolar disorder, attention deficit disorder, and autism affect more than 1 in 4 Americans 18 years or older (26.2%, or 57.7 million people) in any year (National Institute of Mental Health, 2008a). These individual health problems coupled with issues related to life transitions (death of a loved one, loss of job), situations between people (e.g., abuse, discrimination), and external situations (e.g., wars, natural disasters, high unemployment, traffic) contribute to problems at a more macro level as demonstrated by community-based problems such as gangs, violence, high school dropout rates, prostitution, and crime. These individual, familial, and community mental health problems are widespread and have devastating consequences. Yet even with this high prevalence of mental health problems and the problematic consequences at individual and community levels, they continue to be frequently spoken about in whispers. This shame and silence contribute to misunderstandings and stigmas that continue despite the vast amount of knowledge gained in the past three decades about mental illness and its causes. Fortunately, leaders in the mental health field are dedicated to improving the mental health of Americans through their advocacy, educational, and research efforts. These individuals have promoted the need for mental health to become a part of mainstream health. We agree that mental health needs to be integrated into the healthcare system and should no longer be a shameful and embarrassing health problem that often goes untreated.

People with mental illness and their loved ones have experienced devastating consequences for decades, but some of the repercussions could have been avoided or reduced if mental illnesses were viewed in the same light as physical illnesses. Fear and stigma persist and have prevented people with mental health problems from receiving treatment and improving their condition or recovering from the illness. But why has mental health lagged behind advances in physical health and been met with such shame? Part of the reason lies in its history, which is filled with tragic events.

This book will help you understand mental health and illness, dispel the myths and stigma surrounding mental illness, and provide the information you need to effectively prevent mental health problems and/or assist individuals, families, and community members who suffer from them. To accomplish this goal, we include information about mental health at different levels of analysis (individual, family, and community) because the individual is nested in the mental well-being of families and communities. We begin our journey with an overview of mental health and illness and the definitions of key terms. We then describe the history of mental illness and stigmas. We finish the chapter by defining community, how it affects mental health, and why public health professionals need to study the topic.

AN OVERVIEW OF MENTAL HEALTH AND ILLNESS

Mental health and mental illness are on opposite ends of a continuum, and there is no clear-cut boundary between the two. Our state of mental health is dynamic and fluctuates daily and throughout our lifetime. Consider these definitions of mental health and mental illness:

> *Mental health*: "The successful performance of mental function, resulting in productive activities, fulfilling relationships with other people, and the ability to adapt to change and to cope with adversity" (U.S. Department of Health and Human Services [DHHS], 1999).
>
> *Mental illness*: "A term that refers collectively to all diagnosable mental disorders. Mental disorders are health conditions characterized by alterations in thinking, mood, or behavior (or some combination thereof) associated with distress and/or impaired functioning" (DHHS, 1999).

As indicated in the definition, **mental disorders** are health conditions characterized by alterations in thinking, mood, or behavior (or some combination thereof) associated with distress and/or impaired functioning (DHHS, 1999). Examples of the three types of alterations include Alzheimer's disease, which is related to thinking, particularly with memory; attention deficit disorder and kleptomania, which have effects on behavior; and depression, a mental disorder largely marked by alterations in mood. Some disorders can affect more than one of the three areas. For example, mania affects both mood and behavior.

We use the phrase **mental health problems** here to mean the signs and symptoms are of insufficient intensity or duration to meet the criteria for any mental disorder. If left untreated, mental health problems can lead to mental disorders. Unresolved bereavement symptoms that adults experience are a good example of how an untreated mental health problem can manifest into a mental health disorder, and it illustrates the importance of prevention and early intervention. Bereavement symptoms that last for less than 2 months do not qualify as a mental disorder, according to the professional manual for diagnosis of mental health disorders, the ***Diagnostic and Statistical Manual of Mental Disorders* (*DSM*)**. If left untreated, bereavement symptoms can lead to depression. With treatment, the symptoms can be alleviated and the disorder avoided. This example illustrates the importance of early intervention, needed to address a mental health problem and avoid having it become a debilitating disorder.

Preventing and treating mental health problems and disorders is essential, because mental health is a core component of our lives. It is related to our own internal state as well as interpersonal relationships with family, significant others, work colleagues, and others that we encounter, along with being related to our contributions to the community and society. People often do not think of mental health until a problem arises, yet from early childhood until late in life, mental health is the springboard of thinking and communication skills, learning, emotional growth, resilience, and self-esteem (DHHS,

1999). In the United States we are bombarded with messages related to the importance of success in school and in the workplace, of being independent, and of being productive members in society. To accomplish these goals, we need to be mentally healthy.

It is important to take the cultural content of mental health issues into consideration because what it means to be mentally healthy varies among **cultures**. For example, in our dominant culture, being independent is valued, which is in contrast to collectivist cultures where the preference is to behave in a way that benefits the group. In the dominant culture of the United States, one who relies on family too much may be viewed as being too dependent and insecure. We explore culture and mental health further in Chapter 3.

Culture and mental health are integrated, and so are physical and mental health. For centuries, the mind and body have been viewed as separate, but they really are not. The distinction between the mind and body was derived from the work of the philosopher René Descartes (1596–1650). He saw the mind and body as completely separate. Descartes thought that religion should be concerned with the mind and physicians should be concerned with the body (Eisendrath & Feder, 1995).

Language is one reason the public continues to distinguish the difference between mental and physical health (DHHS, 1999). An alternative and improved way of separating physical and mental health is through the distinction between mental and **somatic** health (DHHS, 1999). ***Somatic*** is a medical term that comes from the Greek word *soma*, which means "the body." Mental health refers to the successful performance of mental functions in terms of thought, mood, and behavior, and when one experiences alterations in those functions it is termed **mental disorders**. Somatic conditions are primarily alterations in nonmental functions. The brain carries out all mental and somatic functions, including somatic functions such as movement, touch, and balance. Thus not all brain diseases are mental disorders. For example, a stroke may cause physical problems such as paralysis or blindness as well as impair mental functioning such as speech or memory. The former outcome is considered a somatic problem, but the symptoms related to impaired mental functioning are considered a mental problem. Therefore, the outcome of a problem that affects the brain can be considered a somatic one or a mental one depending on how it impacts the person's functioning.

HISTORY OF MENTAL ILLNESS

It is important to describe the history of the treatment of mental illness to understand the sources of the stigmas and to learn from previous attempts to improve the health of the mentally ill. The history of mental illness includes ambivalence, violence, torture, fear, discrimination, and suffering. These attributes contributed to movements to improve the treatment and services for this population. Four major reform movements occurred, referred to as the moral treatment era, the mental hygiene movement, the community mental health movement, and the community support movement (**Table 1-1**).

Mental illness, now referred to as **psychopathology**, was initially believed to be related to the moon. People who were mentally ill were referred to as *lunatics*, a term derived from the root word *lunar*, which means "moon." The belief was that insanity is caused by a baby being born when there was a full moon or a baby sleeping in the light created by a full moon (Leupo, n.d.). This expanded to the belief that mental illness is caused by demons or bad spirits. Many believed, even as late as the 16th and 17th centuries, that mental illness could only be an act of the devil himself. In an attempt to drive out the demon or evil spirit, many mentally ill people were tortured, now commonly referred to as witch hunts. When the torturous methods failed to return the person to sanity, he or she was deemed eternally possessed and was killed (DHHS, 1999).

In colonial America, the mentally ill were cared for in the home. As the population grew and urbanization developed, state governments stepped in and institutionalization of the mentally ill began to take place. As a result, state governments built institutions to house the mentally ill, known first as **asylums** and later as mental hospitals. In 1751 the first institution for the mentally ill in America was built. The Pennsylvania Hospital provided harsh conditions and treatment of the mentally ill. This inhumane treatment ignited the beginning of the four historical movements in mental health reform.

TABLE 1-1 Historical Reform Movements in Mental Health Treatment in the United States

Reform Movement	Era	Setting	Focus of Reform
Moral treatment	1800–1850	Asylum	Humane, restorative treatment
Mental hygiene	1890–1920	Mental hospital or clinic	Prevention, scientific orientation
Community mental health	1955–1970	Community mental health center	Deinstitutionalization, social integration
Community support	1975–present	Community	Mental illness as a social welfare problem (e.g., housing, employment)

Source: Morrissey, J. P., & Goldman, H. H. (1984). Cycles of reform in the care of the chronically mentally ill. *Hospital and Community Psychiatry*, *35*, 785–793.

Moral Treatment Movement (1800–1850)

The first movement began in the early 1800s and was introduced by William Tuke. He believed that when people were removed from everyday life situations they could restore their moral deterioration. Tuke thought they needed an asylum away from their home environments to heal. Dorothea Dix and Horace Mann, two other important reformers, agreed that mental illness could be treated by relocating the individual to an asylum where the he or she could receive both somatic and psychosocial treatments in a controlled environment. Note that the term *moral* had a different connotation at that time. It meant "the return of the individual to reason by the application of psychologically oriented therapy" (DHHS, 1999). The building of private and public asylums defined the moral treatment period. Almost every state had an asylum, which served the purpose of treating the mentally ill at an early stage to restore mental health and prevent the illness from becoming chronic. These asylums were used and built for untreatable chronic patients. Over time, the quality of care deteriorated in public institutions. Overpopulation and underfunding were growing problems.

Mental Hygiene Movement (1890–1920)

The mental hygiene movement began in the late 1800s. Two prominent people during this time were Adolf Meyer and Clifford Beers. This movement was based on the belief that mental illness could be cured if it was identified and treated early. This approach incorporated the newly emerging concepts of public health (which at the time

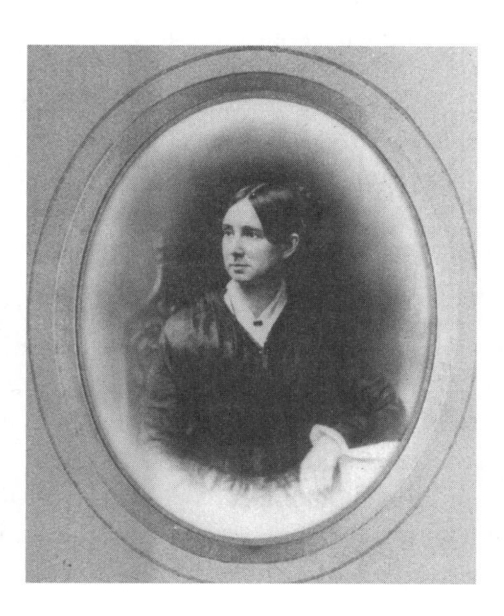

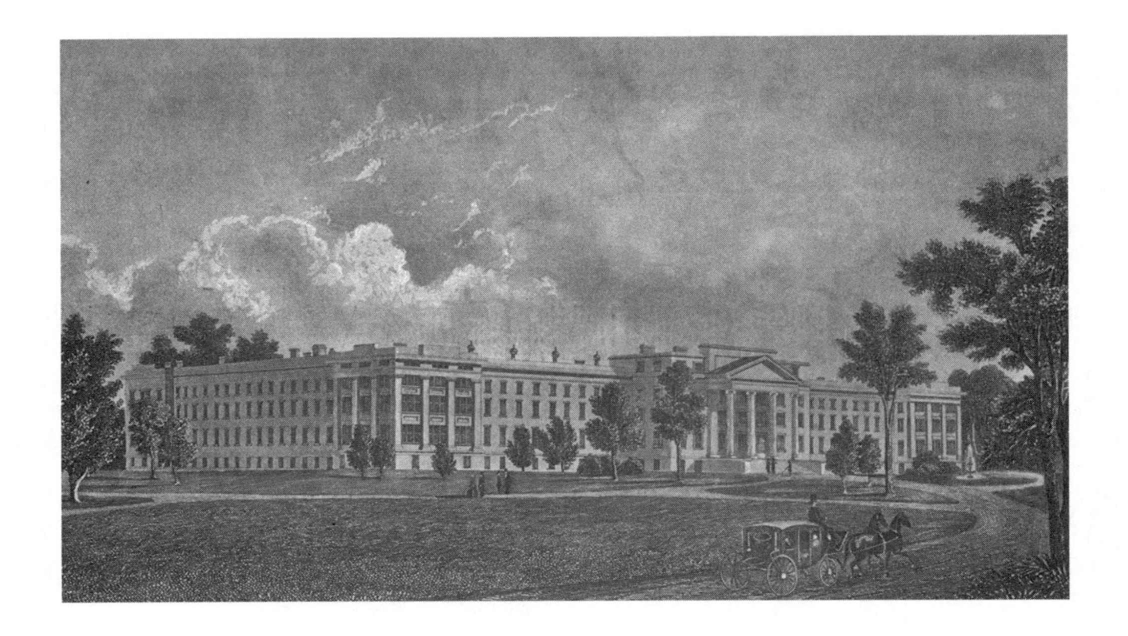

was referred to as *hygiene*). **Electroconvulsive therapy** and the **lobotomy** were developed. Treatments were sometimes effective, but early treatment had not prevented patients from becoming chronically ill.

Although the states built the public asylums, which were renamed mental hospitals, local government was expected to pay for each episode of care. Asylums could not maintain their budgets, and care continued to deteriorate. Newspapers revealed inhumane conditions both in the asylums and local welfare institutions. Care ranged widely, and the best treatment was in facilities that provided humane custodial care. On the other end of the spectrum, care was poor, and staff neglected or abused the patients (DHHS, 1999).

Community Mental Health Movement (1955–1970)

In the mid-20th century, a new concept, community mental health, was born. The idea was initiated by the Joint Commission on Mental Health and Illness report issued in 1961. The report led to the Mental Retardation Facilities and Community Mental Health Centers Act, passed in 1963 under President Kennedy. The goal of the act was to establish full-time community mental health centers throughout the United States.

Community mental health reformers claimed that they could implement services in the communities in part because of the advent of new medications used to treat psychosis and depression. These reformers suggested that long-term institutional care in mental hospitals had not been effective and had even been harmful. The policies of community care and deinstitutionalization led to decreases in the lengths of hospital stays and to the discharge of many patients who were in hospitals (DHHS, 1999).

Another policy affected mental health during this time. In the mid-1960s, limited mental health benefits were provided to recipients of Medicare and Medicaid. This change in benefits helped stimulate "the transfer of many long-term inpatients from public mental hospitals to nursing homes, encouraged the opening of psychiatric units in general hospitals, and ultimately paid for many rehabilitation services for individuals with severe and persistent mental disorders" (DHHS, 1999).

The community mental health centers did provide care, but they were not successful at addressing the needs of those who were deinstutionalized and had chronic mental health problems. The social network and services they needed, such as housing and vocational opportunities, were not available in the community. Also, community members did not welcome the returning mental patients. Many discharged mental patients found themselves on welfare and in criminal justice institutions, as had their predecessors in earlier eras; some became homeless or lived in regimented residential (e.g., board and care) settings in the community (DHHS, 1999).

Community Support Movement (1975–present)

The realization and criticism related to the community mental health centers not meeting the needs of deinstitutionalized patients contributed to the initiation of the fourth reform era, referred to as the community support movement. This movement grew directly out of the community mental health movement, and it called for acute treatment and prevention and assisting people with chronic mental illness. Reformers wanted community support systems that included addressing the social welfare needs of the mentally ill such as housing and job training. A model that developed at this time is called **Assertive Community Training (ACT)**. It is a way of delivering comprehensive and effective services to individuals who are diagnosed with severe mental illness and who have needs that have not been well met by traditional approaches to delivering services. Support services that stemmed from this model were domestic support and training, advocacy, housing assistance, and financial assistance for people who are mentally ill.

The present mental health care system is discussed in detail in Chapter 5. The current system is complex and fragmented. Many problems exist, such as the lack of health insurance for many people in the United States, underinsurance for mental disorders even among those who have health insurance, access barriers to members of many racial and ethnic groups, discrimination, and the stigma of mental illness, which is one of the factors that prevents help-seeking behavior (DHHS, 1999).

STIGMAS, PERCEPTIONS, AND MYTHS ABOUT MENTAL ILLNESS

Stigmatization of people with mental disorders has persisted throughout history. It is manifested by bias, distrust, stereotyping, fear, embarrassment, anger, and/or avoidance. Stigma leads others to avoid living, socializing, or working with, renting to, or employing people with mental disorders, especially severe disorders such as schizophrenia (Corrigan & Penn, 1999; Penn & Martin, 1998). It reduces patients' access to resources and opportunities (e.g., housing, jobs) and leads to low self-esteem, isolation, and hopelessness. It deters the public from seeking and being willing to pay for care and can lead to overt discrimination and various types of abuse. Stigma deprives people of their dignity and interferes with their full participation in society.

Nationally representative surveys have tracked public attitudes about mental illness since the 1950s (Gurin, Veroff, & Feld, 1960; Star, 1952, 1955; Veroff, Douvan, & Kulka, 1981). To permit comparisons over time, several surveys of the 1970s and the 1990s phrased questions exactly as they had been asked in the 1950s (Swindle, Heller, & Pescosolido, 1997).

In the 1950s, the public view of mental illness revealed the stigma and unscientific understanding of mental illness. After viewing vignettes of mentally ill people, survey respondents typically were not able to identify them as mentally ill using the professional standards of the day (DHHS, 1999). The public was not particularly skilled at distinguishing mental illness from ordinary unhappiness and worry and tended to see only extreme forms of behavior—namely psychosis—as mental illness (DHHS, 1999). Mental illness carried great social stigma, especially linked with the fear of unpredictable and violent behavior (Gurin et al., 1960; Star, 1952, 1955; Veroff et al., 1981).

By 1996 the Mental Health America survey revealed that Americans had achieved greater scientific understanding of mental illness, but the increase in knowledge did not defuse social stigma (Phelan, Link, Stueve, & Pescosolido, 1997). The public learned to define mental illness and to distinguish it from ordinary worry and unhappiness. It expanded its definition of mental illness to encompass anxiety, depression, and other mental disorders. The public attributed mental illness to a mix of biological abnormalities and vulnerabilities to social and psychological stress (Link, Phelan, Bresnahan, Stueve, & Pescosolido, 1999). Yet, in comparison with the 1950s, the public's perception of mental illness more frequently incorporated violent behavior (Phelan et al., 1997). This was true primarily among those who defined mental illness to include psychosis (a view held by about a third of the entire sample). Thirty-one percent of this group mentioned violence in its descriptions of mental illness, in comparison with 13% in the 1950s (DHHS, 1999). In other words, the perception of people with psychosis as dangerous is stronger today than in the past (Phelan et al.,

1997). The 1996 Mental Health America survey also showed that only 38% of Americans viewed depression as a health problem rather than a sign of a personal weakness (Mental Health America, 2007).

Conducted 10 years later, in this same Mental Health America survey, nearly three quarters of respondents knew that depression is a real health problem (72%), so nearly a quarter of Americans (22%) still saw depression as a sign of weakness in 2006 (Mental Health America, 2007). Overall, the behavioral health conditions most thought to be a sign of weakness were alcohol or drug problems (57%) and suicide attempts (46%) (Mental Health America, 2007). Ninety-four percent and 92% of respondents said that they feel comfortable interacting with someone with diabetes and cancer, respectively; 63% felt the same way about someone with depression, 45% for someone with bipolar disorder or schizophrenia, 43% for alcohol or drug abuse, and 46% for suicide (Mental Health America, 2007).

Finding ways to reduce and eliminate stigma is critical, but there is likely no simple method. Overall approaches to stigma reduction involve programs of advocacy, research, public education, and contact with persons with mental illness. Research needs to be conducted on effective ways to share research findings and educate the public about mental illness to help reduce and ultimately eliminate stigma and yield increasingly effective treatments for mental disorders. When people understand that mental disorders are not the result of moral failings or weakness and rather are legitimate illnesses responsive to specific treatments, the stigma may decline. As a result, people may be more willing to seek care and to pay for the costs. We hope this will lead to mental health and mental illness becoming integrated into health in general.

ABOUT COMMUNITIES

A **community** is a group of people who share common characteristics. Communities are dynamic and change over time. Individuals are influenced by communities, and individuals influence communities.

Communities may be in a specific geographic location, such as a neighborhood or town, or be geographically disbursed. Dalton, Elias, and Wandersman (2001) define two types of communities: locality and relational. Locality is what people think of as community in the traditional sense. It is related to geographic locations and types such as small towns, urban areas, and city neighborhoods (e.g., Sunset district, Harlem). The second type, relational, is defined by interpersonal relationships and not bound by geographic region. Examples of relational communities include nurses (occupation), gays and lesbians (sexual orientation), Italians (ethnic group), animal advocates (interest in a problem), women (gender), Americans (nationality), homeless people (living situation), members of bowling leagues (activities), and fathers (roles). The Internet has created new forms of communities such as online dating networks, support groups, and chat rooms.

Communities have been defined by possessing the six following elements:

1. Membership: a sense of identity and belonging
2. Common symbol systems: similar rituals, language, ceremonies, or other symbols that identify membership
3. Shared values and norms
4. Mutual influence: members influence the group and the group influences the members
5. Shared needs and commitment to meeting them
6. Shared emotional connection (a spiritual bond, not necessarily religion based) (Israel, Checkoway, Schultz, & Zimmerman, 1994).

Overall, people's sense of community seems to be declining in the United States. There are numerous indicators of this occurring. Results of Harris polls show that people report higher levels of alienation from their communities and lower trust in others now than in the past. This decline in community is due to numerous factors such as an increase in single-parent households, more families in which both parents work, decreases in leisure time, technology, and longer commute times. People are using technology to create new communities, which are on the rise (i.e., social media such as Facebook).

Communities exist at different ecological levels. Dalton et al. (2001) identified and explained these five levels of communities:

1. Individuals: This is the smallest unit nestled within the other levels. Program implementation and research at this level would focus on the relationship between the individual and his or her environment. For example, what changes may have contributed to the person's depression or increase in alcohol consumption? Some examples could be job loss, divorce, having a baby, or other such life transitions.
2. Microsystems: These are communities that the individual directly interacts with over time. Examples include family, coworkers in a small business, friends, neighbors, members of an organization such as professional coalition or workgroup, regulars at the gym, or classmates. These are people with whom the individual person has interpersonal relationships. They see each other regularly and influence each other.
3. Organizations: Organizations are large systems usually made up of smaller units such as departments in a university or large business, prayer groups at a church, or a unit in a hospital. Participation in the organization usually occurs through these smaller units, and individuals often feel a loyalty toward them.

4. Localities: This refers to geographic localities such as rural regions, small towns, section of the country (e.g., the Northeast), and urban areas. Localities can positively or negatively impact the culture of the community, including a positive sense of community or feelings of isolation.
5. Macrosystems: This is a largest level of community. Examples are nations, government, large political groups, and international corporations. Populations categorized by factors such as gender, race, ethnicity, and groups such as people with disabilities, black men, immigrants, homosexuals, homeless, and seniors also are part of macrosystems. People identify with these macrosystems with regard to their strengths and stressors.

Why are these different levels (or systems) important? A system has mutually interrelated parts, called *subsystems*. Each subsystem affects the others, and the whole is made up of the sum of its parts. When you analyze or work in a subsystem, it is important to define the level at which you intend to focus so the intervention is in line with your goals. For example, if you want to reduce violence in a local school, a national media campaign would not be the best approach for achieving your program goal. Because subsystems are interrelated and make up the whole, you still need to consider how your area of focus (the community of interest) affects and is affected by the other systems. This concept of systems and subsystems, referred to as the *general systems theory*, was developed by Ludwig von Bertalanffy. According to Bertalanffy, a system is characterized by the interactions of its components and the nonlinearity of those interactions. When working with communities, it is essential to identify your focus and level of intervention without losing sight that it is part of a larger system and made up of smaller systems. Using the same example of reducing violence in a particular school, you would still need to take into consideration other systems such as the family structure, the school district's policy on violence, and resources available in the town where the school is located.

COMMUNITY EFFECTS ON MENTAL HEALTH

Three main factors affect the health of a community. These factors include social, physical, and cultural issues. The factors can have a negative affect on mental health, called risk factors, or a positive affect on mental health, called protective factors. **Figure 1-1** provides examples of some risk and protective factors.

Social and cultural factors are numerous, complex, and related. These include issues such as socioeconomic status, the fast pace of an urban environment, the availability of social and medical services, crime rates, and informal neighboring. A literature review on the community context of mental and physical health concluded that processes may play out differently in different contexts (Shinn & Toohey, 2003, as cited

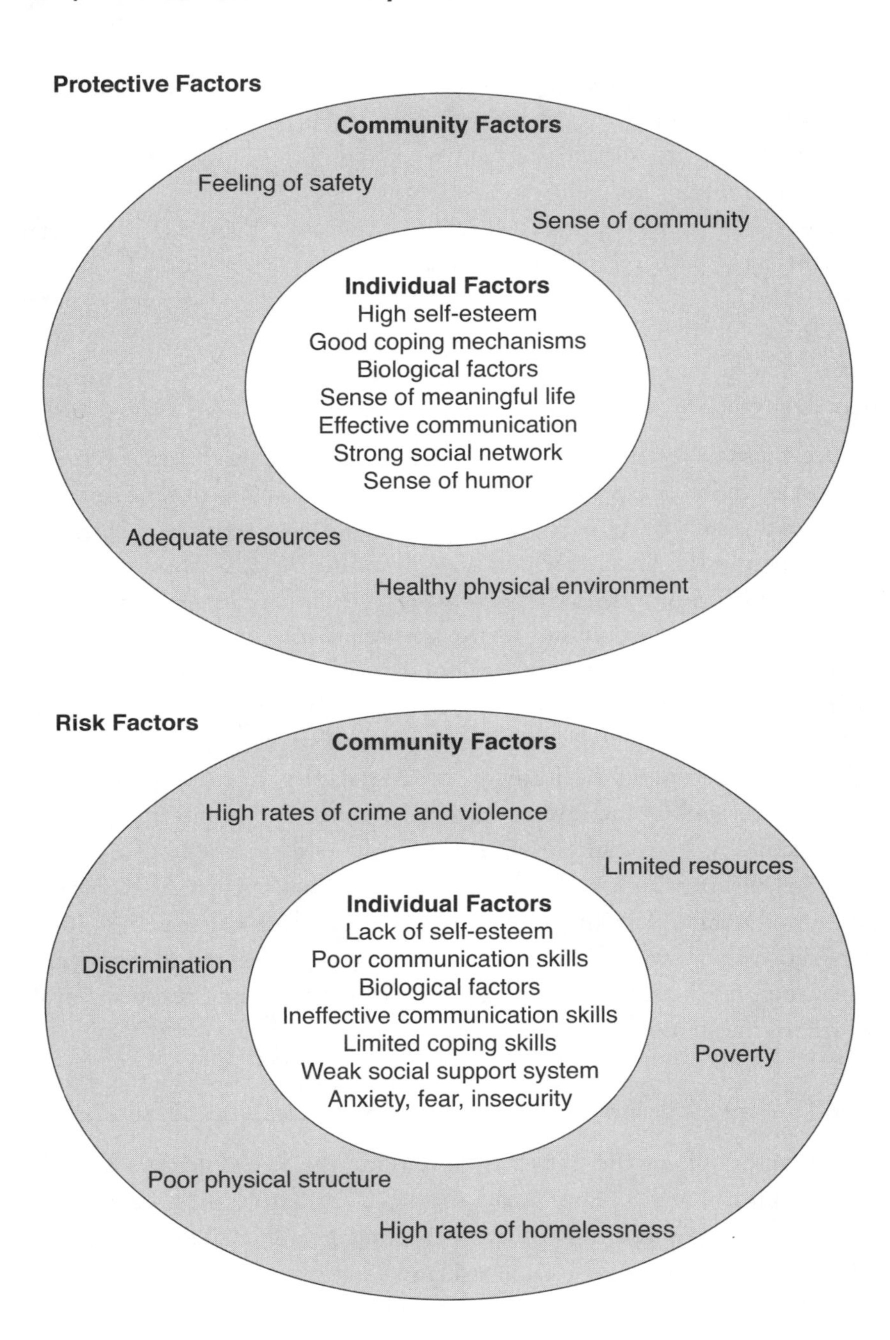

FIGURE 1-1 Examples of Risk and Protective Factors for Mental Health and Illness

in Dupéré and Perkins, 2007). For example, evidence shows that informal ties with neighbors are beneficial in advantaged areas but can be detrimental in disadvantaged areas (Caughy, O'Campo, & Muntaner, 2003; Ceballo & McLoyd, 2002; Warner & Roundtree, 1997; Wen et al., 2005, as cited in Dupéré and Perkins, 2007). In communities where stressors are more common, isolation from neighbors may have a protective effect on mental health (Dupéré and Perkins, 2007).

Neighborhood social and physical disorder have been measured in numerous ways (e.g., dilapidation, litter, graffiti, loitering youth), and they are consistently associated with fear of crime (Dupéré and Perkins, 2007). Living in poor neighborhoods may exacerbate tensions between social groups, magnify workplace stressors, induce maladaptive coping behaviors such as alcohol use, and translate into individual stress.

The stress associated with living in poor neighborhoods that have problems such as crime and physical deterioration can lead to **mental health problems**. Community stressors include crime, noise, traffic, litter, density, and residential crowding. Stress has effects on the physical and psychological state of humans and as a result can lead to mental health problems such as depression, violence, and substance abuse.

As stated previously, physical factors affect mental health as well as social and cultural circumstances. A broken window—or a littered sidewalk, graffiti, abandoned buildings, neglected homes—do not harm a community if they are repaired or eliminated. But if these issues are left untended, they send a message that no one cares about this neighborhood, and these behaviors are the culture and are acceptable. And once these minor problems escalate, they may contribute to other neighborhood problems such as public drunkenness, panhandling, crime, and prostitution. This famous theory, developed by James Q. Wilson and George L. Kelling and published in their article "Broken Windows: The Police and Neighborhood Safety," appeared in the *Atlantic Monthly* in March 1982. It is referred to as the broken-window theory. The developers of the broken-window theory argue that at the community level, disorder and crime are usually inextricably linked, in a kind of developmental sequence. Social psychologists and police officers tend to agree that if a window in a building is broken and is left unrepaired, all the rest of the windows will soon be broken. This is as true in nice neighborhoods as it is in rundown ones. "One unrepaired broken window is a signal that no one cares, and so breaking more windows costs nothing" (Wilson & Kelling, 1982, pp. 2–3). Other physical factors of deterioration can lead to mental health problems. Lead in playgrounds or others areas can cause lead poisoning in children, leading to behavioral and cognitive problems. Even the climate can impact mental health. For example if a person lives in an area that gets a high amount of rain and has many dark days, it can contribute to depression and **seasonal affective disorder**.

WHAT IS COMMUNITY MENTAL HEALTH?

We have defined mental health and community and described the relationship between the two, so how do we define community mental health? From a public health perspective, **community mental health** entails the development and delivery of programs for a defined group of people to promote, protect, and treat mental health and mental health problems. Some examples include programs for new mothers (to prevent postpartum depression), widows (to prevent grieving from escalating into depression), and victims of natural disasters (to prevent or treat posttraumatic stress disorder).

WHY STUDY COMMUNITY MENTAL HEALTH?

You probably have some ideas now why community mental health programs are important, but we have organized them into five primary reasons:

1. Mental health problems are widespread.
2. Mental health problems are disabling.
3. Research has paved the way for identification and treatment of mental illness and will continue to do so.
4. Prevention efforts, primarily through education and public health programs, have been shown to be effective at preventing mental health problems.
5. Mental health problems are costly.

The Widespread Occurrence of Mental Illness

Mental illness is widespread across the globe. The World Health Organization (WHO) reported in 2001 that psychiatric disorders account for 24% of all health-related disability, and when alcohol and drug use and dementias are added, 43% of all health-related disability is directly due to psychiatric disorders (American Nurses Association, 2007). In the United States, an estimated 22.1% of Americans 18 years of age and older suffer from a diagnosable psychiatric disorder in any given year (American Nurses Association, 2007). The overall prevalence of mental disorders among children is not as well documented as it is for adults, but approximately 20% of children are estimated to have mental disorders with at least mild functional impairment (American Nurses Association, 2007). According to the 2003 Epidemiologic Catchment Area study, approximately 20% of older adults have a diagnosable psychiatric disorder during a 1-year period (American Nurses Association, 2007). Mental disorders are the leading cause of disability in the United States and Canada for ages 15 to 44 (National Institute of Mental Health, 2008a), and they are tragic contributors to mortality, with suicide perennially representing one of the leading preventable causes of death. In 2005 suicide was the 11th leading cause of death for all ages (Centers for Disease Control and Prevention, 2008). Many people suffer from more than one mental disorder at a given time (National Institute of Mental Health, 2008a). Approximately 15% of the population with a psychiatric disorder has a co-occurring psychiatric illness (American Nurses Association, 2007). These data underscore the importance and urgency of treating and preventing mental disorders and of promoting mental health in our society.

Mental Health Problems Are Disabling

In the mid-1990s, the World Health Organization began an ambitious research study to determine the burden of disability associated with the whole range of diseases and health conditions suffered by people across the globe. A striking finding was related to the impact of mental illness on overall health and productivity in the United States and throughout the world. The impact had been profoundly underrecognized. In strong market economies, such as the United States, mental illness is the second leading cause of disability and premature mortality (DHHS, 1999). The measure of calculating disease burden in the Global Burden of Disease study, called **disability-adjusted life years (DALYs)**, allows comparison of the burden (**Table 1-2**). These data are strong indicators of the importance and urgency of treating and preventing mental disorders and of promoting mental health in our society (DHHS, 1999).

TABLE 1-2 Disease Burden by Selected Illness Categories in Established Market Economies, 1990 (measured in DALYs*)

Disease Category	Percentage of Total
All cardiovascular conditions	18.6
All mental illness including suicide	15.4
All malignant disease (cancer)	15.0
All respiratory conditions	4.8
All alcohol use	4.7
All infectious and parasitic disease	2.8
All drug use	1.5

* Disability-adjusted life years (DALYs) measure lost years of healthy life regardless of whether the years were lost to premature death or disability.

Source: Murray, C. J. L., & Lopez, A. D. (Eds.). (1996). *The global burden of disease: A comprehensive assessment of mortality and disability from diseases, injuries, and risk factors in 1990 and projected to 2020.* Cambridge, MA: Harvard School of Public Health. Retrieved from http://www.mental-health-matters.com/articles/print.php?artID=332. Accessed July 20, 2010.

DALYs are a measure of the lost years of healthy life caused by premature death or disability. The disability component of this measure is weighted for severity of the disability, but loss of years of healthy life is only one measure of the way in which mental health problems are disabling. The Centers for Disease Control and Prevention and the WHO (2007) have divided the burden into two categories: the undefined burden and the hidden burden.

Undefined Burden

The undefined burden of mental problems refers to the economic and social burden for families, communities, and countries. This burden is challenging because of the lack of quantitative data and the difficulties in measuring and evaluating.

Mental illnesses affect the functioning and thinking processes of the individual, which negatively impacts his or her social role and productivity in the community. Mental illness also affects the family and caregivers as well as the nation due to economic and social costs. Some of the specific economic and social costs include the following:

- Lost productivity due to premature deaths caused by suicide
- Lost productivity from people with mental illness who are unable to work
- Lost productivity from family members caring for the mentally ill person
- Reduced productivity from people who are ill while at work
- Toll of accidents caused by people who are psychologically disturbed, which is especially dangerous in people like train drivers, airline pilots, and factory workers
- Financial and social support for dependents of the mentally ill person
- Direct and indirect financial burdens for families caring for the mentally ill person
- Unemployment, alienation, and crime in young people whose childhood problems, for example, depression or behavior disorder, were not sufficiently well addressed for them to benefit fully from the education available
- Poor cognitive development in the children of mentally ill parents
- Emotional burden and diminished quality of life for family members (DHHS, 1999)

The Hidden Burden

The hidden burden includes the burden associated with stigma and violations of human rights and freedoms. Stigma has been defined as "a mark of shame, disgrace, or disapproval that results in an individual being shunned or rejected by others." The stigma associated with all forms of mental illness is strong but generally increases the more an individual's behavior differs from that of the "norm" (DHHS, 1999). Because of stigma, the mentally ill are often rejected by friends, coworkers, relatives, neighbors, and employers, leading to feelings of rejection and isolation. The mentally ill also are often denied equal participation in family life, normal social networks, and productive employment (DHHS, 1999). A major cause of the stigmas associated with mental illness are the myths, misconceptions, fears, and negative stereotypes about mental illness that many people hold (DHHS, 1999).

There also are burdens related to human rights violations. Persons experiencing mental problems are more vulnerable than others to experience violations of certain human rights and freedoms, such as the following:

- "The right not to be discriminated against (e.g., in access to health care, social services, or employment),
- The right to liberty (e.g., not to have restrictions automatically imposed on freedom of movement through measures such as detention),
- The right to integrity of the person (e.g., not to be unduly subjected to mental or physical harm; typical violations include treatment that ignores the requirement to obtain either the patient's informed consent or a surrogate decision maker's and sexual abuse), and
- The right to control one's own resources (e.g., one should not be automatically removed on the mere grounds of status as a mental patient but should be judged on his or her actual ability to manage resources)." (Centers for Disease Control and Prevention and the World Health Organization, 2007)

Research and the Advancement of Prevention, Detection, and Treatment

Research is an essential component to improving the well-being of people suffering from mental illness and society as a whole because it has, and will continue to, alleviate human suffering and reduce the financial burden created by mental health problems and disorders. This has occurred because of the advances in preventing, diagnosing, and treating mental illness as a result of research.

The U.S. Congress declared the 1990s the decade of the brain because of the increase in mental health problems. As a result, much was learned about mental illness through research during that decade and beyond. The Human Genome Project also has added to the knowledge about mental health problems and their causes. Other advances include improved medications and dosing, diagnosis, and prevention approaches. Improvements have been made with regard to understanding the processes related to thought, emotion, and behavior, and what goes wrong with these processes that leads to mental illness (DHHS, 1999). Research also has led to improved services for diverse population members.

Prevention of Mental Illness

Prevention of health problems is important for people for a variety of reasons, primarily the reduction of the human suffering and the financial burden. Therefore, studying community mental health and illness has the benefit of identifying ways to prevent or minimize mental health problems and illness from occurring or reducing their negative consequences.

In the United States, mental health programs, like general health programs, are rooted in a population-based **public health** model. Public health, which is focused on the prevention of disease and the promotion of health by government agencies, attends to the health of the entire population. A public health approach encompasses a focus on epidemiologic surveillance, health promotion, disease prevention, and access to services and is concerned about the link between health and the physical and psychosocial environment. In the past, mental health was primarily focused on serving people who were severely mentally ill, but using the public health model, mental health and illness are addressed from more of a broad bird's-eye view. As the field of mental health has changed and matured, its focus has been altered to not only focus on the ill but also to respond to the intensifying interest and concerns about disease prevention and health promotion. Because of the more recent consideration of these topic areas, the body of accumulated knowledge regarding them is not as expansive as that for mental illness (DHHS, 1999). As a result, much more is known through research about mental illness than about mental health. Further and continued research is needed to identify public health practices that identify risk and protective factors for mental health problems that are effective preventive interventions that may block the emergence of severe illnesses and effective ways to actively promote good mental health (DHHS, 1999).

The Cost of Mental Illness

The costs of mental illness are exceedingly high. Total cost estimates of mental illness are $318 billion annually (National Institute of Mental Health, 2008b). The direct costs of mental health services in the United States are approximately $100 billion annually (National Institute of Mental Health, 2008b), with the remaining balance spent on indirect costs. Indirect costs can be defined in different ways, but here they refer to lost productivity at the workplace, school, and home due to premature death or disability. The indirect costs of mental illness is estimated to be higher than the direct costs, with 60.8% of total indirect costs in lost wages alone (National Institute of Mental Health, 2008b).

CHAPTER SUMMARY

Mental illness is widespread yet continues to encounter stigmas and feelings of shame, embarrassment, and fear. These perceptions are anchored in its history, and the four major reform movements have certainly improved the social situations and health of people with these disorders. Although much has been accomplished to help understand mental illness and improve treatment, much more work needs to be done. More research is needed to identify effective ways to prevent and treat mental illness at the community level and ways to reduce stigmas.

In this chapter we defined the key terms *community*, *community mental health*, *mental health*, and *mental illness* and explained the history of mental illness. We discussed stigmas and their negative outcomes. Then we described communities and their effects on mental health and ended with a section on the importance of studying community mental health.

REVIEW

1. Define community, community mental health, mental health, and mental illness.
2. Explain the history of mental illness and how that has contributed to the existing stigmas.
3. What are the four reform mental health movements and their prominent characteristics?
4. What are some ways to reduce stigmas, and why is it important to do so?
5. What are the two types of communities?
6. What are the six elements of a community?
7. What are the five levels of communities?
8. Explain the general systems theory.
9. What are the five reasons identified in this chapter for studying community mental health?

ACTIVITY

Describe a few of your communities. Explain your relationship with that community and integrate some or all of the six elements of a community (membership, common symbol systems, shared values and norms, mutual influence, shared needs and commitment to meeting them, shared emotional connection) in your discussion. Describe how these communities impact your mental health.

REFERENCES AND FURTHER READINGS

American Nurses Association. (2007). *Psychiatric mental health nursing scope & standards*. Washington, DC: Author.

Angermeyer, M. C., & Matschinger, H. (1996). The effect of violent attacks by schizophrenic persons on the attitude of the public towards the mentally ill. *Social Science Medicine*, *43*, 1721–1728.

Baum, A., & Posluszny, D. M. (1999). Health psychology: Mapping biobehavioral contributions to health and illness. *Annual Review of Psychology*, *50*, 137–163.

Caughy, M. O., O'Campo, P. J., & Muntaner, C. (2003). When being alone might be better: neighborhood poverty, social capital, and child mental health. *Social Science and Medicine*, *57*, 227–237.

Ceballo, R., & McLoyd, V. C. (2002). Social support and parenting in poor, dangerous neighborhoods. *Child Development*, *73*, 1310–1321.

Centers for Disease Control and Prevention. (2008, Summer). *Suicide*. Retrieved from http://www.cdc.gov/ncipc/dvp/suicide/suicide_data_sheet.pdf

Centers for Disease Control and Prevention and the World Health Organization. (2007). Mental health problems: The undefined and hidden burden. Retrieved from http://www.allcountries.org/health/mental_health_problems_the_undefined_and_hidden_burden.html

Chaffin, A. J. (2001). *Psychiatric nursing teachers*. Retrieved from http://www.scs.unr.edu/~chaffina/

Cooper-Patrick, L., Powe, N. R., Jenckes, M. W., Gonzales, J. J., Levine, D. M., & Ford, D. E. (1997). Identification of patient attitudes and preferences regarding treatment of depression. *Journal of General Internal Medicine*, *12*, 431–438.

Corrigan, P. W., & Penn, D. L. (1999). Lessons from social psychology on discrediting psychiatric stigma. *American Psychologist*, *54*, 765–776.

Dalton, J. H., Elias, M. J., and Wandersman, A. (2001). *Community psychology*. Belmont, CA: Wadsworth/Thomson Learning.

Dupéré, V., & Perkins, D. D. (2007). Community types and mental health: A multilevel study of local environmental stress and coping. *American Journal of Community Psychology*, *39*, 107–119. Retrieved from http://www.people.vanderbilt.edu/~douglas.d.perkins/DuperePerkins.2007.community_types_&_mental_health.AJCP.pdf

Eisendrath, S. J., & Feder, A. (1995). The mind and somatic illness: Psychological factors affecting physical illness. In H. H. Goldman (Ed.), *Review of general psychiatry* (5th ed.). Norwalk, CT: Appleton & Lange.

Eronen, M., Angermeyer, M. C., & Schulze, B. (1998). The psychiatric epidemiology of violent behavior. *Social Psychiatry and Psychiatric Epidemiology*, *33*(Suppl. 1), S13–S23.

Goldman, H. H. (1998). Deinstitutionalization and community care: Social welfare policy as mental health policy. *Harvard Review of Psychiatry*, *6*, 219–222.

Goldman, H. H., & Morrissey, J. P. (1985). The alchemy of mental health policy: Homelessness and the fourth cycle of reform. *American Journal of Public Health*, *75*, 727–731.

Grob, G. N. (1983). *Mental illness and American society, 1875–1940*. Princeton, NJ: Princeton University Press.

Grob, G. N. (1991). *From asylum to community: Mental health policy in modern America*. Princeton, NJ: Princeton University Press.

Grob, G. N. (1994). *The mad among us: A history of the care of America's mentally ill*. New York: Free Press.

Gurin, J., Veroff, J., & Feld, S. (1960). *Americans view their mental health: A nationwide interview survey* (A report to the staff director, Jack R. Ewalt). New York: Basic Books.

Hanson, K. W. (1998). Public opinion and the mental health parity debate: Lessons from the survey literature. *Psychiatric Services*, *49*, 1059–1066.

Heginbotham, C. (1998). UK mental health policy can alter the stigma of mental illness. *Lancet, 352*, 1052–1053.

Hoyt, D. R., Conger, R. D., Valde, J. G., & Weihs, K. (1997). Psychological distress and help seeking in rural America. *American Journal of Community Psychology, 25*, 449–470.

Israel, B. A., Checkoway, B., Schultz, A. & Zimmerman, M. (1994). Health education and community empowerment: Conceptualizing and measuring perceptions of individual, organizational, and community control. *Health Education Quarterly, 21*(2): 149–170.

Jones, A. H. (1998). Mental illness made public: Ending the stigma? *Lancet, 352*, 1060.

Kessler, R. C., Nelson, C. B., McKinagle, K. A., Edlund, M. J., Frank, R. G., & Leaf, P. J. (1996). The epidemiology of co-occurring addictive and mental disorders: Implications for prevention and service utilization. *American Journal of Orthopsychiatry, 66*, 17–31.

Leupo, K. (n.d.). *The history of mental illness*. Retrieved from http://www.toddlertime.com/advocacy/hospitals/Asylum/history-asylum.htm

Link, B., Phelan, J., Bresnahan, M., Stueve, A., & Pescosolido, B. (1999, September). Public conceptions of mental illness: The labels, causes, dangerousness and social distance. *American Journal of Public Health, 89*, 1328–1333.

Mental Health America. (2007). *Mental health attitudinal survey*. Alexandria, VA: Author.

Morrissey, J. P., & Goldman, H. H. (1984). Cycles of reform in the care of the chronically mentally ill. *Hospital and Community Psychiatry, 35*, 785–793.

Murray, C. J. L., & Lopez, A. D. (Eds.). (1996). *The global burden of disease: A comprehensive assessment of mortality and disability from diseases, injuries, and risk factors in 1990 and projected to 2020.* Cambridge, MA: Harvard School of Public Health. Retrieved from http://www.mental-health-matters.com/articles/print.php?artID=332

National Institute of Mental Health. (2008a). *Statistics*. Retrieved from http://www.nimh.nih.gov/health/statistics/index.shtml

National Institute of Mental Health. (2008b). *National Institute of Mental Health strategic plan*. Retrieved from http://www.nimh.nih.gov/about/strategic-planning-reports/nimh-strategic-plan-2008.pdf

Penn, D. L., & Martin, J. (1998). The stigma of severe mental illness: Some potential solutions for a recalcitrant problem. *Psychiatric Quarterly, 69*, 235–247.

Phelan, J., Link, B., Stueve, A., & Pescosolido, B. (1997, August). *Public conceptions of mental illness in 1950 and 1996: Has sophistication increased? Has stigma declined?* Paper presented at the meeting of the American Sociological Association, Toronto, Ontario.

Putnam, R. (1995). Bowling alone: America's declining social capital. *Journal of Democracy, 6*, 65–78.

Regier, D. A., Narrow, W. E., Rae, D. S., Manderscheid, R. W., Locke, B. Z., & Goodwin, F. K. (1993). The de facto US mental and addictive disorders service system: Epidemiologic catchment area prospective 1-year prevalence rates of disorders and services. *Archives of General Psychiatry, 50*, 85–94.

Shinn, M., & Toohey, S. M. (2003). Community contexts of human welfare. *Annual Review of Psychology, 54*, 427–459.

Star, S. A. (November, 1952). *What the public thinks about mental health and mental illness*. Paper presented at the annual meeting of the National Association for Mental Health..

Star, S. A. (1955). *The public's ideas about mental illness*. Paper presented at the annual meeting of the National Association for Mental Health.

Sussman, L. K., Robins, L. N., & Earls, F. (1987). Treatment-seeking for depression by black and white Americans. *Social Science and Medicine*, *24*, 187–196.

Swanson, J. W. (1994). Mental disorder, substance abuse, and community violence: An epidemiological approach. In J. Monahan & H. J. Steadman (Eds.), *Violence and mental disorder: Developments in risk assessment* (pp. 101–136). Chicago: University of Chicago Press.

Swartz, M. S., Swanson, J. W., & Burns, B. J. (1998). Taking the wrong drugs: The role of substance abuse and medication noncompliance in violence among severely mentally ill individuals. *Social Psychiatry and Psychiatric Epidemiology*, *33*(Suppl. 1), S75–S80.

Swindle, R., Heller, K., & Pescosolido, B. (1997, August). *Responses to "nervous breakdowns" in America over a 40-year period: Mental health policy implications*. Paper presented at the meeting of American Sociological Association, Toronto, Ontario.

U.S. Department of Health and Human Services [DHHS]. (1999). *Mental health: A report of the surgeon general*. Rockville, MD: U.S. Department of Health and Human Services, Substance Abuse and Mental Health Services Administration, Center for Mental Health Services, National Institutes of Health, National Institute of Mental Health. Retrieved from http://www.surgeongeneral.gov/library/mentalhealth/home.html

Veroff, J., Douvan, E., & Kulka, R. A. (1981). *Mental health in America: Patterns of help-seeking from 1957 to 1976*. New York: Basic Books.

Warner, B. D., & Roundtree, P. W. (1997). Local social ties in a community and crime model: Questioning the systematic nature of informal social control. *Social Problems*, *44*, 520–537.

Wilson, J. Q., & Kelling, G. L. (1982). *Broken windows: The police and neighborhood safety*. Retrieved from http://www.manhattan-institute.org/pdf/_atlantic_monthly-broken_windows.pdf

Wen, M., Cagney, K. A., & Christakis, N. A. (2005). Effect of specific aspects of community social environment on the mortality of individuals diagnosed with serious illness. *Social Science & Medicine*, *61*, 1119–1134.

CHAPTER 2

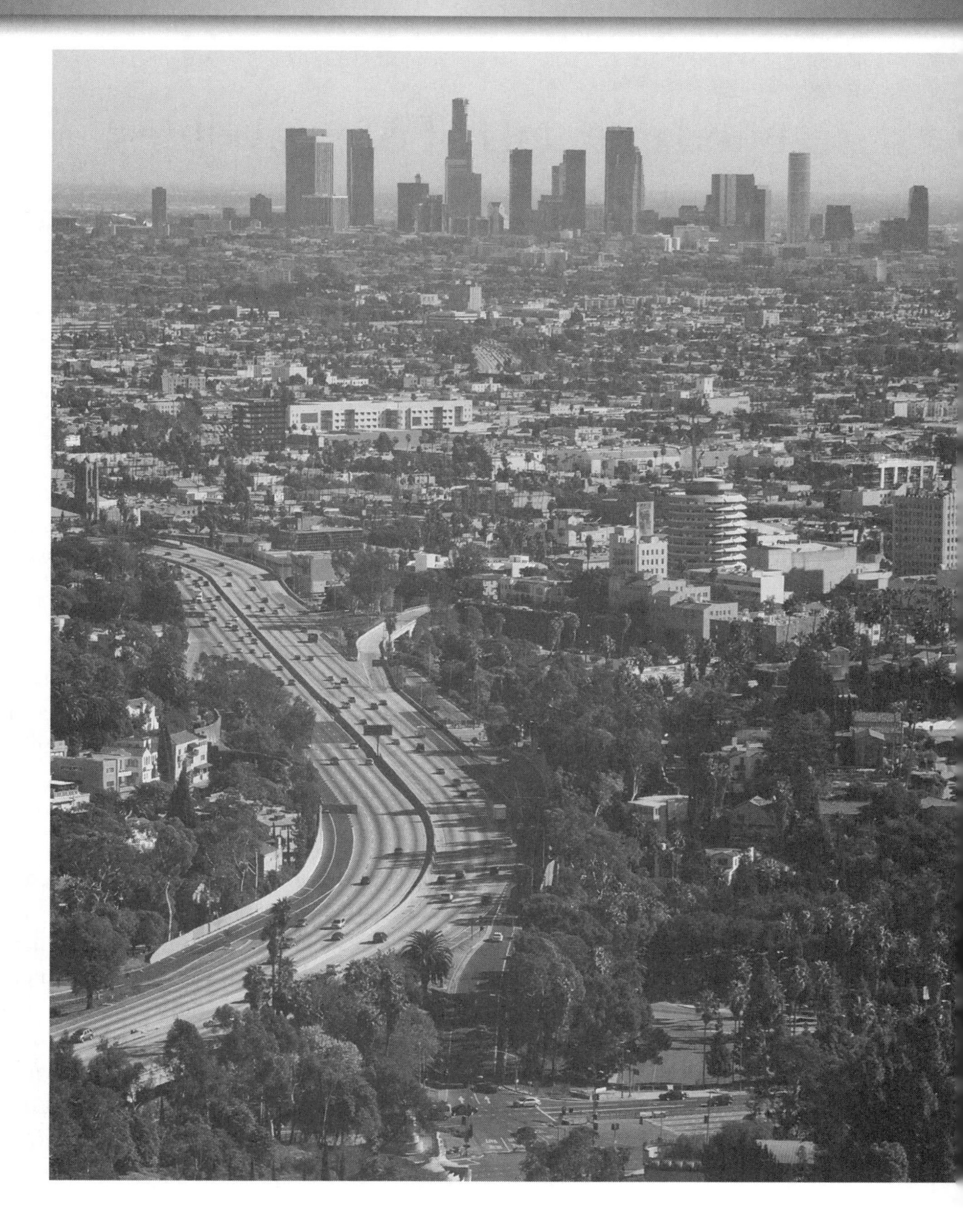

Fundamentals of Mental Illness

CHAPTER OBJECTIVES

1. Explain the etiology of mental illness.
2. List and describe the types of mental illness.
3. List at least six manifestations of mental illness.
4. Describe the process of diagnosing mental illness.
5. Explain the methods that can be used to treat mental illness.

KEY TERMS

- Behavioral therapy
- Biopsychosocial model of disease
- Cognitive therapy
- Crisis hotline
- Curanderismo
- Delusion
- Disease
- Disorder
- Naturopathy
- Pediatric autoimmune neuropsychiatric disorders associated with streptococcus (PANDAS)
- Psychosis
- Tourette syndrome

Mental illness, as stated in Chapter 1, is a term that collectively refers to all diagnosable mental disorders. Mental disorders are a problem that every community encounters. Research on mental disorders is beginning to uncover the origins of mental illness, which are complex, not always understood, and often caused by biological or psychosocial factors or a combination of the two. There are an abundance of signs and symptoms that vary from mild to severe when mental illness occurs. As a result, the diagnosis and treatment can be challenging and imperfect.

The content of this chapter primarily includes information about mental illness on an individual level. Recall that a community is made of up people with common characteristics. Therefore, individuals who have substance abuse problems or an eating disorder collectively make a community. In addition, if you are working with a homeless community or female athletes, for example, some common individual mental illnesses that are more prevalent in these communities are substance abuse disorders and eating disorders, respectively. Therefore, we believe it is essential to understand mental illness at the individual level in order to understand it at the familial and community levels.

This chapter begins with a discussion about the causes of mental illness among individuals, which includes fundamental biological and psychosocial contributions. After we address the etiology of mental illness, we move into discussions about the types of mental illness, the signs and symptoms, how mental illness is diagnosed, and treatment options.

OVERVIEW OF ETIOLOGY

The causes (etiology) of mental disorders can usually be linked to biological or to genetic or psychosocial (environmental) forces or a combination of both influences. Therefore, we begin our discussion of the etiology of mental illness with a description of the biopsychosocial model of disease, followed by sections that address biological and psychosocial influences on mental health and mental illness.

Biopsychosocial Model of Disease

George L. Engel (1977), who proposed the **biopsychosocial model of disease**, is a contributor to the realization that multiple factors contribute to mental health and disease. The biopsychosocial model, commonly known as the mind-body connection, is in contrast to the traditional biomedical model of medicine. Engel's model is a framework for understanding mental health and disease that posits that biological, social, and psychological factors, not just biological factors, all play a significant role in human disease and illness. The model does not provide specific causes of disease. The purpose of the biopsychosocial model is to take a bird's-eye view and assert that simply looking at biological factors alone—which had been the prevailing view of disease at the time Engel was writing—is not sufficient to explain mental health and illness.

According to Engel's model, biopsychosocial factors are involved in the causes, manifestation, course, and outcome of health and disease, including mental disorders. Psychosocial factors can cause a biological effect by predisposing the patient to risk factors. For example, stress can exacerbate asthma or migraines. The link may be less direct as well. For example, depression can cause excess eating, leading to obesity and diabetes. Also, biological problems can lead to mental health problems. For example, a stroke can cause dementia, and a head injury can contribute to depression.

The relative roles of biological, psychological, or social factors also may vary across individuals and across stages of the lifespan. In some people, for example, depression arises primarily as a result of exposure to stressful life events, whereas in others the foremost cause of depression is genetic predisposition.

Biological Influences on Mental Health and Mental Illness

There are numerous biological and physical influences on mental health and mental illness, which can occur before or after birth. Mental deficiencies at birth can be caused by inheritance (genetics), be the result of maternal exposure to agents (e.g., alcohol), or be unknown in origin (idiopathic). Mental problems after birth can be caused by biological factors such as inheritance, trauma, or infections.

The major categories of biological causes of mental illness are genetics, infections, traumatic brain injury, nutrition, hormones, and toxins. This section touches on each of these areas.

Genetics

You may hear that certain problems tend to run in the person's family. This is an indicator that the problem may be genetic. It is difficult to determine at times if a health problem is caused by genes or by life experiences or a combination of both. Twin studies are often conducted to help determine the influence of genes because they help separate the influences of genes and environments. Twin studies often examine children who were not raised by their biological parents to help assess genetic linkages.

Genetic influences on behavior have been known for some time now, but determining which genes are involved and how they influence behavior presents a great challenge. Another challenge is determining how the environment impacts genetic expression. Making the genetic link even more complicated is that research suggests that many mental disorders arise, in part, from defects not in single genes, but in multiple genes. In fact, scientists have discovered that no single gene is responsible for a mental disorder, several susceptibility genes may interact with one another, and the environment influences genetic expression to increase the risk of developing a mental disorder (Kneisl & Trigoboff, 2009).

Because mental illness appears to result from the interaction of multiple genes and the interaction of genes with environmental factors, it means that no gene determines the fate for mental illness. This gives us hope that modifiable environmental risk factors can eventually be identified and become targets for prevention efforts even when someone is genetically prone to the mental illness. The downside is that this makes it challenging to identify which genes are related to the illness. As a result of the Human Genome Project and research on inherited psychiatric illnesses, we know the sequence of each human gene and the common variants for each gene throughout the human race and much more about expressive patterns of genetic expression, gene therapy, mutation detection, and other components of the links of genes and mental illness. With the genetic information, combined with modern technologies, we will be able to better understand the dynamics and interactions of genes, environmental influences, and mental health in the future.

Information from the Human Genome Project will be valuable on individual and community levels. On the individual level, it can identify what time during the development of the brain that a particular gene is active and in which cells and circuits the gene is expressed. The genetic information will provide important information about the critical times for intervention in a disease process and information about what it is that goes wrong. On a community level, genetic information will be invaluable in identifying and modifying environmental risk factors. For example, information from genetics will help us understand how the environmental factors (e.g., psychosocial environment, nutrition, healthcare access) play a role in the development, severity, and course of a disorder and assist with identifying prevention and early intervention strategies.

Because no single gene causes mental health problems, all communities are susceptible to mental health problems caused by genetic factors. When more is known about the environmental contributing factors, then high-risk communities may be identified.

Infectious Influences

It has been known since the early part of the 20th century that infectious agents can affect the brain and cause mental disorders. For example, syphilis, a sexually transmitted infectious disease, can migrate to the brain and cause neurosyphilis. Neurosyphilis can cause numerous symptoms, including mood and personality changes, poor concentration, irritability, depression, and dementia. Another example is the dementia that can be associated with infection by the human immunodeficiency virus (HIV). Other infectious agents that cause mental health problems such as personality changes, anorexia, behavioral symptoms (such as fear, anxiety, and confusion) include herpes simplex encephalitis (inflammation of the brain caused by the herpes virus), measles encephalomyelitis (inflammation of the brain and spinal cord caused by measles), rabies encephalitis (inflammation of the brain and spinal cord caused by rabies), and chronic meningitis (inflammation of the membranes that cover the brain and spinal cord that can be caused by a number of infectious agents including viruses and bacteria). Research also has identified an infectious etiology to one form of obsessive-compulsive disorder, called **pediatric autoimmune neuropsychiatric disorders associated with streptococcus (PANDAS)**. The children who suffer from PANDAS usually have a dramatic and sudden onset of symptoms that are preceded by a streptococcal (strep) throat infection. The symptoms include motor or vocal tics, obsessions and/or compulsions, moodiness, concerns about being separated from loved ones, and irritability.

Communities that are at risk of mental health problems caused by infectious diseases include the same populations that are at risk of the infectious disease. For example, high-risk populations of HIV include groups such as men who have sex with men, injection drug users, and people with multiple sex partners. People at high risk of meningitis include young individuals (infants and young children) and elderly individuals (more than 60 years of age).

Traumatic Brain Injury

A traumatic brain injury (TBI) is a blow or jolt to the head or a penetrating head injury that disrupts the function of the brain. Not all blows or jolts to the head result in a TBI. The severity of such an injury may range from mild (i.e., a brief change in mental status or consciousness) to severe (i.e., an extended period of unconsciousness or amnesia after the injury). TBI can cause a wide range of functional changes affecting thinking, sensation, movement, language, and/or emotions. Causes of trauma are numerous and include motor vehicle accidents, sports injuries, abuse, falls, and violence.

Factors that may adversely influence the mental health of a person with brain injury may be seen in various ways. It may cause direct effects on the person (e.g., cognitive and motor disturbances, emotional disorders, increased impulsivity, depression, rigidity, memory problems, and/or hyperactivity) or have longer term implications, such as profound personality changes. People with TBI have an increase in the likelihood of depression, and suicide rates are higher among people with brain injuries than the general population. Brain injury is often a catastrophic life-changing event for individuals and their families. Many TBI survivors experience dramatic and permanent changes in work status, roles, income, family life, support network, and quality of life. This may predispose them to significant depressive reactions and feelings of social isolation, helplessness, and hopelessness. Given these complex and multiple risk factors for people with brain injury, there is a need for targeted and tailored mental health interventions.

In terms of community health, people in the military encounter high rates of TBI. For example, between 10% and 20% of troops returning from Iraq and Afghanistan are estimated to have suffered a TBI (Institute of Federal Health Care, 2009). Additional high-risk communities include young people, low-income individuals, unmarried individuals, members of ethnic minority groups, residents of inner cities, men (they are approximately twice are likely as women to sustain TBI), individuals with a history of substance abuse, and individuals who have suffered a previous TBI (Dawodu, 2009).

Nutrition

Mental health can be influenced by several nutritional factors, including overall energy intake, intake of the energy-containing nutrients (proteins, carbohydrates, and fats), alcohol intake, and intake of vitamins and minerals (*Gale Encyclopedia of Mental Health*, 2007). Often deficiencies of multiple nutrients rather than a single nutrient are responsible for changes in brain functioning. The list of the affects of nutrition on mental functioning is extensive, but a few include the following:

- Niacin deficiencies may cause irritability, headaches, memory loss, an inability to sleep, and emotional instability.
- People with consistently low energy intake often feel apathetic, sad, and hopeless.
- A magnesium deficiency can cause restlessness, nervousness, apathy, and delirium.
- An iron deficiency can lead to anemia, which can cause fatigue and impair brain functioning.
- A vitamin B_6 deficiency can cause fatigue, insomnia, depression, and irritability.
- Malnutrition early in life has been associated with below-normal intelligence and functional and cognitive defects (*Gale Encyclopedia of Mental Health*, 2007).

As these examples show, diet affects mood, behavior, and brain function.

The human brain has high energy and nutrient needs. Changes in energy or nutrient intake can alter both brain chemistry and the functioning of nerves in the brain. Intake of energy and several different nutrients affect levels of neurotransmitters, which are chemicals in the brain that transmit nerve impulses from one nerve cell to another. Neurotransmitters influence mood, sleep patterns, and thinking. Deficiencies or excesses of certain vitamins or minerals can damage nerves in the brain, causing changes in memory that can limit problem-solving ability and impair brain function (*Gale Encyclopedia of Mental Health*, 2007).

Proper nutrition affects our mental health throughout our lives, even before we are born. Fetal alcohol syndrome is a well-known example. When a pregnant mother consumes alcohol during her pregnancy, it can cause physical, mental, or behavioral problems, including mental retardation, to the fetus. Another example is that male children of mothers who experience inadequate nutrition during pregnancy are 2.5 times as likely to experience antisocial behavior disorder when compared with sons of women with adequate nutrition during pregnancy (Fontaine, 2009).

What we eat affects our mental health, and our mental health can affect what we eat. People eat (or do not eat) when they are sad, angry, lonely, stressed, depressed, or for other emotional reasons. This emotional eating can lead to weight gain (or loss), which can lead to depression and low self-esteem, for example. It can become a damaging cycle. Also, mental health problems such as dementia and mental retardation can make it difficult for people to make sound nutritional choices.

In terms of community mental health, because nutrition is related to mental health it needs to be particularly considered when working with high-risk communities. People who have substance abuse problems, the homeless, and people who are in poverty are at a high risk of nutrient deficiencies.

Hormones

Hormones have physiological effects on the body that can impact mental health. For example, high cortical levels have been associated with violence, testosterone has been associated with male irritable aggression, and decreases in progesterone during a female's menstrual cycle and low levels of serotonin have been linked to irritability. Irregularities of neuroendocrine function (cells in the nervous and endocrine systems that release a hormone into the circulating blood in response to a neural stimulus) have been linked to depression, postpartum psychosis, schizophrenia, or polydipsia (excessive thirst) in people with psychosis, panic disorder, obsessive-compulsive disorder, anorexia nervosa, and dementia of the Alzheimer's type (Kneisl & Trigoboff, 2009).

Aging has an impact on our hormone levels. For example, as men age, their bodies produce fewer male hormones. There's evidence that replacing these hormones can help men stave off some of the effects of aging, including decline in intellectual functioning and Alzheimer's disease. Another example is that feelings of depression or anxiety may be a signs of a thyroid problem. An overactive thyroid can lead to anxiety and panic attacks, whereas an underactive thyroid can contribute to depression. In fact, very minor reductions in thyroid hormone that do not have any important effect on physical health may make one feel depressed.

Hormones also can temporarily fall out of balance during certain points of a woman's life such as during her menstrual cycle and after giving birth. During both of these times, women may suffer from depression, irritability, and other mental health problems.

Because of these links, community planners should consider the age or stage of life of the population. Age brackets at which hormonal changes are particularly high include adolescents, the elderly, pregnancy and postpartum, and perimenopause. At these times, hormones may impact mental health.

Toxins

Heavy metals is the term used for a group of elements that are on the heavier end of the periodic table of elements and weigh more than most other elements. Some heavy metals such as cobalt, copper, iron, manganese, and zinc are essential to health in trace amounts but can be harmful in excess amounts. Other elements are nonessential and can be harmful to health. These include cadmium, antimony, chromium, mercury, lead, and arsenic. These last three are the most common in cases of heavy metal toxicity. As an example of the scope of a heavy metal's toxicity, lead poisoning can cause physical problems as well as mental symptoms such as irritability, aggressiveness, impulsiveness, hyperactivity, problems with concentration and learning, and memory loss. Lead also is being explored in terms of its relationship to attention deficit hyperactivity disorder (ADHD). Mercury toxicity has been linked to irritability, apathy, autism, depression, psychosis, mental deterioration, and anorexia.

Sources of toxicity can include the water supply, industrial exposure, and certain hobbies, among others. Therefore, when working with communities, work, hobbies, and living habits should be considered. For example, if a parent works in an industry that exposes him or her to lead, the contaminated parent may then expose his or her children to lead via physical contact. With regard to lifestyle, lead can be found in clay pots, so cooking with them—which is common in some cultures and geographic regions—may be a source of toxicity. Certain folk remedies also contain lead. Children can be accidentally exposed to toxins via toys, playgrounds, and objects such as lead in jewelry. Individuals working with hobbies using glue or aerosol spray paint may also be exposed to toxic substances. Therefore, high-risk communities for mental health problems related to toxicity include people and their families who work in certain occupations, malnourished populations, people with nutritional deficiencies, and children living in inner-city and urban areas or in old homes.

Psychosocial Influences on Mental Illness

The psychosocial component of mental includes the "thinking" component of health as well as the social component. The thinking component includes the ability to reason and make decisions and to interpret information and events accurately and realistically. The social part refers to interactions with others and the ability to adapt to social situations. Numerous life experiences can lead to problems with psychosocial mental health. These experiences can be both external and internal. Examples of external events that can impair mental health include dysfunctional families, being raped, socioeconomic status, and exposure to violence. Internal factors include issues such as poor coping skills, low self-esteem, and personality attributes.

Another way to look at psychosocial cause of mental health includes (1) individual characteristics; (2) life events, stresses, and relationships; and (3) neighborhoods, society, and culture. These three causes are discussed in the following paragraphs.

Individual Characteristics

Psychosocial characteristics of individuals have been identified as risk factors for mental illness. Individual psychosocial risk factors for mental illness include gender, level of optimism, coping style, personality and temperament, levels of resilience and empathy, feelings of personal control, and level of self-esteem.

Life Events, Stresses, and Relationships

Life events and the related stress can contribute to mental illness. Domestic violence; being bullied, raped, tortured, or abandoned; and exposure to crime, violence, natural disasters, and wars are examples of contributing factors. Negative or stressful life events more generally have been implicated in the development of a range of disorders, including mood and anxiety disorders. The main risks appear to be from a cumulative combination of such experiences over time, although exposure to a single major trauma can sometimes lead to psychopathology.

Relationship issues in the home, at school, and at work have been consistently linked to the development of mental disorders. Family relationships such as severe marital discord; paternal criminality, substance abuse, or mental disorder; admission into foster care; and neglect are examples of family situations that can impact one's mental health. Lack of ongoing harmonious, secure, committed relationships has been implicated both in childhood (including in institutional care) and also through the lifespan in social relations and the experience of loneliness, particularly during adolescence, and the development of mental disorder (Heinrich & Gullone, 2006; Marano, 2003).

Neighborhoods, Society, and Culture

Problems in communities, societies, and cultures have been implicated in the development of a mental disorder. Poverty, unemployment or underemployment, lack of social cohesion, violence, inadequate schools, crime, discrimination, and migration are a few examples. Poverty and socioeconomic position have been linked to the occurrence of major mental disorders, with a lower or more insecure educational, occupational, economic, or social position generally linked to more mental disorders (Muntaner, Eaton, Miech, & O'Campo, 2004). In addition, minority groups have been found to be at greater risk for developing mental disorders because of lack of health insurance, discrimination, social isolation, weakened social ties, and poverty.

TYPES OF MENTAL ILLNESS

Many different conditions are recognized as mental illnesses. The major categories are explained in this section.

Adjustment Disorder

Adjustment disorder occurs when a person develops emotional or behavioral symptoms in response to a stressful event or situation that is a maladaptive reaction that begins within 3 months of the event or situation and has continued for no more than 6 months. The stressors may include natural disasters, such as an earthquake or flood; events or crises, such as an accident, a house being burned down, the diagnosis of a major illness; or interpersonal problems, such as a divorce, death of a loved one, financial problems, relocation, loss of independence, or a problem with substance abuse. Symptoms include a depressed or anxious mood, isolation, and physical complaints.

Anxiety Disorders

Anxiety is an uncomfortable and subjective feeling that occurs in response to fear of certain objects or situations. It can be accompanied by physical signs such as high blood pressure, shortness of breath, eye twitch, sweating, and a rapid heartbeat. In a normal response, anxiety can help people cope with the situation. A person whose response is not appropriate for the situation, who cannot control the response, or whose response adversely affects normal functioning may be diagnosed with an anxiety disorder, which is the most common of all mental illnesses (Kneisl & Trigoboff, 2009). The anxiety may be triggered by an unknown reason as well as a specific object or situation. For example, a person with generalized anxiety disorder may experience anxiety unrelated to a specific event that occurs for no apparent reason. Others may experience anxiety related to certain objects, such as dogs (phobias), or specific situations, such as a fear of being away from home (agoraphobia). Examples of anxiety disorders include generalized anxiety disorder, posttraumatic stress disorder (PTSD), obsessive-compulsive disorder (OCD), panic disorder, agoraphobia, social anxiety disorder, and phobias.

Cognitive Disorders

These mental disorders are a result of mental deterioration. The disorders affect cognitive functions such as memory, perception, and problem solving. The cognitive disorders are delirium, dementia, and amnestic disorder. Symptoms of dementia include impaired memory, judgment, intellectual functioning, and abstract thinking; signs of delirium are a decreased awareness of the environment, attention and memory impairment, and altered perception; characteristics of amnesia are short and long-term memory deficits, an inability to recall previously learned information or to learn new information, and apathy. With the aging population, these problems, in particular, dementia, are becoming more prevalent.

Dissociative Disorders

A common thread of the dissociative disorders is that they are a defense against trauma. There is an alteration in conscious awareness of memories, identity, behavior, or affect, which acts as a defense mechanism. The traumatic events, accidents, or disasters may be experienced or witnessed by the individual. People with these disorders suffer severe disturbances or changes in memory, consciousness, identity, and general awareness of themselves and their surroundings. Sufferers of dissociative disorders often encounter persistent or recurrent feelings of depersonalization, which gives a sense of automation and going through life without experiencing it. They may feel detached from their own body or thoughts. Dissociative identity disorder (formally called multiple personality disorder) is a more commonly known disorder in which the ill person has at least two personalities.

Eating Disorders

Eating disorders involve extreme emotions, attitudes, and behaviors involving weight and food. Anorexia nervosa, bulimia nervosa, and binge eating are the most common eating disorders. Women and athletes are communities particularly at risk of anorexia and bulimia.

Factitious Disorders

Factitious disorders are conditions in which physical and/or emotional symptoms are intentionally experienced in order to place the individual in the role of a patient or a person in need of help. The self-induction of the disease is a conscious act, but the motivation behind it is usually unconscious (Kneisl & Trigoboff, 2009).

Impulse Control and Addiction Disorders

People with impulse control disorders are unable to resist urges, or impulses, to perform acts that could be harmful to themselves or others. Frequently people with these disorders become so focused on their addiction that they begin to ignore responsibilities and relationships. Examples of impulse disorders include pyromania (starting fires), kleptomania (stealing), and compulsive gambling. Alcohol and drugs are common objects of addictions among people with impulse control disorders.

Mood Disorders

Also known as affective disorders, these disorders involve disturbances in emotional, behavioral, and physical patterns. These patterns of affect (mood) range from extreme lows to extreme elations. People encounter persistent feelings of sadness (depression) or periods of feeling overly happy (mania) or fluctuate from extreme happiness to extreme sadness (bipolar). Other symptoms include problems with memory and concentration, fatigue, grandiosity, indecisiveness, apathy, and irritability. Examples of mood disorders are depression, mania, bipolar disorder, and seasonal affective disorder.

Personality Disorders

People with personality disorders have extreme and inflexible personality traits that are distressing to them. The person may not understand the effect of their behavior on others or not accept the consequences of their behavior. They may become manipulative, impulsive, self-centered, and controlling. As a result, the disorder may cause problems in social relationships, school, or work. Examples include antisocial personality disorder, obsessive-compulsive personality disorder, and paranoid personality disorder.

Psychotic Disorders

Psychotic disorders involve distorted awareness and thinking such as hallucinations (a subjective sensory experience of images or sounds that are not real, such as hearing voices) and delusions (a mistaken or false belief about the self or the environment that the ill person accepts as true, despite evidence to the contrary). Schizophrenia and delusion disorder are examples of psychotic disorders.

Sexual and Gender Disorders

These include disorders that affect sexual desire, performance, and behavior. Sexual dysfunction, gender identity disorder, paraphilias (characterized as unconventional sexual behaviors as defined by the dominant culture, such as getting sexually aroused by inflicting emotional or physical pain), and sexual desire disorders are examples.

Sleep Disorders

Disorder in a person's sleep patterns include insomnia, hypersomnia (prolonged or excessive sleep), sleep terror disorder (also known as night terrors), and circadian-rhythm disorders (the sleep-wake cycle is disturbed by factors such as jet lag and shift work).

Somatoform Disorders

Also known as psychosomatic disorders, people experience physical symptoms suggesting a physical disorder but there is no evidence of a physiologic cause. They have a dysfunction related to physical self-awareness and become obsessively interested in diseases and bodily processes. Examples include hypochondriasis, panic disorder, and body dysmorphic disorder (a preoccupation with an imagined or slight defect in physical appearance).

Substance-Related Disorders

These disorders are characterized by the recurrent use of substances that results in a failure to fulfill major role obligations related to work, school, or home or causing other related negative consequences such as encountering legal problems or driving while under the influence. Some substance abuse problems are related to the use of alcohol, opioids (such as heroin and morphine), or cocaine.

Tic Disorders

People with tic disorders make sounds or display body movements that are repeated, quick, sudden, and/or uncontrollable. Sounds that are made involuntarily are called vocal tics; rapid and recurrent movements are called motor tics. **Tourette syndrome** is an example of a tic disorder.

MANIFESTATIONS OF MENTAL ILLNESS

Signs and symptoms of mental illness exist on an individual and community level. In this section we discuss the symptoms of mental illness on both levels.

On an Individual Level

Persons suffering from any of the severe mental disorders present with a variety of symptoms that may include inappropriate anxiety, disturbances of thought and perception, dysregulation of mood, and cognitive dysfunction. Many of these symptoms may be relatively specific to a particular diagnosis or cultural influence. For example, disturbances of thought and perception (**psychosis**) are most commonly associated with schizophrenia. Similarly, severe disturbances in expression of affect and regulation of mood are most commonly seen in depression and bipolar disorder. However, it is not uncommon to see psychotic symptoms in patients diagnosed with mood disorders or to see mood-related symptoms in patients diagnosed with schizophrenia. Symptoms associated with mood, anxiety, thought process, or cognition may occur in any patient at some point during his or her illness.

Anxiety

Anxiety is one of the most understood of the major symptoms of mental disorders. Each of us encounters anxiety in many forms throughout the course of our routine daily activities. It may often take the concrete form of intense fear experienced in response to an immediately threatening experience such as dodging a falling object or oncoming car. Strong emotional responses of fear and dread as well as physical signs of anxiety such as rapid heartbeat and sweating are typically responses of intense fear. Anxiety is aroused most intensely by immediate threats to one's safety, and it also may result from situations that one imagines or anticipates, such as worrying about failing an upcoming examination.

Anxiety is an uncomfortable feeling that occurs from fear or losing something valued. It involves an innate biological response to dangerous situations that prepares one to evade or confront a threat in the environment. The appropriate regulation of anxiety is critical to the survival of virtually every higher organism in every environment. However, the mechanisms that regulate anxiety may break down in a wide variety of circumstances, leading to an excessive or inappropriate expression of anxiety. Examples include phobias, panic attacks, PTSD, and generalized anxiety. In phobias, high-level anxiety is aroused by specific situations or objects that may range from tangible items, such as snakes, to complex circumstances, such as social interactions or public speaking. Panic attacks are brief and very intense episodes of anxiety that often occur without a precipitating event or stimulus. Generalized anxiety is a chronic condition in which the anxiety is not specific. Sufferers often worry about everyday issues, and it may be triggered by stress. Sometimes the trigger is unknown, and the anxiety appears to come out of nowhere.

In addition to these common manifestations of anxiety, OCD and PTSD are generally believed to be related to the anxiety disorders. In the case of OCD, individuals experience a high level of anxiety that drives their obsessional thinking or compulsive behaviors. When such an individual fails to carry out a repetitive behavior such as hand washing or counting, they experience severe anxiety. PTSD occurs from an intense fear caused by an exposure to a dangerous event that often is life threatening. The characteristic symptoms that result from such a traumatic event include the persistent reexperience of the event in dreams and memories, persistent avoidance of stimuli associated with the event, and increased arousal.

Psychosis

A disturbance in the ability to comprehend reality and in relating and communicating with others is referred to as a psychosis. Hallucinations and delusions often accompany psychosis. Hallucinations are said to occur when an individual experiences a sensory impression that has no basis in reality. This impression could involve any of the sensory modalities. Thus hallucinations may be auditory, olfactory, gustatory, kinesthetic, tactile, or visual. For example, auditory hallucinations frequently involve the impression that one is hearing a voice. In each case, the sensory impression is falsely experienced as real. It is important to take culture into consideration with regard to hallucination. In some cultures, for example, hearing voices is perceived as having a connection with a higher being or as part of religious ceremonies and is not viewed as a mental disorder.

A **delusion** is a false belief that an individual holds despite evidence to the contrary. Attempts to persuade the person that these beliefs are unfounded typically fail and may even result in the further entrenchment of the beliefs. A common example is paranoia, in which a person has delusional beliefs that others are trying to harm him or her. Delusions can be dangerous. For example, if a person believes that he or she can fly and attempts to do so by jumping off of a building, the outcome can be life threatening.

Hallucinations and delusions are among the most commonly observed psychotic symptoms. A list of other symptoms seen in psychotic illnesses such as schizophrenia appears in **Table 2-1**. Symptoms of schizophrenia are divided into two broad classes: *positive* symptoms and *negative* symptoms. Positive symptoms are excessive or added behaviors that are not normally seen in mentally healthy adults, and negative symptoms are the loss of normal functions normally seen in mentally healthy adults (Fontaine, 2009). Positive symptoms such as hallucinations are responsible for much of the acute distress associated with schizophrenia, but negative symptoms appear to be responsible for much of the chronic and long-term disability associated with the disorder.

Positive symptoms generally involve the experience of something in consciousness that should not normally be present. For example, hallucinations and delusions

TABLE 2-1 Common Manifestations of Schizophrenia

Positive Symptoms
Hallucinations
Delusions
Disorganized thoughts, behaviors, and/or speech
Hyperactivity
Inappropriate or overreactive affect
Loose or illogical thoughts
Agitation or hostility
Negative Symptoms
Blunted or flat affect
Attention impairment
Concrete thoughts
Memory problems
Social withdrawal
Decreased activity level
Anhedonia (inability to experience pleasure)
Avolition (lack of motivation or initiative)
Alogia (complete lack of speech)

represent perceptions or beliefs that should not normally be experienced. In addition to hallucinations and delusions, patients with psychotic disorders such as schizophrenia frequently have marked disturbances in the logical process of their thoughts. Specifically, psychotic thought processes are characteristically loose, disorganized, illogical, or bizarre, and these thought behaviors may produce observable patterns of behavior that are also disorganized and bizarre (U.S. Department of Health and Human Services [DHHS], 1999).

In contrast to positive symptoms, which represent the presence of something not normally experienced, negative symptoms reflect the absence of thoughts and behaviors that would otherwise be expected. Concreteness of thought represents impairment in the ability to think abstractly. Blunting of affect refers to a general reduction in the ability to express emotion. Motivational failure and inability to initiate activities represent a major source of long-term disability in schizophrenia. Anhedonia reflects a deficit in the ability to experience pleasure and to react appropriately to pleasurable situations.

Disturbances of Mood

Emotions are a very strong component of the human experience and exist on a continuum from very positive to very negative. One's mood is composed of their emotional state. "Mood is defined as a sustained emotional state and how you subjectively feel" (Fontaine, 2009, p. 297). Disorders that impact the regulation of mood represent a major category among mental disorders called mood disorders. There are many subtypes of mood disorders.

Disturbances of mood characteristically manifest themselves as a sustained feeling of sadness or sustained elevation of mood. Disturbances of mood may occur in a variety of patterns associated with different mental disorders. The disorder most closely associated with persistent sadness is major depression, whereas that associated with sustained elevation is referred to as mania. Extreme fluctuations of mood is called bipolar disorder. **Table 2-2** lists the most common signs of these mood disorders. Along with the prevailing feelings of sadness or elation, disorders of mood are associated with a host of related symptoms that include disturbances in appetite, sleep patterns, energy level, concentration, and memory.

Disturbances of Cognition

Cognitive function refers to the general ability to organize, process, and recall information. Cognitive tasks may be subdivided into a large number of more specific functions depending on the nature of the information remembered and the circumstances

TABLE 2-2 Common Signs of Mood Disorders

Symptoms Commonly Associated with Depression
Persistent sadness or despair
Insomnia or hypersomnia
Change in appetite
Psychomotor agitation or retardation
Fatigue or loss of energy
Anhedonia (inability to experience pleasure)
Irritability
Apathy, poor motivation, social withdrawal
Hopelessness
Poor self-esteem; feelings of helplessness, worthlessness, or excessive or inappropriate guilt
Suicidal ideation
Symptoms Commonly Associated with Mania
Elevated or euphoric mood
Grandiosity (inappropriately high self-esteem)
Psychomotor agitation
Decreased need for sleep
Racing thoughts and distractibility
Difficulty with sitting still
Irritability
Impulsivity
Increased sexual interest
Rapid or pressured speech
More talkative than usual
Excessive involvement in pleasurable activities that have a high potential for painful consequences

of its recall. In addition, many functions are commonly associated with cognition, such as the ability to execute complex sequences of tasks.

Disturbances of cognitive function may occur in a variety of disorders. Progressive deterioration of cognitive function is referred to as dementia. Dementia may be caused by a number of specific conditions, including Alzheimer's disease. Mood disturbances such as depression and other mental disorders also can impair cognitive function. Chemical, metabolic, and infectious diseases that exert an impact on the brain also can lead to problems with cognition.

The manifestations of cognitive impairment can vary across an extremely wide range, depending on severity. Short-term memory is one of the earliest functions to be affected and, as severity increases, retrieval of more remote memories becomes more difficult. Attention, concentration, and higher intellectual functions can be impaired as the underlying disease process progresses. Language difficulties range from mild word-finding problems to complete inability to comprehend or use language. Functional impairments associated with cognitive deficits can markedly interfere with the ability to perform activities of daily living such as dressing and bathing.

Other Symptoms

Anxiety, psychosis, mood disturbances, and cognitive impairments are among the most common and disabling manifestations of mental disorders. It is important, however, to appreciate that mental disorders leave no aspect of human experience untouched. Other common manifestations include, for example, somatic or other physical symptoms and impairment of impulse control.

On a Community Level

On the community level, manifestations of mental illness are often found using statistical data. Numerous indicators can be used to assess the communities' mental health. Statistics related to crime, school dropout rates, violence, emergency department admissions, teenage pregnancy rates, divorce rates, child abuse cases, domestic violence cases, employment rates, school attendance and performance, drug arrests, homeless rates, poverty rates, road rage, drunk driving arrests, suicide rates, and lack of mental health services are all symptoms of mental health problems.

DIAGNOSIS OF MENTAL ILLNESS

The discussion in the previous section divided the manifestations of mental disorders into distinct categories. These categories are broad and overlap. Dividing the manifestations into categories such as this is certainly not perfect, but despite these imperfections, this systematic approach is the foundation of how the classification and diagnosis of mental illness has developed. The classification system used to diagnose mental illness is important for treatment, insurance reimbursement, obtaining supportive services, establishing a prognosis, and preventing related disability. Diagnosis also is valuable for research and surveillance.

As we mentioned in Chapter 1, mental illness refers collectively to all of the diagnosable mental disorders. Because the signs and symptoms of mental illness lie on a continuum, there is no clear-cut dividing line between mental health and illness, which makes diagnosis challenging. It is clear when a person has a severe mental illness with prominent symptoms, such as schizophrenia, but for other mental disorders, such as depression or ADHD, it is more difficult to differentiate between distress and disease. In addition, the manifestations of mental disorders vary with age, gender, religion, and culture. The thresholds of mental illness or disorder have, indeed, been set by convention (DHHS, 1999). At what point does one move along a continuum from normal into the realm of illness? Ultimately, the dividing line has to do with severity of symptoms, duration, and functional impairment (DHHS, 1999).

The diagnosis of mental disorders is often more difficult than the diagnosis of somatic problems because there is no physical indicator such as an x-ray or laboratory test that can identify the illness. The diagnosis of mental disorders must rest with the patients' reports of the intensity and duration of symptoms, signs from their mental status examination, and clinician observation of their behavior including functional impairment (DHHS, 1999). These combined indicators can lead the clinician to recognizing patterns known as syndromes. When the syndrome meets all the criteria for a diagnosis, it constitutes a mental disorder. Most mental health conditions are referred to as disorders, rather than as diseases, because diagnosis rests on clinical criteria (DHHS, 1999). The term **disease** generally is reserved for conditions with known pathology (detectable physical change). The term **disorder** is reserved for clusters of symptoms and signs associated with distress and disability (i.e., impairment of functioning), yet the pathology and etiology are unknown (DHHS, 1999).

Assessment of mental illness on an individual level includes a psychiatric and physiologic examination. The psychiatric examination includes looking at the patient's history and current state (i.e., affect, appearance, obsessions). The physical examination includes looking for any biological causes for the symptoms and possibly conducting some clinical tests, such as brain images and intelligence tests.

On a community level, assessment includes looking at indicators of mental health problems, such as high school dropout rates, crime statistics, and divorce rates. Community screening programs also help identify mental health problems. Screening provides a quick way to identify whether the person may be experiencing symptoms commonly associated with an illness and determine whether follow-up with a professional is recommended. Screening is not a substitute for a complete mental health evaluation. It does not result in a diagnosis but rather provides an indication of whether or not a person has symptoms consistent with a particular illness.

Screening for Mental Health, Inc. (SMH) introduced the concept of large-scale mental health screenings with National Depression Screening Day in 1991 (Screening for Mental Health, n.d.). National Depression Screening Day occurs each October and operates a toll-free, year-round phone line that allows callers to find free and confidential screening locations in their local areas. SMH programs include both in-person and online programs for depression, bipolar disorder, generalized anxiety disorder, PTSD, eating disorders, alcohol problems, and suicide prevention (Screening for Mental Health, n.d.). Screening programs are implemented by local clinicians at mental health facilities, hospitals, primary care offices, social service agencies, colleges/ universities, workplaces, schools, and the military.

CLASSIFICATION OF MENTAL ILLNESS

The standard manual used for the classification and diagnosis of mental disorders in the United States is the *Diagnostic and Statistical Manual of Mental Disorders* (*DSM*), which is published by the American Psychiatric Association. The first edition was published in 1952, and the most recent edition was published in 2000 (*DSM-IV-TR*). The *DSM-IV-TR* organizes mental disorders into the major diagnostic classes listed in **Table 2-3**. For each disorder within a diagnostic class, the *DSM* identifies specific criteria for making the diagnosis and diagnostic subtypes for some disorders. A subtype is a subgroup within a diagnosis that confers greater specificity. The *DSM* includes a descriptive listing of symptoms and does not address the causes of the disorders.

The World Health Organization's *International Classification of Diseases* (ICD) is a valuable compendium of all diseases. The 10th edition (ICD-10) is the latest edition. Between revisions, updates are made to the content to keep it current. The ICD is the official classification for mortality and morbidity statistics established by the World Health Organization, and the official classification for the Health Care Financing Administration. The Health Care Financing Administration uses the coding system (each diagnosis is tied to a specific numeric code) as the basis of a uniform language that accurately describes medical, surgical, and diagnostic services. Often health insurance companies use the codes to determine provider reimbursement rates and for decisions related to treatment authorizations. The ICD is the international standard diagnostic classification for all general epidemiologic, many health management purposes, and clinical use. These include the analysis of the general health situation of population groups and monitoring of the incidence and prevalence of diseases and other health problems in relation to other variables such as the characteristics and circumstances of the individuals affected, reimbursement, resource allocation, quality, and guidelines.

Knowledge about diagnosis continues to evolve. Evolution in the diagnosis of mental disorders generally reflects greater understanding of disorders as well as the influence of social norms. Years ago, for instance, addiction to tobacco was not viewed as

TABLE 2-3 Major Diagnostic Classes of Mental Disorders (*DSM-IV-TR*) and Examples

Category	Examples
Disorders usually first diagnosed in infancy, childhood, or adolescence	Mental retardation, learning disorders, autistic disorder, attention deficit disorder, destructive behavior disorder
Delirium, dementia, and amnestic and other cognitive disorders	Alzheimer's, substance-induced dementia, amnestic disorders
Mental disorders due to a general medical condition	Catatonic disorder, personality change due to a general medical condition
Substance-related disorders	Substance-induced persisting dementia, substance-induced sexual dysfunction, hallucinogen persisting perception disorder
Schizophrenia and other psychotic disorders	Paranoid type, delusional disorder, brief psychotic disorder
Mood disorders	Major depressive disorder, bipolar disorders, hypomanic episode
Anxiety disorders	Obsessive-compulsive disorder, social phobia, agoraphobia, panic attack, posttraumatic stress disorder
Somatoform disorders	Pain disorder, body dysmorphic disorder, hypochondriasis
Factitious disorders	Factitious disorder with predominantly psychological signs and symptoms
Dissociative disorders	Dissociative amnesia, dissociative identity disorder (formally multiple personality disorder)
Sexual and gender identity disorders	Sexual dysfunctions, male erectile disorder, orgasmic disorders
Eating disorders	Anorexia nervosa, bulimia nervosa
Sleep disorders	Insomnia, narcolepsy, sleepwalking disorder
Impulse-control disorders not elsewhere classified	Kleptomania, pathological gambling, pyromania
Adjustment disorders	Withdrawal, anxious mood
Personality disorders	Paranoid personality disorder, antisocial personality disorder
Other conditions that may be a focus of clinical attention	Problems related to abuse or neglect, age-related cognitive decline, medication-induced movement disorders

a disorder, but today it falls under the category of substance-related disorders. At one time, homosexuality was considered a mental disorder. Although the *DSM* strives to cover all populations, it is not without limitations. Diagnosis relies on clinician judgment about whether clients' symptom patterns and impairments of functioning meet diagnostic criteria. Cultural differences in emotional expression and social behavior can be misinterpreted as impaired if clinicians are not sensitive to the cultural context and the meaning of exhibited symptoms.

TREATMENT OF MENTAL ILLNESS

Mental health professionals use a variety of approaches to treat those suffering from mental illness. They vary in terms of length and intensity. Treatment may involve a single method or several different methods. The information that follows highlights a few of the more common treatment methods, but note that many more exist. Treatments can occur in a variety of settings such as schools, clinics, and online. Chapter 5 describes the systems in which the treatment methods are provided.

Animal-Assisted Therapy

Animal-assisted therapy (also known as pet therapy) is the use of specially trained animals for specific and therapeutic reasons. The animals can assist with physical, social, emotional, and/or cognitive problems. The animals can reduce stress, anxiety, and feelings of isolation; increase empathy; assist with people socializing with others; improve memory and self-expression; and alleviate feelings of depression and loneliness.

Case Management

Mental health case management is designed to assist mentally ill adults and to shift their care from an inpatient setting to community care. Case management services can be related to medical, social, psychological, educational, financial, vocational, and other services to maintain maximum level of independence and community functioning. The focus of case management is to coordinate and integrate the person's care and to advocate for the patient and his or her family. Case management can prevent unnecessary hospitalization, fragmented care, and care in the least restrictive setting possible (Kneisl & Trigoboff, 2009). A case manager, often a nurse or social worker, is designated to negotiate and navigate through the complex mental health system on the patient's behalf and to work with a variety of healthcare providers to facilitate the person's care.

Complementary and Alternative Therapies

Complementary and *alternative* are broad terms that cover hundreds of therapies from all over the world, many of which are ancient. Studies show that about a third of people in the United States use complementary and alternative medicine. When prayer is included, the number jumps to 62% (Fontaine, 2009). Approximately 43% of people with anxiety attacks and 41% of adults with severe depression use alternative therapies (Fontaine, 2009). Some users use them in isolation (alternative), and some combine them with traditional Western medicine (complementary). Examples include acupuncture, aromatherapy, animal-assisted therapy, traditional Chinese medicine, herbal medicine, **curanderismo**, chiropractic medicine, herbs, prayer, therapeutic touch, hypnotherapy, homeopathy, yoga, spiritual journeys, and **naturopathy**.

Some examples of herbs and supplements used for mental health include chamomile and kava for anxiety; St. John's wort for depression; catnip, passion flower, and melatonin for insomnia; ginkgo for memory; and evening primrose oil, ginseng, and chamomile for alcohol and drug withdrawal (Fontaine, 2009). Examples of aromatherapy essential oils used to treat mental health problems include lavender, sage, and chamomile for insomnia; peppermint for alertness; jasmine for depression; and lemon balm for anxiety (Fontaine, 2009). Other examples of complementary and alternative medicine are tai chi and meditation for stress and anxiety, therapeutic touch and hypnosis for pain and stress relief, and prayer for many types of problems.

Couples Counseling and Family Therapy

These two similar approaches to therapy involve discussions and problem-solving sessions facilitated by a therapist, sometimes with the couple or entire family group, sometimes with individuals. Such therapy can help couples and family members improve both their understanding of one another and the way they respond to each another. This type of therapy can resolve patterns of behavior that might lead to more severe mental illness. Family therapy can help educate the individuals about the nature of mental disorders and teach them skills to cope better with the effects of having a family member with a mental illness, such as how to deal with feelings of anger or guilt.

Crisis Hotlines

A **crisis hotline** is a phone number people can call to get immediate over-the-phone emergency counseling, which is usually provided by trained volunteers. Initially set up to help those contemplating suicide, crisis hotlines have been expanded to provide mental health services in other areas as well. Topics also include child and elder abuse, substance abuse, domestic violence, eating disorders, and many more.

Crisis Response Services

Crisis response services refers to a crisis intervention service that is a short-term intervention of psychiatric care designed to address the immediate presenting symptoms of a psychiatric emergency and ameliorate the client's distress, so that individual, family, and community resources and supports can be mobilized, and planning for further treatment can occur. A crisis intervention service is often the entry point to a course of treatment within a system of services, and thus involves screening, assessment, and disposition to the next appropriate and least restrictive level of service. The purpose of the crisis intervention is to stabilize individuals in psychiatric crisis and prevent further dysfunction.

Mentally ill people with severe or acute illness are the people who typically avail themselves of these services and use the hospital to care for them. There are a variety of reasons why people use these services, including failure to take their medication, relapse from drug abuse, or limited services. The hospital's role is to evaluate, treat, and stabilize the person, but staff usually do not have the resources to help clients transition back into the community after discharge. This contributes to the cycle of crisis and hospitalization, discharge, and recurrent crisis and hospitalization.

Educational Programs

Public health professionals develop and implement a variety of programs in various settings such as schools, hospitals, community centers, and universities. These programs encompass a broad range of topics such as education about drugs, violence prevention, anger and stress management, and cyber bullying.

Electroconvulsive Therapy

Electroconvulsive therapy, also known as ECT, is a highly controversial technique that uses low-voltage electrical stimulation of the brain to treat some forms of major depression, acute mania, and some forms of schizophrenia. This potentially lifesaving technique is considered only when other therapies have failed, when a person is seriously medically ill and/or unable to take medication, or when a person is very likely to commit suicide. Substantial improvements in the equipment, dosing guidelines, and anesthesia have significantly reduced the possibility of side effects.

Group Therapy

This form of therapy involves groups of usually 4 to 12 people who have similar problems and meet face-to-face regularly with a trained therapist. The therapist uses the emotional interactions of the group's members to help them get relief from distress and possibly modify their behavior. Members are encouraged to give feedback and support to others. Feedback includes members of the group expressing their own feelings about what someone says or does. Interaction between group members is highly encouraged and provides each person with an opportunity to try out new ways of behaving; it also provides members with an opportunity for learning more about the way they interact with others. It is a safe environment in which members work to establish a level of trust that allows them to talk personally and honestly. Group members make a commitment to the group and are instructed that the content of the group sessions is confidential. It is not appropriate for group members to disclose events of the group to an outside person.

Interpersonal Psychotherapy

Through one-on-one conversations with a trained therapist, this approach focuses on the patient's current life and relationships within the family, social, and work environments. The goal is to identify and resolve problems with insight, as well as build on strengths.

Several types of therapeutic approaches are used, sometimes in combination. Behavioral therapy and cognitive therapy are two common therapeutic types. **Behavioral therapy** focuses on changing unwanted behaviors through rewards, reinforcements, and desensitization. Behavioral therapy often involves the cooperation of others, especially family and close friends, to reinforce a desired behavior. **Cognitive therapy** is based on the idea that thoughts are directly connected to how people feel. Therapists in the cognitive field work with clients to solve present-day problems by helping them to identify distorted thinking that causes emotional discomfort. The historical root of a problem is not the focus of this type of therapy. The focus is on how the person's present thinking is causing distress. It aims to identify and correct distorted thinking patterns that can lead to feelings and behaviors that may be troublesome, self-defeating, or even self-destructive. The goal is to replace such thinking with a more balanced view that, in turn, leads to more fulfilling and productive behavior. An example is trying to eliminate negative self-talk.

Light Therapy

Seasonal affective disorder (SAD) is a form of depression that appears related to fluctuations in the exposure to natural light. It usually strikes during autumn and often continues through the winter when natural light is reduced. Researchers have found that people with SAD can be helped with the symptoms of their illness if they spend blocks of time bathed in light from a special full-spectrum light source called a light box.

Play Therapy

Geared toward young children, this technique uses a variety of activities such as painting and puppets to establish communication with the therapist and resolve problems. Play allows the child to express emotions and problems that would be too difficult to discuss with another person.

Play therapy is also used as tool of diagnosis. A play therapist observes a client playing with toys (playhouses, pets, dolls, etc.) to determine the cause of the disturbed behavior. The objects and patterns of play, as well as the willingness to interact with the therapist, can be used to understand the underlying rationale for behavior both inside and outside the session.

Psychopharmacology

Several psychotropic medications are on the market today. This assortment of medications provides more options for people with mental illness, but a challenge is to find the best medication or right combination and doses. Medication alone, or in combination with psychotherapy, has proven to be an effective treatment for a number of emotional, behavioral, and mental disorders. The kind of medication that a psychiatrist prescribes varies with the disorder and the individual being treated.

Support Groups

Support groups can be very helpful to people struggling with mental health problems such as substance abuse, grieving, and anger management, and to those coping with disease. In a support group, members share thoughts and feelings related to a particular issue, such as divorce or being a victim of domestic violence. The help given by group members may take the form of providing and evaluating relevant information, sharing related personal experiences, listening to and accepting others' experiences, providing sympathetic understanding, and establishing social networks. Attendance is voluntary, and usually the groups are not led by trained professionals.

CHAPTER SUMMARY

Mental illness is influenced by biological, psychological, and social factors. There are several types of mental illness, and the symptoms range from mild to severe. The diagnosis and treatment can be challenging and must take into consideration issues such as age and culture. Certain mental illnesses tend to run in some communities. Examples include substance abuse among the homeless, eating disorders among athletes, TBI in the military, and cognitive disorders in the elderly.

In this chapter, we discussed the etiology of mental illness. We described the types of illness, common symptoms, and how mental illness is diagnosed and classified. An overview of treatment methods ended the chapter.

REVIEW

1. List examples of clinical features of anxiety, psychosis, mood disturbances, and cognitive disturbances.
2. What are positive and negative symptoms of psychosis?
3. What is the *DSM*?
4. What is *ICD*?
5. What is the biopsychosocial model of disease?
6. How can biological influences (genes, infections, physical trauma, nutrition, hormones, and toxins) affect mental health?
7. How does the social environment affect mental health?
8. What treatment methods are used to assist people with mental problems or disorders?

ACTIVITY

Research what types of mental health care services are provided in your community, and find three Web sites that provide mental health services (e.g., self-assessments, online support groups). Write a paragraph or two about the types of services provided and assess how you feel about the mental health care services that are available in your community.

REFERENCES AND FURTHER READINGS

American Psychiatric Association. (1994). *Diagnostic and statistical manual of mental disorders* (4th ed.). Washington, DC: Author.

Andreasen, N. C. (1997). Linking mind and brain in the study of mental illnesses: A project for a scientific psychopathology. *Science*, *275*, 1586–1593.

Bandura, A. (1977). *Social learning theory*. Englewood Cliffs, NJ: Prentice-Hall.

Barondes, S. (1993). *Molecules and mental illness*. New York: Scientific American Library.

Baum, A., & Posluszny, D. M. (1999). Health psychology: Mapping biobehavioral contributions to health and illness. *Annual Review of Psychology*, *50*, 137–163.

Berrento-Clement, J. R., Schweinhart, L. J., Barnett, W. S., Epstein, A. S., & Weikart, D. P. (1984). *Changed lives: The effects of the Perry Preschool Program on youths through age 19*. (High/Scope Educational Research Foundation, Monograph 8). Ypsilanti, MI: High/Scope Press.

Bowlby, J. (1951). *Maternal care and mental health*. Geneva: World Health Organization.

Brenner, C. (1978). *An elementary textbook of psychoanalysis* (2nd ed.). New York: International Universities Press.

Breslau, N., Kessler, R. C., Chilcoat, H. D., Schultz, L. R., Davis, G. C., & Andreski, P. (1998). Trauma and posttraumatic stress disorder in the community: The 1996 Detroit Area Survey of Trauma. *Archives of General Psychiatry, 55*, 626–632.

Cabaj, R. P., & Stein, T. S. (1996). *Textbook of homosexuality and mental health*. Washington, DC: American Psychiatric Press.

Canino, G. J., Bird, H. R., Shrout, P. E., Rubio-Stipec, M., Bravo, M., Martinez, R., . . . Guevara, L. M. (1987). The prevalence of specific psychiatric disorders in Puerto Rico. *Archives of General Psychiatry, 44*, 727–735.

Center for Mental Health Services. (1998). *Cultural competence standards in managed care mental health services for four underserved/ underrepresented racial/ethnic groups*. Rockville, MD: Author.

Centers for Disease Control and Prevention. (1991). *Strategic plan for the elimination of childhood lead poisoning*. Atlanta, GA: Author.

Chambless, D. L., Baker, M. J., Baucom, D. H., Beutler, L. E., Calhoun, K. S., Crits-Christoph, P., . . . Woody, S. R. (1998). Update on empirically validated therapies II. *Clinical Psychologist, 51*, 3–16.

Chambless, D. L., Sanderson, W. C., Shohman, V., Bennett, J. S., Pope, K. S., Crits-Cristoph, P., . . . McMurry, S. (1996). An update on empirically validated therapies. *Clinical Psychologist, 49*, 5–18.

Cheung, F. K., & Snowden, L. R. (1990). Community mental health and ethnic minority populations. *Community Mental Health Journal, 26*, 277–291.

Ciarlo, J. A. (1998). Estimating and monitoring need for mental health services in rural frontier areas. *Rural Community Mental Health, 24*, 17–18.

Clarke, G. N., Hawkins, W., Murphy, M., Sheeber, L. B., Lewinsohn, P. M., & Seeley, J. R. (1995). Targeted prevention of unipolar depressive disorder in an at-risk sample of high school adolescents: A randomized trial of a group cognitive intervention. *Journal of the American Academy of Child and Adolescent Psychiatry, 34*, 312–321.

Cohen, S., & Herbert, T. B. (1996). Health psychology: Psychological factors and physical disease from the perspective of human psychoneuroimmunology. *Annual Review of Psychology, 47*, 113–142.

Conwell, Y. (1996). *Diagnosis and treatment of depression in late life*. Washington, DC: American Psychiatric Press.

Cooper, C. R., & Denner, J. (1998). Theories linking culture and psychopathology: Universal and community-specific processes. *Annual Review of Psychology, 49*, 559–584.

Cooper, J. R., Bloom, F. E., & Roth, R. H. (1996). *The biochemical basis of neuropharmacology*. New York: Oxford University Press.

Danbom, D. (1995). *Born in the country: A history of rural America*. Baltimore: Johns Hopkins University Press.

Dawodu, S. T. (2009). Traumatic brain injury (TBI)—Definition, epidemiology, pathophysiology. Retrieved from http://emedicine.medscape.com/article/326510-overview

del Pinal, J., & Singer, A. (1997). Generations of diversity: Latinos in the United States. *Population Bulletin*, *52*, 1–44.

Dohrenwend, B. P., Levav, I., Schwartz, S., Naveh, G., Link, B. G., Skodol, A. E., & Stueve, A. (1992). Socioeconomic status and psychiatric disorders: The causation-selection issue. *Science*, *255*, 946–952.

Emerick, R. (1990). Self-help groups for former patients: Relations with mental health professionals. *Hospital and Community Psychiatry*, *41*, 401–407.

Engel, G. L. (1977). The need for a new medical model: A challenge for biomedicine. *Science*, *196*, 129–136.

Erikson, E. (1950). *Childhood and society*. New York: Norton.

Family Process. (2005). Toward a biopsychosocial model for 21st-century genetics. Vol. 44(1), pp. 3–24. Retrieved from http://www.redorbit.com/news/display?id=137821&source=r_health

Farragher, B. (1998). Psychiatric morbidity following the diagnosis and treatment of early breast cancer. *Irish Journal of Medical Science*, *167*, 166–169.

Federation of Families for Children's Mental Health. (1999). *Federation of Families for Children's Mental Health home page*. Retrieved from http://www.ffcmh.org

Feldman, R. S. (1997). *Development across the lifespan*. Upper Saddle River, NJ: Prentice Hall.

Fontaine, K. L. (2009). Mental health nursing. Upper Saddle River, NJ: Pearson-Prentice Hall.

Frese, F. J. (1998). Advocacy, recovery, and the challenges of consumerism for schizophrenia. *Psychiatric Clinics of North America*, *21*, 233–249.

Frese, F. J., & Davis, W. W. (1997). The consumer-survivor movement, recovery, and consumer professionals. *Professional Psychology: Research and Practice*, *28*, 243–245.

Friedman, L. M., Furberg, C. D., & DeMets, D. L. (1996a). *Fundamentals of clinical trials* (3rd ed.). St. Louis: Mosby.

Friedman, R. M., Katz-Levey, J. W., Manderschied, R. W., & Sondheimer, D. L. (1996b). Prevalence of serious emotional disturbance in children and adolescents. In R. W. Manderscheid & M. A. Sonnenschein (Eds.), *Mental health, United States, 1996* (pp. 71–88). Rockville, MD: Center for Mental Health Services.

Friesen, B. J., & Stephens B. (1998). Expanding family roles in the system of care: Research and practice. In M. R. Epstein, K. Kutash, & A. J. Duchnowski (Eds.), *Outcomes for children and youth with behavioral and emotional disorders and their families: Programs and evaluation, best practices* (pp. 231–259). Austin, TX: Pro-Ed.

Gale Encyclopedia of Mental Health. (2007). Nutrition and mental health. Thomson Gale Publisher. Retrieved from http://www.gale.cengage.com/pdf/samples/sp429878.pdf

Gallo, J. J., Marino, S., Ford, D., & Anthony, J. C. (1995). Filters on the pathway to mental health care: II. Sociodemographic factors. *Psychological Medicine*, *25*, 1149–1160.

Garcia, M., & Rodriguez, P. F. (1989). Psychological effects of political repression in Argentina and El Salvador. In D. Koslow & E. Salett (Eds.), *Crossing cultures in mental health* (pp. 64–83). Washington, DC: SIETAR International.

Garmezy, N. (1983). Stressors of childhood. In N. Garmezy & M. Rutter (Eds.), *Stress, coping, and development in children* (pp. 43–84). New York: McGraw-Hill.

Garvey, M. A., Giedd, J., & Swedo, S. E. (1998). PANDAS: The search for environmental triggers of pediatric neuropsychiatric disorders. Lessons from rheumatic fever. *Journal of Child Neurology*, *13*, 413–423.

Gazzaniga, M. S., Ivry, R. B., & Mangun, G. R. (1998). *Cognitive neuroscience: The biology of the mind.* New York: Norton.

Geller, J. L., Brown, J. M., Fisher, W. H., Grudzinskas, A. J., Jr., & Manning, T. D. (1998). A national survey of "consumer empowerment" at the state level. *Psychiatric Services, 49*, 498–503.

General Accounting Office. (1977). *Returning the mentally disabled to the community: Government needs to do more*. Washington, DC: Author.

Goldman, H. H. (1998). Deinstitutionalization and community care: Social welfare policy as mental health policy. *Harvard Review of Psychiatry, 6*, 219–222.

Goldman, H. H., & Morrissey, J. P. (1985). The alchemy of mental health policy: Homelessness and the fourth cycle of reform. *American Journal of Public Health, 75*, 727–731.

Gordon, M. F. (1964). *Assimilation in American life*. New York: Oxford University Press.

Granger, D. A. (1994). Recovery from mental illness: A first person perspective of an emerging paradigm. In Ohio Department of Mental Health, *Recovery: The new force in mental health* (pp. 1–13). Columbus, OH: Author.

Grant, I., Atkinson, J. H., Hesselink, J. R., Kennedy, C. J., Richman, D. D., Spector, S. A., & McCutchan, J. A. (1987). Evidence for early central nervous system involvement in the acquired immunodeficiency syndrome (AIDS) and other human immunodeficiency virus (HIV) infections. Studies with neuropsychologic testing and magnetic resonance imaging. *Annals of Internal Medicine, 107*, 828–836.

Grob, G. N. (1983). *Mental illness and American society, 1875–1940*. Princeton, NJ: Princeton University Press.

Grob, G. N. (1991). *From asylum to community. Mental health policy in modern America*. Princeton, NJ: Princeton University Press.

Grob, G. N. (1994). *The mad among us: A history of the care of America's mentally ill*. New York: Free Press.

Grover, P. L. (1998). *Preventing substance abuse among children and adolescents: Family-centered approaches: Prevention enhancement protocols system reference guide*. Rockville, MD: Center for Substance Abuse Prevention.

Hannan, R. W. (1998). Intervention in the coal fields: Mental health outreach. *Rural Community Mental Health, 24*, 1–3.

Harding, C., Strauss, J. S., & Zubin, J. (1992). Chronicity in schizophrenia: Revisited. *British Journal of Psychiatry, 161*, 27–37.

Harrow, M., Sands, J. R., Silverstein, M. L., & Goldberg, J. F. (1997). Course and outcome for schizophrenia versus other psychotic patients: A longitudinal study. *Schizophrenia Bulletin, 23*, 287–303.

Hatchett, S. J., & Jackson, J. S. (1993). African American extended kin systems: An assessment. In H. P. McAdoo (Ed.), *Family ethnicity: Strength in diversity* (pp. 90–108). Newbury Park, CA: Sage.

Health Care Financing Administration. (1991). *International classification of diseases* (9th revision, clinical modification, ICD-9-CM). Washington, DC: Author.

Heinrich, L. M., & Gullone, E (2006). The clinical significance of loneliness: A literature review. *Clinical Psychology Review, 26*(6):695–718.

Hernandez, M., Isaacs, M. R., Nesman, T., & Burns, D. (1998). Perspectives on culturally competent systems of care. In M. Hernandez & M. R. Isaacs (Eds.), *Promoting cultural competence in children's mental health services* (pp. 1–25). Baltimore: Brookes.

Herring, R. D. (1994). Native American Indian identity: A people of many peoples. In E. Salett & D. Koslow (Eds.), *Race, ethnicity, and self: Identity in multicultural perspective* (pp. 170–197). Washington, DC: National Multicultural Institute.

Holzer, C., Shea, B., Swanson, J., Leaf, P., Myers, J., George, L., . . . Bednarski, P. (1986). The increased risk for specific psychiatric disorders among persons of low socioeconomic status. *American Journal of Social Psychiatry, 6*, 259–271.

Horowitz, M. J. (1988). *Introduction to psychodynamics: A new synthesis*. New York: Basic Books.

Horwitz, A. V. (1987). Help-seeking processes and mental health services. *New Directions for Mental Health Services, 36*, 33–45.

Hough, R. L., Landsverk, J. A., Karno, M., Burnam, M. A., Timbers, D. M., Escobar, J. I., & Regier, D. A. (1987). Utilization of health and mental health services by Los Angeles Mexican Americans and non-Hispanic whites. *Archives of General Psychiatry, 44*, 702–709.

Hoyt, D. R., Conger, R. D., Valde, J. G., & Weihs, K. (1997). Psychological distress and help seeking in rural America. *American Journal of Community Psychology, 25*, 449–470.

Hoyt, D., O'Donnell D., & Mack, K. Y. (1995). Psychological distress and size of place: The epidemiology of rural economic stress. *Rural Sociology, 60*, 707–720.

Hu, T. W., Snowden, L. R., Jerrell, J. M., & Nguyen, T. D. (1991). Ethnic populations in public mental health: Services choice and level of use. *American Journal of Public Health, 81*, 1429–1434.

Hubel, D., & Wiesel T. (1970). The period of susceptibility to the physiological effects of unilateral eye closure in kittens. *Journal of Physiology, 206*, 419–436.

Hunt, D. (1984). Issues in working with Southeast Asian refugees. In D. Koslow & E. Salett (Eds.), *Crossing cultures in mental health* (pp. 49–63). Washington, DC: SIETAR International.

Indian Health Service. (1997). *Trends in Indian health 1997*. Retrieved from http://www.ihs.gov/PublicInfo/Publications/trends97/trends97.asp

Inhelder, B., & Piaget, J. (1958). *The growth of logical thinking from childhood to adolescence: An essay on the construction of formal operational structures*. New York: Basic Books.

Institute of Federal Health Care. (2009). *Exploring advances in research to improve TBI outcomes*. Retrieved from http://www.usminstitute.org/pdf/TBIResearchSumm.pdf

Institute of Medicine. (1990). *Broadening the base of treatment for alcohol problems: Report of a study by a committee of the Institute of Medicine, Division of Mental Health and Behavioral Medicine*. Washington, DC: National Academy Press.

Institute of Medicine. (1994a). *Reducing risks for mental disorders: Frontiers for preventive intervention research*. Washington, DC: National Academy Press.

Institute of Medicine. (1994b). *Adverse events associated with childhood vaccines: Evidence bearing on causality*. Washington, DC: National Academy Press.

Institute of Medicine & Committee for the Study of the Future of Public Health. (1988). *The future of public health*. Washington, DC: National Academy Press.

Interagency Council on the Homeless. (1991). *Reaching out: A guide for service providers*. Rockville, MD: The National Resource Center on Homelessness and Mental Health.

Jenkins, E. J., & Bell, C. C. (1997). Exposure and response to community violence among children and adolescents. In J. Osofsky (Ed.), *Children in a violent society* (pp. 9–31). New York: Guilford Press.

Jimenez, A. L., Alegria, M., Pena, M., & Vera, M. (1997). Mental health utilization in depression. *Women & Health, 25*(2), 1–21.

Kandel, E. R. (1998). A new intellectual framework for psychiatry. *American Journal of Psychiatry, 155*, 457–469.

Kandel, E. R., Schwartz, J. H., & Jessell, T. M. (1995). *Essentials of neural sciences and behavior*. Stanford, CT: Appleton and Lange.

Kaplan, G. A., Roberts, R. E., Camacho, T. C., & Coyne, J. C. (1987). Psychosocial predictors of depression. Prospective evidence from the human population laboratory studies. *American Journal of Epidemiology, 125*, 206–220.

Kaplan, H. I., & Saddock, B. J. (1998). *Synopsis of psychiatry* (8th ed.). Baltimore: Williams and Wilkins.

Karno, M., Jenkins, J. H., de la Selva, A., Santana, F., Telles, C., Lopez, S., & Mintz, J. (1987). Expressed emotion and schizophrenic outcome among Mexican-American families. *Journal of Nervous and Mental Disease, 175*, 143–151.

Kazdin, A. E. (1996). Cognitive behavioral approaches. In M. Lewis (Ed.), *Child and adolescent psychiatry: A comprehensive textbook* (2nd ed., pp. 115–126). Baltimore: Williams and Wilkins.

Kazdin, A. E. (1997). Behavior modification. In J. M. Weiner (Ed.), *Textbook of child and adolescent psychiatry* (2nd ed., pp. 821–842). Washington, DC: American Academy of Child and Adolescent Psychiatry.

Kellam, D. G., & Rebok, G. W. (1992). Building developmental and etiological theory through epidemiologically-based preventive intervention trials. In J. McCord & R. E. Tremblay (Eds.), *Preventing antisocial behavior: Interventions from birth through adolescence* (pp. 162–195). New York: Guilford Press.

Kessler, R. C., Berglund, P. A., Zhao, S., Leaf, P. J., Kouzis, A. C., Bruce, M. L., . . . Schneier, M. (1996). The 12-month prevalence and correlates of serious mental illness. In R. W. Manderscheid & M. A. Sonnenschein (Eds.), *Mental health, United States, 1996* (DHHS Publication No. [SMA] 96-3098, pp. 59–70). Washington, DC: U.S. Government Printing Office.

Kessler, R. C., McGonagle, K. A., Zhao, S., Nelson, C. B., Hughes, M., Eshleman, S., . . . Kendler, K. S. (1994). Lifetime and 12-month prevalence of DSM-III-R psychiatric disorders in the United States. Results from the National Comorbidity Survey. *Archives of General Psychiatry, 51*, 8–19.

Kimmel, W. A. (1992). *Rural mental health policy issues for research: A pilot exploration*. Rockville, MD: National Institute of Mental Health, Office of Rural Mental Health Research.

Klerman, G. L., Weissman, M. M., Rousaville, B. J., & Sherron, E. S. (1984). *Interpersonal psychotherapy of depression*. New York: Basic Books.

Kneisl, C. R., and Trigoboff, E. (2009). *Contemporary psychiatric-mental health nursing*. Upper Saddle River, NJ: Pearson Education.

Knitzer, J. (1982). *Unclaimed children: The failure of public responsibility to children and adolescents in need of mental health services*. Washington, DC: Children's Defense Fund.

Kosslyn, S. M., & Shin, L. M. (1992). The status of cognitive neuroscience. *Current Opinions in Neurobiology, 2*, 146–149.

Lamb, H. R. (1994). A century and a half of psychiatric rehabilitation in the United States. *Hospital and Community Psychiatry, 45*, 1015–1020.

La Mendola, W. (1997). *Telemental health services in U.S. frontier areas* (Frontier Mental Health Services Resource Network, Letter to the Field, No. 3). Retrieved from http://www.du.edu/frontier-mh/ letter3.html

Larson, D. B., Hohmann, A., Kessler, L. G., Meador, K. G., Boyd, J. H., & McSherry, E. (1988). The couch and the cloth: The need for linkage. *Hospital and Community Psychiatry, 39*, 1064–1069.

Lawson, W. B., Hepler, N., Holladay, J., & Cuffel, B. (1994). Race as a factor in inpatient and outpatient admissions and diagnosis. *Hospital and Community Psychiatry, 45*, 72–74.

Lebowitz, B. D., & Rudorfer, M. V. (1998). Treatment research at the millennium: From efficacy to effectiveness. *Journal of Clinical Psychopharmacology, 18*, 1.

Lee, S. M. (1998). Asian Americans: diverse and growing. *Population Bulletin, 53*, 1–39.

Leete, E. (1989). How I perceive and manage my illness. *Schizophrenia Bulletin, 8*, 605–609.

Lefley, H. P. (1996). Impact of consumer and family advocacy movement on mental health services. In B. L. Levin & J. Petrila (Eds.), *Mental health services: A public health perspective* (pp. 81–96). New York: Oxford University Press.

Lefley, H. (1997). Mandatory treatment from the family's perspective. *New Directions in Mental Health Services, 75*, 7–16.

Lehman, A. F., & Steinwachs, D. M. (1998). Translating research into practice: The Schizophrenia Patient Outcomes Research Team (PORT) treatment recommendations. *Schizophrenia Bulletin, 24*, 1–10.

Leong, F. T., & Lau, A. S. (2001, December). Barriers to providing effective mental health services to Asian Americans. *Mental Health Services Research, 3*(4), 201–214. Retrieved from http://www.aasc.ucla.edu/policy/leong_lau_2001.pdf.

Levine, J. D., Gordon, N. C., & Fields, H. L. (1978). The mechanism of placebo analgesia. *Lancet, 2*, 654–657.

Lin, K. M., Anderson, D., & Poland, R. E. (1997). Ethnic and cultural considerations in psychopharmacotherapy. In D. Dunner (Ed.), *Current psychiatric therapy II* (pp. 75–81). Philadelphia: Saunders.

Lin, K., Inui, T. S., Kleinman, A. M., & Womack, W. M. (1982). Sociocultural determinants of the help-seeking behavior of patients with mental illness. *Journal of Nervous and Mental Disease, 170*, 78–85.

Lombroso, P., Pauls, D., & Leckman, J. (1994). Genetic mechanisms in childhood psychiatric disorders. *Journal of the American Academy of Child and Adolescent Psychiatry, 33*, 921–938.

Lu, F. G., Lim, R. F., & Mezzich, J. E. (1995). Issues in the assessment and diagnosis of culturally diverse individuals. In J. Oldham & M. Riba (Eds.), *Review of psychiatry* (Vol. 14, pp. 477–510). Washington, DC: American Psychiatric Press.

Marano, H. E. (2003, July 1). The dangers of loneliness. *Psychology Today*. Retrieved from http://www.psychologytoday.com/articles/200308/the-dangers-loneliness.

McArthur, J. C., Hoover, D. R., Bacellar, H., Miller, E. N., Cohen, B. A., Becker, J. T. . . . Saah, A. (1993). Dementia in AIDS patients: Incidence and risk factors. Multicenter AIDS Cohort Study. *Neurology, 43*, 2245–2252.

McGauhey, P., Starfield, B., Alexander, C., & Ensminger, M. E. (1991). Social environment and vulnerability of low birth weight children: A social-epidemiological perspective. *Pediatrics, 88*, 943–953.

McLeod, J. D., & Kessler, R. C. (1990). Socioeconomic status differences in vulnerability to undesirable life events. *Journal of Health and Social Behavior, 31*, 162–172.

Melaville, B., & Asayesh, G. (1993). *Together we can: A guide for crafting a profamily system of education and human services*. Washington, DC: U.S. Department of Education.

Mezzich, J. E., Kleinman, A., Fabrega, H., & Parron, D. L. (Eds.). (1996). *Culture and psychiatric diagnosis: A DSM-IV perspective*. Washington, DC: American Psychiatric Press.

Milburn, N. G., & Bowman, P. J. (1991). Neighborhood life. In J. S. Jackson (Ed.), *Life in black America* (pp. 31–45). Newbury Park, CA: Sage.

Minneman, K. (1994). Pharmacological organization of the central nervous system. In T. M. Brody, J. Larner, K. Minneman, & H. Neu (Eds.), *Human pharmacology: Molecular to clinical*. St. Louis: Mosby-Year Book.

Miranda, J., & Green, B. L. (1999). The need for mental health services research focusing on poor young women. *Journal of Mental Health Policy and Economics*, *2*, 73–89.

Mohatt, D., & Kirwan, D. (1995). *Meeting the challenge: Model programs in rural mental health*. Rockville, MD: Office of Rural Health Policy.

Mollica, R. F. (1989). Developing effective mental health policies and services for traumatized refugee patients. In D. Koslow & E. Salett (Eds.), *Crossing cultures in mental health* (pp. 101–115). Washington, DC: SIETAR International.

Morrissey, J. P., & Goldman, H. H. (1984). Cycles of reform in the care of the chronically mentally ill. *Hospital and Community Psychiatry*, *35*, 785–793.

Mowbray, C., Moxley, D., Thrasher, S., Bybee, D., McCrohan, N., Harris, S., & Clover, G. (1996). Consumers as community support providers: Issues created by role innovation. *Community Mental Health Journal*, *32*, 47–67.

Munoz, R. F., Hollon, S. D., McGrath, E., Rehm, L. P., & VandenBos, G. R. (1994). On the AHRQ depression in primary care guidelines. Further considerations for practitioners. *American Psychologist*, *49*, 42–61.

Munoz, R. F., Ying, Y., Arman, R., Chan, F., & Gurza, R. (1987). The San Francisco depression prevention research project: A randomized trial with medical outpatients. In R. F. Munoz (Ed.), *Depression prevention: Research directions* (pp. 199–215). Washington, DC: Hemisphere Press.

Muntaner, C., Eaton, W. W., Miech R., & O'Campo, P. (2004). Socioeconomic position and major mental disorders. *Epidemiology Review*, *26*, 53–62.

National Advisory Mental Health Council. (1993). Health care reform for Americans with severe mental illnesses: Report of the National Advisory Mental Health Council. *American Journal of Psychiatry*, *150*, 1447–1465.

National Alliance for the Mentally Ill. (1999). *State mental illness parity laws*. Arlington, VA: Author.

National Association of State Mental Health Program Directors. (1993). *Putting their money where their mouths are: SMHA support of consumer and family-run programs*. Arlington, VA: Author.

National Institute of Mental Health. (1998). *Genetics and mental disorders: Report of the National Institute of Mental Health's Genetics Workgroup*. Rockville, MD: Author.

National Mental Health Association. (1987). *Invisible Children Project. Final report and recommendations of the Invisible Children Project*. Alexandria, VA: Author.

National Mental Health Association. (1993). *A guide for advocates to all systems failure. An examination of the results of neglecting the needs of children with serious emotional disturbance*. Alexandria, VA: Author.

National Resource Center on Homelessness and Mental Illness. (1989). *Self-help programs for people who are homeless and mentally ill*. Delmar, NY: Policy Research Associates.

Navia, B. A., Jordan, B. D., & Price, R. W. (1986). The AIDS dementia complex: I. Clinical features. *Annals of Neurology*, *19*, 517–524.

Neighbors, H. W., Bashshur, R., Price, R., Donavedian, A., Selig, S., & Shannon, G. (1992). Ethnic minority health service delivery: A review of the literature. *Research in Community and Mental Health*, 7, 55–71.

Nelson, S. H., McCoy, G. F., Stetter, M., & Vanderwagen, W. C. (1992). An overview of mental health services for American Indians and Alaska Natives in the 1990s. *Hospital and Community Psychiatry*, *43*, 257–261.

Nemeroff, C. B. (1998). Psychopharmacology of affective disorders in the 21st century. *Biological Psychiatry*, *44*, 517–525.

Olds, D. L., Henderson, C. R., Jr., Tatelbaum, R., & Chamberlin, R. (1986). Improving the delivery of prenatal care and outcomes of pregnancy: A randomized trial of nurse home visitation. *Pediatrics*, 77, 16–28.

Olweus, D. (1991). Bullying/victim problems among school children: Basic facts and effects of an intervention program. In K. Rubin & D. Pepler (Eds.), *Development and treatment of childhood aggression* (pp. 411–448). Hillsdale, NJ: Erlbaum.

O'Sullivan, M. J., Peterson, P. D., Cox, G. B., & Kirkeby, J. (1989). Ethnic populations: Community mental health services ten years later. *American Journal of Community Psychology*, *17*, 17–30.

Padgett, D. K., Patrick, C., Burns, B. J., & Schlesinger, H. J. (1995). Use of mental health services by black and white elderly. In D. K. Padgett (Ed.), *Handbook of ethnicity, aging, and mental health*. Westport, CT: Greenwood Press.

Pargament, K. I. (1997). *The psychology of religion and coping: Theory, research, practice*. New York: Guilford Press.

Pasamanick, B. A. (1959). *The epidemiology of mental disorder*. Washington, DC: American Association for the Advancement of Science.

Penninx, B. W., Guralnik, J. M., Pahor, M., Ferrucci, L., Cerhan, J. R., Wallace, R. B., & Havlik, R. J. (1998). Chronically depressed mood and cancer risk in older persons. *Journal of the National Cancer Institute*, *90*, 1888–1893.

Perry, P., Alexander, B., & Liskow, B. (1997). *Psychotrophic drug handbook* (7th ed.). Washington, DC: American Psychiatric Press.

Pierce, C. M. (1992). Contemporary psychiatry: Racial perspectives on the past and future. In A. Kales, C. M. Pierce, & M. Greenblatt (Eds.), *The mosaic of contemporary psychiatry in perspective* (pp. 99–109). New York: Springer-Verlag.

Pirkle, J. L., Brody, D. J., Gunter, E. W., Kramer, R. A., Paschal, D. C., Flegal, K. M., & Matte, T. D. (1994). The decline in blood lead levels in the United States. The National Health and Nutrition Examination Surveys. *Journal of the American Medical Association*, *272*, 284–291.

Plomin, R., DeFries, J. C., McClearn, G. E., & Rutter, M. (1997). *Behavioral genetics* (3rd ed.). New York: Freeman.

Plomin, R., Owen, M. J., & McGuffin, P. (1994). The genetic basis of complex human behaviors. *Science*, *264*, 7133–7139.

Porter, R. (1987). *A social history of madness: Stories of the insane*. London: Weidenfeld and Nicholson.

Potter, W. Z., Scheinin, M., Golden, R. N., Rudorfer, M. V., Cowdry, R. W., Calil, H. M. . . . Linnoila, M. (1985). Selective antidepressants and cerebrospinal fluid. Lack of specificity on norepinephrine and serotonin metabolites. *Archives of General Psychiatry*, *42*, 1171–1177.

President's Commission on Mental Health. (1978). *Report to the President from the President's Commission on Mental Health* (4 vols.). Washington, DC: Superintendent of Documents, U.S. Government Printing Office.

Priest, R. (1991). Racism and prejudice as negative impacts on African American clients in therapy. *Journal of Counseling and Development*, *70*, 213–215.

Primm, A. B., Lima, B. R., & Rowe, C. L. (1996). Cultural and ethnic sensitivity. In W. R. Breakey (Ed.), *Integrated mental health services: Modern community psychiatry* (pp. 146–159). New York: Oxford University Press.

Rauch, K. D. (1997, December 9). Mental health care scarce in rural areas. *The Washington Post Health*, pp. 7–9.

Regier, D. A., Farmer, M. E., Rae, D. S., Myers, J. K., Kramer, M., Robins, L. N. . . . Locke, B. Z. (1993a). One-month prevalence of mental disorders in the United States and sociodemographic characteristics: The Epidemiologic Catchment Area study. *Acta Psychiatrica Scandinavica*, *88*, 35–47.

Regier, D. A., Narrow, W. E., Rae, D. S., Manderscheid, R. W., Locke, B. Z., & Goodwin, F. K. (1993b). The de facto US mental and addictive disorders service system. Epidemiologic Catchment Area prospective 1-year prevalence rates of disorders and services. *Archives of General Psychiatry*, *50*, 85–94.

Resnick, H. S., Kilpatrick, D. G., Dansky, B. S., Saunders, B. E., & Best, C. L. (1993). Prevalence of civilian trauma and posttraumatic stress disorder in a representative national sample of women. *Journal of Consulting and Clinical Psychology*, *61*, 984–991.

Rice, D. P., & Miller, L. S. (1996). The economic burden of schizophrenia: Conceptual and methodological issues, and cost estimates. In M. Moscarelli, A. Rupp, & N. Sartorious (Eds.), *Handbook of mental health economics and health policy: Vol. 1. Schizophrenia* (pp. 321–324). New York: Wiley.

Rogers, C. (1961). *On becoming a person*. Boston: Houghton Mifflin.

Rogers, E. S., Chamberlin, J., Ellison, M. L., & Crean, T. (1997). A consumer-constructed scale to measure empowerment among users of mental health services. *Psychiatric Services*, *48*, 1042–1047.

Rogler, L. H., Malgady, R. G., Costantino, G., & Blumenthal, R. (1987). What do culturally sensitive mental health services mean? The case of Hispanics. *American Psychologist*, *42*, 565–570.

Rutter, M. (1979). Protective factors in children's responses to stress and disadvantage. *Annals of the Academy of Medicine, Singapore*, *8*, 324–338.

Sapolsky, R. M. (1996). Stress, glucocorticoids, and damage to the nervous system: The current state of confusion. *Stress*, *1*, 1–19.

Scheffler, R. M., & Miller, A. B. (1991). Differences in mental health service utilization among ethnic subpopulations. *International Journal of Law and Psychiatry*, *14*, 363–376.

Schloss, P., & Williams, D. C. (1998). The serotonin transporter: A primary target for antidepressant drugs. *Journal of Psychopharmacology*, *12*, 115–121.

Schweizer, E., & Rickels, K. (1997). Placebo response in generalized anxiety: Its effect on the outcome of clinical trials. *Journal of Clinical Psychiatry*, *58*(Suppl. 11), 30–38.

Screening for Mental Health. (n.d.). Retrieved from http://www.mentalhealthscreening.org/

Segal, S. P., Bola, J. R., & Watson, M. A. (1996). Race, quality of care, and antipsychotic prescribing practices in psychiatric emergency services. *Psychiatric Services*, *47*, 282–286.

Segal, S. P., Silverman, C., & Temkin, T. (1995). Measuring empowerment in client-run self-help agencies. *Community Mental Health Journal*, *31*, 215–227.

Seligman, M. E. (1995). The effectiveness of psychotherapy. The Consumer Reports study. *American Psychologist*, *50*, 965–974.

Shaffer, D., Fisher, P., Dulcan, M. K., Davies, M., Piacentini, J., Schwab-Stone, M. E. . . . Regier, D. A. (1996). The NIMH Diagnostic Interview Schedule for Children Version 2.3 (DISC 2.3): Description, acceptability, prevalence rates, and performance in the MECA Study. Methods for the Epidemiology of Child and Adolescent Mental Disorders Study. *Journal of the American Academy of Child and Adolescent Psychiatry*, *35*, 865–877.

Shalev, A. Y. (1996). Stress vs. traumatic stress: From acute homeostatic reactions to chronic psychopathology. In B. A. Van der Kolk, A. C. MacFarlane, & L. Weisaeth (Eds.), *Traumatic stress* (pp. 77–101). New York: Guilford Press.

Shatz, C. J. (1993). The developing brain. In *Readings from Scientific American*: *Mind and brain* (pp. 15–26). New York: Freeman.

Short, P., Feinleib, S., & Cunningham, P. (1994). *Expenditures and sources of payment for persons in nursing and personal care homes* (AHRQ Publication No. 9400-0032). Rockville, MD: Agency for Healthcare Research and Quality (AHRQ).

Silverman, P. R. (1988). Widow to widow: A mutual help program for the widowed. In R. Price, E. Cowen, R. P. Lorion, & J. Ramos-McKay (Eds.), *Fourteen ounces of prevention*: *A case-book for practitioners* (pp. 175–186). Washington, DC: American Psychological Association.

Size, T. (1998, March/April). Would John Wayne ask for Prozac? *Rural Health FYI*, pp. 5–7.

Snowden, L. R. (1999a). *Mental health system reform and ethnic minority populations*. Manuscript submitted for publication.

Snowden, L. R. (1999b). Inpatient mental health use by members of ethnic minority groups. In J. M. Herrera, W. B. Lawson, & J. J. Sramek (Eds.), *Cross cultural psychiatry*. Chichester, UK: Wiley.

Snowden, L. R. (2000). Social embeddedness and psychological well-being among African Americans and whites. *American Journal of Community Psychology*, *29*, 519–537.

Snowden L. R. (2001). Barriers to effective mental health services for African Americans. *Mental Health Services Research*, *3*(4), pp. 181–187.

Snowden, L. R., & Cheung, F. K. (1990). Use of inpatient mental health services by members of ethnic minority groups. *American Psychologist*, *45*, 347–355.

Snowden, L. R., & Hu, T. W. (1996). Outpatient service use in minority-serving mental health programs. *Administration and Policy in Mental Health*, *24*, 149–159.

Snowden, L. R., Hu, T. W., & Jerrell, J. M. (1995). Emergency care avoidance: Ethnic matching and participation in minority-serving programs. *Community Mental Health Journal*, *31*, 463–473.

Snowden, L., Storey, C., & Clancy, T. (1989). Ethnicity and continuation in treatment at a black community mental health center. *Journal of Community Psychology*, *17*, 111–118.

South Carolina SHARE (1995). *National directory of mental health consumer and ex-patient organizations and resources*. Charlotte, SC: Author.

Spaniol, L. J., Gagne, C., & Koehler, M. (1997). *Psychological and social aspects of psychiatric disability*. Boston: Center for Psychiatric Rehabilitation, Sargent College of Allied Health Professions, Boston University.

Specht, D. (Ed.). (1998). *Highlights of the findings of a national survey on state support of consumer/ex-patients activities*. Holyoke, MA: Human Resource Association of the Northeast.

Srole, L. (1962). *Mental health in the metropolis*: *The Midtown Manhattan study*. New York: McGraw- Hill.

Stocks, M. L. (1995). In the eye of the beholder. *Psychiatric Rehabilitation Journal*, *19*, 89–91.

Sue, S., Fujino, D. C., Hu, L. T., Takeuchi, D. T., & Zane, N. W. (1991). Community mental health services for ethnic minority groups: A test of the cultural responsiveness hypothesis. *Journal of Consulting and Clinical Psychology*, *59*, 533–540.

Sue, S., & McKinney, H. (1975). Asian Americans in the community mental health care system. *American Journal of Orthopsychiatry*, *45*, 111–118.

Sue, S., Zane, N., & Young, K. (1994). Research on psychotherapy with culturally diverse populations. In A. E. Bergin & S. L. Garfield (Eds.), *Handbook of psychotherapy and behavior change* (4th ed., pp. 783–817). New York: Wiley.

Sullivan, G. M., Coplan, J. D., & Gorman, J. M. (1998). Psychoneuroendocrinology of anxiety disorders. *Psychiatric Clinics of North America*, *21*, 397–412.

Sullivan, W. P. (1994). A long and winding road: The process of recovery from severe mental illness. *Innovations and Research*, *3*, 19–27.

Sussman, L. K., Robins, L. N., & Earls, F. (1987). Treatment-seeking for depression by black and white Americans. *Social Science and Medicine*, *24*, 187–196.

Takeuchi, D. T., Sue, S., & Yeh, M. (1995). Return rates and outcomes from ethnicity-specific mental health programs in Los Angeles. *American Journal of Public Health*, *85*, 638–643.

Takeuchi, D. T., & Uehara, E. S. (1996). Ethnic minority mental health services: Current research and future conceptual directions. In B. L. Levin & J. Petrila (Eds.), *Mental health services: A public health perspective* (pp. 63–80). New York: Oxford University Press.

Taylor, O. (1989). The effects of cultural assumptions on cross-cultural communication. In D. Koslow & E. Salett (Eds.), *Crossing cultures in mental health* (pp. 18–27). Washington, DC: SIETAR International.

Taylor, R. J. (1986). Religious participation among elderly blacks. *Gerontologist*, *26*, 630–636.

Turner, J., & TenHoor, W. (1978). The NIMH community support program: Pilot approach to a needed social reform. *Schizophrenia Bulletin*, *4*, 319–348.

U.S. Department of Health and Human Services [DHHS]. (1999). *Mental Health: A report of the surgeon general—Executive Summary*. Rockville, MD: U.S. Department of Health and Human Services, Substance Abuse and Mental Health Services Administration, Center for Mental Health Services, National Institutes of Health, National Institute of Mental Health. Retrieved from http://www.surgeongeneral.gov/library/mentalhealth/home.html

Werner, E. E., & Smith, R. S. (1992). *Overcoming the odds: High risk children from birth to adulthood.* New York: Cornell University Press.

World Health Organization. (1992). *International statistical classification of diseases and related health problems* (10th revision, ICD-10). Geneva, Switzerland: Author.

Yehuda, R. (1999). Biological factors associated with susceptibility to post-traumatic stress disorder. *Canadian Journal of Psychiatry*, *44*, 34–39.

Zhang, A. Y., & Snowden, L. R. (1999). Ethnic characteristics of mental disorders in five U.S. communities. *Cultural Diversity and Ethnic Minority Psychology*, *5*, 134–146.

Zhang, A. Y., Snowden, L. R., & Sue, S. (1998). Differences between Asian and white Americans' help-seeking patterns in the Los Angeles area. *Journal of Community Psychology*, *26*, 317–326.

Zinman, S., Harp, H. T., & Budd, S. (1987). *Reaching across*. Riverside, CA: California Network of Mental Health Clients.

Zunzunegui, M. V., Beland, F., Laser, A., & Leon, V. (1998). Gender difference in depressive symptoms among Spanish elderly. *Social Psychiatry Psychiatric Epidemiology*, *5*, 175–205.

CHAPTER 3

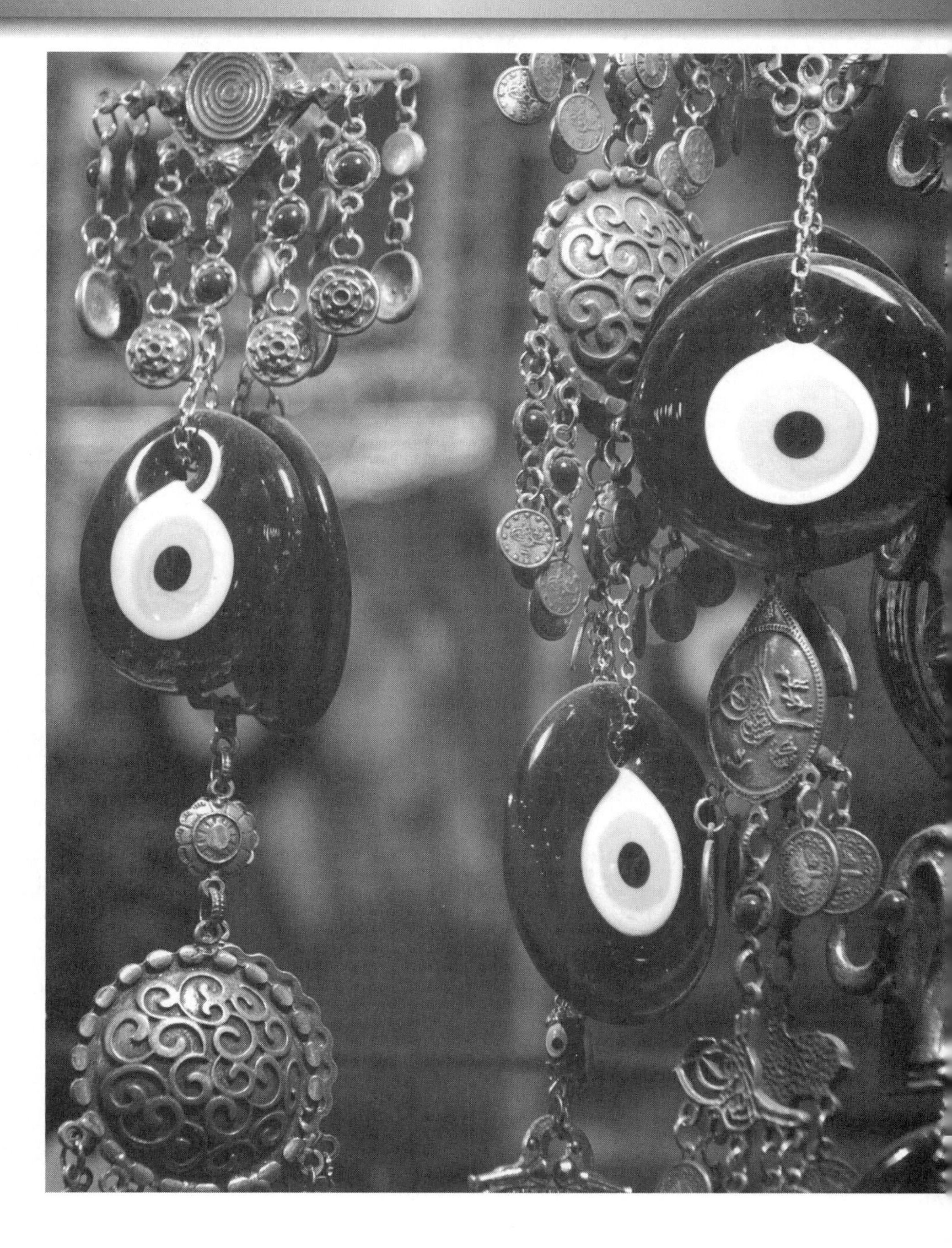

Culture and Mental Health

CHAPTER OBJECTIVES

1. Define culture, ethnicity, and race.
2. Describe the beliefs about personalistic and naturalistic ethnomedical systems.
3. Explain the nature and extent of mental health disparities.
4. Describe at least six culture-bound mental health illnesses.
5. Describe promising directions toward the elimination of mental health disparities and the promotion of mental health.

KEY TERMS

- Acculturation
- Cultural competence
- Culture
- Culture-bound syndromes
- Dominant culture
- Ethnicity
- Ethnocentricity
- Ethnopsychiatry
- Ethnopsychopharmacology
- Ghost sickness
- Idioms of distress
- Mal de ojo
- Minority
- Naturalistic system
- Personalistic system
- Race
- Somatization
- Susto

The diversity of our people is a great strength of the United States, which is home to an array of cultures, races, and ethnicities. This diversity has enriched our nation by bringing together traditions, languages, perspectives, and ideas that benefit all of us. But diversity has not come without a price. Cultural conflicts, discrimination, hate crimes, and other negative aspects of our diverse landscape have caused great suffering. These negative outcomes have contributed to mental health problems, particularly among minorities, and the mental health needs of many people in the United States are not being met.

The reasons for the problems related to diversity and mental health are numerous and complex. Awareness of the problem dates back to the 1960s and 1970s with the rise of the civil rights and community mental health movements (Rogler, Malgady, Costantino, & Blumenthal, 1987) and with successive waves of immigration from

Central America, the Caribbean, and Asia (Takeuchi & Uehara, 1996). These historical forces triggered recognition of the difficulties that minority groups confront in relation to mental health problems and services.

But this is not to say that white people in the United States do not experience mental health problems as a result of their culture. Gays and lesbians, Jews, Muslims (particularly after 9/11), and other whites have been the victims of hate crimes and discrimination. Race and ethnicity are irrelevant when it comes to suffering mental health problems from events such as a lost loved one, war, natural disaster, and divorce because those factors contributing to mental health problems do not discriminate. We are all vulnerable.

The main message here is that culture, including race and ethnicity, are important considerations when it comes to mental health. Understanding the wide-ranging roles of culture and society enables mental health professionals to design and deliver services that are more responsive to the needs of a variety of groups.

This chapter focuses on culture, and the health disparities that exist among minorities, races, and ethnicities are specifically addressed. We begin with clarifying terminology. Then we move on to the topic of the influence that culture has on mental health, some reasons for the health disparities among certain racial and ethnic groups, the need for mental health services to be culturally sensitive, and ways that professionals can provide services in a way that better meets the needs of various cultural groups.

TERMINOLOGY

You are probably familiar with the terms **culture**, **ethnicity**, and **race**, but we briefly describe them here along with definitions of racial and ethnic groups to help ensure understanding and prevent misinterpretations. But first, note that this chapter employs the phrase *racial and ethnic minorities* to refer collectively to people who identify as African Americans, American Indians, Alaska Natives, Asian Americans, Pacific Islanders, and Hispanic Americans. The term **minority** is used to signify the groups' limited political power and social resources, as well as their unequal access to opportunities, social rewards, and social status. The term is not meant to connote inferiority or to indicate small demographic size when used in this textbook.

Culture

There are countless definitions of culture. The simple definition often used by anthropologists is that culture is a system of shared meanings. E. B. Tylor, considered the founder of cultural anthropology, provided the classical definition of culture.

Tylor stated in 1871, "Culture, or civilization, taken in its broad, ethnographic sense, is that complex whole which includes knowledge, belief, art, morals, law, custom, and any other capabilities and habits acquired by man as a member of society" (Tylor, 1871/1924, p. 1). Tylor's definition is still widely cited today. Here is a more current definition: "The thoughts, communications, actions, customs, beliefs, values, and institutions of racial, ethnic, religious, or social groups" (Office of Minority Health, 2001, p. 131).

Culture is learned, changes over time, and is passed on from generation to generation. It is a very complex system, and many subcultures exist within the **dominant culture**. For example, universities, businesses, neighborhoods, age groups, refugees, homeless, women, homosexuals, athletic teams, and musicians are subcultures of the American dominant culture (Ritter & Hoffman, 2010). People simultaneously belong to numerous subcultures because we are students, fathers or mothers, and employees at the same time.

What follows is a discussion about race and ethnicity, which are common frames and ways of defining cultural practice among groups of people. It is important to note that this is an ineffective way to categorize people because there is a vast amount of diversity within these groups, **acculturation** levels are not considered, and these categories (as we describe shortly) are arbitrary. So why do we do this here then? The reason is that this frame is primarily used in research, so most of the knowledge about mental health and culture has been gathered using these categories, which is why it is replicated in this chapter. As you will see later in the chapter, we recommend that this methodology be changed.

Race and Ethnicity

Race refers to a person's physical characteristics and/or genetic or biological makeup, but the reality is that race is not a scientific construct; it is a social construct (Ritter & Hoffman, 2010). Race was developed to be able to categorize people and is based on the notion that some races are superior to others (also referred to as **ethnocentricity**). Many professionals in the fields of biology, sociology, and anthropology have determined that race is a social construct and not a biological one because not one characteristic, trait, or gene distinguishes all the members of one so-called race from all the members of another so-called race. In the United States both scholars and the general public have been conditioned to view human races as natural and separate divisions within the human species based on visible physical differences (American Anthropological Association, 1998). Science shows that human populations are not clearly demarcated, biologically distinct groups. Evidence from the analysis of genetics (e.g., DNA) indicates that most physical variation, about 94%, lies *within* so-called racial groups (American Anthropological Association, 1998). Conventional geographic "racial" groupings differ from one another only in about 6% of their genes (American Anthropological Association, 1998). This means that there is greater variation within "racial" groups than between them.

So why is race so important, if it does really exist? Race is important because society makes it important (Ritter & Hoffman, 2010). Race shapes social, cultural, political, ideological, and legal functions in society. The result is that race is an institutionalized concept that has had devastating consequences. Race has been the basis for deaths from wars and murders and suffering caused by discrimination, violence, torture, and hate crimes. The ideology of race has been the root of suffering and death for centuries even though it has no scientific merit.

So what is ethnicity? Ethnicity refers to a group of human beings whose members identify with each other on the basis of a boundary that distinguishes them from other groups. This boundary may take any of a number of forms—racial, cultural, linguistic, economic, religious, or political. For example, Hispanics are an ethnicity, not a race. The different Latino American ethnic subgroups such as Cubans, Dominicans, Mexicans, Puerto Ricans, and Peruvians include individuals of all so-called races. They identify with each other through their common language, Spanish, but they are geographically and culturally diverse. Think of an African who just recently immigrated to the United States. Although the new immigrant would be categorized as black, the person may be totally ethically distinct from most black Americans who have lived here for centuries. So you may ask what the difference is between ethnicity and culture. The difference is that ethnicity is tied to one's background and the way of the person's family, whereas culture is the way you live and how you live. For example, someone who is a homosexual is a part of the gay and lesbian culture, which is tied to the way the person lives his or her life and not to the family.

How is race different from culture? One can belong to a culture without having ancestral roots to that culture. For example, a person can belong to the hip-hop culture, but he or she is not born into the culture (Ritter & Hoffman, 2010). People usually are classified as belonging to one or two races or ethnicities but are members of numerous cultures (e.g., students, musicians, seniors). For example, Native Hawaiians and Vietnamese Americans were classified together in the racial category of "Asian and Pacific Islander Americans" in the U.S. census, but their cultures differ.

Categorizations Used in the United States for Racial and Ethnic Groups

Race was asked differently in the 2000 U.S. census because respondents were given the option of selecting one or more race categories to indicate their racial identities. These were the racial categories and their related definitions:

White: A person having origins in any of the original peoples of Europe, the Middle East, or North Africa.
Black or African American: A person having origins in any of the black racial groups of Africa.
American Indian or Alaska Native: A person having origins in any of the original peoples of North and South America (including Central America) who maintain tribal affiliation or community attachment.
Asian: A person having origins in any of the original people of the Far East, Southeast Asia, or the Indian subcontinent including, for example, China, India, and the Philippine Islands.
Native Hawaii or other Pacific Islander: A person having origins in any of the original peoples of Hawaii, Guam, Samoa, or other Pacific Islands.

The U.S. government declared that Hispanics and Latinos are an ethnicity and not a race. The government defines Hispanic or Latino as a person of Cuban, Mexican, Puerto Rican, South or Central American, or other Spanish culture or origin regardless of race.

United States Census 2010

This is the official form for all the people at this address.
It is quick and easy, and your answers are protected by law.

U.S. DEPARTMENT OF COMMERCE
Economics and Statistics Administration
U.S. CENSUS BUREAU

Use a blue or black pen.

Start here

The Census must count every person living in the United

Number of people =

2. Were there any additional people staying here April 1, 2010 that you did not include in Question 1?
Mark ☒ all that apply.

☐ Children, such as newborn babies or foster children
☐ Relatives, such as adult children, cousins, or in-laws
☐ Nonrelatives, such as roommates or live-in baby sitters
☐ People staying here temporarily
☐ No additional people

3. Is this house, apartment, or mobile home —
Mark ☒ ONE box.

☐ Owned by you or someone in this household with a mortgage or loan? *Include home equity loans.*
☐ Owned by you or someone in this household free and clear (without a mortgage or loan)?
☐ Rented?
☐ Occupied without payment of rent?

5. Please provide information for each person living here. Start with a person living here who owns or rents this house, apartment, or mobile home. If the owner or renter lives somewhere else, start with any adult living here. This will be Person 1.
What is Person 1's name? *Print name below.*

Last Name

9. What is Person 1's race? *Mark ☒ one or more boxes.*

☐ White
☐ Black, African Am., or Negro
☐ American Indian or Alaska Native — *Print name of enrolled or principal tribe.*

☐ Asian Indian ☐ Japanese ☐ Native Hawaiian
☐ Chinese ☐ Korean ☐ Guamanian or Chamorro
☐ Filipino ☐ Vietnamese ☐ Samoan
☐ Other Asian — *Print race, for example, Hmong, Laotian, Thai, Pakistani, Cambodian, and so on.*
☐ Other Pacific Islander — *Print race, for example, Fijian, Tongan, and so on.*

☐ Some other race — *Print race.*

CULTURE AND ITS INFLUENCE ON MENTAL HEALTH

Culture has a strong influence on health behaviors. It influences how health problems are believed to occur and how they are expressed, experienced, treated, prevented, and assessed. The stigmas surrounding mental health problems are much stronger in some cultures than in others. Although one can never become familiar with all cultural practices, being aware of some of the key variations is helpful. Therefore, the remainder of this chapter is just the beginning of understanding culture because it is a lifelong journey to learn about the relationship between mental health and culture.

In this section we discuss how culture shapes beliefs about how mental illness is caused along with how culture affects how it is experienced and treated.

Culture's Impact on Beliefs About the Causes of Mental Illness

Beliefs about ways to maintain health and the causes of illness, including mental illness, is deeply ingrained in our cultural beliefs and varies among cultures. Every culture in the world has a medical system, and anthropologists distinguish between personalistic and naturalistic ethnomedical systems. In a **personalistic system**, illness is seen as being caused by the intentional intervention of an agent who may be a supernatural being (a deity or ancestral spirits) or a human being with special powers (a witch or sorcerer). In **naturalistic system**, illness is explained in terms of a disturbed equilibrium of the physical body (e.g., germs, hormones). When the body is in balance with the natural environment, a state of health is achieved. When the balance no longer exists, then illness occurs. People often invoke both types of causation in explaining an episode of illness, and treatment may entail types of therapy related to both systems.

Personalistic illnesses may be caused by the person's misbehavior, which could be related to not adhering to social norms, religious beliefs, or rituals. The illness is often caused by a supernatural being or spirit possession. Healers usually are a means to understand what is wrong with their patients and to return them to health. An example is ***susto***, which literally means fright or sudden fear in Spanish. The fear leads to the person's soul being separated from the body. The symptoms of *susto* related to mental health can include lack of motivation, anxiety, and insomnia. Preventing personalistic illness includes avoiding situations that can provoke jealousy or envy, wearing certain amulets, adhering to social norms and moral behaviors, adhering to food taboos and restrictions, and performing certain rituals.

Naturalistic theories of disease causation often define health as a state of harmony between the person and his or her environment; when this balance is upset, illness results (Breslow, 2002). The naturalistic explanation assumes that illness is due to impersonal, mechanistic causes in nature that can be potentially understood and cured by the application of the scientific method. Examples of causes of illness include an imbalance of hot and cold, an energy imbalance, and parasites. The disturbance of our balance can cause physical and mental illness. Naturalistic illness can be prevented in some cases through preventive measures such as hand washing, proper nutrition, dental flossing, and avoiding falls and other injuries. Some causes may not be preventable, such as hormone imbalances, but they can be managed.

Culture's Impact on How Mental Illness Is Experienced

Culture affects mental health by influencing whether and how individuals experience the discomfort associated with mental illness. For example, some cultures, such as some Asian groups, emphasize restraint, control, and social harmony. These same cultures also tend not to dwell on morbid or upsetting thoughts or to overtly express emotional pain. African Americans, for example, emphasize willpower, minimizing the significance of stress, and trying to prevail in the face of adversity through increased striving (Broman, 1996). Other cultures are much more overt about their feelings.

Cultural norms provide characteristic modes of expressing suffering. **Idioms of distress** is the phrase used to describe specific illnesses that occur in some societies and are recognized by members of those societies as expressions of distress. They often reflect values and themes found in the societies in which they originate and have an impact on the way that distress is experienced and communicated in that culture. An example is the Korean folk syndrome known as *hwa-byung*, which literally translates into English as "anger syndrome" and is attributed to the suppression of anger (Agostinelli, 2008). Koreans commonly describe anger as fire, and this imbalance can cause sickness and disease. According to patients' explanations, those with *hwa-byung* have experiences that "cause hurt, damaging, boiling, exploding sensations inside the chest and body" (Agostinelli, 2008). Korean patients' cultural inclinations to keep the family in peaceful harmony and not to jeopardize social relationships dictate that anger must be suppressed, pent up, and accumulated. The anger becomes like a dense mass "pushing up" in the chest (Agostinelli, 2008).

Somatization, one of the common idioms of distress, is the expression of mental distress in terms of physical suffering. For example, in some cultures distress is expressed through an upset stomach or gas; in others it is expressed through symptoms such as dizziness and blurred vision (U.S. Department of Health and Human Services [DHHS], 2001).

A number of idioms of distress are well recognized as **culture-bound syndromes**, which are clusters of symptoms that are more common in some cultures than in others (DHHS, 2001). Numerous culture-bound syndromes have been identified in the *DSM* (**Table 3-1**). According to the publisher of the *DSM*, culture-bound syndromes

TABLE 3-1 Culture-Bound Syndromes

Category and Cultural Ties	**Symptoms**
Amok (behavior patterns found in Malaysia, Laos, Polynesia (cafard or cathard), Philippines, Papua New Guinea, Puerto Rico (*mal de pelea*), and Navajo (*iich'aa*)	A dissociative episode featuring a period of brooding followed by an outburst of aggressive, violent, or homicidal behavior aimed at people and objects. It seems to occur only among males and is often precipitated by a perceived slight or insult.
Ataque de nervios (Latin America, Latin Mediterranean, Caribbean)	Reported symptoms often include "uncontrollable shouting, attacks of crying, trembling, heat in the chest rising into the head, and verbal and physical aggression" (p. 899). May also experience dissociative episodes, seizure-like or fainting episodes, and suicidal gestures. A key feature is a sense of being out of control, and it is usually triggered by a stressful event within the family (e.g., news of a death, divorce). Symptoms are similar to panic attacks.
Bilis or *colera* or *muina* (Latinos)	The experience of anger or rage is thought to be the cause of these symptoms. Core body balances, such as between hot and cold, are caused by the anger. Symptoms may include acute nervous tension; headache; trembling; screaming; stomach disturbances such as nausea, vomiting, or diarrhea; and even loss of consciousness. An acute episode may lead to chronic fatigue.
Bouffée délirante (West Africa, Haiti)	A sudden outburst of agitated and aggressive behavior, marked confusion, and psychomotor excitement. It may be accompanied by visual and auditory hallucinations or paranoid ideation. Symptoms are similar to a brief psychotic disorder.
Brain fag (West Africa)	This disorder is usually associated with high school or college students and is caused by the challenges of school. Students refer to it as brain fatigue or brain tiredness. Symptoms may include difficulty with concentrating, thinking, or remembering; pain or feelings of pressure and tightness in the head or neck; and blurred vision. Symptoms may be similar to depression, anxiety, and somatoform disorders.
Dhat (India), *jiryan* (India), *sukra pameha* (Sri Lanka), *shen-k'uei* (China)	Refers to severe anxiety or hypochondriacal concerns associated with the discharge of semen, feelings of weakness and exhaustion, and whitish urine.
Falling-out or blacking out (southern United States, Caribbean)	The individual experiences dizziness and a spinning sensation before a sudden collapse. Although the eyes may be open, the person reports being unable to see, although he or she hears and understands what is happening around them without being able to move. Symptoms are similar to conversation and dissociative disorder.

(*continued*)

TABLE 3-1 Culture-Bound Syndromes (*Continued*)

Category and Cultural Ties	Symptoms
Ghost sickness (American Indian tribes)	Symptoms include bad dreams, feelings of danger, confusion, feelings of futility, loss of appetite, feelings of suffocation, fainting, dizziness, hallucinations, and loss of consciousness. A preoccupation with death or with someone who died is often observed.
Koro (Asia and Africa)	An intense anxiety that the penis (the vulva and nipples in females) will be retracted into the body, shrink, be removed, or disappear. The belief is that these changes can be fatal.
Hwa-byung or *wool-hwa-byung* (Korea)	It is believed to be caused by suppressed anger. Sleeplessness, panic, a fear of death, anorexia, panic, and general aches and pains are some of the symptoms.
Latah (Malaysia); *amurakh*, *irkunii*, *olan*, *myriachit*, or *menkeiti* (Siberian groups); *bah tschi*, *bah-tsi*, or *baah-ji* (Thailand); *imu* (Ainu, Sakhalin, Japan); *mali-mali* or *Silok* (Philippines)	An exaggerated startle response to sudden fright. Symptoms can include a trancelike state, echopraxia (automatic imitation of another's movements without conscious control), and echolalia (repetition of vocalizations made by another person). Typically found among middle-aged women in Malaysia.
Locura (Latin America, Latinos in United States)	A chronic state of severe psychosis caused by multiple life stressors, an inherited vulnerability, or both factors. Symptoms include agitation, incoherence, audio and visual hallucinations, inability to follow the rules of social interaction, unpredictability, and possible violence.
Mal de ojo (Mediterranean, Latin, and many other places in the world)	Translated into English, *mal de ojo* means "evil eye." Children, infants, and women are at high risk of getting evil eye. Symptoms include fitful sleep, crying without apparent cause, diarrhea, vomiting, headaches, concentration and sleep difficulties, and trembling. Symptoms can be similar to those of depression, anxiety disorders, somatoform, dissociative disorder, and psychotic disorders.
Nervios (Latinos and other groups in the United States and Latin America)	Refers to a sense of vulnerability to stressful life experiences. Symptoms include emotional distress, somatic complaints, inability to function, headaches, irritability, stomach disturbances, sleep difficulties, nervousness, inability to concentrate, easy tearfulness, trembling, tingling sensations, and *mareos* (dizziness with vertigo-like sensations). Symptoms are similar to those of adjustment and anxiety disorder, depression, psychotic disorders, somatoform, and dissociative disorder.

(*continued*)

TABLE 3-1 Culture-Bound Syndromes (*Continued*)

Category and Cultural Ties	Symptoms
Pibloktoq (Arctic and subarctic Eskimo communities)	This is an abrupt dissociative disorder. Feelings of extreme excitement for up to 30 minutes accompany the dissociative disorder, and they may be followed by convulsive seizures and coma lasting up to 12 hours.
Qi-gong psychotic reaction (China)	Qi-gong is an exercise of vital energy. It is a Chinese method of meditation, based on traditional Chinese medicine. Qi-gong psychotic reaction is an acute and time-limited episode in which the suffer experiences dissociative, paranoid, or other psychotic and nonpsychotic symptoms that occur after participating in qi-gong.
Rootwork (southern United States, Caribbean), also known as *mal puesto* or *brujeria* in Latino societies	The conviction that illnesses are brought about by supernatural means, such as witchcraft, voodoo, or evil influence. Roots, spells, and hexes can be put or placed on other people causing psychological and emotional problems. Symptoms include anxiety, gastrointestinal complaints, and fear of being poisoned or killed.
Sangue dormido (Portuguese Cape Verde Islanders), referred to as sleeping blood	The symptoms include "pain, numbness, tremor, paralysis, convulsions, stroke, blindness, heart attack, infection and miscarriage" (p. 902).
Shenjing Shuairuo (China), referred to as neurasthenia	Symptoms of the disorder include physical and mental fatigue, dizziness, headaches, gastrointestinal problems, difficulty concentrating, sleep disturbance, memory loss, sexual dysfunction, irritability, and excitability. Symptoms would meet the criteria for mood and anxiety disorder.
Shen-k'uei (Taiwan), *shenkui* (China)	Believed to be caused by excessive semen loss from frequent masturbation, sexual intercourse, nocturnal emission, or passing of urine (white urine) believed to contain semen. Symptoms include anxiety or panic symptoms with somatic complaints for which no physical cause can be determined. Backache, dizziness, fatigue, weakness, sleeplessness, sexual dysfunction, and frequent dreams.
Shin-byung (Korean)	Anxiety and somatic complaints, such as general weakness, dizziness, fear, loss of appetite, insomnia, and gastrointestinal problems, followed by dissociation and possession by ancestral spirits
Spell (southern United States)	Individuals communicate with deceased relatives or spirits. They may show distinct personality changes. Spell is not considered pathological in the culture of origin.

(*continued*)

TABLE 3-1 Culture-Bound Syndromes (*Continued*)

Category and Cultural Ties	Symptoms
Susto (Latino societies)	*Susto*, "fright illness," is believed to be caused by a sudden intense fear. It is believed to occur because the soul leaves the body during the frightful episode. Symptoms include nervousness, anorexia, insomnia, listlessness, fatigue, despondency, muscle tics, and diarrhea.
Taijin kyofusho (Japan)	The term *taijin kyofusho* literally means the disorder (*sho*) of fear (*kyofu*) of interpersonal relations (*taijin*). The sufferer dreads and avoids social contact and has a fear of offending or harming other people. *Taijin kyofusho* is divided into four categories: *sekimen-kyofu* (phobia of blushing), *shubo-kyofu* (phobia of a deformed body), *jikoshisen-kyofu* (phobia of eye-to-eye contact), and *jikoshu-kyofu* (phobia of a foul body odor). The illness is seen as social phobia (social anxiety) in Western societies.
Zar (African and Middle Eastern societies)	Those affected experience dissociative episodes and believe they are possessed by a spirit. During the episode they may shout, laugh, weep, sing, or hit their heads on the wall. They also may become apathetic, withdrawn, and unable to carry out daily tasks. Some develop a relationship with the possessing spirit. It may not be considered pathological.

Note: The suggestion has been made that eating disorders such as anorexia and bulimia are culturally specific to the Western world or parts of the world with heavy exposure to Western media.

Source: Adapted from the American Psychiatric Association (2000).

are "recurrent, locality-specific patterns of aberrant behavior and troubling experience that may or may not be linked to a particular DSM-IV diagnostic category" (American Psychiatric Association, 2000, p. 898). It is not well known how applicable *DSM* diagnostic criteria are to culturally specific symptom expression and culture-bound syndromes. Researchers have taken initial steps to examine the interrelationships between culture-bound syndromes and the diagnostic classifications of the *DSM*. In past research, there was an effort to fit culture-bound syndromes into variants of *DSM* diagnoses. Rather than assume that *DSM* diagnostic entities or culture-bound syndromes are the basic patterns of illness, current investigators are interested in examining how the social, cultural, and biological contexts interact to shape illnesses and reactions to them. This is an important area of research in a field known as cultural psychiatry or **ethnopsychiatry**.

Culture's Impact on Treatment Seeking and Approaches

When and if a person seeks treatment depends partially on cultural beliefs. Research shows that racial and ethnic minorities in the United States are less likely to seek treatment for mental illness as well as delay seeking treatment. This is in part due to culturally related factors such as stigma, mistrust in clinicians and the healthcare system, and communication barriers, discussed in more detail later in this chapter. As a result of the cultural barriers, they often turn to other pathways of care, described in this section.

Religion and Spirituality

Culture can be tied to religious beliefs and spirituality, and these beliefs affect where people seek care. Many people seek guidance through religious figures and/or support systems that exist in their place of worship. Through religion and spirituality many find hope, support, and meaning in their lives, thereby reducing stress and suffering.

Family and Community as Resources

The definition of family varies among cultures. Some think of the nuclear family (mother, father, sibling), whereas others also include aunts, uncles, in-laws, grandparents, and nonblood family members. Some cultures, such as the African, Latino, Asian, and Native American communities, have close ties with family. As a result, some cultures may turn to family members for assistance and support more than others.

Healers

A variety of types of healers assist with mental health concerns, such as shamans, medicine men, acupuncturists, religious leaders, and herbalists. For example, American Indians and Alaska Natives often rely on traditional healers, and African Americans rely on ministers. Community mental health professionals should be aware of the types of healers that the community members are using so the users' cultural beliefs can be incorporated into the program plan to improve the mental health of that community.

Complementary and Alternative Treatments

As discussed in Chapter 2, people of different cultures use a variety of complementary and alternative therapies for healing. African Americans, as well as other minority groups, are believed to use alternative treatments extensively (DHHS, 2001). Some of the treatments used straddle both physical and mental health. For example, massage and yoga help reduce muscle tension (physical health) as well as induce relaxation (mental health). What is important to note is that the use of complementary medicine is widespread, and some types may impact treatments provided by Western practices, altering medication responses. Many people do not reveal their use of folk or complementary practices.

MINORITIES AND MENTAL HEALTH

As stated previously, the federal government officially designates four major racial or ethnic minority groups in the United States, but many other racial or ethnic minorities and considerable diversity within each of the four groupings exists. In this section we discuss each of these groups, but realize that a great degree of diversity occurs within each of them. The level of acculturation also has an impact on mental health, and the categories are arbitrary.

African Americans

The prevalence of mental disorders among African Americans is similar to that of whites (DHHS 2001), but the prevalence rates may be understated. This is because many high-risk populations also are ones with a high representation of African Americans. Examples include people who are incarcerated, are in psychiatric hospitals, or live in inner cities. These populations are difficult to incorporate into studies that rely on household surveys; therefore, the higher rates of mental illness among African Americans may not be detected (DHHS, 2001). What we are sure of is that African Americans are more likely than whites to use the emergency department for mental health problems (DHHS, 2001).

Owing to a long history of oppression and the cumulative impact of economic hardship, African Americans are significantly overrepresented in the most vulnerable segments of the population. More African Americans than whites or members of other racial and ethnic minority groups are homeless, incarcerated, or are children in foster care or otherwise supervised by the child welfare system. African Americans are especially likely to be exposed to violence-related trauma, as were the large number of African American soldiers assigned to war zones in Vietnam. Exposure to trauma leads to increased vulnerability to mental disorders. Some statistics highlighting these facts include the following:

- People who are homeless. Although representing only 12% of the U.S. population, African Americans make up about 40% of the homeless population.

- People who are incarcerated. Nearly half of all prisoners in state and federal jurisdictions and almost 40% of juveniles in legal custody are African Americans.
- Children in foster care and the child welfare system. African American children and youth constitute about 45% of children in public foster care and more than half of all children waiting to be adopted.
- People exposed to violence. African Americans of all ages are more likely to be victims of serious violent crime than are non-Hispanic whites. One study reported that more than 25% of African American youth exposed to violence met diagnostic criteria for posttraumatic stress disorder (PTSD). Among Vietnam War veterans, 21% of black veterans, compared to 14% of non-Hispanic white veterans, suffer from PTSD, apparently because of the greater exposure of blacks to war-zone trauma (DHHS, 1999).

Also, the high rates of HIV/AIDS among this group poses special challenges because HIV/AIDS can lead to mental health problems such as dementia, depression, mood disorders, and psychosis.

Somatization (the person reports physical symptoms that cannot be explain in medical terms and is thought to mask mental illness) is more common among African Americans (15%) than among whites (9%) (DHHS, 2001). Moreover, African Americans experience culture-bound syndromes such as isolated sleep paralysis (an inability to move while falling asleep or waking up) and falling out (a sudden collapse sometimes preceded by dizziness) (DHHS, 2001).

Asian Americans/Pacific Islanders

The prevalence of mental illness among Asian Americans is difficult to determine. Some studies suggest higher rates of mental illness, but there is wide variance across different groups of Asian Americans. For example, Speller (2005, p. 70) reports,

> Asian Americans do experience mental illness and have an equally high, if not higher, need for appropriate mental health services as any other racial or ethnic group. Asian American adolescent boys are twice as likely to have been physically abused and are three times more likely to report abuse than their white American counterparts. Asian American women aged 15 to 24 and 65+ have the highest suicide rates in the United States out of all racial and ethnic groups. Asian American college students have been found to report higher levels of depressive symptoms than white students.

It is not well known how applicable *DSM* diagnostic criteria are to culturally specific symptom expression and culture-bound syndromes. With respect to treatment-seeking behavior, Asian Americans are distinguished by extremely low levels of seeking treatment for mental health problems. Asian Americans have proven less likely than whites, African Americans, and Hispanic Americans to seek care. However, low demand for mental health care is not necessarily reflective of low need. The reasons for the underutilization of services include the stigma and loss of face over mental health problems, limited English proficiency among some Asian immigrants, different cultural explanations for the problems, and the inability to find culturally competent services.

Refugees include a high number of Asians and Pacific Islanders, and they also have high rates of mental disorders. Given the relative economic status of Asian Americans and Pacific Islanders, it is not surprising that they are not present in large numbers among the nation's homeless. In its 2006 survey of 25 cities, the U.S. Conference of Mayors document reported that the homeless population is estimated to be only 2% Asian (U.S. Conference of Mayors, 2006). Furthermore, they make up less than 2% of the national incarcerated population (Federal Bureau of Prisons, 2010). Asian Americans are less likely to have substance abuse problems than are other Americans (DHHS, 2008). In sum, Asian Americans and Pacific Islanders are not heavily represented in many of the groups known to have a high need for mental health care. However, many do experience difficulties, such as the lack of English proficiency, acculturative stress, prejudice, discrimination, and racial hate crimes, which place them at risk for emotional and behavioral problems. Southeast Asian refugees, in particular, are considered to be at high risk.

With regard to somatization, Western culture makes a distinction between the mind and body, but many Asian cultures do not. Therefore, it has long been hypothesized that Asians express more somatic symptoms of distress than white Americans. The influence of the teachings and philosophies of a Confucian collectivist tradition discourages open displays of emotions, in order to maintain social and familial harmony or to avoid exposure of personal weakness. Mental illness is highly stigmatizing in many Asian cultures. In these societies, mental illness reflects poorly on one's family lineage and can influence others' beliefs about how suitable someone is for marriage if he or she comes from a family with a history of mental illness. Thus, either consciously or unconsciously, Asians are thought to deny the experience and expression of emotions. Even if Asian Americans are not at high risk for a few of the psychiatric disorders that are common in the United States, they may experience culture-bound syndromes, such as neurasthenia and *hwa-byung*.

The portion of Asian Americans among those who use psychiatric clinics and hospitals is lower than their proportion of the general population. Many studies demonstrate that Asian Americans who use mental health services are more severely ill than white Americans who use the same services. Two explanations for this finding are that (1) Asian Americans are reluctant to use mental health care so they seek care only when they have severe illness, and (2) families tend to discourage the use of mental health facilities among family members until disturbed members become unmanageable. The reluctance to use services is attributable to factors such as the shame and stigma accompanying use of mental health services, cultural conceptions of mental health and treatment that may be inconsistent with Western forms of treatment, and cultural or language barriers.

Hispanic Americans

Several epidemiologic studies revealed few differences between Hispanic Americans and whites in lifetime rates of mental illness, and research suggests that immigrants have lower rates than Mexican Americans born in the United States. Although rates of mental illness may be similar to those of whites in general, the prevalence of particular mental health problems, the manifestation of symptoms, and help-seeking behaviors within Hispanic subgroups need attention and further research.

Given that poverty is associated with homelessness and that many Hispanic American subgroups experience high rates of poverty, high rates of homelessness might be anticipated. However, the fact is that an estimated 13% of homeless individuals are Hispanics (U.S. Conference of Mayors, 2006). Likewise, the need to place children in foster care is related to socioeconomic factors. Again, few Hispanic children are in the foster care system (DHHS, 1999). The fact that Hispanics are more likely to live with extended family members and with unrelated individuals suggests that family or friends may be taking care of those in need. Although Hispanics are relatively underrepresented among persons who are homeless or in foster care, they are present in high numbers within other vulnerable, high-need populations, such as incarcerated individuals, war veterans, survivors of trauma, and persons who abuse drugs or alcohol.

As noted previously, the *DSM* recognizes culture-bound syndromes. Relevant examples of these syndromes for Latinos are **susto** (fright illness), as mentioned earlier, *nervios* (nerves), and **mal de ojo** (evil eye). One expression of distress most commonly associated with Caribbean Latinos but recognized in other Latinos as well is *ataques de nervios*. Symptoms of an *ataque de nervios* include screaming uncontrollably, crying, trembling, and verbal or physical aggression. Dissociative experiences, seizure-like or fainting episodes, and suicidal gestures are also prominent in some *ataques*.

There is value in identifying specific culture-bound syndromes such as *ataques de nervios* because it is critical to recognize the existence of conceptions of distress and illness outside traditional psychiatric classification systems. Some of these popular conceptions may have what appear to be definable boundaries, whereas others are more fluid and cut across a wide range of symptom clusters. Although it is valuable for researchers and clinicians alike to learn about specific culture-bound syndromes, it is more important that they assess variable local representations of illness and distress. The latter approach casts a wider net around understanding the role of culture in illness and distress. In the treatment setting, integrating consumers' popular or commonsense notions of health and illness with biomedical notions has the potential to enhance treatment alliances and, in turn, treatment outcomes.

Two specific strengths have been noted among this population that may help protect them from mental disorders and substance abuse. First, as noted, Latino adults who are immigrants have lower prevalence rates of mental disorders than those born in the United States. Among the competing explanations of these findings is that Latino immigrants may be particularly resilient in the face of the hardships they encounter in settling in a new country. If this is the case, then the identification of what these immigrants do to reduce the likelihood of mental disorders could be of value for all Americans. One of many possible factors that might contribute to their resilience is what Suarez-Orozco and Suarez-Orozco (1995) refer to as a "dual frame of reference." Investigators found that Latino immigrants in middle school frequently used their families back home as reference points in assessing their lives in the United States. Given that the social and economic conditions are often much worse in their homelands than in the United States, they may experience less distress in handling the stressors of their daily lives than those who lack such a basis of comparison. U.S.-born Latinos are more likely to compare themselves with their peers in the United States. Suarez-Orozco and Suarez-Orozco argue that these Latino children are more aware of what they do not have and thus may experience more distress. A second factor noted by the Suarez-Orozcos that might be related to the resilience of Latino immigrants is their high aspiration to succeed. Particularly noteworthy is that many Latinos want to succeed to help their families rather than for their own personal benefit. Because the Suarez-Orozcos did not include measures of mental health, it is not certain whether their observations about school achievement apply to mental health. Nevertheless, a dual frame of reference and collective achievement goals are part of a complex set of psychological, cultural, and social factors that may explain why some Latino immigrants function better than Latinos of later generations.

A second type of strength noted in the literature is how Latino families cope with mental illness. Many Latinos are very spiritual, and these strong beliefs in God give some family members a sense of hope. The spirituality of Latino families, their conceptions of mental illness, and their warmth contribute to the support they offer in coping with serious mental illness.

Although limited, the attention given to Latinos' possible strengths is an important contribution to the study of Latino mental health. Strengths are protective factors against distress and disorder and can be used to develop interventions to prevent mental disorders and to promote well-being. Such interventions could be used to inform interventions for all Americans, not just Latinos. In addition, redirecting attention to strengths helps point out the overemphasis researchers and practitioners give to pathology, clinical entities, and treatment, rather than to health, well-being, and prevention.

American Indians and Alaska Natives

American Indians/Alaska Natives have been studied in few epidemiologic surveys of mental health and mental disorders. The indications are that depression is a significant problem in many American Indian/Alaska Native communities (Office of Minority Health, 2005). Alcohol abuse and dependence appear also to be especially problematic, occurring at perhaps twice the rate found in any other population group. Relatedly, suicide occurs at alarmingly high levels (Office of Minority Health, 2005).

Because American Indians and Alaska Natives compose such a small percentage of U.S. citizens in general, nationally representative studies do not generate sufficiently large samples of this special population to draw accurate conclusions regarding their need for mental health care. Even when large samples are acquired, findings are constrained by the marked heterogeneity that characterizes the social and cultural ecologies of Native people. There are 561 federally recognized tribes with over 200 indigenous languages spoken. Similar differences abound among Native customs, family structures, religions, and social relationships. The magnitude of this diversity among Indian people has important implications for research observations.

Language is important when assessing the mental health needs of individuals and the communities in which they reside. Approximately 280,000 American Indians and Alaska Natives speak a language other than English at home; more than half of Alaska Natives who are Eskimos speak either Inuit or Yup'ik. Consequently, evaluations of need for mental health care often have to be conducted in a language other than English. Yet the challenge can be more subtle than that implied by stark differences in language. Cultural differences in the expression and reporting of distress are well established among American Indians and Alaska Natives, and these differences can make it difficult to assess mental illness. Words such as *depressed* and *anxious* are absent from some American Indian and Alaska Native languages. Other research has demonstrated that certain *DSM* diagnoses, such as major depressive disorder, do not correspond directly to the categories of illness recognized by some American Indians. Thus evaluating the need for mental health care among American Indians and Alaska Natives requires careful clinical inquiry that attends closely to culture.

American Indians and Alaska Natives are the most impoverished ethnic minority group in the United States. Although no causal links have yet been demonstrated, there is good reason to suspect that the history of oppression, discrimination, and removal from traditional lands experienced by Native people has contributed to their current lack of educational and economic opportunities and their significant representation among populations with a high need for mental health care. The high-risk populations include individuals who are homeless, incarcerated, have drug and alcohol problems, and are exposed to trauma, as well as children in foster care.

With regard to somatization, the distinction between mind and body common among individuals in industrialized Western nations is not shared throughout the world. Many ethnic minorities do not discriminate bodily from psychic distress and may express emotional distress in somatic terms or bodily symptoms. Relatively little empirical research is available concerning this tendency among American Indians and Alaska Natives so there is not enough information to report and make any generalizations.

Culture-bound syndromes have been shown to exist among this group. A large body of ethnographic work reveals that some American Indians and Alaska Natives, who may express emotional distress in ways that are inconsistent with the diagnostic categories of the *DSM*, may conceptualize mental health differently. Many unique expressions of distress shown by American Indians and Alaska Natives exist, such as **ghost sickness**. The question becomes how to elicit, understand, and incorporate such expressions of distress and suffering within the assessment and treatment process of the *DSM*.

BARRIERS TO THE RECEIPT OF TREATMENT FOR ALL MINORITIES

Several factors affect the use of mental health treatment. These include cultural, financial, and geographic factors. These factors stem from historical and current social elements that impact help-seeking behavior.

Among adults, the evidence is considerable that persons from minority backgrounds are less likely than are whites to seek outpatient treatment in the specialty mental health sector. This is not the case for emergency department care. African Americans are less likely than whites to seek care for mental health problems. Limited English proficiency, immigration status, and seeking treatment from nontraditional approaches (such as clergy and traditional healers) are a few reasons for lower utilization levels. Others include mistrust, stigma, cost, and clinical bias.

Mistrust

Mistrust has been identified as a major barrier to receiving mental health treatment, yet there are few studies that document it (DHHS, 2001). Mistrust among African Americans may stem from their experiences of segregation, racism, and discrimination. Lack of trust is likely to operate among other minority groups, according to research about their attitudes toward government-operated institutions rather than toward mental health treatment per se. This is particularly pronounced for immigrant families with relatives who may be undocumented, and hence they are less likely to trust authorities for fear of being reported and having the family member deported.

American Indians' past experience in this country also imparted lack of trust of government. Those living on Indian reservations are particularly fearful of sharing any information with white clinicians employed by the government. As with African Americans, the historical relationship of forced control, segregation, racism, and discrimination has affected their ability to trust a white majority population.

Stigma

The stigma of mental illness is another factor preventing people from seeking treatment. Stigma, denial, and self-reliance are likely explanations why other minority groups do not seek treatment, but their contribution has not been evaluated empirically, owing in part to the difficulty of conducting this type of research.

Cost

Cost is yet another factor discouraging utilization of mental health services. Minority persons are less likely than whites to have private health insurance. Also, hourly workers or workers who get paid by their production (e.g., farm workers) may not want to take time off from work to seek care because of the decrease in wages.

Clinician Bias

Bias in clinician judgment is thought to be reflected in overdiagnosis or misdiagnosis of mental disorders. Because diagnosis relies heavily on behavioral signs and patients' reporting of the symptoms, rather than on laboratory tests, clinician judgment plays an enormous role in the diagnosis of mental disorders.

PROVIDING MORE CULTURALLY SENSITIVE CARE

The previous paragraphs have documented underutilization of treatment, less help-seeking behavior, inappropriate diagnosis, and other problems that have beset racial and ethnic minority groups with respect to mental health treatment. This kind of evidence has fueled the widespread perception of mental health treatment as uninviting, inappropriate, or not as effective for minority groups as for whites. In Chapter 14, we describe ways to improve mental health services, but here we describe two ways that are specifically tied to culture: the need for more research on cultural influences on medications and training providers in cultural competence.

Ethnopsychopharmacology

There is mounting awareness that ethnic and cultural influences can alter an individual's responses to medications (pharmacotherapies). The relatively new field of **ethnopsychopharmacology** investigates cultural variations and differences that influence the effectiveness of pharmacotherapies used in the mental health field. These differences are both genetic and psychosocial. They range from genetic variations in drug metabolism to cultural practices that affect diet, medication adherence, placebo effect, and the simultaneous use of traditional and alternative healing methods (Lin, Anderson, & Poland, 1997).

Pharmacotherapies given by mouth usually enter the circulation after absorption from the stomach. From the circulation they are distributed throughout the body and then metabolized. The rate of metabolism affects the amount of the drug in the circulation. A slow rate of metabolism leaves more of the drug in the circulation. Too much medication in the circulation typically leads to heightened side effects. A fast rate of metabolism, in contrast, leaves less drug in the circulation. Too little drug in the circulation reduces its effectiveness.

There is wide racial and ethnic variation in drug metabolism due to genetic variations in drug-metabolizing enzymes (which are responsible for breaking down drugs in the liver). These genetic variations alter the activity of several drug-metabolizing enzymes. Each drug-metabolizing enzyme normally breaks down not just one type of pharmacotherapy but usually several types. Because most of the ethnic variation comes in the form of inactivation or reduction in activity in the enzymes, the result is higher amounts of medication in the blood, triggering untoward side effects.

For example, 33% of African Americans and 37% of Asians are slow metabolizers of several antipsychotic medications and antidepressants (such as tricyclic antidepressants and selective serotonin reuptake inhibitors) (Lin et al., 1997), and studies have shown Asian Americans to be slow metabolizers of cytochrome P-450 enzymes, rendering them much more sensitive to pharmacotherapy (Speller, 2005). This awareness should lead to more cautious prescribing practices, which usually entail starting patients at lower doses in the beginning of treatment. Unfortunately, just the opposite typically had been the case with African American patients and antipsychotic drugs. The combination of slow metabolism and overmedication of antipsychotic drugs in African Americans can yield very uncomfortable extrapyramidal side effects (Lin et al., 1997).

Psychosocial factors also can play an important role in ethnic variation. Compliance with dosing may be hindered by communication difficulties, side effects can be misinterpreted or carry different connotations, some groups may be more responsive to placebo treatment, and reliance on psychoactive traditional and alternative healing methods (such as medicinal plants and herbs) may result in interactions with prescribed pharmacotherapies. The result could be greater side effects and enhanced or reduced effectiveness of the pharmacotherapy, depending on the agents involved and their concentrations (Lin et al., 1997). Greater awareness of ethnopsychopharmacology is expected to improve treatment effectiveness for racial and ethnic minorities, and more research is needed on this topic across racial and ethnic groups.

Cultural Competence in the Healthcare Workforce

Research and clinical practice have propelled advocates and mental health professionals to press for linguistically and culturally competent services to improve utilization and effectiveness of treatment for different cultures. Being culturally competent in health care means providing health services in a sensitive, knowledgeable, and nonjudgmental manner, with respect for people's health beliefs and practices when they are different from the providers. It entails challenging one's own assumptions, asking the right questions, and working with the patient and/or community in a manner that takes into consideration their lifestyle and approach to maintaining health and treating illness. Culturally competent healthcare delivery integrates different approaches to care and incorporates the culture and belief system of the healthcare recipient while providing care within the legal, ethical, and medically sound practices of the practitioner's medical system.

Cultural competence comprises four components: awareness of one's own cultural worldview, attitude toward cultural differences, knowledge of different cultural practices and worldviews, and cross-cultural skills. As illustrated in the Purnell model for cultural competence (**Figure 3-1**), cultural competence occurs on multiple levels. The model includes 12 domains, which determine variations in values, beliefs, and practices of an individual's cultural heritage.

Cultural awareness allows the healthcare professional to see the entire picture and improves the quality of care and health outcomes (Fernandez & Fernandez, 2005). To be culturally competent, providers need to understand their own worldviews and those of the patient and community while avoiding stereotyping and misapplication of scientific knowledge (Fernandez & Fernandez, 2005).

Adapting to different cultural beliefs and practices requires flexibility, respect for other viewpoints, challenging assumptions, and asking the right questions. This entails really listening to the person, finding out and learning about the person's and community's beliefs about health and illness, and being open to other ideas. To provide culturally appropriate care, healthcare professionals need to know and to understand culturally influenced health behaviors (Fernandez & Fernandez, 2005) and provide care that is respectful of these different beliefs.

Because the perception of illness and disease and their causes varies by culture, these individual preferences affect the approaches to health care. Culture also influences how people seek health care, adherence to treatment plans, and how they behave toward healthcare providers. Healthcare providers must possess the ability and knowledge to communicate and to understand health behaviors influenced by culture. Having this ability and knowledge can eliminate barriers to the delivery of health care and improve the quality of care and clinical outcomes. These issues illustrate the need for healthcare organizations to develop policies, practices, and procedures to deliver culturally competent care (Fernandez & Fernandez, 2005). Implementing cultural competence programs is a nonlinear, multilevel, complex process. The paths to progression toward cultural competence are varied. Cultural competence is related to policies, human resource development, and services.

One common approach to educating practitioners about the links between health and culture and the different cultural practices and beliefs is cultural competency training classes. The problem with this approach lies in that knowing the health practices and cultural beliefs of all groups is not possible, and teaching cultural competency can enhance stereotypes (Kleinman & Benson, 2006). Stereotypes can contribute to wrong assumptions and do not take into account differences in acculturation levels and subculture variances. Another concern with the cultural competency approach is that it is usually taught by addressing differences in races and ethnicities and ignores other cultural attributes such as gender, age, religion, geographic region of origin (e.g., rural versus urban and North versus Southeast), and sexual orientation. Therefore, teaching healthcare providers how to conduct a cultural assessment, as mentioned

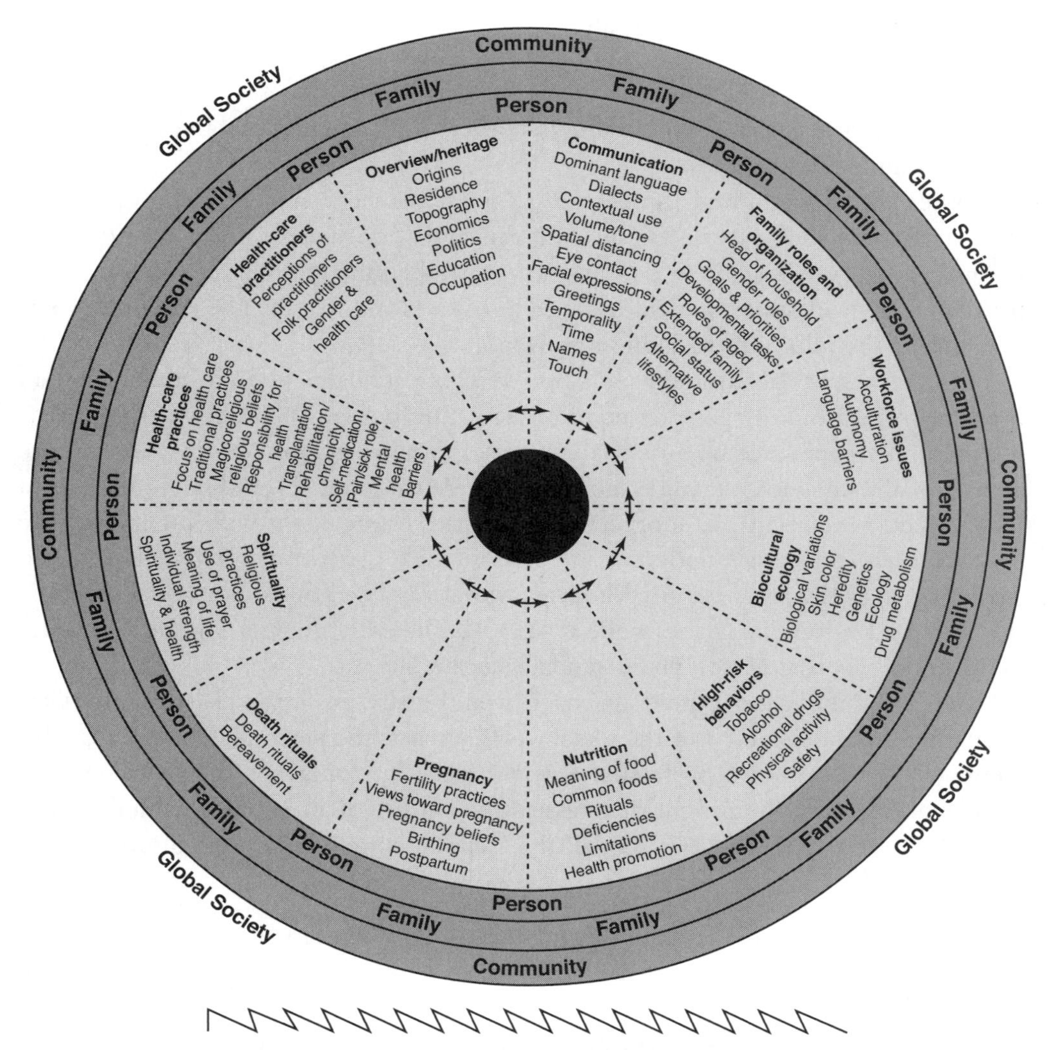

Unconsciously incompetent – Consciously incompetent –
Consciously competent – Unconsciously competent

Primary characteristics of culture: age, generation, nationality, race, color, gender, religion
Secondary characteristics of culture: educational status, socioeconomic status, occupation, military status, political beliefs, urban versus rural residence, enclave identity, marital status, parental status, physical characteristics, sexual orientation, gender issues, and reason for migration (sojourner, immigrant, undocumented status)
Unconsciously incompetent: not being aware that one is lacking knowledge about another culture
Consciously incompetent: being aware that one is lacking knowledge about another culture
Consciously competent: learning about the client's culture, verifying generalizations about the client's culture, and providing culturally specific interventions
Unconsciously competent: automatically providing culturally congruent care to clients of diverse cultures

FIGURE 3-1 The Purnell Model for Cultural Competence
Source: Reprinted with permission from Dr. Larry Purnell, University of Delaware.

previously, in a reasonable time frame is needed. This entails teaching providers to conduct mini-ethnographies.

When teaching cultural competence, it is important to not enhance stereotypes with statements such as "the Chinese do this and Mexicans do that." It also would not portray culture as static or tied only to race and ethnicity, which is usually the approach taken by existing multicultural health courses and videos. The authors recommend using the mini-ethnographic approach.

Ethnographies are an anthropological research modality used to understand an event or belief from the person's point of view. Ethnography is different from teaching cultural competence because the latter uses a trait-list approach and sees culture as a set of already known factors, such as "Chinese eat pork," even though millions of Chinese are vegetarians. Ethnography emphasizes engagement with others and the practices that individuals undertake. It is sensitive to people who live between two worlds (such as the Japanese girl who lives with a very traditional family yet practices the dominant culture behaviors while at school). The ethnographic approach provides insight into how that person understands his or her illness.

Using a mini-ethnographic approach would assist professionals with interview techniques to understand how the social world impacts the person's illness. Using this approach, the healthcare professional would basically conduct a mini-ethnography while working with the patient or to assess the culture of an individual and/or community. Using the explanatory model, the steps to comprehend the culture include understanding:

1. Ethnic identity (ask about ethnic identity and if it matters to the patient),
2. What is at stake (evaluate what is at stake as patients and their loved ones face an episode of illness),
3. The illness narrative (reconstruct the patient's illness by understanding the meaning of the illness),
4. Psychosocial stressors (consider ongoing stressors and social supports),
5. Influence of culture on clinical relationships (examine culture in terms of its influence on clinical relationships), and
6. The problems of a cultural competency approach (assess if the intervention will work in that particular case). (Kleinman & Benson, 2006)

Using this approach enables the researcher or clinician to understand the mental health problem from the individual's or the community's perspective. It avoids stereotypes and helps understand cultural influences while taking acculturation levels into consideration.

Some additional suggestions for achieving a culturally competent organization include maximizing diversity among the workforce; involving community representatives in the organization's planning and quality improvement meetings; establishing a Cultural Competence Board to help guide the implementation of culturally sensitive prevention and treatment efforts; providing ongoing training to staff; developing health materials for the target population that are written at the appropriate literacy level, in a variety of languages and with culturally appropriate images—this includes materials such as educational brochures, consent forms, signage, postprocedural directions, and advance directives; making on-site interpretation services available when possible and ensuring that all appropriate staff is educated about how to use telephone interpretation services; assessing customer satisfaction and clinical outcomes regularly; and considering the health disparities that exist in the community when planning outreach efforts.

The approach to accomplishing these tasks is complex and will depend on the organization's resources and existing level of cultural competence. Once an individual, organization, or system has implemented change to progress toward cultural competence, the change process should be measured. Measurement is important because it can indicate the progress that has been made and areas in need of improvement. The measurement process itself can be a catalyst for change.

CHAPTER SUMMARY

This chapter presents compelling evidence that racial and ethnic minorities collectively experience a disproportionately high disability burden from unmet mental health needs. Despite the progress in understanding the causes of mental illness and the tremendous advances in finding effective mental health treatments, far less is known about the mental health of African Americans, American Indians and Alaska Natives, Asian American and Pacific Islanders, and Hispanic Americans.

The United States has far to go to eliminate racial and ethnic disparities in mental health. The demographic changes anticipated over the next decades magnify the importance of eliminating differences in mental health burden and access to services. Ethnic minority groups are expected to grow as a proportion of the total U.S. population. Therefore, the future mental health of America as a whole will be enhanced substantially by improving the health of racial and ethnic minorities.

It is necessary to expand and improve programs to deliver culturally, linguistically, and geographically accessible mental health services. Financial barriers, including discriminatory health insurance coverage of treatment for mental illness, need to be surmounted. Programs to increase public awareness of mental illness and effective treatments must be developed for racial and ethnic minority communities, as must efforts to overcome shame, stigma, discrimination, and distrust. The time is right for a commitment to expand or redirect resources to support evidence-based, affordable, and culturally appropriate mental health services for racial and ethnic minorities, particularly in settings where those with the highest need are not being adequately served, such as jails, prisons, homeless shelters, and foster care. Where gaps exist in the evidence base about the prevalence, perception, course, detection, and treatment of mental illness in racial and ethnic minority populations, individuals must be trained and supported to carry out systematic programs of research.

As noted in this chapter, community mental health professionals need to be aware of the cultural influences on mental health. The terminology related to race, ethnicity, and culture was clarified along with identifying specific cultural issues for four racial and ethnic categories. We discussed culture-bound syndromes and barriers to care and adequate services. This chapter is just the beginning of your journey to becoming culturally competent because there is a lot to learn about this area. We conclude this chapter and section of the book and move on to a discussion of the legal and healthcare systems in which mental health and illness is prevented and treated.

REVIEW

1. What is cultural competence?
2. Define culture, ethnicity, and race.
3. What are personalistic and naturalistic ethnomedical systems?
4. Explain the extent of mental health disparities and the reasons for them.
5. Why is there a need for mental health services to take culture into consideration?
6. List at least two mental health challenges and high-risk populations for each of the four minority groups discussed in this chapter.
7. What barriers exist for minorities in seeking out treatment?
8. What progress has been made toward the elimination of mental health disparities and the promotion of mental health?

ACTIVITY

Select a mental health problem that exists in a specific culture. Research the topic and write a three-page paper on the status of the problem, the factors related to the cause of the problem, and what could be done to reduce or eliminate the problem.

REFERENCES AND FURTHER READINGS

Acosta, F. X., Yamamoto, J., & Evans, L. A. (1982). *Effective psychotherapy for low-income and minority patients*. New York: Plenum.

Agostinelli, F. Y. (2008). Cross-cultural comparison of mental disorders (1). Retrieved from http://www.webspawner.com/users/pakli/crossculturalco.html

American Anthropological Association. (1998). Statement on "race." Retrieved from http://www.aaanet.org/stmts/racepp.htm

American Psychiatric Association. (2000). *Diagnostic and statistical manual of mental disorders*. Washington, DC: Author.

Bacote, J. C. (1994). Transcultural psychiatric nursing: Diagnostic and treatment issues. *Journal of Psychosocial Nursing*, *32*, 42–46.

Belle, D. (1990). Poverty and women's mental health. *American Psychologist*, *45*, 385–389.

Bowman, P. J. (1996). Naturally occurring psychological expectancies: Theory and measurement among African Americans (pp. 553–578). In R. L. Jones (Ed.), *Handbook of tests and measurements for black populations*. Berkeley, CA: Cobbs & Henry.

Brody, T. M. (1994). Absorption, distribution, metabolism, and elimination. In T. M. Brody, J. Larner, K. Minneman, & H. Neu (Eds.), *Human pharmacology: Molecular to clinical* (2nd ed., pp. 49–61). St. Louis: Mosby-Year Book.

Cabaj, R. P., & Stein, T. S. (1996). *Textbook of homosexuality and mental health*. Washington, DC: American Psychiatric Press.

Canino, G. J., Bird, H. R., Shrout, P. E., Rubio-Stipec, M., Bravo, M., Martinez, R., . . . Guevara, L. M. (1987). The prevalence of specific psychiatric disorders in Puerto Rico. *Archives of General Psychiatry*, *44*, 727–735.

Center for Mental Health Services. (1998). *Cultural competence standards in managed care mental health services for four underserved/ underrepresented racial/ethnic groups*. Rockville, MD: Author.

Centers for Disease Control and Prevention. (1991). *Strategic plan for the elimination of childhood lead poisoning*. Atlanta, GA: Author.

Centers for Disease Control and Prevention. (2008, August 29). Alcohol-Attributable Deaths and Years of Potential Life Lost Among American Indians and Alaska Natives—United States, 2001–2005. *MMWR*, *57*(34), 938–941. Retrieved from http://www.cdc.gov/mmwr/preview/mmwrhtml/mm5734a3.htm?s_cid=mm5734a3_x

Chamberlin, J. (1978). *On our own: Patient-controlled alternatives to the mental health system*. New York: McGraw-Hill.

Chamberlin, J. (1990). The ex-patient's movement: Where we've been and where we're going. *Journal of Mind and Behavior*, *11*, 323–336.

Chamberlin, J. (1995). Rehabilitating ourselves: The psychiatric survivor movement. *International Journal of Mental Health*, *24*, 39–46.

Chamberlin, J. (1997). Confessions of a non-compliant patient. *National Empowerment Center Newsletter*. Lawrence, MA: National Empowerment Center.

Chamberlin, J., & Rogers, J. A. (1990). Planning a community-based mental health system. Perspective of service recipients. *American Psychologist*, *45*, 1241–1244.

Cheung, F. K., & Snowden, L. R. (1990). Community mental health and ethnic minority populations. *Community Mental Health Journal*, *26*, 277–291.

Ciarlo, J. A. (1998). Estimating and monitoring need for mental health services in rural frontier areas. *Rural Community Mental Health, 24*, 17–18.

Clarke, G. N., Hawkins, W., Murphy, M., Sheeber, L. B., Lewinsohn, P. M., & Seeley, J. R. (1995). Targeted prevention of unipolar depressive disorder in an at-risk sample of high school adolescents: A randomized trial of a group cognitive intervention. *Journal of the American Academy of Child and Adolescent Psychiatry, 34*, 312–321.

Cohen, S., & Herbert, T. B. (1996). Health psychology: Psychological factors and physical disease from the perspective of human psychoneuroimmunology. *Annual Review of Psychology, 47*, 113–142.

Coie, J., & Krehbiel, G. (1984). Effects of academic tutoring on the social status of low-achieving, socially rejected children. *Child Development, 55*, 1465–1478.

Comas Diaz, L. (1989). Culturally relevant issues and treatment implications for Hispanics. In D. Koslow & E. Salett (Eds.), *Crossing cultures in mental health* (pp. 31–48). Washington, DC: SIETAR International.

Commission on Chronic Illness. (1957). *Chronic illness in the United States* (Vol. 1). Cambridge, MA: Harvard University Press.

Conwell, Y. (1996). *Diagnosis and treatment of depression in late life*. Washington, DC: American Psychiatric Press.

Cook, J. A., & Jonikas, J. A. (1996). Outcomes of psychiatric rehabilitation service delivery. *New Directions in Mental Health Services, 71*, 33–47.

Cook, K., & Timberlake, E. M. (1989). Cross-cultural counseling with Vietnamese refugees. In D. Koslow & E. Salett (Eds.), *Crossing cultures in mental health* (pp. 84–100). Washington, DC: SIETAR International.

Cooper, C. R., & Denner, J. (1998). Theories linking culture and psychopathology: Universal and community-specific processes. *Annual Review of Psychology, 49*, 559–584.

Cooper, J. R., Bloom, F. E., & Roth, R. H. (1996). *The biochemical basis of neuropharmacology*. New York: Oxford University Press.

Cross, T., Bazron, B., Dennis, K., & Isaacs, M. (1989). *Towards a culturally competent system of care: A monograph on effective services for minority children who are severely emotionally disturbed*. Washington, DC: Georgetown University Child Development Center.

Danbom, D. (1995). *Born in the country: A history of rural America*. Baltimore: Johns Hopkins University Press.

Davidson, L., & Strauss, J. S. (1992). Sense of self in recovery from severe mental illness. *British Journal of Medical Psychology, 65*, 131–145.

del Pinal, J., & Singer, A. (1997). Generations of diversity: Latinos in the United States. *Population Bulletin, 52*, 1–44.

Dixon, L. B., Lehman, A. F., & Levine, J. (1995). Conventional antipsychotic medications for schizophrenia. *Schizophrenia Bulletin, 21*, 567–577.

Dohrenwend, B. P., Levav, I., Schwartz, S., Naveh, G., Link, B. G., Skodol, A. E., & Stueve, A. (1992). Socioeconomic status and psychiatric disorders: The causation-selection issue. *Science, 255*, 946–952.

Duran, D. (1995). *Impact of depression, psychological factors, cultural determinants and patient/care provider relationship on somatic complaints of the distressed Latina*. Unpublished doctoral dissertation, University of Denver.

Dyer, J. (1997). *Harvest of rage: Why Oklahoma City is only the beginning*. Boulder, CO: Westview Press.

Emerick, R. (1990). Self-help groups for former patients: Relations with mental health professionals. *Hospital and Community Psychiatry*, *41*, 401–407.

Engel, G. L. (1977). The need for a new medical model: A challenge for biomedicine. *Science*, *196*, 129–136.

Epstein, L. G., & Gendelman, H. E. (1993). Human immunodeficiency virus type 1 infection of the nervous system: Pathogenetic mechanisms. *Annals of Neurology*, *33*, 429–436.

Erikson, E. (1950). *Childhood and society*. New York: Norton.

Federal Bureau of Prisons. (2010). *Quick facts about the Bureau of Prisons*. Retrieved from http://www.bop.gov/news/quick.jsp

Federation of Families for Children's Mental Health. (1999). *Federation of Families for Children's Mental Health home page*. Retrieved from http://www.ffcmh.org

Feldman, R. S. (1997). *Development across the lifespan*. Upper Saddle River, NJ: Prentice Hall.

Fernandez, V., & Fernandez, K. (2005). *Transcultural nursing: Basic concepts & case studies*. Retrieved from http://www.culturediversity.org/

Fischbach, G. D. (1992). Mind and brain. *Scientific American*, *267*, 48–57.

Frasure-Smith, N., Lesperance, F., & Talajic, M. (1993). Depression following myocardial infarction. Impact on 6-month survival. *Journal of the American Medical Association*, *270*, 1819–1825.

Frasure-Smith, N., Lesperance, F., & Talajic, M. (1995). Depression and 18-month prognosis after myocardial infarction. *Circulation*, *91*, 999–1005.

Friedman, L. M., Furberg, C. D., & DeMets, D. L. (1996a). *Fundamentals of clinical trials* (3rd ed.). St. Louis: Mosby.

Friedman, R. M., Katz-Levey, J. W., Manderschied, R. W., & Sondheimer, D. L. (1996b). Prevalence of serious emotional disturbance in children and adolescents. In R. W. Manderscheid & M. A. Sonnenschein (Eds.), *Mental health, United States, 1996* (pp. 71–88). Rockville, MD: Center for Mental Health Services.

Friesen, B. J., & Stephens B. (1998). Expanding family roles in the system of care: Research and practice. In M. R. Epstein, K. Kutash, & A. J. Duchnowski (Eds.), *Outcomes for children and youth with behavioral and emotional disorders and their families: Programs and evaluation, best practices* (pp. 231–259). Austin, TX: Pro-Ed.

Fukuyama, F. (1995). *Trust*. New York: Free Press.

Garcia, M., & Rodriguez, P. F. (1989). Psychological effects of political repression in Argentina and El Salvador. In D. Koslow & E. Salett (Eds.), *Crossing cultures in mental health* (pp. 64–83). Washington, DC: SIETAR International.

Garmezy, N. (1983). Stressors of childhood. In N. Garmezy & M. Rutter (Eds.), *Stress, coping, and development in children* (pp. 43–84). New York: McGraw-Hill.

Garvey, M. A., Giedd, J., & Swedo, S. E. (1998). PANDAS: The search for environmental triggers of pediatric neuropsychiatric disorders. Lessons from rheumatic fever. *Journal of Child Neurology*, *13*, 413–423.

Gazzaniga, M. S., Ivry, R. B., & Mangun, G. R. (1998). *Cognitive neuroscience: The biology of the mind*. New York: Norton.

General Accounting Office. (1977). *Returning the mentally disabled to the community: Government needs to do more*. Washington, DC: Author.

Goldman, H. H. (1998). Deinstitutionalization and community care: Social welfare policy as mental health policy. *Harvard Review of Psychiatry*, *6*, 219–222.

Goldman, H. H., & Morrissey, J. P. (1985). The alchemy of mental health policy: Homelessness and the fourth cycle of reform. *American Journal of Public Health*, *75*, 727–731.

Gordon, M. F. (1964). *Assimilation in American life*. New York: Oxford University Press.

Granger, D. A. (1994). Recovery from mental illness: A first person perspective of an emerging paradigm. In Ohio Department of Mental Health (Ed.), *Recovery: The new force in mental health* (pp. 1–13). Columbus, OH: Author.

Grob, G. N. (1983). *Mental illness and American society, 1875–1940*. Princeton, NJ: Princeton University Press.

Grob, G. N. (1991). *From asylum to community. Mental health policy in modern America*. Princeton, NJ: Princeton University Press.

Grob, G. N. (1994). *The mad among us: A history of the care of America's mentally ill*. New York: Free Press.

Grover, P. L. (1998). Preventing substance abuse among children and adolescents: Family-centered approaches. In *Prevention Enhancement Protocols System Reference Guide*. Rockville, MD: Center for Substance Abuse Prevention.

Hannan, R. W. (1998). Intervention in the coal fields: Mental health outreach. *Rural Community Mental Health*, *24*, 1–3.

Harding, C., Strauss, J. S., & Zubin, J. (1992). Chronicity in schizophrenia: Revisited. *British Journal of Psychiatry*, *161*, 27–37.

Harrow, M., Sands, J. R., Silverstein, M. L., & Goldberg, J. F. (1997). Course and outcome for schizophrenia versus other psychotic patients: A longitudinal study. *Schizophrenia Bulletin*, *23*, 287–303.

Hatchett, S. J., & Jackson, J. S. (1993). African American extended kin systems: An assessment. In H. P. McAdoo (Ed.), *Family ethnicity: Strength in diversity* (pp. 90–108). Newbury Park, CA: Sage.

Health Care Financing Administration. (1991). *International classification of diseases* (9th revision, clinical modification, ICD-9-CM). Washington, DC: Author.

Hernandez, M., Isaacs, M. R., Nesman, T., & Burns, D. (1998). Perspectives on culturally competent systems of care. In M. Hernandez & M. R. Isaacs (Eds.), *Promoting cultural competence in children's mental health services* (pp. 1–25). Baltimore: Brookes.

Herring, R. D. (1994). Native American Indian identity: A people of many peoples. In E. Salett & D. Koslow (Eds.), *Race, ethnicity, and self: Identity in multicultural perspective* (pp. 170–197). Washington, DC: National Multicultural Institute.

Holzer, C., Shea, B., Swanson, J., Leaf, P., Myers, J., George, L., . . . Bednarski, P. (1986). The increased risk for specific psychiatric disorders among persons of low socioeconomic status. *American Journal of Social Psychiatry*, *6*, 259–271.

Horowitz, M. J. (1988). *Introduction to psychodynamics: A new synthesis*. New York: Basic Books.

Horwitz, A. V. (1987). Help-seeking processes and mental health services. *New Directions for Mental Health Services*, *36*, 33–45.

Hough, R. L., Landsverk, J. A., Karno, M., Burnam, M. A., Timbers, D. M., Escobar, J. I., & Regier, D. A. (1987). Utilization of health and mental health services by Los Angeles Mexican Americans and non-Hispanic whites. *Archives of General Psychiatry*, *44*, 702–709.

Hoyt, D. R., Conger, R. D., Valde, J. G., & Weihs, K. (1997). Psychological distress and help seeking in rural America. *American Journal of Community Psychology, 25*, 449–470.

Hoyt, D., O'Donnell D., & Mack, K. Y. (1995). Psychological distress and size of place: The epidemiology of rural economic stress. *Rural Sociology, 60*, 707–720.

Hu, T. W., Snowden, L. R., Jerrell, J. M., & Nguyen, T. D. (1991). Ethnic populations in public mental health: Services choice and level of use. *American Journal of Public Health, 81*, 1429–1434.

Hubel, D., & Wiesel T. (1970). The period of susceptibility to the physiological effects of unilateral eye closure in kittens. *Journal of Physiology, 206*, 419–436.

Hunt, D. (1984). Issues in working with Southeast Asian refugees. In D. Koslow & E. Salett (Eds.), *Crossing cultures in mental health* (pp. 49–63). Washington, DC: SIETAR International.

Institute of Medicine. (1990). *Broadening the base of treatment for alcohol problems: Report of a study by a committee of the Institute of Medicine, Division of Mental Health and Behavioral Medicine*. Washington, DC: National Academy Press.

Institute of Medicine. (1994a). *Reducing risks for mental disorders: Frontiers for preventive intervention research*. Washington, DC: National Academy Press.

Institute of Medicine. (1994b). *Adverse events associated with childhood vaccines: Evidence bearing on causality*. Washington, DC: National Academy Press.

Institute of Medicine & Committee for the Study of the Future of Public Health. (1988). *The future of public health*. Washington, DC: National Academy Press.

Interagency Council on the Homeless. (1991). *Reaching out: A guide for service providers*. Rockville, MD: The National Resource Center on Homelessness and Mental Health.

Jenkins, E. J., & Bell, C. C. (1997). Exposure and response to community violence among children and adolescents. In J. Osofsky (Ed.), *Children in a violent society* (pp. 9–31). New York: Guilford Press.

Jimenez, A. L., Alegria, M., Pena, M., & Vera, M. (1997). Mental health utilization in depression. *Women & Health, 25*(2), 1–21.

Kaplan, G. A., Roberts, R. E., Camacho, T. C., & Coyne, J. C. (1987). Psychosocial predictors of depression. Prospective evidence from the human population laboratory studies. *American Journal of Epidemiology, 125*, 206–220.

Kaplan, H. I., & Saddock, B. J. (1998). *Synopsis of psychiatry* (8th ed.). Baltimore: Williams and Wilkins.

Karno, M., Jenkins, J. H., de la Selva, A., Santana, F., Telles, C., Lopez, S., & Mintz, J. (1987). Expressed emotion and schizophrenic outcome among Mexican-American families. *Journal of Nervous and Mental Disease, 175*, 143–151.

Kazdin, A. E. (1996). Cognitive behavioral approaches. In M. Lewis (Ed.), *Child and adolescent psychiatry: A comprehensive textbook* (2nd ed., pp. 115–126). Baltimore: Williams and Wilkins.

Kazdin, A. E. (1997). Behavior modification. In J. M. Weiner (Ed.), *Textbook of child and adolescent psychiatry* (2nd ed., pp. 821–842). Washington, DC: American Academy of Child and Adolescent Psychiatry.

Kellam, D. G., & Rebok, G. W. (1992). Building developmental and etiological theory through epidemiologically-based preventive intervention trials. In J. McCord & R. E. Tremblay (Eds.), *Preventing antisocial behavior: Interventions from birth through adolescence* (pp. 162–195). New York: Guilford Press.

Kessler, R. C., Berglund, P. A., Zhao, S., Leaf, P. J., Kouzis, A. C., Bruce, M. L., . . . Schneier, M. (1996). The 12-month prevalence and correlates of serious mental illness. In R. W. Manderscheid & M. A. Sonnenschein (Eds.), *Mental health, United States, 1996* (DHHS Publication No. (SMA) 96-3098, pp. 59–70). Washington, DC: U.S. Government Printing Office.

Kessler, R. C., McGonagle, K. A., Zhao, S., Nelson, C. B., Hughes, M., Eshleman, S., . . . Kendler, K. S. (1994). Lifetime and 12-month prevalence of DSM-III-R psychiatric disorders in the United States. Results from the National Comorbidity Survey. *Archives of General Psychiatry, 51*, 8–19.

Kimmel, W. A. (1992). *Rural mental health policy issues for research: A pilot exploration*. Rockville, MD: National Institute of Mental Health, Office of Rural Mental Health Research.

Kleinman, A., & Benson, P. (2006). *Anthropology in the clinic. The problem of cultural competency and how to fix it*. Boston: Public Library of Science.

Knitzer, J. (1982). *Unclaimed children: The failure of public responsibility to children and adolescents in need of mental health services*. Washington, DC: Children's Defense Fund.

La Mendola, W. (1997). *Telemental health services in U.S. frontier areas* (Frontier Mental Health Services Resource Network, Letter to the Field, No. 3). Retrieved from http://www.du.edu/frontier-mh/ letter3.html

Larson, D. B., Hohmann, A., Kessler, L. G., Meador, K. G., Boyd, J. H., & McSherry, E. (1988). The couch and the cloth: The need for linkage. *Hospital and Community Psychiatry, 39*, 1064–1069.

Lawson, W. B., Hepler, N., Holladay, J., & Cuffel, B. (1994). Race as a factor in inpatient and outpatient admissions and diagnosis. *Hospital and Community Psychiatry, 45*, 72–74.

Lebowitz, B. D., & Rudorfer, M. V. (1998). Treatment research at the millennium: From efficacy to effectiveness. *Journal of Clinical Psychopharmacology, 18*, 1.

Lee, S. M. (1998). Asian Americans: Diverse and growing. *Population Bulletin, 53*, 1–39.

Lehman, A. F., & Steinwachs, D. M. (1998). Translating research into practice: The Schizophrenia Patient Outcomes Research Team (PORT) treatment recommendations. *Schizophrenia Bulletin, 24*, 1–10.

Leong, F. T., & Lau, A. S. (1998). *Barriers to providing effective mental health services to Asian Americans*. Manuscript submitted for publication.

Levine, J. D., Gordon, N. C., & Fields, H. L. (1978). The mechanism of placebo analgesia. *Lancet, 2*, 654–657.

Lin, K. M., Anderson, D., & Poland, R. E. (1997). Ethnic and cultural considerations in psychopharmacotherapy. In D. Dunner (Ed.), *Current psychiatric therapy II* (pp. 75–81). Philadelphia: Saunders.

Lin, K., Inui, T. S., Kleinman, A. M., & Womack, W. M. (1982). Sociocultural determinants of the help-seeking behavior of patients with mental illness. *Journal of Nervous and Mental Disease, 170*, 78–85.

Lombroso, P., Pauls, D., & Leckman, J. (1994). Genetic mechanisms in childhood psychiatric disorders. *Journal of the American Academy of Child and Adolescent Psychiatry, 33*, 921–938.

Long, A. E. (1994). Reflections on recovery. In Ohio Department of Mental Health (Ed.), *Recovery: The new force in mental health* (pp.1–16). Columbus, OH: Author.

Long, L., & Van Tosh, L. (1988). *Program descriptions of consumer-run programs for homeless people with mental illness*. Rockville, MD: National Institute of Mental Health.

Lu, F. G., Lim, R. F., & Mezzich, J. E. (1995). Issues in the assessment and diagnosis of culturally diverse individuals. In J. Oldham & M. Riba (Eds.), *Review of psychiatry* (Vol. 14, pp. 477–510). Washington, DC: American Psychiatric Press.

Manson, S. M. (1998). *Mental health services for American Indians: Need, use, and barriers to effective care.* Manuscript submitted for publication.

McArthur, J. C., Hoover, D. R., Bacellar, H., Miller, E. N., Cohen, B. A., Becker, J. T., . . . Saah, A. (1993). Dementia in AIDS patients: Incidence and risk factors. Multicenter AIDS Cohort Study. *Neurology, 43*, 2245–2252.

McEwen, B. S. (1998). Protective and damaging effects of stress mediators. *New England Journal of Medicine, 338*, 171–179.

McEwen, B. S., & Magarinos, A. M. (1997). Stress effects on morphology and function of the hippocampus. *Annals of the New York Academy of Sciences, 821*, 271–284.

McGauhey, P., Starfield, B., Alexander, C., & Ensminger, M. E. (1991). Social environment and vulnerability of low birth weight children: A social-epidemiological perspective. *Pediatrics, 88*, 943–953.

McLeod, J. D., & Kessler, R. C. (1990). Socioeconomic status differences in vulnerability to undesirable life events. *Journal of Health and Social Behavior, 31*, 162–172.

Meadows, M. (1997). Mental health and minorities: Cultural considerations in treating Asians. *Closing the Gap*, 1–2.

Melaville, B., & Asayesh, G. (1993). *Together we can: A guide for crafting a profamily system of education and human services.* Washington, DC: U.S. Department of Education.

Milburn, N. G., & Bowman, P. J. (1991). Neighborhood life. In J. S. Jackson (Ed.), *Life in black America* (pp. 31–45). Newbury Park, CA: Sage.

Miranda, J., & Green, B. L. (1999). The need for mental health services research focusing on poor young women. *Journal of Mental Health Policy and Economics, 2*, 73–89.

Mollica, R. F. (1989). Developing effective mental health policies and services for traumatized refugee patients. In D. Koslow & E. Salett (Eds.), *Crossing cultures in mental health* (pp. 101–115). Washington, DC: SIETAR International.

Morrissey, J. P., & Goldman, H. H. (1984). Cycles of reform in the care of the chronically mentally ill. *Hospital and Community Psychiatry, 35*, 785–793.

Munoz, R. F., Hollon, S. D., McGrath, E., Rehm, L. P., & VandenBos, G. R. (1994). On the AHRQ depression in primary care guidelines. Further considerations for practitioners. *American Psychologist, 49*, 42–61.

Munoz, R. F., Ying, Y., Arman, R., Chan, F., & Gurza, R. (1987). The San Francisco depression prevention research project: A randomized trial with medical outpatients. In R. F. Munoz (Ed.), *Depression prevention: Research directions* (pp. 199–215). Washington, DC: Hemisphere Press.

National Advisory Mental Health Council. (1993). Health care reform for Americans with severe mental illnesses: Report of the National Advisory Mental Health Council. *American Journal of Psychiatry, 150*, 1447–1465.

National Alliance for the Mentally Ill. (1999). *State mental illness parity laws.* Arlington, VA: Author.

National Association of State Mental Health Program Directors. (1993). *Putting their money where their mouths are: SMHA support of consumer and family-run programs.* Arlington, VA: Author.

National Coalition for the Homeless (2008). How many people experience homelessness? Retrieved from http://www.nationalhomeless.org/publications/facts/How_Many.pdf

National Institute of Mental Health. (1998). *Genetics and mental disorders: Report of the National Institute of Mental Health's Genetics Workgroup*. Rockville, MD: Author.

National Mental Health Association. (1987). *Invisible Children Project. Final report and recommendations of the Invisible Children Project*. Alexandria, VA: Author.

National Mental Health Association. (1993). *A guide for advocates to all systems failure. An examination of the results of neglecting the needs of children with serious emotional disturbance*. Alexandria, VA: Author.

National Resource Center on Homelessness and Mental Illness. (1989). *Self-help programs for people who are homeless and mentally ill*. Delmar, NY: Policy Research Associates.

Navia, B. A., Jordan, B. D., & Price, R. W. (1986). The AIDS dementia complex: I. Clinical features. *Annals of Neurology, 19*, 517–524.

Neighbors, H. W., Bashshur, R., Price, R., Donavedian, A., Selig, S., & Shannon, G. (1992). Ethnic minority health service delivery: A review of the literature. *Research in Community and Mental Health*, 7, 55–71.

Nelson, S. H., McCoy, G. F., Stetter, M., & Vanderwagen, W. C. (1992). An overview of mental health services for American Indians and Alaska Natives in the 1990s. *Hospital and Community Psychiatry, 43*, 257–261.

Office of Minority Health. (2001). *National standards for culturally and linguistically appropriate services in health care*. Washington, DC: U.S. Department of Health and Human Services.

Office of Minority Health. (2005). Mental Health and American Indians/Alaska Natives. Retrieved from http://omhrc.gov/templates/content.aspx?lvl=3&lvlID=9&ID=6475

O'Hare, W. P. (1996). A new look at poverty in America. *Population Bulletin, 51*, 1.

O'Hare, W. P., Pollard, K. M., Mann, T. L., & Kent, M. M. (1991). African-Americans in the 1990s. *Population Bulletin, 46*, 1–40.

Olds, D. L., Henderson, C. R., Jr., Tatelbaum, R., & Chamberlin, R. (1986). Improving the delivery of prenatal care and outcomes of pregnancy: A randomized trial of nurse home visitation. *Pediatrics*, 77, 16–28.

Olweus, D. (1991). Bullying/victim problems among school children: Basic facts and effects of an intervention program. In K. Rubin & D. Pepler (Eds.), *Development and treatment of childhood aggression* (pp. 411–448). Hillsdale, NJ: Erlbaum.

O'Sullivan, M. J., Peterson, P. D., Cox, G. B., & Kirkeby, J. (1989). Ethnic populations: Community mental health services ten years later. *American Journal of Community Psychology, 17*, 17–30.

Padgett, D. K., Patrick, C., Burns, B. J., & Schlesinger, H. J. (1995). Use of mental health services by black and white elderly. In D. K. Padgett (Ed.), *Handbook of ethnicity, aging, and mental health*. Westport, CT: Greenwood Press.

Pargament, K. I. (1997). *The psychology of religion and coping: Theory, research, practice*. New York: Guilford.

Pasamanick, B. A. (1959). *The epidemiology of mental disorder*. Washington, DC: American Association for the Advancement of Science.

Penninx, B. W., Guralnik, J. M., Pahor, M., Ferrucci, L., Cerhan, J. R., Wallace, R. B., & Havlik, R. J. (1998). Chronically depressed mood and cancer risk in older persons. *Journal of the National Cancer Institute, 90*, 1888–1893.

Perry, P., Alexander, B., & Liskow, B. (1997). *Psychotrophic drug handbook* (7th ed.). Washington, DC: American Psychiatric Press.

Pierce, C. M. (1992). Contemporary psychiatry: Racial perspectives on the past and future. In A. Kales, C. M. Pierce, & M. Greenblatt (Eds.), *The mosaic of contemporary psychiatry in perspective* (pp. 99–109). New York: Springer-Verlag.

Plomin, R. (1996). Beyond nature vs. nurture. In L. L. Hall (Ed.), *Genetics and mental illness: Evolving issues for research and society* (pp. 29–50). New York: Plenum Press.

Plomin, R., DeFries, J. C., McClearn, G. E., & Rutter, M. (1997). *Behavioral genetics* (3rd ed.). New York: Freeman.

Plomin, R., Owen, M. J., & McGuffin, P. (1994). The genetic basis of complex human behaviors. *Science*, *264*, 7133–7139.

Porter, R. (1987). *A social history of madness: Stories of the insane*. London: Weidenfeld and Nicholson.

Potter, W. Z., Scheinin, M., Golden, R. N., Rudorfer, M. V., Cowdry, R. W., Calil, H. M., . . . Linnoila, M. (1985). Selective antidepressants and cerebrospinal fluid. Lack of specificity on norepinephrine and serotonin metabolites. *Archives of General Psychiatry*, *42*, 1171–1177.

President's Commission on Mental Health. (1978). *Report to the president from the President's Commission on Mental Health* (4 vols.). Washington, DC: Superintendent of Documents, U.S. Government Printing Office.

Priest, R. (1991). Racism and prejudice as negative impacts on African American clients in therapy. *Journal of Counseling and Development*, *70*, 213–215.

Primm, A. B., Lima, B. R., & Rowe, C. L. (1996). Cultural and ethnic sensitivity. In W. R. Breakey (Ed.), *Integrated mental health services: Modern community psychiatry* (pp. 146–159). New York: Oxford University Press.

Rauch, K. D. (1997, December 9). Mental health care scarce in rural areas. *The Washington Post Health*, pp. 7–9.

Regier, D. A., Farmer, M. E., Rae, D. S., Myers, J. K., Kramer, M., Robins, L. N., . . . Locke, B. Z. (1993a). One-month prevalence of mental disorders in the United States and sociodemographic characteristics: The Epidemiologic Catchment Area study. *Acta Psychiatrica Scandinavica*, *88*, 35–47.

Regier, D. A., Narrow, W. E., Rae, D. S., Manderscheid, R. W., Locke, B. Z., & Goodwin, F. K. (1993b). The de facto US mental and addictive disorders service system. Epidemiologic Catchment Area prospective 1-year prevalence rates of disorders and services. *Archives of General Psychiatry*, *50*, 85–94.

Resnick, H. S., Kilpatrick, D. G., Dansky, B. S., Saunders, B. E., & Best, C. L. (1993). Prevalence of civilian trauma and posttraumatic stress disorder in a representative national sample of women. *Journal of Consulting and Clinical Psychology*, *61*, 984–991.

Rice, D. P., & Miller, L. S. (1996). The economic burden of schizophrenia: Conceptual and methodological issues, and cost estimates. In M. Moscarelli, A. Rupp, & N. Sartorious (Eds.), *Handbook of mental health economics and health policy. Vol. 1: Schizophrenia* (pp. 321–324). New York: Wiley.

Ritter, L. A., & Hoffman, N. A. (2010). *Multicultural health: Promoting health within a cultural context*. Boston: Jones & Bartlett.

Robins, L. N. (1970). Follow-up studies investigating childhood disorders. In E. H. Hare & J. K. Wayne (Eds.), *Psychiatric epidemiology* (pp. 29–68). London: Oxford University Press.

Robins, L. N., & Regier, D. A. (1991). *Psychiatric disorders in America: The Epidemiologic Catchment Area study*. New York: Free Press.

Rogers, C. (1961). *On becoming a person*. Boston: Houghton Mifflin.

Rogers, E. S., Chamberlin, J., Ellison, M. L., & Crean, T. (1997). A consumer-constructed scale to measure empowerment among users of mental health services. *Psychiatric Services, 48*, 1042–1047.

Rogler, L. H., Malgady, R. G., Costantino, G., & Blumenthal, R. (1987). What do culturally sensitive mental health services mean? The case of Hispanics. *American Psychologist, 42*, 565–570.

Sapolsky, R. M. (1996). Stress, glucocorticoids, and damage to the nervous system: The current state of confusion. *Stress, 1*, 1–19.

Scheffler, R. M., & Miller, A. B. (1991). Differences in mental health service utilization among ethnic subpopulations. *International Journal of Law and Psychiatry, 14*, 363–376.

Schloss, P., & Williams, D. C. (1998). The serotonin transporter: A primary target for antidepressant drugs. *Journal of Psychopharmacology, 12*, 115–121.

Shaffer, D., Fisher, P., Dulcan, M. K., Davies, M., Piacentini, J., Schwab-Stone, M. E., . . . Regier, D. A. (1996). The NIMH Diagnostic Interview Schedule for Children Version 2.3 (DISC-2.3): Description, acceptability, prevalence rates, and performance in the MECA Study. Methods for the Epidemiology of Child and Adolescent Mental Disorders Study. *Journal of the American Academy of Child and Adolescent Psychiatry, 35*, 865–877.

Shalev, A. Y. (1996). Stress vs. traumatic stress: From acute homeostatic reactions to chronic psychopathology. In B. A. Van der Kolk, A. C. MacFarlane, & L. Weisaeth (Eds.), *Traumatic stress* (pp. 77–101). New York: Guilford.

Short, P., Feinleib, S., & Cunningham, P. (1994). *Expenditures and sources of payment for persons in nursing and personal care homes* (AHRQ Publication No. 9400-0032). Rockville, MD: Agency for Healthcare Research and Quality (AHRQ).

Silverman, P. R. (1988). Widow to widow: A mutual help program for the widowed. In R. Price, E. Cowen, R. P. Lorion, & J. Ramos-McKay (Eds.), *Fourteen ounces of prevention: A case-book for practitioners* (pp. 175–186). Washington, DC: American Psychological Association.

Size, T. (1998, March/April). Would John Wayne ask for Prozac? *Rural Health FYI*, pp. 5–7.

Smith, H., & Allison, R. (1998). *The national telemental health report*. Washington, DC: Department of Health and Human Services, Center for Mental Health Services and the Office of Rural Health Policy.

Snowden L. R. (1998). *Barriers to effective mental health services for African Americans*. Manuscript submitted for publication.

Snowden, L. R. (1999a). *Mental health system reform and ethnic minority populations*. Manuscript submitted for publication.

Snowden, L. R. (1999b). Inpatient mental health use by members of ethnic minority groups. In J. M. Herrera, W. B. Lawson, & J. J. Sramek (Eds.), *Cross cultural psychiatry*. Chichester, UK: Wiley.

Snowden, L. R. (2000). Social embeddedness and psychological well-being among African Americans and whites. *American Journal of Community Psychology, 29*, 519–537.

Snowden, L. R., & Cheung, F. K. (1990). Use of inpatient mental health services by members of ethnic minority groups. *American Psychologist, 45*, 347–355.

Snowden, L. R., & Hu, T. W. (1996). Outpatient service use in minority-serving mental health programs. *Administration and Policy in Mental Health, 24*, 149–159.

Snowden, L. R., Hu, T. W., & Jerrell, J. M. (1995). Emergency care avoidance: Ethnic matching and participation in minority-serving programs. *Community Mental Health Journal, 31*, 463–473.

Snowden, L., Storey, C., & Clancy, T. (1989). Ethnicity and continuation in treatment at a black community mental health center. *Journal of Community Psychology, 17*, 111–118.

South Carolina SHARE. (1995). *National directory of mental health consumer and ex-patient organizations and resources*. Charlotte, SC: Author.

Spaniol, L. J., Gagne, C., & Koehler, M. (1997). *Psychological and social aspects of psychiatric disability*. Boston: Center for Psychiatric Rehabilitation, Sargent College of Allied Health Professions, Boston University.

Specht, D. (Ed.). (1998). *Highlights of the findings of a national survey on state support of consumer/ex-patients activities*. Holyoke, MA: Human Resource Association of the Northeast.

Speller, H. (2005, Spring). Asian Americans and mental health: Cultural barriers to effective treatment. Retrieved from http://www.bc.edu/research/elements/issues/2005s/elements-spring2005-article8.pdf

Stocks, M. L. (1995). In the eye of the beholder. *Psychiatric Rehabilitation Journal, 19*, 89–91.

Suarez-Orozco, C. & Suarez-Orozco, M. (1995). *Transformations: Migration, family life, and achievement motivation among Latino adolescents*. Stanford, CA: Stanford University Press.

Sue, S., Fujino, D. C., Hu, L. T., Takeuchi, D. T., & Zane, N. W. (1991). Community mental health services for ethnic minority groups: A test of the cultural responsiveness hypothesis. *Journal of Consulting and Clinical Psychology, 59*, 533–540.

Sue, S., & McKinney, H. (1975). Asian Americans in the community mental health care system. *American Journal of Orthopsychiatry, 45*, 111–118.

Sue, S., Zane, N., & Young, K. (1994). Research on psychotherapy with culturally diverse populations. In A. E. Bergin & S. L. Garfield (Eds.), *Handbook of psychotherapy and behavior change* (4th ed., pp. 783–817). New York: Wiley.

Sullivan, G. M., Coplan, J. D., & Gorman, J. M. (1998). Psychoneuroendocrinology of anxiety disorders. *Psychiatric Clinics of North America, 21*, 397–412.

Sullivan, W. P. (1994). A long and winding road: The process of recovery from severe mental illness. *Innovations and Research, 3*, 19–27.

Sussman, L. K., Robins, L. N., & Earls, F. (1987). Treatment-seeking for depression by black and white Americans. *Social Science and Medicine, 24*, 187–196.

Takeuchi, D. T., Sue, S., & Yeh, M. (1995). Return rates and outcomes from ethnicity-specific mental health programs in Los Angeles. *American Journal of Public Health, 85*, 638–643.

Takeuchi, D. T., & Uehara, E. S. (1996). Ethnic minority mental health services: Current research and future conceptual directions. In B. L. Levin & J. Petrila (Eds.), *Mental health services: A public health perspective* (pp. 63–80). New York: Oxford University Press.

Taylor, O. (1989). The effects of cultural assumptions on cross-cultural communication. In D. Koslow & E. Salett (Eds.), *Crossing cultures in mental health* (pp. 18–27). Washington, DC: SIETAR International.

Taylor, R. J. (1986). Religious participation among elderly blacks. *Gerontologist, 26*, 630–636.

Thompson, J. (1997). The help-seeking behavior of minorities. *Closing the Gap*, p. 8.

Turner, J., & TenHoor, W. (1978). The NIMH community support program: Pilot approach to a needed social reform. *Schizophrenia Bulletin, 4*, 319–348.

Tylor, Sir E. B. (1924). *Primitive culture: Researches into the development of mythology, philosophy, religion, language, art, and custom*. 7th ed. New York: Brentano's. (Original work published 1871)

Uba, L. (1994). *Asian Americans: Personality patterns, identity, and mental health*. New York: Guilford.

U.S. Conference of Mayors. (2006). Hunger and homelessness survey. Retrieved from http://usmayors.org/hungersurvey/2006/report06.pdf

U.S. Department of Education. (1990). Training students with learning disabilities for careers in the human services. *OSERS News in Print! III*(3).

U.S. Department of Health and Human Services [DHHS]. (1999). *Mental health: A report of the surgeon general—executive summary*. Rockville, MD: U.S. Department of Health and Human Services, Substance Abuse and Mental Health Services Administration, Center for Mental Health Services, National Institutes of Health, National Institute of Mental Health. Retrieved from http://www.surgeongeneral.gov/library/mentalhealth/home.html

U.S. Department of Health and Human Services [DHHS]. (2001). *Mental health: Culture, race, and ethnicity*. Rockville, MD: U.S. Department of Health and Human Services, Substance Abuse and Mental Health Services Administration, Center for Mental Health Services.

U.S. Department of Health and Human Services [DHHS]. (2008). Results from the 2002 National Survey on Drug Use and Health: National Findings. Retrieved from http://www.oas.samhsa.gov/nhsda/2k2nsduh/Results/2k2Results.htm#chap2

U.S. Government Accountability Office. (2007). African American children in foster care. Retrieved from http://www.gao.gov/new.items/d07816.pdf

Vega, W. A., & Kolody, B. (1998). *Hispanic mental health at the crossroads*. Manuscript submitted for publication.

Vega, W. A., Kolody, B., Aguilar-Gaxiola, S., Alderete, E., Catalano, R., & Caraveo-Anduaga, J. (1998). Lifetime prevalence of DSM-III-R psychiatric disorders among urban and rural Mexican Americans in California. *Archives of General Psychiatry*, *55*, 771–778.

Waldrop, M. M. (1993). Cognitive neuroscience: A world with a future. *Science*, *261*, 1805–1807.

Weissman, M. M., Myers, J. K., & Harding, P. S. (1978). Psychiatric disorders in a U.S. urban community: 1975–1976. *American Journal of Psychiatry*, *135*, 459–462.

Wells, K. B., & Sturm, R. (1996). Informing the policy process: From efficacy to effectiveness data on pharmacotherapy. *Journal of Consulting and Clinical Psychology*, *64*, 638–645.

Werner, E. E., & Smith, R. S. (1992). *Overcoming the odds: High risk children from birth to adulthood*. New York: Cornell University Press.

Williams, D. R., Lavizzo-Mourey, R., and Warren, R. C. (1994). The concept of race and health status in America. Retrieved from http://www.pubmedcentral.nih.gov/picrender.fcgi?artid=1402239&blobtype=pdf

Wolfe, B. E., & Goldfried, M. R. (1988). Research on psychotherapy integration: Recommendations and conclusions from an NIMH workshop. *Journal of Consulting and Clinical Psychology*, *56*, 448–451.

World Health Organization. (1992). *International statistical classification of diseases and related health problems* (10th revision, ICD-10). Geneva, Switzerland: Author.

Yalom, I. D. (1995). *The theory and practice of group psychotherapy* (4th ed.). New York: Basic.

Yeh, M., Takeuchi, D., & Sue, S. (1994). Asian American children in the mental health system: A comparison of parallel and mainstream outpatient service centers. *Journal of Clinical Child Psychology*, *23*, 5–12.

Zhang, A., & Snowden, L. R. (1999). Ethnic characteristics of mental disorders in five U.S. communities. *Cultural Diversity and Ethnic Minority Psychology*, *5*, 134–146.

Zhang, A. Y., Snowden, L. R., & Sue, S. (1998). Differences between Asian and white Americans' help-seeking patterns in the Los Angeles area. *Journal of Community Psychology*, *26*, 317–326.

Zunzunegui, M. V., Beland, F., Laser, A., & Leon, V. (1998). Gender difference in depressive symptoms among Spanish elderly. *Social Psychiatry Psychiatric Epidemiology*, *5*, 175–205.

UNIT II Governance and the Mental Health System

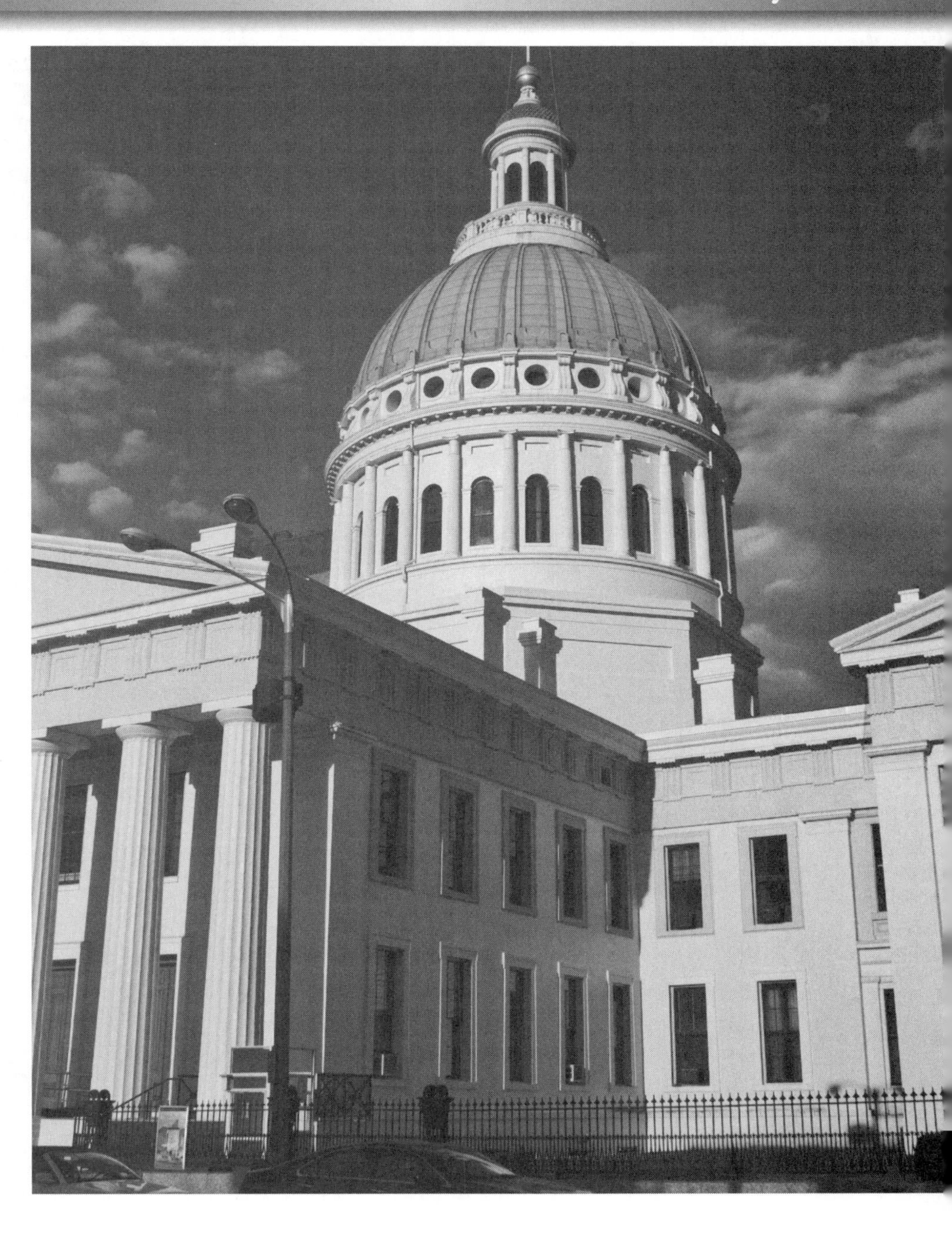

CHAPTER 4

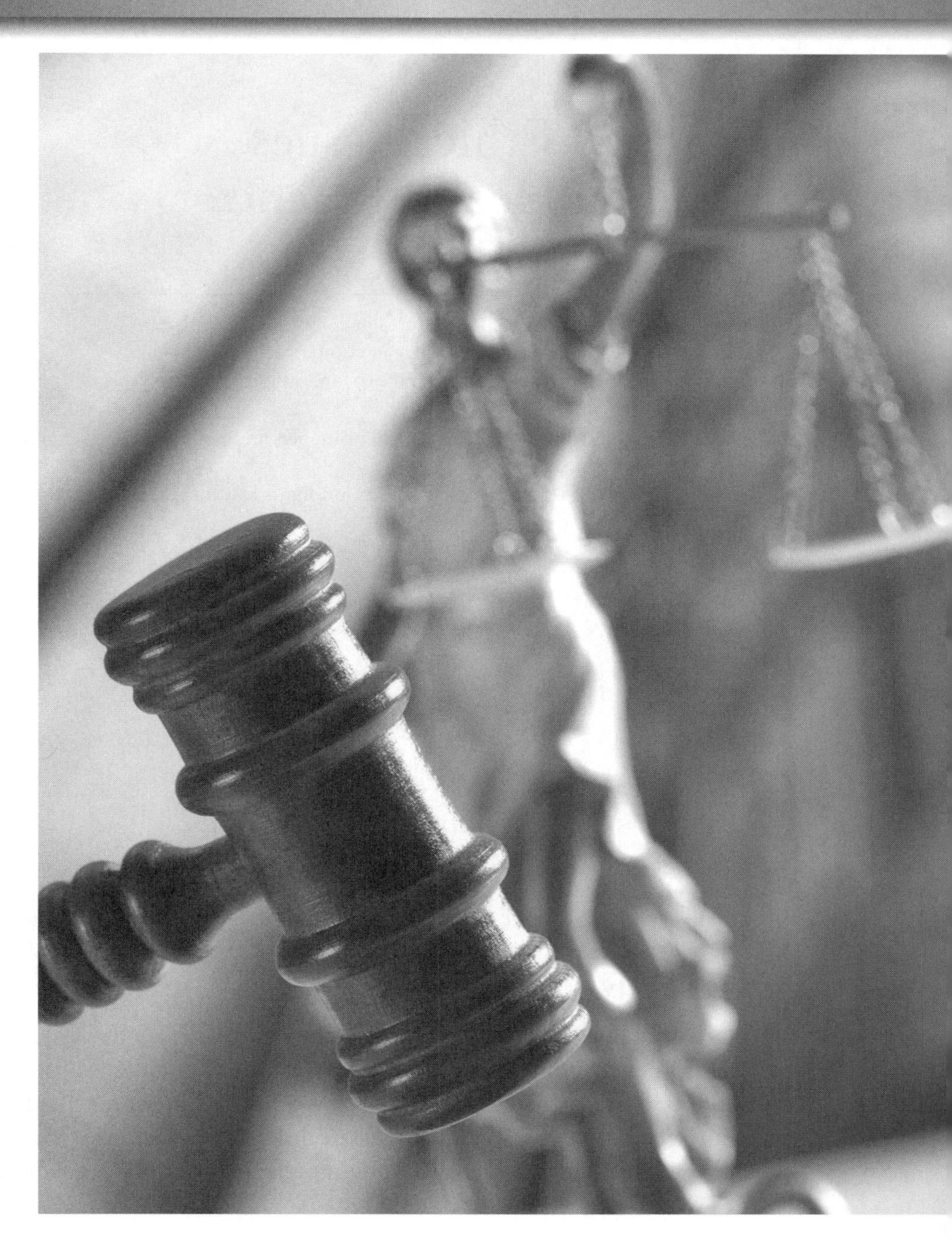

Legal and Ethical Issues in Mental Health Practice

CHAPTER OBJECTIVES

1. Describe the professional responsibilities in community health care.
2. Describe the meaning of accountability in community mental health.
3. Identify how ethical theories, rules, and principles interact in the decisions of community mental health professionals.
4. Discuss the application and role of ethical principles and potential conflicts in community mental health practice.
5. Discuss the rights of mental health patients in today's healthcare environment.

KEY TERMS

- Accountability
- Advanced directives
- Advocacy
- Aggregate
- Autonomy
- Beliefs
- Beneficence
- Block grant
- Caring
- Client's rights
- Code of ethics
- Confidentiality
- Duty of disclosure/protect
- Ethical decision making
- Ethics
- Grant
- Informed consent
- Justice
- Mental Health Services Act (MHSA)
- Nonmaleficence
- Right to health care
- Rule of utility
- Ryan White Care Act
- Value
- Veracity

We all make choices and medical decisions with some uncertainty. Having a mental health disorder makes the decision-making process more daunting and might affect a person's safety, behavior, and thinking, ultimately impacting his or her ability to make informed decisions about personal health and well-being. Mental health professionals (nurses, health educators, community health outreach workers, medical social workers, public health workers, peer advocates, substance abuse counselors, and support group facilitators) promote health, prevent illness, restore health, and alleviate suffering. The need for community mental health care is universal, and the stress, hustle, and bustle of today's society, as well as the economic downturn, have only increased the need for community mental health services in today's society. Inherent in the mental health profession is respect for human rights, including cultural rights, the right to life, choice, and dignity, and the right to be treated with respect. Mental health care is respectful of and unrestricted by considerations of age, color, creed, culture, disability or illness, gender, sexual orientation, nationality, politics, race, or social status. This chapter explains that community health professionals are responsible and accountable for the delivery of services to the individual, the family, and the community, and that they must coordinate their services with those of other related mental health programs and organizations.

It is equally important for you, as community mental health professional, to become familiar with the historical progression of mental health laws in the United States as well as state and federal laws related to working with individuals with mental illness. Mental health professionals have always advocated for the needs and rights of individuals with mental illness as well as the communities they serve. With the many challenges that people face in our communities (e.g., economic concerns, time constraints, and traffic), there are increasing mental health problems. As a result, mental health professionals have an increased role to develop, deliver, and implement therapeutic mental healthcare services to high-risk and vulnerable populations including communities plagued by mental illness. Due to the complex behavioral and emotional problems experienced by individuals with a mental health diagnosis and their limited access to inpatient mental health services, community mental health professionals may face and observe many ethical dilemmas in the community health setting. This chapter provides a historical overview of mental health laws, as well as an understanding of the ethical, legal, and policy issues that affect health professionals in general and specifically community mental health workers.

We analyze the traditional ethics of mental health professionals and apply these principles to the practice of community mental health professionals. A discussion about client rights appears first because patients are the focus of the mental health professional's ethos and actions. We examine patients' rights to health and health care, as well as other rights, from the mental health patient perspective, well-being, and rights in community health settings. We also discuss moral rules and various theories of social justice. These principles, their definitions, and applications as well as discussions of their priority in community mental health are addressed.

Finally, the priority of ethical principles in community mental health practice, including the definition of **accountability**, is discussed. Accountability—being answerable to someone for what had been done in the mental health professional role—is a strong **value** in mental health practice and directs the mental health professional. It is a vital priority in community mental health because mental health professionals must demonstrate that services in promoting health, preventing illness, and meeting the requirements of professional practice will improve the community's health status and the mental health professional's accountability.

RIGHTS OF THE MENTAL HEALTH CLIENT AND PROFESSIONAL RESPONSIBILITY IN COMMUNITY MENTAL HEALTH

From the National Convention of the French Revolution in 1793 came one of the earliest recognitions of patients' rights concerning health. Following the underlying theme of basic human rights, the leaders of the revolution declared there should be only one patient to a bed in the hospital (the usual practice at that time was to assign two to eight patients per bed). The hospital beds were to be placed at least 3 feet apart (Annas, 1978). A right to health and a right to health care are often thought to be a basic human right; however, it is not clear that they are. Other patient rights, such as rights to informed consent, to refusal of treatment, or to privacy, have been affirmed by consumer groups and healthcare providers such as the American Hospital Association (Annas, 1996).

A Right to Health

"Of all the forms of inequality, injustice in health care is the most shocking and inhumane." Dr. Martin Luther King, Jr., spoke these words over 40 years ago at a time when African Americans and other people of color could not expect to receive the same treatment as white Americans. Segregation and racism were rampant and overt. Men and women were killed simply for speaking out in support of basic human rights for themselves and their families. A right to health has been historically recognized as one of the basic human rights. In the United States, 19th-century public health measures, such as sanitation and water supply regulations to protect human health and hygiene and to control the spread of disease, provide examples of early protective laws. However, most of these protective measures also safeguarded a negative right to health: the right *not* to have an individual's health endangered by the actions of others. The negative right to be free to enjoy good health might lead to the positive right to obtain certain services or enact community health safeguards. The negative right not to have one's health endangered by others has led to the following legislation:

- Housing safety measures protecting children's health.
- Federally supported programs to protect citizens against preventable diseases, mental and physical abuse and disability (such as child and elderly abuse, alcoholism, HIV/AIDS, and smoking-related illness), such as driving under the influence of alcohol, mandatory reporting laws, and smoke-free laws.
- Mental health laws like Section 5150, which is a legal hold imposed on a person who is believed to be in need of involuntary psychiatric treatment in the state of California. The section 5150 stipulates that a person is believed to meet the criteria if one or more of the following exist: (1) is a danger to self, (2) is a danger to others, or (3) is gravely disabled.

Advocacy on the pretext of protecting a negative right to health also has helped open the door to consideration of the right to health as a positive right. It has been aided by documents such as the *Universal Declaration of Human Rights of the United Nations Assembly*. Noting the right of all persons to a standard of living adequate to provide for health and well-being and the right "to food, clothing, housing and medical care" (UNESCO, 1949), this document suggests that persons not only have a strong negative right to health but a strong positive right to health (or medical) care as well. The contents of the UNESCO declaration suggest that persons are entitled to certain services, programs, and goods in order to maintain or achieve health as a basic human right. "Even though it is claimed that the right to health is an elliptical term for the expression 'the right to health care'" (Daniels, 1979), the two terms symbolize different kinds of rights and must be addressed separately. The right to health is a negative right to natural human good that can be expressed in various degrees. It is the right not to have one's health interfered with by others. However, the **right to health care** is a positive right to goods and services to maintain and improve whatever state of health exists. It is a specific claim against the state or its agencies to provide specific healthcare services that one is entitled to, that one requests, or those that protect the safety of the community from environmental toxins as well as services and laws that help individuals with mental illness from harming themselves and others. For example, immunizations, medication education, home healthcare services for Medicare and Medicaid recipients, and federally funded prenatal and family planning programs all recognize the right to certain services. The differences between the two terms are often imprecise for the following reasons. First, the World Health

Organization (WHO) defines *health* as "a state of complete physical, mental, and social well-being and not purely the absence of disease or infirmity" (World Health Organization, 1958, p. 459). The emphasis on complete physical, mental, and social well-being in this definition suggests that one is unhealthy without complete well-being. Because individuals experience, as a result of genetics and environmental conditions, various degrees of health (however, not they are not necessarily unhealthy), this would mean that healthcare and psychosocial services must be provided to bring about physical, mental, and social well-being for one to possess complete health. Therefore, in recognizing a right to health, the right to healthcare services to achieve complete health also would have to be recognized. The WHO definition should be viewed as an ideal state of health, one that very few persons actually experience long term. As a definition of an ideal state of health, it does not dictate that healthcare services are a right for all persons.

A second reason the distinction between the terms *right to health* and *right to health care* has become blurred stems from the recent advances of modern medicine. Moreover, the willingness of government to support medical treatment for specific disorders such as renal disease (Public Law 92-603, 1972), genetic disorders like sickle-cell anemia (Public Law 92-278, 1976), and HIV/AIDS was established via the **Ryan White Care Act** (1990). This propensity has created an increase of expectations for services to achieve optimal health, however. Therefore, by supporting the treatment of some diseases and genetic disorders, the government has created a vision that the right to health care means a right to good health, a state that can be achieved only through providing healthcare services that meet the needs of all persons. This vision, however, is not accurate. Recognizing the right to health does not necessarily mean that the government is obligated to offer healthcare services to maintain heath or improve it. Although there may be other reasons why the differences between the right to health and the right to health care are not clear, these two reasons are certainly important.

Historical Overview of Other Mental Health Rights

1975: The CMCH Act Amendments of 1975 (P.L. 94-63) implemented a more comprehensive community mental health center definition for private health plans emphasizing comprehensiveness and accessibility to all persons regardless of ability to pay, through the creation of a community governing board and quality assurance. The law required core services to be expanded from the 1963 level of 5 services to 12. The core services added were children's services, elderly services, screening services, follow-up care, transitional services, alcohol abuse services, and drug abuse services.

1978: Due to the increased number of outpatient and day treatment programs, medical assistance was added to community mental health services.

1980: The Mental Health Systems Act (P.L. 96-398) was reorganized, strengthening the links between the federal, state, and local governments with the federal community mental health center program. The act was born out of recommendations made by President Jimmy Carter's Mental Health Commission. The Mental Health Systems Act is an array of grant programs mandated for the community mental health centers to assist in expanding services to meet a group of priority populations. The act covers services for the following: services for the severely mentally ill population, services for the severely emotionally disturbed population, and non-revenue-producing services aimed at expanding education and consulting needs. The commission also recommended that consumer input and involvement in service and treatment be covered through the grant.

1981–1982: The Federal Mental Health Systems Act was rescinded and replaced by the Alcohol, Drug Abuse and Mental Health Services (ADMS) **Block Grant**. In 1982, dramatic service reductions occurred because the ADMS Block Grant decreased by 30%, and the federal share of funding decreased to 11%.

1985: By 1985, federal funds through the ADMS Block Grant dropped by 11%, whereas state funding grew substantially, to 42%, while local government sources increased to 13% (NCCMHC Profile Data). During the same time frame, Medicaid decreased slightly, to 8%, Medicare remained at 2%, and patient fees doubled to 8% (NCCMHC Profile Data).

Sen. Lowell P. Weicker, Jr., of Connecticut and Rep. Henry Waxman of California held congressional hearings about conditions in state mental hospitals and other treatment programs during this era. Under their leadership, a bill was passed to create advocacy programs in each state and territory to serve individuals with psychiatric disabilities. The majority of the programs, called Protection and Advocacy for Individuals with Mental Illness (PAIMI), became a critical part of the existing advocacy programs for people with developmental disabilities, which were established in the mid-1970s. Some of the programs became part of state agencies; others became independent freestanding agencies. Minimal funding was allocated to this program and was limited to currently hospitalized individuals or persons hospitalized within the past 90 days. This legislation also required that at least 50% of the membership of the advisory councils to each PAIMI program be current or former recipients of mental health services or their family members. Some states tried to get around working with mental patients and recruited only family members rather than the patients. The regulations required participation from consumers, psychiatric survivors, and ex-patients (NCCMHC Profile Data, 1985).

1986: Understanding the need to improve rehabilitative services, and expanded clinical services to the homeless, case management services were established as a benefit under the Mental Health Planning Act of 1986.

1987: Medicare added services to the outpatient mental health benefit; however, large patient copayments and cost sharing remained in place.

1988: Behavioral health managed care progressed from theory to practice. Massachusetts was the first state to use a managed care platform for behavioral healthcare needs, "carve out" mental health from physical health care needs, and award the mental health benefits portion to a private company responsible for authorization, utilization, quality management, a provider network, claims processing, and interagency coordination. The foundation of the managed care proposal was efficiency and effectiveness. The proposal wanted to take advantage of emerging technologies. Capturing cost savings for this program was difficult as managed care programs expanded to other states. Health disparities, failure to implement technology, budget cuts, decreasing social and mental health service in the states, along with decreased access and quality services, had a major effect on managed care systems.

1988: State grants were provided for community residential treatment facilities.

1990: Other basic human rights of patients recognized by the healthcare delivery system include the basic human rights of all clients to refuse treatment. In the Omnibus Budget Reconciliation Act (OBRA) of 1990, the Patient Self-Determination Act (PSDA) was passed. This act requires all healthcare agencies that receive Medicare or Medicaid funds to inform clients they have a right to refuse medical surgical care. Patients also have a right to a written advance directive. The PSDA is a written or oral statement by which competent individuals make their own treatment preferences. They also can employ a proxy decision maker if they are unable to make a medical decision on their own. **Box 4-1** lists specific mandates of the PSDA.

1991: Partial hospitalization services under Medicare were authorized for community mental health centers.

1993: To place more emphasis on the word *community* and focus on the continuum of care, the National Council for Community Mental Healthcare Centers changed its name to the National Community Mental Healthcare Council.

1997: To reflect the growing membership base, the National Community Mental Healthcare Council made another name change, to the National Council for Community Behavioral Healthcare, to include organizations that provided services aimed at treating addictive disorders. As the need for mental health services became more apparent, a crucial statute was defined in Minnesota. Another milestone occurred in 1998; the term *medical necessity for mental health* was defined in a Minnesota statute.

BOX 4-1 Federal Patient Self-Determination Act Final Regulations

Part 489: Provider and Supplier Agreements
The authority citation for part 489 continues to read as follows:
Authority: Secs. 1102,1861. 1864. 1866. 1867, and 1871 of the Social Security Act (42 U.S.C. 1302.1395x.
1395aa. 1395cc. 1395dd. and 1395hh) and sec. 602 (k) of Pub. L. 9621 (42 U.S.C 1395ww note).

Subpart 1 Advance Directives
Section 489.100
Definitions

For the purposes of this part "advance directive" means a written instruction, such as a living will or durable power of attorney for health care, recognized under state law (whether statutory or as recognized by the courts of the State), relating to the provision of health care when the individual is incapacitated.

Section 489.102
Requirements for providers

(a) Hospitals, rural primary care hospitals, skilled nursing facilities, nursing facilities, home health agencies, providers of home health-care (and for Medicaid purposes, providers of personal care services), and hospices must maintain written policies and procedures concerning advance directives with respect to all adult individuals receiving medical care by or through the provider and are required to:
    (1) Provide written information to such individuals concerning:
        (i) An individual's rights under State law (whether statutory or recognized by courts of the State) to make decisions concerning such medical cars, including the right to accept or refuse medical or surgical treatment and the right to formulate, at the individual's option, advance directives. Providers are permitted to contract with other entities to furnish this information but are still legally responsible for ensuring that the requirements of this section are met. Providers are to update and disseminate amended information as soon as possible, but no later than 90 days from the effective date of the changes to State law; and
        (ii) The written policies of the provider or organization respecting the implementation of such rights, including a clear and precise statement of limitation if the provider cannot implement an advance directive on the basis of conscience. At a minimum, a provider's statement of limitation should:
            (A) Clarify any differences between institution-wide conscience objections and those that may be raised by individual physicians:
            (B) Identify the state legal authority permitting such objections.
            (C) Describe the range of medical conditions or procedures affected by the conscientious objection.

(continued)

(Continued)

(2) Document in the individual's medical record whether or not-the individual has executed an advance directive.

(3) Not condition the provision of care or otherwise discriminate against an individual based on whether or not the individual has executed an advance directive.

(4) Ensure compliance with requirements of State law (whether statutory- or recognized by the courts of the State) regarding advance directives. The provider must inform individuals that complaints concerning the advance directive requirements may be filed with the State survey and certification agency.

(5) Provide education for staff concerning its policies and procedures on advance directive; and,

(6) Provide for community education regarding issues concerning advance directives that may include material required in paragraph (a)(1) of this section, either directly or in concert with other providers and organizations. Separate community education materials may be developed and used, at the discretion of providers. The same written materials do not have to be provided in all settings, but the material should define what constitutes an advance directive, emphasizing that an advance directive is designed to enhance an incapacitated individual's control over medical treatment, and describe applicable State law concerning advance directives. A provider must be able to document its community education efforts.

(b) The information specified in paragraph (a) of this section is furnished:

(1) In the case of a hospital, at the time of the individual's admission as an inpatient.

(2) In the case of a skilled nursing facility at the time of the individual's admission as a resident.

(3) (i) In the case of a home health agency, in advance of the individual coming under the care of the agency. HHA may furnish advance directives information to a patient at the time of the first home visit, as long as the information is furnished before care is provided.

(ii) In the case of personal care services, in advance of the individual coming under the care of the personal care services provider. The personal care provider may furnish advance directives information to a patient at the time of the first home visit, as long as the information is furnished before care is provided.

(4) In the case of a hospice program, at the time of initial receipt of hospice care by the individual in the program.

(c) The providers listed in paragraph (a) of this section:

(1) Are not required to provide care that conflicts with an advance directive.

(2) Are not required to implement an advance directive if, as a matter of conscience, the provider cannot implement an advance directive and State law allows any health care provider or any agent of such provider to conscientiously object.

(d) Prepaid or eligible organizations (as specified in sections 1883 (a)(1)(A) and 1876 (b) of the Act) must meet the requirements specified in 417.436 of this chapter.**

(e) If an adult individual is incapacitated- at the time of admission or at the start of care and is unable to receive information-(due to the incapacitating conditions or a mental disorder) or articulate whether or not he or she has executed an advance directive, then the provider may give advance directive information to the individual's family or surrogate in the same manner that it issues other material about policies and procedures to the family of the incapacitated individual or to a surrogate or other concerned persons in accordance with State law. The provider is not relieved of its obligation to provide this information to the individual once he or she is no longer incapacitated or unable to receive such information. Follow up procedures must be in place to provide the information to the individual directly at the appropriate time.

** The Regulations governing prepaid organizations (HMOs) mirror this part. Information is to be provided to individuals at the time of enrollment.

Source: Federal Patient Self-Determination Act, Final Revisions: Vol. 60. No. 123, Tuesday. June 27, 1995, page 33294 forward Interim Final Rule: Vol. 57 No. 45, Friday March 6, 1992, pages 8194-8204.

1999: The Supreme Court issued its judgment on *Olmstead v. L.C.* The Court stipulated it is a violation of the Americans with Disabilities Act to hold individuals in restrictive inpatient settings when more appropriate community services are available.

The National Council for Community Behavioral Healthcare helped secure passage of the Ticket to Work and Work Incentives Improvement Act (TWWIIA, P.L. 106-170). TWWIIA removed several barriers facing people with disabilities receiving Social Security Income (SSI) or Social Security Disability Insurance (SSDI) benefits desiring to return to full-time employment. The law includes presumed eligibility for immediate continuation of SSI or SSDI cash payments if a recurrence of an acute episode occurred. In 1999, the Clinton administration held a conference on mental health issues that focused on dispelling myths about mental illness and criticized prejudices against behavioral health consumers, especially insurance agencies with polices that excluded behavioral health services. The conference also brought together the mental health community in anticipation of *Mental Health: A Report of the Surgeon General*, published in late 1999. The Clinton administration also wanted to eradicate the stigma surrounding mental health and simultaneously encourage the use of innovative pharmaceutical and psychotherapy treatments.

2000: By the 21st century, behavioral health providers' revenue streams were different from those 40 years ago. A key example of the change has been Medicaid funding, which currently accounts for 80% of revenue. Medicaid funding accounted for only 16% of the average revenue in the late 1980s (NCCMHC Profile Data).

In 2000, President Clinton also signed into law the Children's Health Act (P.L.106-310). The law established national standards that restrict the use of seclusion and restraint in all psychiatric facilities that receive federal funds and in "non-medical community-based facilities for children and youth." The act also mandated that a report be submitted to Congress on co-occurring disorders. The Minnesota attorney general sued Blue Cross/Blue Shield of Minnesota; they agreed to a settlement aiming to improve/reform the mental health system.

2001: Minnesota advocates proposed the Mental Health Act of 2001, which led to additional or expanded mental health services and funding for adults and children. In August, the Department of Health and Human Services (DHHS) provided guidance to states on Medicaid 1115 demonstration waivers, which allowed them to expand the program to include uninsured individuals by incorporating unspent State Children's Health Insurance Program (SCHIP) block grant funds through a new demonstration initiative: the Health Insurance Flexibility and Accountability (HIFA) Waiver. Chief among the National Council's concerns was the role that behavioral health consumers played as the waivers were comprised in each state.

2002: An in-depth study on co-occurring disorders, mandated under the Children's Health Act of 2000, was delivered to Congress. Because of the report, President Bush increased funding to community health centers to construct additional centers and those that offered more services, including behavioral health care. In addition, President Bush formed the New Freedom Commission on Mental Health, which sought "to conduct a comprehensive study of the United States mental health service delivery system, including both private and public sector providers" (New Freedom Commission on Mental Health, 2003). The objectives of the commission were to review the quality and effectiveness of private and public providers, identify best treatment practices and technologies, and make a report on its recommendations for future programs. The Minnesota State Legislature approved copayments and adjusted General Assistance Medical Care (GAMC) eligibility, decreasing eligible populations.

2003: President Bush's New Freedom Commission on Mental Health issued a final report on the mental health service delivery system.

2004: In November, voters in the California passed Proposition 63, the **Mental Health Services Act (MHSA)**, designed to expand and transform California's county mental health service systems by increasing the taxes of high-income individuals. The voter-approved MHSA initiative provided a comprehensive approach to providing community-based mental health services and supports for California residents. The MHSA addresses six components of building a better mental health system to guide policies and programs: (1) community program planning, (2) services and supports, (3) capital (buildings) and information technology (IT), (4) education and training (human resources), (5) prevention and early intervention, and (6) innovation.

Finally, in 2008 an effort was made to end health insurance benefits inequity between mental health/substance use disorders and medical/surgical benefits for group health plans with more than 50 employees. The Paul Wellstone and Pete Domenici Mental Health Parity and Addiction Equity Act of 2008 (the Wellstone-Domenici Parity Act) was enacted into law on October 3, 2008, and the law became effective on January 1, 2010. Under this law U.S. citizens have the right to nondiscriminatory mental health coverage, including individuals enrolled in self-funded plans who cannot be assisted by state parity laws.

Knowledge of the history of mental health rights and laws will help increase your understanding of laws and mental health priorities of the past as well as potential future challenges for mental health services. Having an understanding of past laws and rights will help you learn how health policies are developed and how laws are used to make decisions to create or eliminate services.

Responsibility to Society

Ensuring that **clients' rights** are protected can be difficult because society does not clearly state its obligations regarding health to the American public, resulting in healthcare providers failing to recognize and protect patient's basic rights. To correct this problem, healthcare professionals must consider what society's obligations are to citizens regarding health and the kind of responsibilities that healthcare providers have in response to client rights.

Many healthcare disparities such as race, income, or community were reported by the President's Commission for the Study of Ethical Problems in Medical, Biomedical and Behavioral Research in a comprehensive report entitled *Securing Access to Health Care* (President's Commission, 1983): "The commission reached several conclusions concerning current patterns of access to health care and made significant recommendations for changes noting that 'society' has an ethical and moral obligation to ensure equal access to health care for all" (President's Commission, 1983, p. 4) and that this obligation "rests on the special importance of health care and is derived from its role in relieving suffering, preventing premature death and restoring functioning" (President's Commission, 1983, p. 29).

PROFESSIONAL RESPONSIBILITIES

Healthcare professionals have duties and responsibilities that are supported by professional codes of ethics, as illustrated in **Figure 4-1**. In addition, community mental health professionals must adhere to mandated reporting laws. In the United States, it is required to report cases of child abuse, neglect, and elder abuse (discussed in Chapter 10).

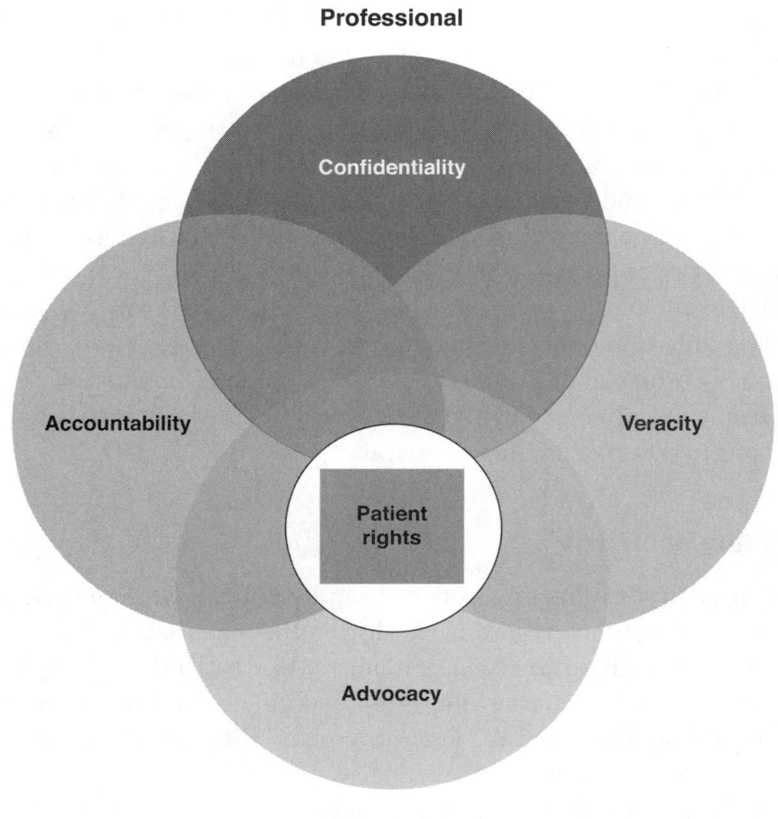

FIGURE 4-1 Clients' Rights and Professional Responsibilities

Additionally, it is mandatory for healthcare professionals to warn potential victims that a client has made a credible threat to kill them: the **duty of disclosure/protect**. Some states and jurisdictions also mandate that healthcare professionals include threats against personal property as part of the duty to disclose law. If a mental health professional assesses a client showing signs of violence or making threats to harm himself, spouse, girlfriend, boyfriend, coworker, or a staff member, he or she must take appropriate action to protect others from danger (Edwards, 2010). This law has become vital in recent years, as we have witnessed more murder suicides of families due to the economic downturn and increased stress levels and of employers by former employees or coworkers, as well as broken relationships and marriages. Failure to report an actual or suspected abuse can lead to civil liabilities, criminal penalties, and loss of licensure.

Code of Ethics for Mental Health Professionals

In response to patients' rights, healthcare professionals have particular duties or responsibilities. Some of these duties are supported by professional codes of ethics and correlate with the patients' rights. Professional **codes of ethics** are statements of rules that apply to individuals in professional roles. This section provides an introduction to thinking ethically. We all have an image of our better selves—of how we are when we act ethically or are "at our best." We probably also have a vision of what we believe to be an ethical community, an ethical business, an ethical government, or an ethical society and what we believe is an ethical mental health professional. **Ethics** relates to the following levels: acting ethically as individuals, creating ethical organizations and governments, and making our society as a whole ethical in the way it treats everyone. Some ethical codes have legal ties to licensure requirements concerning professional acts. For example, the rules of accountability, as well as protecting and respecting a patient's **confidentiality**, are both obligatory and legally mandated. Codes of ethics also stipulate specific duties that are required of the professional in response to patients' rights (Fry & Damrosch, 1994).

Duty of Veracity

Being truthful and honest is a fundamental foundation for trust among human beings. **Veracity** is a duty to tell the truth, not to lie or deceive others. In healthcare relationships, several arguments are usually given in support of veracity (Beauchamp & Childress, 1994).

- Veracity is respect that is owed other persons, including the right to be told the truth and not be lied to or deceived. An example is being truthful to clients regarding the nature of the care they are receiving.
- The duty of veracity is derived from, or is a way of expressing, the duty of keeping promises.
- Relationships of trust are necessary for cooperation between clients and healthcare professionals.

Community mental health professionals often have difficulty paying attention to or considering a duty of veracity. At times, mental health professionals believe they must withhold certain information from a client or community because they feel that certain information might cause more harm or anxiety. On an individual level, community health professionals also withhold information because they think that clients, particularly those who are terminally ill or dying, do not really want to know the truth about their condition. However, this information is not substantiated by recent research on persons with a terminal illness and individuals who have signed an advanced directive. An **advanced directive** is a written or oral statement by which competent persons make known their desired course of treatment if they are unable to make decisions for themselves. They also name a surrogate decision maker if they should become unable to make medical decisions on their own behalf.

In the community setting, and in light of tragedies such as 9/11, the Columbine High School massacre, child kidnappings, and Hurricane Katrina, communities in imminent danger are quickly notified via television, radio, the Amber Alert system, the Weather Channel, 24-hour news channels, and the Homeland Security Advisory color code system. The advisories contain required information about an independent incident or a threat targeting critical national networks, infrastructures, or key assets. They could, for example, relay newly developed procedures that, when implemented, would significantly improve security or protection. They also could suggest a change in readiness posture, protective actions, or response. Advisories target federal, state, and local governments, private sector organizations, and international partners.

Rule of Confidentiality

Generally, social interaction contains some information regarded as confidential, that is, information that should not be disclosed. Information regarded as confidential enables us to control the discourse of personal information and to limit others' access to certain information (Fry, 1994). In community mental health, the relationship between confidentiality and information is preserved for several reasons:

- First, if healthcare professionals do not follow the rules of confidentiality, clients might not seek help when they need it (for example, an individual might not want his or her HIV status revealed to family or friends).
- It helps to maintain provider–client relationships.
- Privacy is recognized as a basic human right. Because of respect for persons, mental health professionals respect clients' rights to privacy by maintaining the moral rule of confidentiality.

Duty of Advocacy

Mental health professionals recognize a strong duty of **advocacy** for the care and safety of clients and the communities they serve. In the role of advocate, the mental health professional speaks in support of the best interests of the individual client, the underserved, vulnerable populations, and communities.

Caring

The value of **caring** is extremely important to the mental health professional/client relationship in the community setting (Fry, 1994). Because mental health professionals have unique relationships with their clients, mental health patients often seek their assistance and expect them to provide caring behaviors to those in need. Caring is a form of involving self with others that is directly related to concern about how other individuals experience their world.

Accountability

According to Fry (1994), mental health professionals are recognized for moral accountability in responding to basic human rights practice.

- Accountability includes giving an explanation to oneself, the client, the employing agency, and the individual's health professional for his or her actions in the role as a health professional.
- The mental health professional's role is an obligation that has both moral and legal components and implies that a contract exists between two parties.
- When a mental health professional enters into an agreement to perform a service for a client, the professional is accountable for the performance according to agreed upon terms and conditions, within a determined time period, and with use of specified resources and performance standards. The mental health professional as a contractor is responsible for the quality of the service and is accountable to the individual client, the health services agency, their individual profession, and to his or her own conscience for what has been done.

THE PRIVACY RULE

In recent years, the shift of medical records from paper to electronic formats and to patients seeing multiple healthcare providers because of several chronic medical conditions has increased the potential for individuals to access, use, and disclose sensitive personal health data. Although protecting individual privacy is a long-standing tradition among healthcare providers and public health practitioners in the United States, the protections at the federal, tribal, state, and local levels were inconsistent and inadequate.

In 1996, the U.S. DHHS addressed concerns with new privacy standards that set a national minimum of basic protections. The Health Insurance Portability and Accountability Act of 1996 (HIPAA) was adopted to ensure that workers would be able to maintain health insurance coverage after leaving an employer and also to provide standards for facilitating healthcare-related electronic transactions between and among healthcare providers. To improve the efficiency and effectiveness of the healthcare system, HIPAA included administrative simplification provisions that required DHHS to adopt national standards for electronic healthcare transactions (Amoroso & Middaugh, 2003). In 2003, Congress acknowledged that advances in electronic medical records might potentially violate the privacy of an individual's health information. Therefore, Congress integrated mandated protection of federal privacy identifiable health information into the HIPAA provisions.

The HIPAA Privacy Rule is the first national set of standards for protecting the privacy of health information in the United States. The Privacy Rule regulates how certain entities use and disclose certain individually identifiable health information, defined as protected health information (PHI). PHI is individually identifiable health information that is transmitted or maintained in any form or medium (e.g., electronically, on paper, or orally), but it excludes certain educational records and employment records. Among other provisions, the Privacy Rule:

- Allows patients to have more control over their health information.
- Sets boundaries on the use and release of health records by healthcare providers.
- Establishes appropriate safeguards that the majority of healthcare providers and others must accomplish to protect the privacy of an individual's health information.
- Imposes civil and criminal penalties on an organization or individual if they violate a patient's privacy rights.
- Provides a balance to support disclosure of specific forms of data for public health departments.
- Allows the patient to make informed choices on how individual health information may be used and what information has been requested.
- Limits the amount of information to the minimum reasonably needed for the purpose of the disclosure.
- Gives patients the right to obtain a copy of health records and request corrections if warranted.
- Offers control to individuals for certain uses and disclosures of their health information.

The deadline to meet the terms of the Privacy Rule was April 14, 2003, for most of the three types of covered entities specified by the rule (45 CFR §160.102). The covered entities include health plans, healthcare clearinghouses, and healthcare providers who transmit health information in electronic form in connection with certain transactions. At DHHS, the Office for Civil Rights has oversight and enforcement responsibilities for the Privacy Rule.

TYPES OF HEALTH INFORMATION

Protected Health Information

The Privacy Rule protects specific information used and disclosed by an entity. The PHI is generally individually identifiable health information that is transmitted by, or maintained in, electronic media or any other form or medium. The information must relate to (1) the past, present, or future physical or mental health or condition of an individual; (2) provision of health care to an individual; or (3) payment for the provision of health care to an individual. If the information identifies or provides a reasonable basis to believe it can be used to identify a person, it is considered individually identifiable health information.

De-Identified Information

De-identified data (e.g., **aggregate** statistical data or data removing individual identifiers) does not require privacy protections and are not covered by the Privacy Rule. De-identifying can be conducted through statistical de-identification—a methodology used by statisticians substantially limiting information that might be used alone or in combination with other reasonably available information to identify the subject of the information (45 CFR §164.514[b]), or the safe-harbor method—a covered entity or its business associate de-identifies information by removing 18 identifiers (**Box 4-2**), and the covered entity does not have actual knowledge that the remaining information can be used alone or in combination with other data to identify the subject (45 CFR §164.514[b]); HIPAA Privacy Rule and Public Health Guidance from the Centers for Disease Control and Prevention (CDC) and the U.S. Department of Health and Human Services (Health Insurance Portability and Accountability Act of 1996.)

In certain instances, working with de-identified data may have limited value to clinical research and other activities. When that is the case, a limited data set may be useful.

Impact on Public Health

Public health practice and research use PHI to identify, monitor, and respond to disease, death, and disability among populations. Public health authorities have a long history of protecting and preserving the confidentiality of health information. They also recognize and understand the importance of protecting individual privacy and respecting individual dignity to maintain the quality and integrity of health data.

It is important to share PHI in certain circumstances. For example, PHI is required to accomplish essential public health objectives, protect the public, and meet

BOX 4-2 Individual Identifiers Under the Privacy Rule

The following 18 identifiers of a person, or of relatives, employers, or household members of a person must be removed, and the covered entity must not have actual knowledge that the information could be used alone or in combination with other information to identify the individual, for the information to be considered de-identified and not protected health information (PHI):

- names;
- all geographic subdivisions smaller than a state, including county, city, street address, precinct, zip code,* and their equivalent geocodes;
- all elements of dates (except year) directly related to an individual; all ages >89 and all elements of dates (including year) indicative of such age (except for an aggregate into a single category of age >90);
- telephone numbers;
- fax numbers;
- electronic mail addresses;
- Social Security numbers
- medical record numbers;
- health-plan beneficiary numbers;
- account numbers;
- certificate and license numbers;
- vehicle identifiers and serial numbers, including license plate numbers;
- medical device identifiers and serial numbers;
- Internet universal resource locators (URLs);
- Internet protocol (IP) addresses;
- biometric identifiers including fingerprints and voice prints;
- full-face photographic images and any comparable images; and
- any other unique identifying number, characteristic, or code, except that covered identities may, under certain circumstances, assign a code or other means of record identification that allows de-identified information to be re-identified.

* The first three digits of a zip code are excluded from the PHI list if the geographic unit formed by combining all zip codes with the same first three digits contains >20,000 persons.

Source: Reprinted from HIPAA Privacy Rule and Public Health Guidance from CDC and the U.S. Department of Health and Human Services; retrieved from http://www.cdc.gov/mmwr/preview/mmwrhtml/m2e411a1.htm. Accessed July 15, 2010.

other societal needs (e.g., administration of justice and law enforcement). Therefore, the Privacy Rule expressly permits sharing PHI for specified public health purposes. PHI cannot be disclosed without individual authorization to a public health authority legally authorized to collect or receive the information for the purpose of preventing or controlling disease, injury, or disability (45 CFR §164.512[b]; **Box 4-3**). The Privacy Rule also permits covered entities to make disclosures that are required by law, including those that require disclosures for public health purposes.

BOX 4-3 Protected Health Information (PHI) Disclosures by Covered Entities for Public Health Activities Requiring No Authorization Under the Privacy Rule

Without individual authorization, a covered entity may disclose PHI to a public health authority* that is legally authorized to collect or receive the information for the purposes of preventing or controlling disease, injury, or disability including, but not limited to

- reporting of disease, injury, and vital events (e.g., birth or death); and
- conducting public health surveillance, investigations, and interventions.

PHI may also be disclosed without individual authorization to

- report child abuse or neglect to a public health or other government authority legally authorized to receive such reports;
- a person subject to jurisdiction of the Food and Drug Administration (FDA) concerning the quality, safety, or effectiveness of an FDA-related product or activity for which that person has responsibility;
- a person who may have been exposed to a communicable disease or may be at risk for contracting or spreading a disease or condition, when legally authorized to notify the person as necessary to conduct a public health intervention or investigation; and
- an individual's employer, under certain circumstances and conditions, as needed for the employer to meet the requirements of the Occupational Safety and Health Administration, Mine Safety and Health Administration, or a similar state law.

* Or to an entity working under a grant of authority from a public health authority, or when directed by a public health authority, to a foreign government agency that is acting in collaboration with a public health authority.

Source: Reprinted from HIPAA Privacy Rule and Public Health Guidance from CDC and the U.S. Department of Health and Human Services; retrieved from http://www.cdc.gov/mmwr/preview/mmwrhtml/m2e411a1.htm. Accessed July 15, 2010.

The Privacy Rule provides for the continued functioning of the U.S public health system. An entity covered by the Privacy Rule must be familiar with the scope of permissible disclosures for public health activities as well as state and local reporting laws and regulations. A public health agency that operates a health clinic, providing essential healthcare services and performing covered transactions electronically, is a covered entity.

The following sections provide guidance to public health authorities and their authorized agents, researchers, and healthcare providers in interpreting the Privacy Rule as it affects public health.

Who Is Covered

Congress via HIPAA limited the authority of the DHHS to issue health-information privacy regulations to a defined set of covered entities. Covered entities are as follows:

- *Health plans*. An individual or group plan that provides or covers medical care that includes the diagnosis, cure, mitigation, treatment, or prevention of disease as well as diagnosis of mental illness. Health plans include health insurers, managed care organizations, and government organizations such as Medicaid, Medicare, and the Veterans Health Administration.

- *Healthcare clearinghouses.* Includes billing services and re-pricing companies. A re-pricing company takes bills, matches them with a specific hospital contract, and adjusts them to the prenegotiated price or community health information system that processes nonstandard data or transactions received from another entity into standard transactions or data elements, or vice versa.
- *Healthcare providers.* A provider of healthcare services and any other individual or organization that supply, bills, or is reimbursed for healthcare services. Healthcare providers (e.g., nurses, physicians, hospitals, and clinics) are covered entities if they transmit health information in electronic form.

Sharing certain PHI among healthcare providers is important. Therefore, the Privacy Rule establishes requirements allowing nonemployee business associates (e.g., nurse consultants, lawyers, accountants, billing companies, and other contractors) to use PHI. The Privacy Rule also allows a covered provider or health plan to disclose PHI to a business associate if written assurance is obtained that the business associate will use the information only for the purposes for which it was engaged and will safeguard the information from misuse.

We are all fascinated with celebrities and sports figures. Thus, when they enter our healthcare facilities, we might be tempted to look at their medical records even if we are not assigned to them, despite the consequences. Moreover, some employees of healthcare institutions have been willing to sell private medical information to tabloid magazines for personal financial gain. California legislators responding to unauthorized peeping by employees at several medical records, including those of celebrities such as California First Lady Maria Shriver, Britney Spears, and Farrah Fawcett, implemented the passage of two bills, Senate Bill 541 and Assembly Bill 211, which took effect January 1, 2009:

> Senate Bill (SB) 541 authored by Senator Elaine Alquist (D-Santa Clara) sets health facility fines for privacy breaches and increases the fines for serious medical errors in hospitals. The new law ensures that health care providers face strict penalties when they fail to protect patients. Facility fines for disclosing private medical information range from $25,000 to $250,000 per reported event. The California Department of Public Health (CDPH) will assess an administrative penalty of $25,000 per patient incident whose medical information is breached and a penalty of $17,500 per subsequent breach. Based on SB 541, if several individuals access the same patient's file, for example, the penalty would be $25,000 plus $17,500 for each additional person who violated the same file, up to a maximum of $250,000.

AB 211, authored by Assembly member Dave Jones (D-Sacramento), requires health providers to prevent unlawful access, use, or disclosure of patients' medical information and hold healthcare providers and other individuals accountable for ensuring the privacy of patients. The legislation calls for the development of the Office of Health Information Integrity within the California Health and Human Services Agency. The purpose of the agency is to assess administrative penalties against individuals up to $250,000. The legislation will also refer individuals, if licensed, to appropriate licensing boards. In SB 541, in addition to the fines, many employers can terminate employees involved in the unauthorized access to a patient's medical record.

The discussion of autonomy, justice, beneficence, nonmaleficence, and fidelity are important ethical considerations in the provision of mental health services. In the next section, we discuss the rules, principles, and ethical theories that guide the mental health professionals in the community health setting and assist them in making appropriate decisions.

ETHICAL PRINCIPLES IN COMMUNITY MENTAL HEALTH

As stated earlier, *ethics* refers to standards of behavior that tell us how we should act in the many situations in which we find ourselves—as friends, parents, children, citizens, businesspeople, teachers, professionals, and patients. In making moral decisions, various rules, principles, or theories apply. Moral judgments are evaluations of what is good or bad, right or wrong, and have certain characteristics that separate them from nonmoral evaluations such as personal preferences, **beliefs**, or matters of taste. Moral judgments are commonly made about human actions, character traits, or institutions. Mental health professionals make moral judgments, for example, in the following situations:

- When organizing a home visiting schedule on the basis of a mental illness requiring home visits
- When deciding to refer a client to a physician for further evaluation based on findings from a mental heath assessment, based on requests expressed by the client and his or her condition
- When refusing to take part in political activities that might reduce healthcare coverage for vulnerable populations

Rules state that certain actions should or should not be performed given that they may or may not be correct. One example would be that a mental health professional must always tell a client the truth. Principles are more abstract than rules and serve as the foundation of rules. For example, the ethical principle of autonomy is the foundation for rules such as "Always support the right to informed consent, tell the truth, and protect the privacy of the client." The principle of justice serves as the foundation of rules such as "Treat equals equally and divide your time on the basis of needs."

Moral Principles

According to Kitchener (1984), five moral principles are viewed as the cornerstone of our ethical guidelines: autonomy, justice, beneficence, nonmaleficence, and fidelity (duties or obligation). Ethical guidelines cannot address all situations that a mental health professional might face. However, reviewing these ethical principles often helps to clarify and guide the issues involved in a given situation. The five principles are each absolute truths in and of themselves. By exploring the dilemma regarding these principles, you may come to a better understanding of conflicting issues. Beneficence, autonomy, and justice are discussed in detail in the next section, with examples of the rules that relate to them. The principle of fidelity (professional responsibilities) was discussed earlier in the chapter.

First, **beneficence** reflects the principles to contribute to the welfare of the client. It is the duty to do good, to be affirmative, and to do no harm, or **nonmaleficence** (Forester-Miller & Rubenstein, 1992). Beneficence is the duty to help others gain assets of benefit to them and not to risk one's own well-being or interests in assisting others. Treatment should not be expected if clients' needs violate either mental health professionals' personal lives or their responsibilities to other clients, their own families, or the community at large. A service that brings about the greatest balance of good over evil, or benefit over harm, is in accordance with a rule of utility (Beauchamp & Childress, 1994). In community mental health, a **rule of utility** may be the basis for deciding whether to conduct screening programs for mental cognizance, for example. Decisions might be made by balancing the possible harm and the benefit of the course of action. You should accurately assess the known benefits and problems to clients from the standpoint of mental health care and present them with other relevant facts that might influence the decision-making process. For example, the benefit of taking a medication for depression may be the reduced possibility of being depressed, whereas the harm may be a mild adverse side effect from the medication or an allergic reaction to the medication.

Second, **autonomy** addresses the concept of independence. The spirit of this principle is allowing an individual the freedom of choice and action. It also addresses your responsibility to encourage clients, when appropriate, to make their own decisions and to act on their own values and beliefs. Two important aspects must be considered in encouraging clients to be autonomous. First, it involves helping clients to understand how their decisions and values may or may not be received within the context of the society in which they live and how their decisions and values may impose on the rights of others. The second consideration is related to the client's ability to make sound and rational decisions. Persons incapable of making competent choices, such as children and some persons with mental illness or elderly individuals, might be incapable of making rational decisions. Thus they should not be allowed to act on decisions that could harm themselves or others. Respecting a person as an autonomous individual is to acknowledge his or her personal rights to make choices and act accordingly (Fry, 1994).

The principle of autonomy is used in rules related to the following issues:

1. Respect for persons
2. Protections of privacy
3. Provision of informed consent
4. Freedom of choice including refusal of treatment
5. Protection of diminished autonomy

Respect for Persons

Clients are respected because they are persons and have the right to determine their own life plan. Community mental health professionals must show acknowledgment and respect by genuinely considering the opinions and choices of clients and not impeding their actions unless those actions are harmful to themselves or others. A community mental health professional demonstrates a lack of respect if clients are prevented from expressing themselves or acting on their judgments or if essential information vital to the client's making an informed decision is withheld.

Mental health clients living in community settings provide an example. Community health professionals often find it easier and quicker to communicate with family members rather than with the client. Having a mental illness does not make a client less worthy of respect. Disabled and mentally ill persons have the right to determine their life and health plans as long as they have the capacity to do so.

Protections of Privacy

Community mental health care often involves close observations of clients, physical touching, and access to personal health and economic information about clients and their families. All of these aspects of mental health care may invade the privacy of clients or threaten their right to control personal information.

The mental health professional client relationship is built on trust, but the care provider has the responsibility to protect the privacy of clients and their families to the extent that the clients' health is concerned. This means that personal information gathered in the initial community mental health assessment of clients must be recorded in a manner that acknowledges respect for clients' privacy and is communicated only to those directly concerned with the clients' care. When personal economic information must be shared with third parties for payment of mental health services, clients have the right to authorize or withhold information. Even though the information may be essential for continuity of care services, the client maintains control of his or her information.

Using medical records to determine funding levels for community mental health services does not justify using the information gathered by the provider about the clients without their knowledge and permission. Currently, medical record information can be used only for quality assurance proposes. Individual health information, in contrast, can be used for research if the internal review board has approved the study and the client has given written consent to participate in a research study. Healthcare information in this circumstance can be shared only under clearly defined policies and written guidelines protecting client privacy.

Provision of Informed Consent

Clients *must* be provided with the opportunity to choose what type of treatment will or will not happen when adequate disclosure standards for **informed consent** are included in the contract for mental health services. The following are elements essential for an acceptable informed consent:

- *Information.* Must disclose the type of treatment and procedures, their purpose, any discomforts and anticipated benefits, alternative procedures for therapies, procedures, or interventions, and options for questioning procedures or ending the agreement at any time during the treatment phase.
- *Comprehension.* The manner and context in which information is conveyed to clients also is required and is important for informed consent requirements. Clients must be allowed sufficient time to consider information provided to them and time to ask questions. If the client is unable to comprehend the information because of a language barrier, an interpreter must be provided. The client should be capable of understanding the information and be able to make rational decisions.
- *Voluntariness.* All informed consents or agreements with a client constitute a valid consent only if given voluntarily, free of coercion or undue influences. Voluntariness includes the freedom to choose one's own health goals and treatment

regimen without the influence of another person or certain conditions, such as debilitating disease, psychiatric disorders, or drug addictions (Beauchamp & Childress, 1994).

These three essential elements constitute an informed consent. An informed consent is not valid if it does not include all three components. More important, no formal contract between a client and provider is ethically acceptable without a valid informed consent.

Freedom of Choice Including Refusal of Treatment

Respecting the client's right to self-determination and freedom of choice includes respecting his or her decision to refuse treatment. The mental health provider must consider the client's personal freedom, the potential harm to the client or to others if critical treatment is refused, the cost of treatment refusal, and the values of society. The right of the client to refuse treatment and the right to initiate written advance directives are protected by the Patient Self-Determination Act Omnibus Budget Reconciliation Act of 1990 (OBRA, 1990).

When a client's competency is questionable, decisions have generally been made by opting for the preservation of life (Beauchamp & Childress, 1994). Mental health professionals however, must recognize that respect for individuals may involve allowing clients, their legal guardians, or a conservator to make decisions concerning their lives and health that might be difficult to accept.

Protection of Diminished Autonomy

In general, the principle of autonomy is applied to persons able to make reliable choices. Factors such as immaturity or physical or psychological inabilities may diminish one's autonomy. The mental health professional might have difficulty recognizing when diminished competence portrays clients incapable of self-determination. The capacity for dependable self-determination is related to maturity, chronological age, presence, or absence of illness, mental disability, and social factors as depicted in **Figure 4-2**.

Respect for the principle of autonomy requires the mental health professional to recognize when persons lack the capacity to act autonomously and are thus entitled to protection in healthcare delivery.

To protect the health of vulnerable populations, a mental health professional might infringe on the rights to privacy rule by actively gathering private information. For instance, a rise in venereal disease rates in a homeless population might require

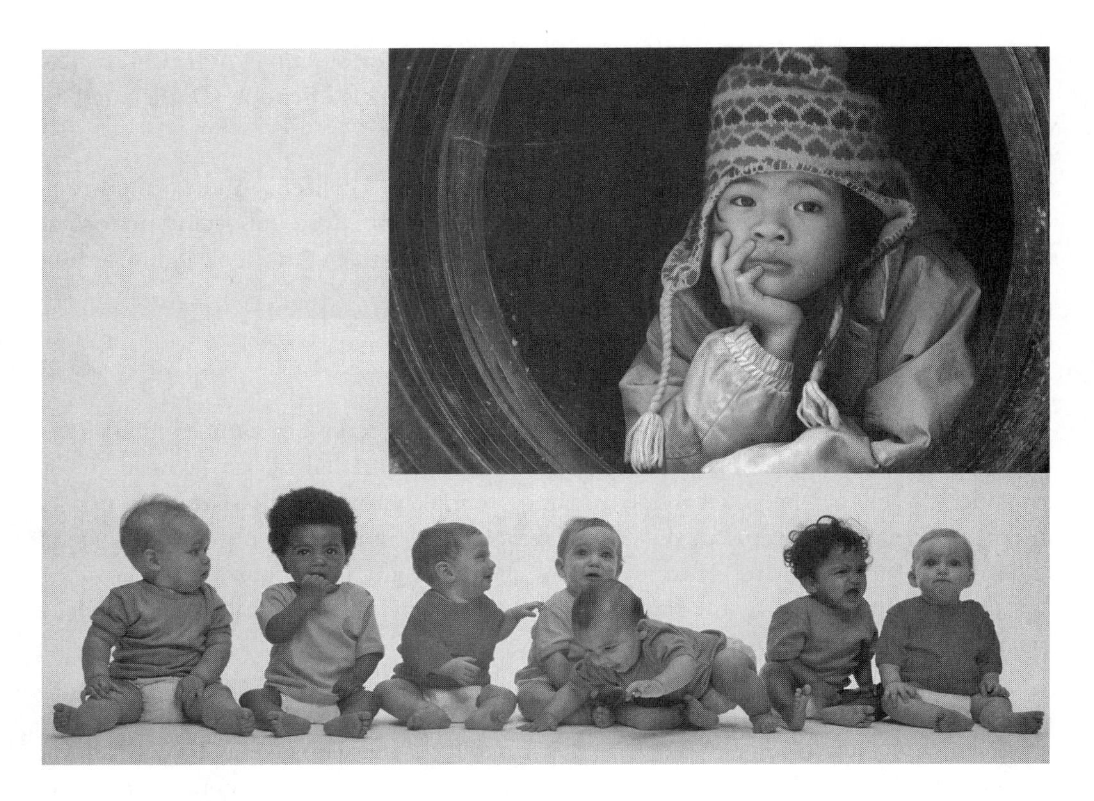

FIGURE 4-2 Samples of Group with Diminished Autonomy

interviewing homeless persons diagnosed with the disease and following up with all named contacts. This action might lead to an invasion of individual privacy through discussion of sexual habits and preferences of potential disclosers, including friends of the informants.

Privacy also might be invaded by the assessment and recording of personal client information. For example, the community mental health professional might record information about the social habits, lifestyles, and beliefs of pregnant women who are mentally ill. Subsequently, the lifestyle information might be used in areas of research correlating neonatal mortality and morbidity with the social habits and lifestyle of mentally ill women during pregnancy. Personal information in this instance is often communicated because of the trust relationship between the provider and client. Additionally, the information might be recorded in the client's medical record without understanding the potential effect of the information if, in fact, a child is born with anomalies related to social habits or lifestyles during pregnancy. Recording information about the lifestyle of pregnant women in the prenatal medical records means it might eventually be shared with other health professionals and members of the client's family, constituting further invasion of the client's right to privacy of personal information. The actions just described infringe on self-determining behavior; however, they are considered justifiable because of the potential harm to others.

Finally, **justice** is the principle of fairness (Beauchamp & Childers, 1994). According to Kitchener (1984), justice does not mean treating all individuals equally. Kitchener points out that the formal meaning of *justice* is "treating equals equally and unequals unequally but in proportion to their relevant differences" (p. 49). If an individual is to be treated differently, the provider must be able to offer a rationale explaining the necessity and appropriateness of treating an individual differently. The application of a principle of justice creates conflicts in two areas. It first creates a challenge about priorities for distributing basic goods and health services in the community. Second, justice creates conflicts in determining which population or individual should obtain available health goods and mental health services. Healthcare reform is a major subject of discussion for the most Americans as it relates to deciding how to distribute health services. In the next section, we discuss a framework for distributing basic mental health services.

DISTRIBUTING BASIC HEALTH SERVICES

Several decisions must be made when deciding how to apply the rule to distribute basic healthcare goods or resources within a community. What follows is a list of factors that must be considered:

1. How should mental heath priorities be determined? Should health protection and promotion be the main consideration or should resources be set aside for other social goods, such as housing or education?
2. What are the most effective, efficient methods of meeting this basic right while preventing catastrophic events (leading to death or disability) that need immediate attention that is more concentrated? One might ask whether the emphasis should be placed on direct health services to care for people with mental illness (e.g., community mental health clinics, programs) or on indirect services, such as programs that prevent illness or promote health (e.g., health education or transportation services).
3. What is the appropriate relationship between rescue services and preventive services? Would it be more effective to concentrate on organ transplant and terminal cancer services or to concentrate efforts and economic resources to prevent disease and disability through hypertension, diabetes screening, and mental health screening programs?

4. Is it essential to provide more emphasis to one disease category over another? Should a priority be the prevention and treatment of sexually transmitted infections, the prevention and treatment of coronary disease, or the provision of mental health services?
5. When establishing priorities, will they compromise important values or principles? Preventive strategies aimed at discouraging alcohol use or smoking, for example, may involve emphasis on behavioral change or altering of lifestyles. Mental public health professionals might question whether these preventive strategies would have a significant effect on the autonomy of community members, particularly regarding their choice to engage in risky behaviors.

Distributing Resources in Mental Health

Once health priorities are known, community mental health professionals in collaboration with local, state, and national mental health officials must decide how to deliver health care equally according to client needs. Several strategies can be implemented:

1. Focus services on individuals who have the most practical chance of benefiting from services. One prime example would be providing services to children and childbearing families. The goal would be to provide the greatest overall benefit.
2. Provide basic healthcare services in all categories in limited amounts and accommodate requests for mental healthcare services on a first-come, first-served basis. This approach might not be cost effective in terms of the services provided in the community. Although providing limited mental health services meets the basic requirement of providing the opportunity for everyone to have equal access to services, individuals might have a long wait time before being served.
3. Focus mental health services on persons who are able to pay for the service or who have healthcare insurance that covers mental health services. In today's healthcare delivery system, this is the approach currently being used and has been fostered by legislation and funding by government agencies. This approach, however, has limits when looking at services for vulnerable populations and for persons in need of mental health services who are underinsured or uninsured.
4. Categorize community services according to health needs, and then decide which population or services should be prioritized. Persons who cannot survive without resources (those receiving kidney dialysis or respiratory therapy at home, for example) might have first priority. Individuals who can be assisted to prevent long-term disability (e.g., populations at high risk of mental disorders, preeclamptic clients, and children with minor cardiac anomalies) would come next. The last priority would be given to those without an acute disabling illness or who are not

at risk of long-term disability (e.g., school-age children or some persons with chronic illness). Other high-priority groups are those whose health needs can be easily met and benefit the health of others (e.g., women with uncomplicated pregnancy, mothers with children with mental health disorders). Using this approach limits the access to mental health services from some groups according to their priority (**Figure 4-3**).

As demonstrated by the various approaches to distributing mental health care resources, the moral requirements of justice can create numerous conflicts of interest for healthcare providers when they face specific choices.

MAKING DECISIONS

Good ethical decisions require a trained sensitivity to ethical issues in the mental health field. Making good ethical decisions requires a method for exploring the ethical characteristics of a decision and weighing the considerations that should affect our choice of action. Having a method for **ethical decision making** is essential. When

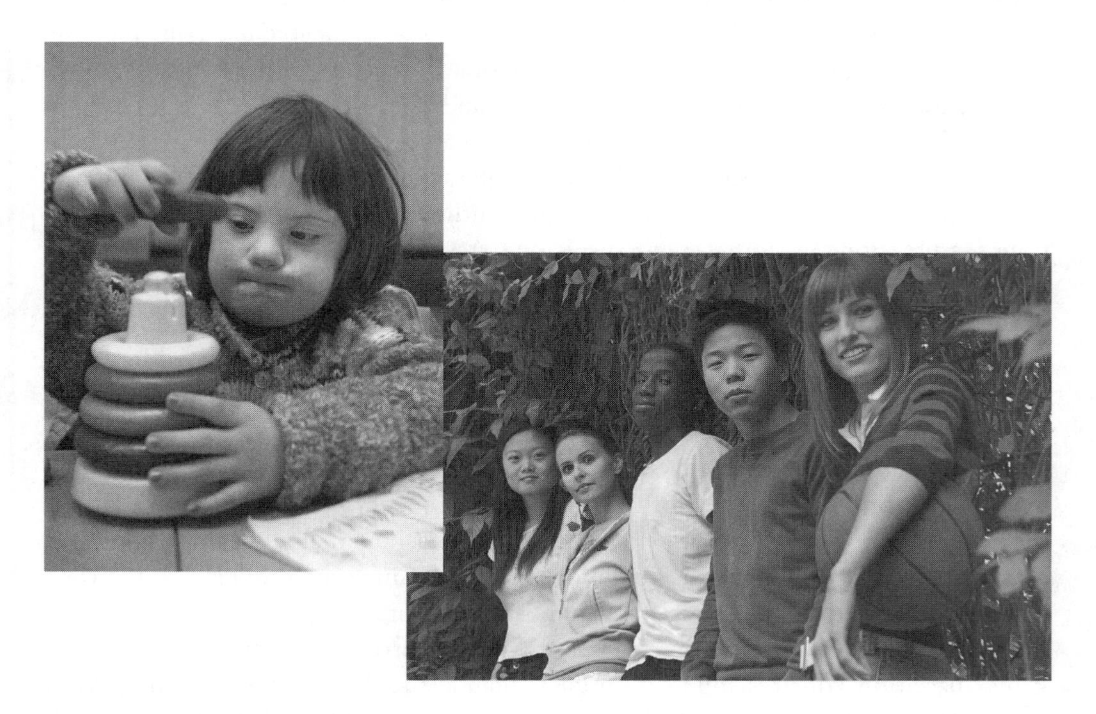

FIGURE 4-3 Pictures of Individuals with Low Priority in Allocation of Nursing Services: Elderly, Homeless, Adolescents

practiced regularly, the method becomes so familiar that we work through it automatically without consulting the specific steps. We have found that following a framework for ethical decision making is a useful method for exploring ethical dilemmas and identifying ethical courses of action.

When exploring an ethical dilemma, it is important to examine the situation in detail and determine how each of the ethical principles described in this chapter may relate to that particular case. At times, these principles by themselves will clarify the ethical dilemmas enough that the means for resolving the dilemma becomes apparent. In more complicated cases it is helpful to work through the steps of an ethical decision-making model and assess which of these moral principles may be in conflict. To assist you with the ethical decision process, we discuss the integrated ethical decision-making model developed by several researchers.

Ethical Decision-Making Model

Based on the work of Van Hoose and Paradise (1979), Kitchener (1984), Stadler (1986), Haas and Malouf (1989), Forester-Miller and Rubenstein (1992), and Sileo and Kopala (1993), we present seven practical sequential steps of decision-making principles you can use to help guide the decisions you make or will make in difficult clinical, community, and individual situations. A description and discussion of the steps follows.

1. *Identify the problem.* Gather as much information as possible that will shed light on the situation. Be as specific and objective as possible. Writing the scenario out also may help you gain clarity about the problem. Outline the facts, separating out allegations, assumptions, hypotheses, or suspicions. Ask the following questions: Is it an ethical, legal, professional, or clinical problem? Is it a combination of more than one of these problems? If a legal question exists, seek legal advice.

Other useful questions might include the following: Is the issue related to what I am or am not doing? Is the mental health crisis related to a client and/or the client's significant others and what they are or are not doing? Is it related to the institution or agency and their policies, practices, and procedures? Can the problem be resolved by implementing a new policy for the institution or agency? It is important to look at the agency's guidelines. Remember that dilemmas faced by mental health professionals are often complex. Thus a useful guideline is to examine the problem from several perspectives and avoid searching for a simplistic solution.

2. *Apply the Code of Ethics.* After clarifying the problem, refer to the Code of Ethics based on your discipline. Examples include the American Counseling Association (ACA), 2005; American Nurses Association (2001) Code of Ethics; American Psychological Association (APA), *APA Ethics Code: Commentary and Case Illustrations*; Campbell, Vasquez, Behnke, and Kinscherff (2010); and American Mental Health

Counseling Association (AMHCA) (2010). Determine if the issue is addressed. If there is an applicable standard or several standards and they are specific and clear, following the course of action indicated should lead to a resolution of the problem. Applying the ethical standards is essential. Read them carefully and understand their implications.

If the mental health problem is more complex and a resolution does not seem apparent, a true ethical dilemma exists, and further steps in the ethical decision-making process should be followed.

3. *Determine the nature and dimensions of the dilemma.* There are several avenues to follow to ensure that the mental health problem has been fully examined in all its various dimensions.

- Consider reviewing the moral principles of autonomy, nonmaleficence, beneficence, and justice. Decide which principles apply to the specific circumstances, as they relate to the individual and/or the community and determine which principle takes priority over the current situation. In theory, each principle is of equal value, which means it can be a challenge to determine the priorities when two or more of them are in conflict.
- Review the relevant professional literature to ensure that up-to-date professional thinking and literature are used to help in reaching a decision.
- Seek advice from experienced professional colleagues and/or supervisors. During the review process, they may see other issues that are relevant or that provide a perspective you have not contemplated. They also may be able to identify aspects of the dilemma that you are not viewing objectively.
- Consult your state or national professional associations for assistance with the dilemma.

4. *Generate potential courses of action.* Brainstorm as many possible courses of action as possible. Be creative and consider all options. If possible, enlist the assistance of colleagues to help you produce alternatives.

5. *Consider the potential consequences of all options, and determine a course of action.* Review the information gathered, set priorities, evaluate each option, and assess the potential consequences for all involved. Think about the implications of each course of action for the client, for others who will be affected, and for yourself as a mental health professional. Eliminate the options that will not give the desired outcomes or will cause more problems.

6. *Evaluate the selected course of action.* Determine if the crisis presents any new ethical considerations. Stadler (1986) suggests applying three easy tests to the selected course of action to ensure it is appropriate. Applying the test of justice assesses your own sense of fairness by determining whether to treat others the same way in this situation. The test of publicity should be completed first. Ask yourself whether you would

want your behavior reported in the press. Secondly, the test of universality asks you to assess whether you could recommend the same course of action to another mental health provider in the same situation.

If the course of action you have selected seems to present new ethical issues, you will need to go back to the beginning of the process and reevaluate each step of the process. Perhaps your chose the wrong option or identified the problem incorrectly. If there is a positive answer to each of the questions suggested by Stadler (you must pass the tests of justice, publicity, and universality), you should be satisfied that you have selected an appropriate course of action, and moving to the implementation phase is appropriate at this point.

7. *Implement the course of action.* Taking the appropriate action in an ethical dilemma is often difficult. The final step involves strengthening your ego, allowing you to carry out the implementation plan. After implementing the course of action, follow up on the situation to assess whether your actions had the anticipated outcomes.

Remember that different professionals may implement different courses of action for the same scenario. Therefore, there is rarely one right answer to any complex ethical dilemma. However, following a systematic model assures that a proficient explanation for the course of action selected is explained and validated. Van Hoose and Paradise (1979) suggest that a health professional "is probably acting in an ethically responsible way concerning a client if: (1) he or she has maintained personal and professional honesty, coupled with (2) the best interests of the client, (3) without malice or personal gain, and (4) can justify his or her actions as the best judgment of what should be done based upon the current state of the profession" (Van Hoose et al., 1979, p. 58). If the community mental health nurse follows this model, it will help to ensure that all four of these conditions have been met (Van Hoose et al., 1979).

APPLICATION OF ETHICS TO COMMUNITY MENTAL HEALTH PRACTICE

In community mental health, ethical principles guide and direct mental health professionals' actions with individuals and aggregates. The professional ethic in mental health practice places a greater emphasis on observing the principles of autonomy, freedom of choice, and beneficence (do good, and do no harm) as it relates to the principle of justice (treat everyone equally). The actions of mental health professionals are guided by the professional's ethic, priority of ethical principles, as well as by a public ethic, which has a different priority of principles. This ethic is strongly shaped on the priority principle of beneficence—do good, and do not do harm—and it follows the rule of utility (the greatest good for the greatest number of people), in the detection and prevention of disease, as well as health maintenance. Following the rule of utility in health issues might influence the practice of community mental health services. The rule of utility, for example, might encourage you to identify the needs of aggregates (specific populations or defined groups). The rule of utility provides population groups with net benefit over possible health harms, such as in the case of spending money for a flu vaccine program rather than facing the prospect of increased deaths among the elderly from respiratory infections and pneumonia in a mental health shelter (Fry, 1994).

CHAPTER SUMMARY

Practicing community mental health professionals are influenced by traditional ethics of professional practice for the individual as well as the aggregate focus of community health. When providing care to the individual or aggregate groups within the community, you must balance both of these influences. Clients' rights to equal access to healthcare services and aggregate group needs and interests in matters of health often compete for the attention and services of practicing community mental health workers. Therefore, you must be familiar with the moral mental health services in general and community mental health practice specifically.

Community mental health practice, as a combination of both public health science and the individual mental health discipline's science, is theoretically responsive to our prevailing ideas of social justice and the methods of distributing healthcare resources as chosen by the community. Community mental health professionals also are responsive to the moral requirements of ethical principles as prioritized within the individual ethic of their discipline and the aggregate ethic of public health. How the individual community mental health provider and community mental health services view the moral requirements may determine the future direction and influence of the discipline in meeting the health needs of the community.

REVIEW

1. Because clients have rights, healthcare professionals have responsibilities to tell the truth, respect confidentiality, function as an advocate, and accept accountability for providing proper health care. How do these attributes impact community mental health professionals?
2. How are the methods to measure accountability in community mental health defined?
3. Is the right to health care a basic human right?

4. Explain how the negative right to be free to enjoy good health led to the positive right to obtain certain services or community mental health safeguards.
5. Explain the differences and similarities in the terms "Right to health" and "right to health care."
6. Does "Society have an ethical obligation to ensure equitable access to health care for all?"
7. What are the ethical principles operable in community mental health?
8. What are the four major theories of justice used to decide how to allocate health-care resources?

ACTIVITIES

1. Search the Internet or newspaper for a problem facing the mentally ill or homeless in your community. Use the decision-making framework and ethical principles in this chapter to discuss and identify ethically important aspects of the situation and to justify controversial or difficult decisions.
2. What situations have placed you in an ethical conflict? Write a two-page paper describing the situation, how you handled it, and what influenced your decision.
3. Write a two-page paper describing how your cultural background affects your decision making.

REFERENCES AND FURTHER READINGS

American Counseling Association [ACA]. (2005). *ACA Code of ethics*. Alexandria, VA: Author.

American Mental Health Counseling Association [AMHCA]. (2010). Principles for AMHCA Code of Ethics. Retrieved from http://www.amhca.org/assets/content/AMHCA_Code_of_Ethics_11_30_09b1.pdf

American Nurses Association. (2001). *Code of ethics for nurses with interpretive statements*. Washington, DC: Author.

American Psychiatric Association [APA]. (1999). *Mandatory outpatient treatment: A resource document of the American Psychiatric Association*. Washington DC: Author.

Amoroso, P. J., & Middaugh, J. P. (2003). Research vs. public health practice: When does a study require IRB review? *Preventive Medicine*, *36*(2), 250–253.

Annas, G. J. (1978). Patient's rights movement. In W. T. Reich (Ed.), *Encyclopedia of bioethics* (Vol. 3, pp. 1201–1205). New York: Free Press.

Annas, G. J. (1996). Patient's rights movement. In W. T. Reich (Ed.), *Encyclopedia of bioethics* (2nd ed.). New York: Simon & Schuster.

Beauchamp, T. L., & Childress, J. F. (1994). *Principles of biomedical ethics* (4th ed.). New York: Oxford University Press.

Campbell, L., Vasquez, M., Behnke, S., & Kinscherff, R. (2010). *APA Ethics Code: Commentary and case illustrations*. Washington, DC: American Psychological Association.

Centers for Disease Control and Prevention [CDC]. (1999). *Guidelines for defining public health research and public health non-research.* Retrieved from http://www.cdc.gov/od/science/regs/hrpp/researchdefinition.htm

Daniels, N. (1979, June). Rights to health care and distributive justice: programmatic worries. *Journal of Medical Philosophy*, *4*, 174–191.

Department of Health and Human Services. (2003). *Protecting personal health information in research: Understanding the HIPAA privacy rule*. Washington, DC: Author.

Edwards, Griffin Sims. (2010). *Doing their duty: An empirical analysis of the unintended effect of* Tarasoff v Regents *on homicidal activity*. Retrieved from: http://userwww.service.emory.edu/~gsedwar/research.html

Forester-Miller, H., & Rubenstein, R. L. (1992). Group counseling: Ethics and professional issues. In D. Capuzzi & D. R. Gross (Eds.), *Introduction to group counseling* (pp. 307–323). Denver, CO: Love Publishing.

Fry, S. T. (1994). *Ethics in nursing practice: A guide to ethical decision making*. Geneva, Switzerland: International Council of Nurses.

Fry, S. T., & Damrosch S. (1994). Ethics and human rights issues in nursing practice: a survey of Maryland nurses. *Maryland Nurse*, *13*(7):11.

Haas, L. J., & Malouf, J. L. (1989). *Keeping up the good work: A practitioner's guide to mental health ethics*. Sarasota, FL: Professional Resource Exchange.

Health Insurance Portability and Accountability Act of 1996. (1996). Pub. L. No. 104-191, 110 Stat. 1936.

Human Rights: Comments and Interpretations, UNESCO. London: Allan Wingate.

Kitchener, K. S. (1984). Intuition, critical evaluation and ethical principles: The foundation for ethical decisions in counseling psychology. *Counseling Psychologist*, *12*(3), 43–55.

Mental Health Treatment Preference Declaration Act, Illinois Stat. Public Act 86-1190 (1990).

National Alliance for the Mentally Ill. (1995). *NAMI's principles for managed care* [Brochure]. Arlington, VA: Author.

National Alliance for the Mentally Ill. (1997, September). *About mental illness: Obsessive-compulsive disorder*. Retrieved from www.nami.org/helpline/ocd.htm

National Commission for the Protection of Human Subjects of Biomedical and Behavioral Research, Department of Health, Education and Welfare. (1979). *Belmont report: Ethical principles and guidelines for the protection of human subjects of research*. Retrieved from http:// ohsr.od.nih.gov/guidelines/belmont.html.

National Council for Community Behavioral Healthcare [NCCBH] (n.d.). Commemorating forty years (1963–2003) of community mental health for people in need. *Health*. Retrieved from http://www.trinityqc.com/documents/mentalhealthtimeline.pdf

National Council of Community Mental Health Centers [NCCMHC]. (1984, February). *Membership Profile Report*. National Council of Community Mental Health Centers.

New Freedom Commission on Mental Health. (2003). *Achieving the promise: Transforming Mental healthcare in America. Final Report*. DHHS Pub. No. SMA-03-3832. Rockville, MD. Retrieved from http://www.mentalhealthcommission.gov/reports/reports.htm

Office for Civil Rights, Department of Health and Human Services. (2001). Standards for privacy of individually identifiable health information; Final rule, 45 CFR Parts 160 and 164. Retrieved from http://aspe.hhs.gov/ADMNSIMP/final/FR010226.pdf

Office for Civil Rights, Department of Health and Human Services. (2002). OCR guidance explaining significant aspects of the privacy rule. Available at http://www.hhs.gov/ocr/hipaa

Office for Protection from Research Risks, National Institutes of Health, Department of Health and Human Services. (2001). Public welfare: Protection of human subjects, 45 CFR 46. Retrieved from http://www.hhs.gov/ohrp/documents/OHRPRegulations.pdf

P.L. 92-603. Approved October 30, 1972 (86 Stat. 1329) Social Security Amendments of 1972. The Ryan White Comprehensive AIDS Resources Emergency (CARE) Act (Ryan White Care Act, Ryan White, Pub. L. 101-381, 104 Stat. 576, enacted August 18, 1990)

Policy Research Associates, Inc. (1998, December 4). *Final report: Research study of the New York City Involuntary Outpatient Commitment Pilot Program, prepared for the New York City Department of Mental Health, Mental Retardation and Alcoholism Services*. New York: Policy Research Associates.

President's Commission for the Study of Ethical Problems in Medicine and Biomedical and Behavioral Research. (1983). *Securing access to health care. Vol. 1: Report on the ethical implications of differences in the availability in health services*. Washington, DC: U.S. Government Printing Office.

Sileo, F., & Kopala, M. (1993). An A-B-C-D-E worksheet for promoting beneficence when considering ethical issues. *Counseling and Values, 37*, 89–95.

Stadler, H. A. (1986). Making hard choices: Clarifying controversial ethical issues. *Counseling & Human Development, 19*, 1–10.

Universal Declaration of Human Rights. (2009). ohchr.org. Retrieved from http://www.ohchr.org/EN/UDHR/Pages/Introduction.aspx.-12-18

Van Hoose, W. H. (1980). Ethics and counseling. *Counseling & Human Development, 13*(1), 1–12.

Van Hoose, W. H., & Paradise, L. V. (1979). *Ethics in counseling and psychotherapy: Perspectives in issues and decision-making*. Cranston, RI: Carroll Press.

World Health Organization. (1958). *The first ten years of the World Health Organization*. New York: World Health Organization.

CHAPTER 5

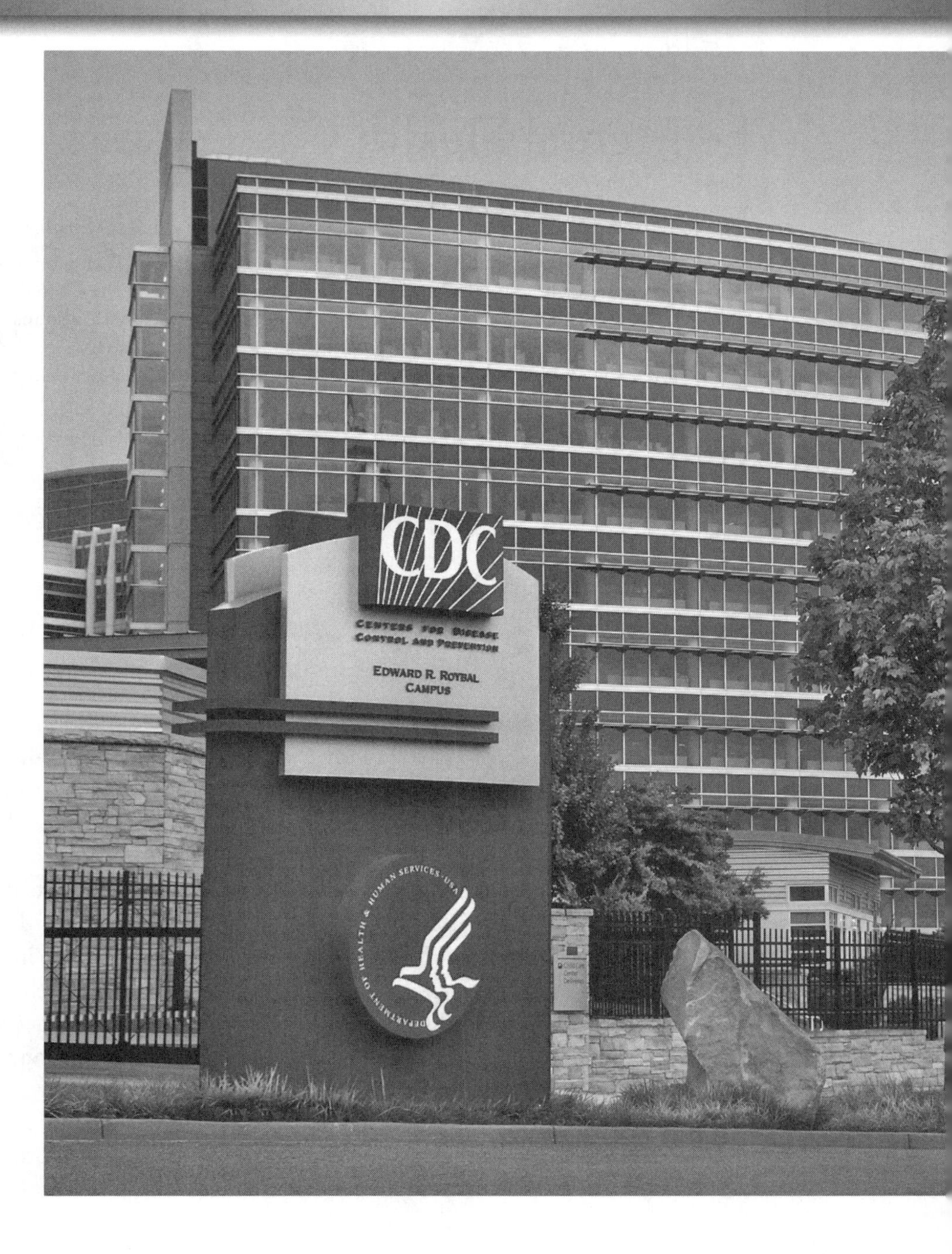
CDC
CENTERS FOR DISEASE
CONTROL AND PREVENTION
EDWARD R. ROYBAL
CAMPUS
DEPARTMENT OF HEALTH & HUMAN SERVICES·USA

The Mental Health Care System

CHAPTER OBJECTIVES

1. Describe the de facto mental health service system and the four major components.
2. Compare, contrast, and describe the current mental health system in the United States.
3. Contrast the responsibilities of the federal, state, and local mental health systems.
4. Discuss the impact of the New Freedom Act on the mental health system.
5. Identify how the historical changes in American society have impacted the mental health care system.
6. Define the types of mental health services that are available in the United States.

KEY TERMS

- Catchment area
- Child protective services
- De facto mental health service system
- Housing plan
- Individualized treatment plan
- National Institute of Mental Health (NIMH)
- Recovery orientation
- Specialty mental health

Mental disorders in 2006 were one of the five most costly conditions in the United States with expenditures at $57.5 billion (Soni, 2009). In addition, according to Kessler and colleagues (2008), major mental health disorders lead to at least $193 billion annually in lost earnings. These costs include but are not limited to lost earning potential, costs associated with treating coexisting conditions, Social Security payments, homelessness, and incarceration. Persons with problems related to mental health and special needs are often clients of community mental health programs or become clients of healthcare professionals. The problems that these individuals face are often complex and result from the interaction of many factors, including heredity, family relationships, living conditions, disasters, and social as well as economic barriers. Because the mentally ill are often discharged back to the community following inpatient treatment, returning from the war, or from the criminal justice system, with conditions such as posttraumatic stress syndrome, bipolar disease, or depression, community mental health professionals are well positioned to assess symptoms associated with mental illness, to plan and implement best practice interventions, and to make referrals to appropriate programs in the community. This chapter provides a historical and current overview of the mental health system in the United States from federal, state, and local perspectives.

Understanding the mental health system and how it is organized will help you navigate mental health patients and their families appropriately through the system. Having an understanding of the mental health system also will assist you in designing and implementing effective community health programs, knowing how community health policies are made and advocating for policy changes, establishing effective partnerships with organizations, and using resources effectively. The first section of this chapter provides an overview of the mental health system. The second section spotlights mental health service delivery, and the third part of the chapter examines the role of community mental health professionals and discusses the kind of community mental health care system needed in today's environment to provide cost-efficient culturally and linguistically appropriate community mental health services.

Over the past 40 years, there have been dramatic changes in the financing and organization of the mental health system from a relatively simple single-facility system to a current system characterized by a multiplicity of providers that exists in a highly complex and often fragmented environment (Grob, 1991; Hadley, Schinnar, & Rothbard, 1991; Rothbard, Hadley, Schinnar, Morgan, & Whitehill, 1989; Schlesinger, 1986). Because financing models often drive the organization of care, it is important to understand how the changes in financing have shaped the structure of the mental health system over time. Since 1950, the mental health system has been through what can be described as five major phases of financing mental health services: phase 1, operation of psychiatric hospitals; phase 2, community mental health centers; phase 3, fee-for-services federal and state healthcare finance systems; phase 4, private insurance expanded coverage; and phase 5, parity of mental health benefits (Hadley et al., 1991).

Throughout the 1950s, the mental health system was relatively simple, with most funding coming from the states and the federal government to operate state psychiatric hospitals and Veterans Administration hospitals. The first major change in this system began in the early 1960s with the advent of community mental health center grants funded by the federal government's Alcohol, Drug Abuse and Mental Health Administration (ADAMHA). Funds flowed through grants from the **National Institute of Mental Health (NIMH)** to local provider agencies termed *community mental health centers* whose existence often depended on the grant (Beigel, 1982). In the 1970s, the beginning of the fee-for-service (FFS) federal and state healthcare finance systems, Medicaid and Medicare, created further complexity in the system. These programs simultaneously expanded the number of persons receiving service and supported the creation of new general hospital psychiatry services (McGuire & Fairbank, 1988). At around the same time a small but increasing number of private health insurers began to expand coverage for mental illness. This growth in the privately insured sector helped create the for-profit private psychiatric hospital system and the ever-growing private practice of psychiatrists and other mental health professionals. In recent years, the pressures to achieve "parity" of mental health benefits and the enormous growth of the care system have increasingly led to a wide variety of managed mental health-care services (National Advisory Mental Health Council, 1998; Strum, McCulloch, & Goldman, 1999; Strum & Sherbourne, 1999; Substance Abuse and Mental Health Services Administration, 1998, 1999).

OVERVIEW OF THE MENTAL HEALTH SERVICE SYSTEM

The U.S. federal government became involved in the financing of mental health services with the passage of the Social Security Act of 1935. This paradigm shift grew out of the notion that if local governments could not take care of mentally ill individuals during the Depression, the federal government should take on the responsibility. The impact of World War II on community health was extraordinary: 875,000 draftees of 15 million, or approximately 6%, were disqualified from the military because of existing mental health problems (Snow & Newton, 1976). At the end of the war, the role of the government with the mentally ill increased significantly, leading to the enactment of the National Mental Health Act in 1946, giving grants to states to develop programs outside of a state mental health facility. The goal of the 1946 legislation was to develop a community-based approach to the treatment based on a medical model. In 1949 the act also led to the NIMH, an agency that would be responsible and oversee the mental health services for Americans. The next phase of legislation to affect mental health from 1955 to 1980 is chronicled here.

- 1955: The creation of the Joint Commission on Mental Health illness was established. Under the leadership of this commission the historical document *Action for Mental Health* was published in 1961. This 338-page report emphasized the need for better training for personnel providing early and intensive treatment for the acutely mentally ill and for professionals carrying out research. In addition, the report suggested the development of facilities such as general hospitals, clinics, programs for aftercare, rehabilitation, and mental health education (Joint Commission, 1961).
- 1963: Congress enacted Public Law 88-164, the Mental Health Retardation Facilities, and Community Mental Health Centers Construction Act of 1963. Under this act, a $150 million matching fund grant award was released over a

3-year period to build comprehensive mental health centers. The purpose of the grant was to provide comprehensive mental health services in a specific area known as a **catchment area**. A catchment area consisted of 75,000 to 200,000 people.

- 1964: To keep the centers operational, Congress extended P.L. 89-105 to establish funds to finance mental health centers over a 51-month period.
- 1975: Congress passed the Community Mental Health Centers Amendments of 1975 (P.L. 94-63). These amendments provided a stable steam of funding for mental health centers, made more grants available, and extended the funding cycle of a grant to a maximum of 12 years. The grants also included areas such as child care, aging, court screening, and care for discharged mentally ill people, transitional services, and substance abuse services. The amendments also defined and stipulated the service components that a community mental health center must provide.
- 1977: The President's Commission on Mental Health report was released recommending strengthening the community mental health system and again extended funding for mental health services. The report included 117 recommendations, which were divided in these eight categories: community support systems, service delivery, financing, personnel, patient's rights, research, prevention, and public understanding (President's Commission, 1978).
- Because of the lack of flexibility in previous laws, legislation was passed in 1980 emphasizing the need for communities to be flexible in planning services to meet their unique needs. The legislation also gave states greater authority over mental health funds and allowed flexible and innovative program planning, as well as development of new approaches to meet the mental health needs of priority populations. More important, communities were able to plan according to the needs of the community, and they were not restricted to federally mandated services.

Mental health care has changed drastically during the past five decades. Prior to the 1960s, most clients with mental disorders were institutionalized in long-term care facilities, some never leaving the institution in their lifetime. The passage of the 1963 act generated the first community mental health movement based on the philosophy that individuals would receive better care if they remained in their communities and were not separated from their families and friends. The plan proposed to make an array of community-based services available to all individuals seeking mental health care. Each community mental health center was expected to provide five basic services to the community: inpatient care, outpatient care, emergency care, partial hospitalization, and consultation and education.

The Public and Private Sectors

Mental disorders and mental health problems are treated by a variety of caregivers who work in diverse, relatively independent, and coordinated facilities and services both public and private, referred to as the **de facto mental health service system** (Regier, Goldberg, & Taube, 1978; Regier, Narrow, Rae, Manderscheid, Locke, & Goodwin, 1993). The term *public sector* refers both to services directly operated by government agencies (e.g., state and county mental hospitals) and to services financed with government resources (e.g., Medicaid, a federal and state program for financing healthcare services for people who are poor and disabled, and Medicare, a federal health insurance program primarily for older Americans and people who retire early due to disability). Publicly financed services may be provided by private organizations. The term *private sector* refers both to services directly operated by private agencies and to services financed with private resources (e.g., employer-provided insurance). The public and private parts of the de facto mental health system treat distinct populations with some overlap. The system is usually described as having four major components or sectors:

1. The **specialty mental health** sector consists of mental health professionals such as psychiatrists, psychologists, psychiatric nurses, community mental health outreach workers, and psychiatric social workers who are trained specifically to treat people with mental disorders. The great bulk of specialty treatment is provided in outpatient settings such as private office-based practices or in private or public clinics. Most acute hospital care for the mentally ill is now provided in special psychiatric units of public health hospitals or beds scattered throughout private hospitals. Private psychiatric hospitals and residential treatment centers for children and adolescents provide additional intensive care in the private sector. Public sector facilities include state/county mental hospitals and multiservice mental health facilities, which often coordinate a wide range of outpatient, intensive case management, partial hospitalization, and inpatient services.
2. The *general medical/primary care* sector consists of healthcare professionals such as general internists, pediatricians, physician assistants, and nurse practitioners in office-based practice, clinics, acute medical/surgical hospitals, and nursing homes. The general medical sector has long been identified as the initial point of contact for many adults with mental disorders; for some, these providers may be their only source of mental health services.
3. The *human services sector* consists of social services, school-based counseling services, residential rehabilitation services, vocational rehabilitation, criminal justice/prison-based services, and religious professional counselors.

4. The *voluntary support network* sector includes self-help and social support groups such as breast cancer support groups, caregiver support groups, 12-step programs, and peer counselors and is a rapidly growing component of the mental health care, stress management, and addictive disorder treatment system.

State and local governments have been the major payers for public mental health services historically and remain so today. Since the mid-1960s, however, the role of the federal government has increased. In addition to Medicare and Medicaid, the federal government funds special programs for adults with serious mental illness and children with serious emotional disabilities. Although small in relation to state and local funding, these federal programs provide resources that include the Community Mental Health Block Grant, community support programs, and the PATH program for people with mental illness who are homeless, the Knowledge Development and Application Program, and the Comprehensive Community Mental Health Services for Children and their families program.

These federally funded public sector programs support the traditional responsibility of state and local mental health systems and serve as the mental health service "safety net" and "catastrophic insurer" for individuals with the most severe mental problems and the fewest resources in the United States. The public sector serves individuals with no health insurance, those who have insurance but no mental health coverage, and those who limited mental health benefits as part of their health insurance benefit.

Each sector of the de facto mental health service system has different types of care and different patterns of funding. Within the specialty mental health sector, state- and county-funded mental health services have long served as a safety net for people unable to obtain or retain access to privately funded mental health services. The general medical sector, for example, receives a large proportion of federal Medicaid funds; the voluntary support network sector, staffed principally by people with mental illness and their families, is mainly funded by private donations of time and money to social support and educational groups.

Effective functioning of the mental health service system requires connections and coordination among many sectors (public and private, specialty and general health, health and social welfare, housing, criminal justice, and education systems). Without coordination, services can become organizationally fragmented, creating barriers to access. Adding to the system's complexity is its dependence on many streams of funding. At times, these funding sources have competing incentives. For example, as part of Medicaid reform, a financial incentive leads to the reduction in inpatient admissions to the psychiatric unit in a public health hospital, and patients are sent to state mental hospitals instead. This cost containment policy possibly could conflict with a policy directive to reduce the census of state mental hospitals.

A broad array of services and treatments exists to help people with mental illnesses as well as prevention services targeting a particular group of individuals at risk of developing a mental illness go through less emotional pain and disability and live healthier, longer, and more productive lives.

A System in Disarray

The mental health system in the United States is fragmented and in a state of disarray. The rate of unemployment is at an all-time high, and as a result people are anxious and most people with mental illness are impoverished, with 71% reporting an annual income of $20,000 (Hall, Graf, Fitzpatrick, Lane, & Birkel, 2003) or less, and many suffer posttraumatic syndrome because of their wartime experiences. Moreover, because of the poor economic market, large number of layoffs, furloughs, and increased demand to complete assignments with a smaller workforce, more individuals are taking more time off work, report they are more stressed, and are using more employee-assisted mental health services than in previous years. Additionally, individuals who are laid off work, living on unemployment or disability benefits, might not be able to afford an apartment, and as a result, those with persistent mental illness might live in shelters or have rooms in cheap single-occupancy hotels (Gruttadaro, 2005).

Services for individuals with severe and persistent mental illness are often disorganized and poorly funded. This is especially true for individuals who are dually diagnosed with substance abuse. People with a history substance abuse who are dually diagnosed with mental illness are frequently unable to cope with complex public mental health systems of care. When a person has disorganized thoughts, it is difficult and frustrating to try to locate appropriate help. Oftentimes these individuals have multiple hospitalizations to manage their medications. If they become a danger to themselves or to others, they might be court ordered to a long-term community treatment center, only to be discharged back to the same environment to start the cycle over again. Barriers to effective treatment of mental illness include lack of recognition of the seriousness of a mental illness and failure to understand the benefits of services. Policymakers, insurance companies, health and labor policies, as well as the public at large, all discriminate between physical and mental problems. If there are any funding shortages, funding of mental health services is usually cut before funding of services to primary care or communicable disease. Most middle- and low-income countries devote less than 1% of their health expenditure to mental health (World Health Organization, 2005). Consequently, mental health policies, legislation, community care facilities, and treatments for people with mental illness are not given the priority they deserve.

EXPLORING THE CURRENT MENTAL HEALTH SYSTEM IN THE UNITED STATES

In 2002, President George W. Bush appointed a 15-member commission to examine the mental health system in the United States. The charge to the president's New Freedom Commission on Mental Health was to undertake an in-depth review of the public/private mental health system and make recommendations on steps to achieve an effective mental health system in the United States. The commission included seven ex-officio federal participants who spent a year examining all aspects of the U.S. mental health delivery system. The commission used public hearings, site visits, written and oral testimony from experts, and comments and concerns received via the Internet to hear concerns about the mental system from U.S. citizens. After 6 months, an interim report to the president stated that "the system was in shambles" and identified substantial fragmentation as a barrier to access to care for children, adults, and older adults. Analysis of all the reports and findings seemed to suggest that the only way to create an effective and efficient mental health system was to fundamentally transform the system, not just to make minor changes to the existing system.

To achieve the transformation, the commission developed a plan that included 6 goals and 19 recommendations (described in detail in Chapter 14). It was the commission's belief that these recommendations needed to be seen in totality because they were interrelated. The overarching principles in the findings emphasized that the mental health system needed to be equivalent to the public health system, with better access, equity in treatment and funding, and a reduction of stigma. Findings suggested that the mental health system was built around a delivery and payment system instead of the needs of mental health service recipients and their families, resulting in unsatisfactory outcomes. Further findings pointed to the public mental health system's failure to employ evidence-based practices or the newest technologies and confirmed that a person's race, ethnicity, or geographic location could compromise his or her access to services. The commission's findings and recommendations pointed out the benefits of early detection and the need for community-based services and support, as opposed to a crisis-oriented system that responds several years after the first appearance of mental symptoms.

The report's six goals were broad-based visionary expressions of how a transformed mental health system would appear. Nineteen supporting recommendations were drafted to apply to those with a stake in the public system, whether at the local, state, or federal level. The commission's goals were meant to change the perception about mental health care service delivery as well as certain mental health care practices. Since the report was drafted, the commission's work has had an impact on the language of several agencies involved with publicly funded mental health services.

In particular, the concept that "recovery is possible" and the recommendation of a "consumer- and family-driven" system have captured considerable attention.

For practical application of the recommendations, the commission looked to the federal government for leadership but to local and state governments and advocacy groups at all levels to ensure that the transformation of the mental health service delivery system took place in the nation. The recommendation targeting the federal government was recommendation 2.3: *Align relevant federal programs to improve access and accountability for mental health services*. Under the direction of the Substance Abuse and Mental Health Services Administration's (SAMHSA) Center for Mental Health Services, federal agencies have developed programs that impact the delivery of mental health services. A workgroup of federal agency representatives meets regularly to examine ways to ensure consistency in the government's approach to meeting the needs of consumers and families affected by mental illness and mental health disorders.

The most concrete recommendation of the commission was the creation of a comprehensive mental health plan in each state. The commission saw the comprehensive state mental health plan as binding disparate elements of mental health services that in most states contribute to the fragmentation highlighted in the commission's report. The commission envisioned several purposes for developing a comprehensive plan in each state, for example promoting partnerships between state agencies and among the broad range of stakeholders in the mental health care delivery system. Developing a plan would help mental health providers ensure a more coordinated use of existing resources. Most important, it would enable stakeholders to assess the strengths and weakness of the existing array of services and provide a framework for creating a robust set of relationships and develop the full range of services contemplated by the commission.

Although some of the commission's goals were geared to be acted on by the federal government, many were developed to be put in place by state governments and specifically by state mental health authorities (SMHAs) or the lead agencies on mental health services in each state. SMHAs are responsible for developing comprehensive mental health systems and serve as the nation's safety net for the provision of mental health services to adults with serious mental illnesses and children with serious emotional disturbances. Collectively, the SMHAs serve 6 million individuals with mental illnesses each year (CMHS, 2004) and expend $26 billion each year to pay for these mental health services (National Association of State Mental Health Program Directors Research Institute [NASMHPD], 2005).

Most SMHAs have embraced the commission's report and recommendations as a road map for their own efforts to improve the quality of their mental health systems and to guide their transformation activities. After the commission released its final report, the SMHAs, through the National Association of State Mental Health Program

Directors (NASMHPD), collectively endorsed the goals in an official policy statement (NASMHPD, 2003). To help states initiate the development of the comprehensive plans, the federal government invited applications for states to apply for the Mental Health Transformation State Incentive Grants (MHT-SIG). Administered by CMHS, this grant program requires governors' offices to oversee planning and system development through creation of Transformation Working Groups. The MHT-SIG program places a premium on collaboration, with a clear goal in mind:

> The intended outcome of Comprehensive State Mental Health Plans is to encourage States and localities to develop a comprehensive strategy to respond to the needs and preferences of consumers or families. The final result should be an extensive and coordinated State system of services and supports that work to foster consumer independence and their ability to live, work, learn, and participate fully in their communities. (New Freedom Commission on Mental Health, 2003, p. 44)

As SMHAs have embraced the commission's principles and goals and begun to fundamentally overhaul their mental health systems based on principles of recovery, client and family-centered services, and emphasis on coordinated services in the community, they have encountered the critical issue of collection and appropriate use of data. SMHAs realize the importance of information and data in both program development and in delivery of quality services. Therefore, SMHAs must make conscientious decisions to view data and information as a product that should be readily available, proactive, and transparent. Since the release of the commission's report, the states have made a concerted effort to collect and disseminate data to help support and illuminate the report's six goals.

SMHAs are making substantial progress toward achieving the major goals of the New Freedom Commission on Mental Health. Seventy-one percent of SMHAs are collaborating with Medicaid and state health departments to promote the diagnosis and treatment of mental health. Almost all states are working to reduce fragmentation across state agencies providing mental health services, and they are providing prevention/early intervention services and propose to implement at least one evidence-based practice (EBP) service. SMHAs also are investing in technology to enhance quality and accountability of mental health services.

The National Association of State Mental Health Program Directors Research Institute, Inc. (NRI) and NASMHPD have been working with the states to document their efforts to transform their systems and implement the commission's goals. The information being compiled by NRI through its CMHS-supported State Profiles System is publicly accessible to help states and advocates who would like to track how SMHAs are transforming systems.

State Profiling System

The SMHA Profiling System, funded under a contract from CMHS, provides a central database of information describing the organization, funding, operation, services, policies, statutes, and consumers of SMHAs. This database describes each SMHA's organization and structure, service systems, eligible populations, emerging policy issues, number of consumers served, fiscal resources, consumer issues, information management structures, and the research and evaluation the SMHA conducts. Questions within each component are designed to address specific needs of SMHA managers and others interested in public mental health systems, and to support decision making, policy analysis, research, and evaluation. To minimize the response burden on SMHAs, the following criteria were developed to determine what information should be maintained in the Profiling System: Sufficient detail to answer important state-level questions, state-level information is maintained, not individual program or sub-state levels. Items are not duplicative of existing information systems. Profiling information should help develop a better understanding of existing information systems, not replace them. The Profiling Systems also document the profiles focused on the New Freedom Commission's six goals for transforming mental health. The Profiles have compiled information on the activities of SMHAs to implement major portions of each of the six goals. Individual state responses to the Profiles are available on NRI's Web site at www.nri-inc.org. On the Profiles Web site, users can access state responses by keyword, by state, and by special topical reports.

BARRIERS TO MENTAL HEALTH CARE

There are a number of barriers to receiving adequate mental health care in the community. Many individuals will not seek care because of the perceived stigma; they are uninsured or if they are insured, many employers cover mental illness; however, benefits are more restricted for mental health as compared to primary care and chronic disease (Zuvekas, Banthin, & Selden, 1998). Mental health care is delivered through a variety of local, state, and national programs, all of which have different criteria for allocating and prioritizing funds for mental health services.

The commission's report has provided considerable activity in the mental health community. Not only has it created a road map for the CMHS and its sister federal agencies, it has simultaneously provided a standard for state-initiated activity, and it has given the notably fractious mental health advocacy community a set of principles on which many key organizations can agree in order to decrease barriers to mental health care.

Most publicly, CMHS has been tasked and funded by Congress to develop a program of MHT-SIGs for which states, territories, and federally recognized tribes could apply. The MHT-SIG was funded in the federal budget for fiscal year 2005, and it is anticipated that the program will continue to be a centerpiece of CMHS efforts until 2010. In the first year of funding there were enough funds (approximately $18.5 million) for six to eight grantees to receive $2 to $3 million each (President's New Freedom Commission on Mental Health, 2003).

The purpose of the MHT-SIG is to enable states, territories, and tribes to plan for and develop infrastructure that will enable them to create the Comprehensive State Mental Health Plans recommended by the commission. The MHT-SIG asks states to create Mental Health Transformation Working Groups chaired by appointees answerable directly to the office of the governor or, in the case of territories or tribes, the entity's designated chief executive. The idea is that it will take the attention of the chief executive to bring the disparate players in the mental health field to the table with the purpose of coordinating mental health service delivery in that jurisdiction. In their applications for the grants, states were asked to demonstrate the degree to which appropriate parties already were collaborating and working toward development of a comprehensive state plan, as well as to lay out in detail how a grant award would help them move forward with the planning process.

The campaign partners embraced the commission report as a platform on which to continue to build the mental health system. The campaign provided considerable advocacy in support of the MHT-SIG program as well as the Mentally Ill Offender Treatment and Crime Reduction Act, which created a grant program within the Department of Justice for the diversion and reintegration of persons with mental illness who come into contact with the criminal justice system. The campaign's collaborative approach signaled to the broader field and to policymakers that the transformation agenda has found acceptance among the mental health system's stakeholders and, more important, that they are willing to set aside their differences to work on its behalf.

As described earlier, the 2004 cycle of NRI's State Profiling System was redesigned to compile information from the SMHAs about their activities related to each of the six goals. The state responses to each of the goals are listed here:

Goal 1: Americans Understanding Mental Health Is Essential to Overall Health Care

The commission's first goal is to reduce the stigma and discrimination related to mental illnesses and increases the public's understanding of mental illnesses. With the elimination of stigma and a better understanding of the fundamental role of mental health to overall health care, the public will seek care earlier and more often.

Fundamental to increased access is providing better information to Americans about mental illness and better recognition of mental illnesses among primary care ıers. SMHAs are traditionally specialty systems that focus their attention on the sion of mental health (and often other disability services). However, many states a. ıow actively working across state governments to increase the recognition and treatment of mental illnesses. For example, 71% of SMHAs (32 of 45 reporting states) are collaborating with their state health department and/or Medicaid agency to increase the recognition and treatment of persons with mental illness by primary care providers. These initiatives include providing psychiatric consultation (three states) and providing training and education to primary care providers (seven states).

In addition to the efforts to make primary care workers accurately identify and treat mental illnesses, more than half of the states are working with primary care systems to improve the quality of physical healthcare treatment for individuals with mental illness. Several studies have recently found that the physical conditions of persons with mental illnesses are often not adequately addressed and major medical conditions are often not treated (Cradock-O'Leary, Young, Yano, Wang, & Lee, 2002). More than half (56%) of SMHAs are working with primary care providers to improve the physical health treatment of persons with mental illnesses (the second area of focus by more than half the SMHAs is the development of public awareness and information efforts). Sixty percent of SMHAs (27 of 45) have public information campaigns to promote better understanding of the role of mental health in overall health care of the adult.

The commission found that stigma related to mental illnesses remains a major impediment to many people seeking mental health treatment: 33 SMHAs (73%) report they have public health information campaigns designed to combat stigma with mental illnesses. Ensuring that private health insurance coverage addresses the needs of persons to receive mental health services is an additional component of ensuring access to services, although health plans are not required to include mental health in their benefits package. Building on the 1996 Mental Health Parity Act, employers who offer mental health or substance abuse benefits must equate the same aggregate lifetime and annual limits for mental health benefits like medical and surgical benefits. Enacted on October 3, 2008, the act (P.L. 110-343) was voted on to end health insurance benefits' inequity between mental health/substance use disorders and medical/surgical benefits for group health plans with more than 50 employees. The law is projected to provide parity protection to 113 million people across the country, including 82 million individuals enrolled in self-funded plans (regulated under the Employment Retirement Income Security Act [ERISA] and, under its terms, not subject to state parity laws). The act will apply to plans beginning in the first plan coverage year that begins 1 year after the date of enactment. For most plans, the effective date begins January 1, 2010 (Glantz, 2008).

Goal 2: Mental Health Care Is Consumer and Family Driven

The commission promulgated the objective that all mental health care should be recovery oriented, organized, and driven by consumer and family needs, and that every consumer should have an individualized plan of care. Per **Recovery Orientation**, all of the 45 reporting SMHAs have adopted a mission statement or policy about the potential of consumers to recover from their illnesses and is seeking to reorient the mental health system to be more recovery oriented. SMHA recovery initiatives include drafting recovery mission statements, changing the array of services funded by the SMHA, working with consumers and families to promote recovery concepts, and moving toward EBP.

Individualized Treatment Plans

SMHAs are taking action to reduce fragmentation and to move their systems to reflect the desires of mental health consumers to recover and direct their own care. Ninety-five percent of SMHAs (39 states) have initiatives to ensure that every consumer receives an **individualized treatment plan** that meets his or her unique needs. To monitor the development and implementation of these person-centered individualized treatment plans, 29 SMHAs receive information on individualized treatment plans from community mental health providers. SMHAs involve consumers and family members in the SMHA's policymaking, quality assurance, and research and evaluation activities.

Reducing Fragmentation

The commission identified as a major problem the provision of comprehensive consumer-directed mental health services. That is, mental health services are fragmented among many different funding and service delivery systems. As a result, the provision of mental health care is often driven more by eligibility and funding considerations than by the desires and needs of families and consumers in need of mental health services. Consumers often are subject to multiple eligibility determinations to receive services, and the services they receive may be determined more by what funding sources will pay for instead of what the consumer actually needs or wants.

Over half the SMHAs (24 of 25) developed a comprehensive state mental health plan that spans multiple state government agencies and addresses the mental health services and essential supports provided by state agencies other than the SMHA. All SMHAs include representatives of other state government agencies in the SMHA's mental health planning council. Most SMHAs are working with other major state government agencies to reduce fragmentation in mental health services and improve access to services. Thirty-nine states are working with housing, 39 with Medicaid, 37 with juvenile justice, and 37 with corrections.

Housing for Persons with Mental Illnesses

Persons with mental illness often need more than just mental health services to live productive lives in the community. As a result, many SMHAs are working with consumers to provide vocational and housing support to assist them in their recovery and healing process. Finding clean, safe, and affordable housing is a major issue for most SMHAs. SMHAs identified the following major barriers to addressing consumer housing needs:

- Insufficient availability of subsidized housing (41 states)
- Consumer income insufficient to afford private market housing (41 states)
- Insufficient funding for development of affordable housing (37 states)
- Insufficient funding for necessary support services (26 states)
- Community opposition—"not in my backyard" (NIMBY) (20 states)

Most SMHAs (65%) have a **housing plan** (a delineated set of strategies to address the housing needs of persons with mental illness). Housing specialists/coordinators are responsible for increasing affordable housing opportunities for persons with serious mental illnesses within the SMHA in 32 states, within the state housing agency in 11 states, and within both agencies in nine states. In 38 states, the SMHA supports or collaborates with community development corporations or local housing authorities. In 26 states, the local mental health authority works with these local housing authorities.

SMHAs have established working interagency relationships with the other major state agencies responsible for the development of housing: 90% (35 states) with the state housing finance agency, 31 states with the state department of housing/community development, 25 with the state affordable housing coalition, and 38 with the state coalition for homeless persons (New Freedom Commission on Mental Health, 2003).

Custody Relinquishment of Children/Foster Care

A major barrier for seeking services for children with mental disorders identified by the commission was the requirement that many parents have to relinquish the custody of their children to the state government so their child can receive publicly funded mental health services. The commission called for policy changes to eliminate the need for parents to relinquish custody of their children in order for them to receive services. States working to ensure this change have laws or policies designed to keep parents from having to relinquish custody of children in this situation.

Goal 3: Disparities in Mental Health Services Are Eliminated

The commission found that minority populations are underserved and "that the mental health system has not kept pace with the diverse needs of racial and ethnic minorities, often underserving or inappropriately serving them" (New Freedom Commission on Mental Health, 2003). SMHAs report taking many steps to address the needs of ethnic and minority populations, as well as rural and geographically remote persons with mental illnesses.

Rural and Geographically Remote Mental Health Services

Seventy-eight percent of SMHAs (36 of 46) have initiatives to increase access to mental health services in rural and geographically remote areas. In addition, 42% (18 of 43) have initiatives to recruit and train mental health professionals to work in rural and remote areas. Seventy-four percent of SMHAs (35 of 47) have initiatives to provide transportation for mental health clients so they can access needed mental health services (New Freedom Commission on Mental Health, 2003).

Cultural Competence Issues

To improve cultural competence in SMHAs, one of the first steps essential to the provision of culturally appropriate services to ethnic and cultural minorities is identifying the needs of these consumers and planning to develop the appropriate mental health services and staff training required to meet these needs. The NASMHPD task force has been working on cultural competence issues for several years. The task force has developed a self-assessment instrument for SMHAs and mental health programs to use in moving their cultural competence planning and implementation forward (NASMHPD, 2004).

Seventy-eight percent of SMHAs (28 of 42) have a cultural competence plan; 23% of them have established measurable objectives in their cultural competence plan and have conducted a cultural competence assessment of their mental health system. Twenty-two SMHAs address linguistic competence in their cultural competence plan. When 32 SMHAs report, they have a staff person with overall responsibility for cultural competence, and 25 SMHAs have a cultural competence advisory committee (New Freedom Commission on Mental Health, 2003).

Minority Staffing Issues

Having a mental health services workforce that understands and can provide culturally competent mental health services are an important step to reduce disparities and barriers to care. Many SMHAs are undertaking initiatives to recruit and train minority mental health workers into the public mental health system. Twenty-one SMHAs have initiatives to recruit and train members of minority groups, ethnic groups, or other special populations for work in state-funded mental health programs: Ten have staff recruitment initiatives for African Americans, seven for Hispanics, six for Asians, five for Native Americans, and four for Pacific Islanders.

In addition to efforts to recruit more minorities into the public mental health system, SMHAs are fostering initiatives to increase the training they provide to minorities in their system: Eight SMHAs have staff training initiatives for blacks/African Americans, six for Hispanics, eight for Asians, six for Native Americans, and seven for Pacific Islanders (New Freedom Commission on Mental Health, 2003).

Staffing Shortages

A significant barrier for SMHAs in providing quality mental health services is a universal shortage of mental health staff. Of SMHAs reporting, 44 of 45 are currently experiencing shortages of mental health staff. Psychiatrists, social workers, community health outreach workers, and registered nurses were the professional disciplines for which the largest numbers of SMHAs reported shortages (New Freedom Commission on Mental Health, 2003).

Many SMHAs (29) report they have initiatives to address these staffing shortages: Twenty-four SMHAs are working with universities to increase the training of future staff and increase recruitment into the public sector, 19 are increasing salaries paid in the SMHA system, 17 are providing training at mental health providers, and 14 are providing recruitment bonuses or other financial incentives (New Freedom Commission on Mental Health, 2003).

Goal 4: Early Mental Health Screening, Assessment, and Referral to Services Are Common Practice

The commission report found that "emerging research indicates that intervening early can interrupt the negative course of some mental illnesses and might, in some cases, lessen long-term disability" (New Freedom Commission on Mental Health, 2003, p. 57). As a result, the commission called for a major increase in the early identification of mental health problems and for making mental health screening and assessment part of routine practice in health care. SMHAs are undertaking a number of efforts to meet these goals.

Early Detection

Thirty-nine of 50 SMHAs (78%) have initiatives for the early detection of mental health problems: 39 states for children, 17 for adults, and 17 for older adults. Thirty-three SMHAs (67%) operate or fund prevention/early intervention programs for children, 16 operate or fund such programs for adults, and 10 operate or fund them for elderly persons. Thirty-four of 44 SMHAs (82%) work with schools to expand and improve mental health services for children (New Freedom Commission on Mental Health, 2003).

Persons with co-occurring mental illnesses and substance abuse disorders often experience difficulty having both of their illnesses appropriately recognized and treated. Thirty-seven of 46 SMHAs (80%) require mental health providers to screen for co-occurring mental health and substance abuse disorders. Thirty-one SMHAs operate or fund separate specialized treatment programs for persons with co-occurring mental health and substance abuse disorders. In addition, 28 of 47 SMHAs (60%) require or work with mental health providers to screen for histories of trauma in persons served in the public mental health system (New Freedom Commission on Mental Health, 2003).

Criminal Justice System Issues

Many persons with mental illness unfortunately fall into the criminal justice system, where their mental health needs are either unrecognized or often inadequately treated. SMHAs have undertaken a variety of initiatives to work with the criminal justice system to help divert persons with mental illness out of corrections programs and into treatment. Forty-six of 48 of the states (96%) reported having at least one mental health court or other criminal justice diversion program for persons with mental illnesses. Sixty-seven percent of SMHAs (31 of 45) have at least one mental health court designed to divert persons with mental illnesses from the criminal justice system into mental health treatment (Morrissey, Fagan, & Cocozza, 2009). Mental health courts, which are modeled after drug courts, are special courts designed to handle criminal cases of persons with mental illnesses and divert them out of jail or prison and into treatment. These states reported on 178 courts that served 5251 persons in 2003. Ten of the states have the courts control dedicated resources for services totaling over $1.7 million (President's New Freedom Commission on Mental Health, 2003).

Diversion Programs

According to the CMHS-funded GAINS Center, "diversion" programs refer to "programs that divert individuals with serious mental illness (and often co-occurring substance use disorders) in contact with the justice system from jail and provide linkages to community-based treatment and support services. The individual thus avoids or spends a significantly reduced time period in jail and/or lockups on the current charge" (gainscenter.samhsa.gov/flash/default).

Thirty-one states have pre-booking diversion programs to help divert adults with mental illnesses into treatment. Pre-booking diversion programs aim to move people out of the criminal justice system and into treatment before formal criminal charges are made against them. Twenty-eight SMHAs have funded or otherwise promoted pre-booking programs for adults in the past 2 years. Twenty-seven SMHAs have plans to fund or otherwise promote pre-booking programs in the next fiscal year.

Twenty-seven SMHAs have post-booking pre-adjudication programs to help divert adults with mental illnesses into treatment. These programs are designed to move persons with mental illnesses out of the criminal justice system and into community treatment after charges have been filed but before they go to court. SMHAs have funded or otherwise promoted criminal justice diversion programs for adults in the last 2 years. Twenty-four SMHAs have plans to fund or promote any criminal justice diversion programs in the next fiscal year.

Twenty-nine of 45 SMHAs support diversion programs for youth with mental illnesses from the juvenile justice system into treatment. Nineteen SMHAs have juvenile justice diversion programs at the intake level, 17 at the adjudication level, and 15 at pre-arrest stages.

Sixty-one percent of SMHAs (27 of 44) have reentry programs to support prisoners or jail detainees with mental illness and/or co-occurring substance abuse disorders who are returning to the community (President's New Freedom Commission on Mental Health, 2003).

Goal 5: Excellent Mental Health Care Is Delivered and Research Is Accelerated

The commission set a goal that persons with mental illnesses receive the highest quality mental health services demonstrated effective by research. One major impediment to the provision of quality mental health services is the long delay between the advances in knowledge from research to the implementation of these advances into common clinical practice. The commission called for concerted action to accelerate research to promote recovery and resilience and to advance the use of evidence-based practices in mental health services.

Most SMHAs, approximately 76%, are working with academia to move research results into better mental health services. States report a number of initiatives between SMHAs and academia to accelerate the movement of research findings into practice.

Examples of these initiatives include establishing "centers for excellence" to work with mental health providers, establishing joint appointments with mental health researchers and mental health policy and clinical providers, and using local academic institutions to provide training to mental health providers. In addition to activities to move research into practice, 61% of SMHAs have initiatives to help academia and other researchers to study mental health issues identified by the SMHA (President's New Freedom Commission on Mental Health, 2003).

Ninety-two percent of SMHAs are measuring client outcome measures. The most common client outcome measures being routinely measured by SMHAs for community services are as follows (49 SMHAs reporting):

Consumer perception of care: 42
Consumer functioning: 40
Family involvement/satisfaction: 35
Change in employment status: 30
Change in living situation: 31
Consumer symptoms: 26
Strength-based measures: 17
Consumer recovery: 15

Evidence-Based Practices

The commission recommended an increase in the implementation of mental health services that have been demonstrated to be effective (EBPs). The NRI's State Profiles System compiles information on the implementation by SMHAs of the six adult EBPs for which CMHS has developed "toolkits," as well as for several child/adolescent services that many researchers have identified as having strong research evidence.

Every reporting SMHA is implementing at least one adult EBP, and most States are implementing multiple EBPs, with three EBPs being implemented in most states: assertive community treatment teams: 37 SMHAs; supported employment: 37 SMHAs; and integrated dual diagnosis programs for persons with co-occurring mental health and substance abuse: 34 SMHAs. SMHAs are increasingly offering these EBPs throughout the states and are working to increase the training of mental health providers to deliver EBPs according to practice standards. For example, assertive community treatment (ACT) is being provided by more than 485 programs to 64,242 consumers (32 SMHAs reporting). Twenty-six of these SMHAs measure the fidelity of ACT programs to the model on which studies were conducted (President's New Freedom Commission on Mental Health, 2003).

Supported employment (SE) was provided statewide in 20 states and in parts of 16 states and was provided to 39,513 persons by 650 programs in 29 states. Fourteen states reported they measure the fidelity of their SE programs to the model. SMHAs are using a number of initiatives to promote the adoption of EBPs across their systems.

Goal 6: Technology Is Used to Access Mental Health Care and Information

The commission established a goal of increasing the use of technology to improve the quality of mental health services and to promote better information about services among consumers and family members. SMHAs are investing in technology to implement this goal.

Forty-seven percent of SMHAs (23) have implemented electronic medical records in either state hospitals or community programs. Most of these initiatives are in the community (18), and 13 are in state psychiatric hospitals. Seventeen SMHAs have implemented electronic medication ordering systems for their state psychiatric hospitals, and four states have implemented them with community mental health providers (President's New Freedom Commission on Mental Health, 2003).

Telemedicine Initiatives

Health information technology shows tremendous promise for improving mental health care delivery. Electronic communications, for example, will allow mental health care providers to follow mental health clients throughout their mental health treatment regimen. For example, a child suffering a mental health crisis can be followed from the inpatient hospital setting, to protective custody, or crisis center to various mental healthcare providers in the community setting. A health information exchange can aid in coordination of care as well as sharing important information via electronic health records and telepsychiatry. Telepsychiatry has been shown to improve access to therapy for veterans suffering from combat-related posttraumatic stress syndrome. Frueh and colleagues in a 2007 randomized trial found that veterans who received 14 weekly 90-minute treatment sessions by telepsychiatry via videoconferencing or in a room with a psychiatrist had similar outcomes and satisfaction within 3 months after treatment. Improvement was seen in overall psychiatric function, depression, and the quality of social relationships.

Eighty-one percent of SMHAs (38 of 47) promote the use of telemedicine to provide mental health services. To help promote the use of telemedicine services,

10 SMHAs reimburse providers for providing telemedicine services, and 25 state Medicaid agencies reimburse for mental health telemedicine services. In addition, three states have changed state licensure or scope-of-practice restrictions to promote and encourage the use of telemedicine.

Providing Consumers Access to Data on Mental Health Services

SMHAs have many initiatives to make information about recovery, self-help services, and data on services available to consumers, family members, and advocates via the Internet:

- Information about self-help services, education, and supports to consumers and family members: 26
- Information about identifying mental illnesses: 21
- Information about mental health treatments: 20
- Information about EBPs: 20
- Information about outcomes of SMHA providers: 16
- Information about specific recovery initiatives by the SMHA: 15
- Performance measures about SMHA providers: 12

Seventy-two percent of SMHAs (33) survey consumers to assess the extent to which services did or did not achieve the self-defined goals of recipients. Twenty-five SMHAs make these survey data public, and 23 SMHAs use these data in policy decisions.

NEXT STEPS/FUTURE

The Profiles information about SMHA activities related to the commission goals demonstrates that the states have embraced the goals and challenges of the commission report as a road map to transform their systems. States are in the midst of major changes in the way they organize, fund, and deliver mental health services.

The Profiles Technical Advisory Group met during the spring of 2005 and refined the information compiled by the NRI related to the six goals. The NRI updated the Profiles information on state implementation of the commission goals during the fall of 2005. The updated information became available on the NRI's Web site as of spring 2006. The NASMHPD commissioners have committed to making information and data more accessible to consumers, family members, and advocates, to allow all interested groups to better understand systems and work toward achieving quality and appropriate mental health services for all who need them. The full State Mental Health Agency Profiles, a database on the implementation of the six commission goals is available via the NRI's Web site at www.nri-inc.org. Using the Profiles Web site, interested users can search by state or by keyword to find out what each of the states is accomplishing on the specific issues described previously.

Schools

A large amount of the research on the mental health status of children and youth indicate that public schools are the major providers of mental health services for school-aged children. In the 1999 *Surgeon General's Report on Mental Health* (U.S. Department of Health and Human Services [DHHS], 1999) several prevalence studies found that approximately a fifth of the children and adolescents in the United States experience signs and symptoms of a mental health problem sometime in the course of a school year. The report also suggests that schools are the primary setting for identifying mental disorders in children and youth.

The National data on childhood mental illness describe the prevalence of a range of mental health problems in children and youth. The *Surgeon General's Report on Mental Health* (DHHS, 1999) cites that 3–5% of school-aged children are diagnosed with attention deficit hyperactivity disorder in a 6-month period; 5% of children 9 to 17 years are diagnosed with major depression; and approximately 13% of children 9 to 17 years old experience a variety of anxiety disorders. Based on findings from the 1999 Youth Risk Behavior Survey (Centers for Disease Control and Prevention [CDC], 2000), a national survey of youth, found problems covering a range of severity, from daily sadness and hopelessness (experienced by over a quarter of students) to thoughts of suicide (nearly 20%) to attempted suicide (8%). Many of the children with these conditions had not been identified, and many had not received services, as displayed in **Figure 5-1**.

According to the literature, there are diverse staffing structures, types of professionals, roles, and levels of service in school systems. Staffing structures might comprise individuals and groups of professionals that work in programs operated by single schools, individual districts, and/or in collaboration with the community, city, and/or county agencies. Mental health providers typically provide direct and indirect services to the students, their families, education staff, and school administrators. National data on staffing of school mental health services is provided by the School Health Policies and Programs Study (SHPPS) (CDC, 2000) as shown in graph 2. The SHPPS found that school guidance counselors, school psychologists, and school social workers usually provide school mental health services. The 2006 study found that 77.9%

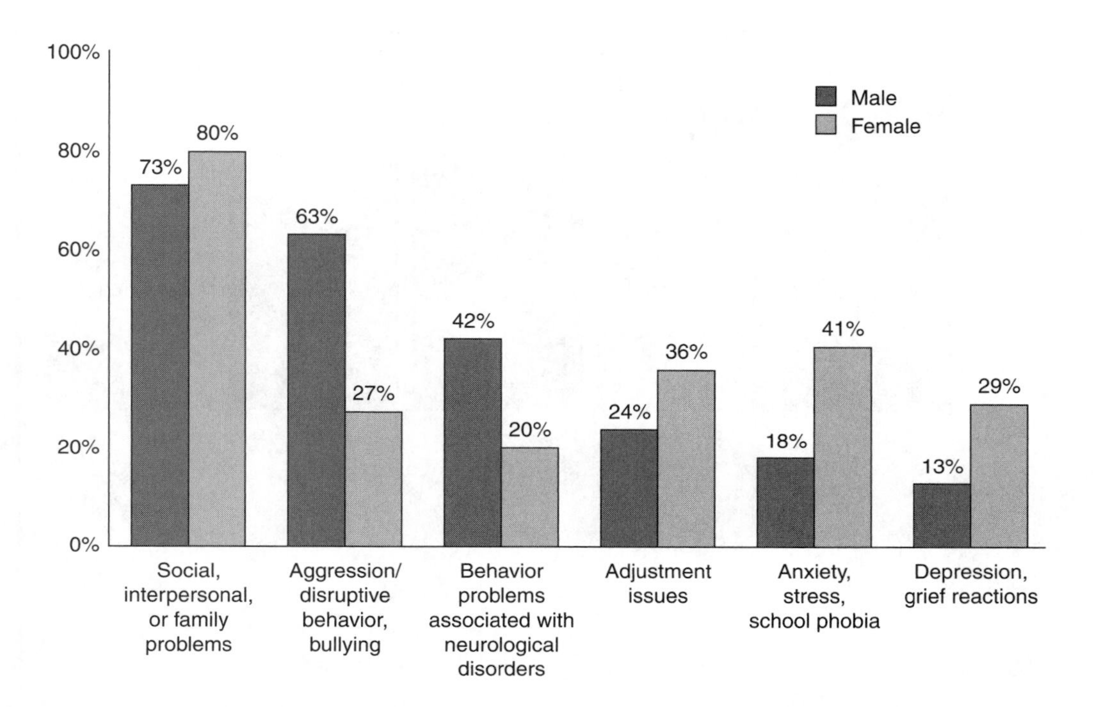

FIGURE 5-1 Percentage of Schools That Ranked the Following Mental Health Problems as Among Their Top Three Problems for Male and Female Students, 2002–2003

Source: *School Mental Health Services in the United States, 2002–2003*. SAMHSA, U.S. Department of Health and Human Services. School Questionnaire, Item 27, Appendix C, School Tables 15, 15A.

of schools had a part-time or full-time school counselor, 61.4% of the nation's schools had a part-time or full-time school psychologist, and 41.7% of schools had a part-time or full-time school social worker. Moreover, 55.6% of states and 73.0% of districts had adopted a policy stating that student assistance programs will be offered to all students, and 57.4% of schools offered such programs as displayed in **Figure 5-2** (Kann, Brener & Wechsler, 2007).

Although school nurses, special education teachers, and other health staff (e.g., resource teachers, rehabilitation, and occupational therapists) are mentioned in the literature, it is not clear to what degree these professionals provide traditional mental health services in the school setting (Flaherty et al., 1998).

Community mental health professionals also may provide services to students, either in the school or in the community setting. These staff may function independently or as teams to deliver services to students. Some approaches (Weist, Lowie,

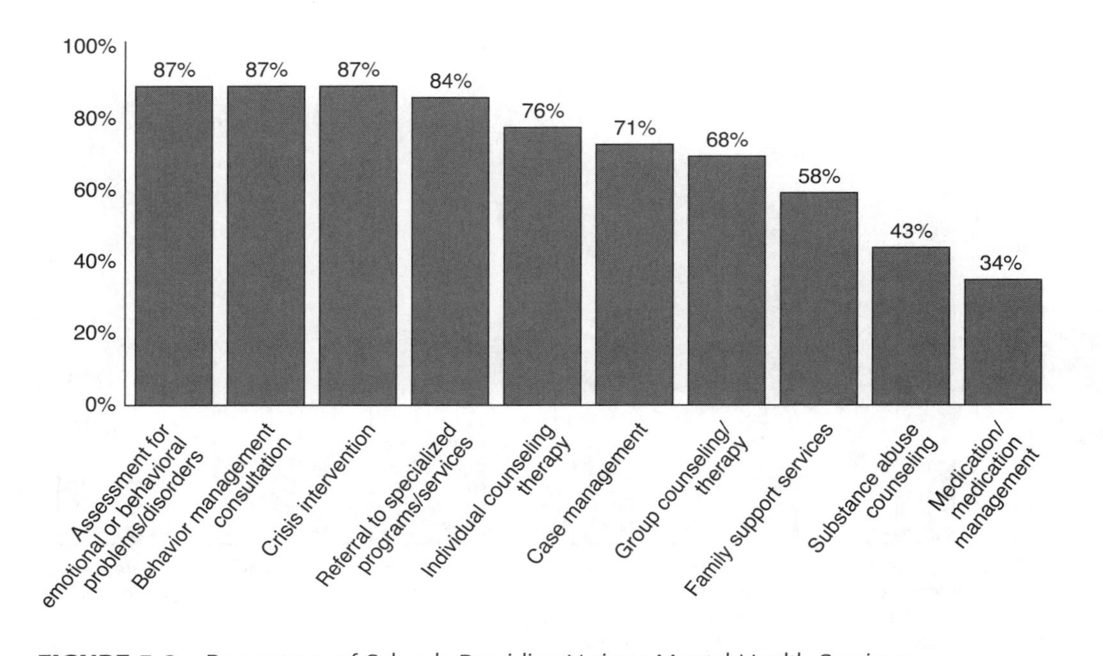

FIGURE 5-2 Percentage of Schools Providing Various Mental Health Services, 2002–2003

Source: *School Mental Health Services in the United States, 2002–2003*. Substance Abuse and Mental Health Services Administration, U.S. Department of Health and Human Services. School Questionnaire, Item 29, Appendix C, School Table 17.

Flaherty, & Pruitt, 2001) involve partnerships between school and community providers to deliver a comprehensive continuum of mental health and social services, including prevention, referral, diagnostic evaluation, treatment, and case management. Moreover, the survey described the problems most frequently presented by students in their school by gender. The list covered a broad spectrum of concerns, from relatively mild, commonly seen problems such as difficulty adjusting to a new school, to more significant behavior problems such as bullying, to serious psychiatric and developmental disorders. The complete list of problem categories is presented in **Table 5-1**.

Although schools reported providing a wide array of services, they also described barriers to ensuring that children and youth receive the services they need. Financial constraints of families (defined in the survey instrument as "can't afford services or lack of insurance") and insufficient school and community-based resources were the factors most often reported as barriers or serious barriers. This finding suggests that even if some mental health services are provided free of charge by school staff, families must pay for other services. Competing priorities for use of funds and difficulties

TABLE 5-1 Psychosocial and Mental Health Problem Categories

Mental Health Problem	Elementary School Students (%)		Middle School Students (%)		High School Students (%)	
	Males	Females	Males	Females	Males	Females
Social, interpersonal, or family	72	80	77	83	66	74
Aggression or disruptive behavior	64	30	69	30	54	18
Behavior problems associated with neurological disorders	51	26	35	15	20	6
Adjustment issues	24	37	27	37	23	27
Depression, grief reaction	8	21	12	31	23	47
Anxiety	17	42	22	12	17	36
Substance use or abuse	**	**	4	3	34	19
Delinquency and gang-related problems	2	**	11	4	10	5

** Value <1%

Source: *School Mental Health Services in the United States, 2002–2003*. Substance Abuse and Mental Health Services Administration, U.S. Department of Health and Human Services.

with transportation were also considered barriers to services. Least often reported as serious barriers were protection of student confidentiality and language and cultural barriers. A large number of students are not able to access mental health services in the community due to linguistic and insurance barriers; in these cases, counseling provided by the school might be the only service available.

Increasingly, education and mental health experts recognize a definition of mental health in schools that includes not only treatment but promotion of social and emotional development and efforts to address psychosocial and mental health problems as barriers to learning (Policy Leadership Cadre for Mental Health in Schools, 2001). Schools have begun to direct resources to schoolwide and/or curriculum-based programs intended to reach the broader student population, not just those individual students identified with mental health problems. Early intervention by mental health staff or multidisciplinary teams is gaining ground as a means to address mild psychosocial problems quickly and thereby prevent unnecessary entry into special education.

Although the focus of the current survey was on traditional mental health treatment, schools were also asked to report on the types of prevention and early intervention programs that they offer.

Although schoolwide screening for behavioral and emotional problems is uncommon, many schools have implemented prevention and prereferral interventions (e.g., team and family meetings for students with behavioral problems) and curriculum-based programs. Schoolwide strategies to promote safe and drug-free schools include programs like the Safe Schools/Healthy Students Initiative (SSHSI). The SSHSI goals are to prevent alcohol, tobacco, or drug use in the schools and receive a wide variety of funds to operate the program. Less frequently reported approaches to prevention and early intervention included peer counseling, mediation, peer support groups, and outreach to parents regarding mental health issues prevalent in the school setting.

Systems of Care: Children, Youth, and Adolescents

A system of care is a wide range of mental health and related services and supports organized to work together to provide care. Systems of care are designed to help children or adolescents with serious emotional disturbances get the services they need in or near their home and community. Youth care, for example, includes service plans that are driven by their families.

In systems of care, local public and private organizations work in teams to plan and implement a tailored set of services for each individual child's physical, emotional, social, educational, and family needs. Teams include family advocates and may be composed of representatives from mental health, health, education, child welfare, juvenile justice, vocational counseling, recreation, substance abuse, or other organizations (see **Figure 5-3** depicting the "Components of Systems of Care"). Mental health care teams find and build on the strengths of a child and his or her family, rather than focusing solely on their problems. Mental health care teams work with individual families, including the children, and with other caregivers as partners when developing a plan for the child and when making decisions that affect the child's care.

Why Are "Systems of Care" Needed?

A serious emotional disturbance touches every part of a child's life. Therefore, children and adolescents with serious emotional disturbances and their families need many kinds of services from a variety of sources, such as schools, community mental health centers, and social service organizations.

Unfortunately, many state and community organizations do not work together to coordinate the services that children with serious emotional disturbances and their

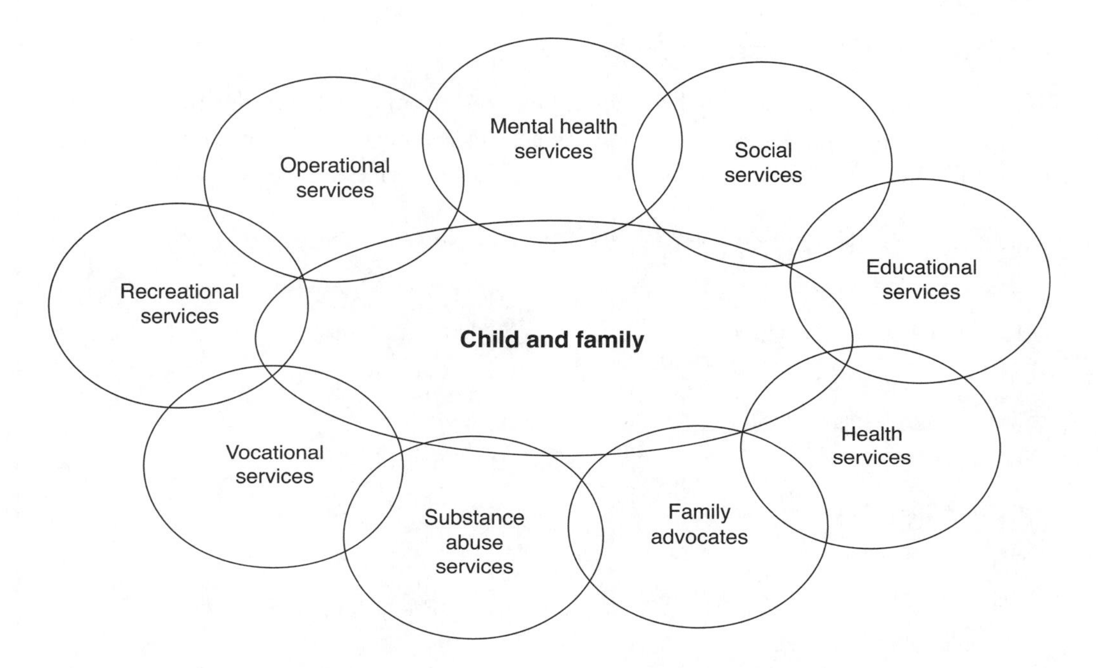

FIGURE 5-3 Components of Systems of Care for Adolescents and Children
Source: Substance Abuse and Mental Health Services Administration: Systems of Care, Children and Adolescents With Serious Emotional Disturbances. Retrieved from: http://mentalhealth.samhsa.gov/publications/allpubs/CA-0014/default.asp. Accessed July 20, 2010.

families need. For example, while children might be attending special education classes at school, they may not have access to after-school or recreation programs. Families might not receive the support they need to care for their children. To get needed services, some families have to give up custody or agree to place their children in a hospital or residential treatment center.

Today, with a much better understanding of serious emotional disturbances, many mental health providers know that children and their families can receive effective, accessible treatment and support through community-based systems of care.

Cultural competence is an important goal in systems of care working with children. It means that each provider organization must show respect for, and respond to, individual differences and special needs. Services must be provided in the appropriate cultural context and without discrimination related to race, national origin, income level, religion, gender, sexual orientation, age, or physical disability, to name a few. Culturally competent caregivers are aware of the impact of their own culture on their relationships with consumers and know about and respect cultural and ethnic differences. They adapt their skills to meet each family's values and customs.

What Kinds of Services Are Included?

The ranges of service that may be included in a system of care fall under the categories shown in Figure 5-3. A young person with a serious emotional disturbance and his or her family may be referred for one or more of these services:

Case management (service coordination)	Protection and advocacy
Community-based inpatient psychiatric care	Psychiatric consultation
Counseling (individual, group, and youth)	Recreation therapy
Crisis residential care	Residential treatment
Crisis outreach teams	Respite care
Day treatment	Self-help or support groups
Education/special education services	Small therapeutic group care
Family support	Therapeutic foster care
Health services	Transportation
Independent living supports	Tutoring
Intensive family-based counseling (in the home)	Vocational counseling
Legal services	

Source: U.S. Department of Health and Human Services (2003).

Integrated Health Models

In the past decade, privatization of mental health care delivery has resulted in the diminishing role of government in administering publicly funded mental health care programs for persons with severe mental illness (SMI). Most states today are contracting out mental health services to nongovernmental, private sector managed behavioral care entities in order to contain costs and reduce fiscal risk. A managed care tracking project funded by the Substance Abuse and Mental Health Services Administration (SAMHSA) documented that 97 managed care programs operating in 47 states include some form of mental health and drug abuse benefits. Most integrated programs (which include mental health and physical health) contract with private sector organizations, whereas carve-out arrangements for behavioral health are equally divided between private and governmental agencies. Almost all contracts place the managed care entity at financial risk through capitated arrangements where the providers are usually paid on a FFS basis (Babigian, Cole, Brown, & Lehman, 1992).

From Unmanaged Care Systems to Managed Care Organizations

How persons with SMI fare under managed care has been a policy concern, particularly when the care has been managed by for-profit companies. Whether the cost reductions and administrative efficiencies associated with managed care in the private health sector can be realized in the public mental health sector is uncertain, given that these persons have the most severe and long-standing psychiatric conditions, often overlaid with a variety of co-occurring medical and substance abuse problems, poverty, inadequate housing, and the lack of social supports. Due to the recurrent nature of their illnesses and the associated high volume of service use, persons with SMI may not fare as well under managed care programs that emphasize cost reductions, substitute high-intensity services for low-intensity services, and cost-shift or outright cost-avoid, whenever possible. Moreover, the variety of social rehabilitative needs that historically were attended to by state funding and by tacit use of insurance reimbursements may be ignored when the criteria of stringent medical necessity is applied. It has been argued that managed care arrangements under a for-profit organizational structure put persons with SMI at a disadvantage.

Studies of managed care programs in the private sector and in some public sector populations have been able to document substantial reductions in the costs of mental health treatment by reducing hospitalization and substituting less expensive and less intensive outpatient services for more costly approaches. Additionally, access to care is increased in that a larger number of enrollees in managed care plans receive mental health services compared to those in FFS plans; however, fewer receive extended treatment in managed care (Rothbard, 1999). Nevertheless, direct application of private sector models to public sector populations is likely to be unsuccessful for persons with SMI unless cost-containment goals are integrated with performance measures involving quality of care. In addition, there needs to be community involvement and oversight through advising boards and consumer groups (Bartsch & Shern, 1990; Stuart & Weinrich, 1998).

However, there is reason for cautious optimism. Preliminary results of a SAMHSA multisite study on managed care for persons with SMI find little difference in satisfaction or clinical outcomes for adults with SMI in managed care versus FFS programs. Five sites have collected data using a common protocol, including common outcome measures. Additionally, the SAMHSA study offers a large amount of person-level administrative data that is equal to or greater than all that exists from individual studies that have been completed to date. Also, information on a variety of managed care programs used by persons with SMI will enable researchers to associate which mechanisms relate to access, utilization, cost, and outcomes of care.

Service System Integration

One promising organizational change is the increased attention paid to addressing service fragmentation, duplication, and restricted array of services available to address effectively the needs of adults with mental illness. Systems-level integration efforts have been aimed at five important areas outlined by Konrad (1996): information sharing and communication, cooperation and coordination, collaboration, consolidation, and integration (single authority, operates collectively, activities fully blended). Changes in these areas are hypothesized to increase the array of available services, increase access to these services, improve service-delivery patterns (e.g., fewer hospital services and more rehabilitation services), and increase service efficiency and effectiveness. One review (Salzer, Kamis-Gould, & Hadley, 2001) indicates that the few system intervention demonstration projects have been undertaken in the adult area, such as the Robert Wood Johnson Foundation Program on Chronic Mental Illness and the Access to Community Care and Effective Services and Supports (ACCESS) study, have produced changes in critical areas like access to services, the development of a continuum of services, decreased use of expensive inpatient services, enhanced service coordination and continuity of care, and consumer satisfaction. However, these interventions have not had a convincing impact on clinical outcomes. Interestingly, similar results are found for systems interventions in the children's area, such as the Fort Bragg Demonstration Project (Bickman et al., 1995) and Stark County Evaluation Project (Bickman, Noser, & Summerfelt, 1999; Bickman, Summerfelt, & Noser, 1997).

Clinical effectiveness is arguably a result of the potency of the services that are delivered. One explanation for why systems integration efforts might not impact clinical effectiveness is that delivered services are not sufficiently improved by increased integration (Goldman, Morrissey, & Ridgely, 1994; Ridgely, Morrissey, Paulson, Goldman, & Calloway, 1998; Salzer & Bickman, 1997). It is noteworthy that, to date, no system integration demonstrations have focused on ensuring that delivered services are more effective. For example, financial incentives for using EBPs or performance-based contracting may lead to the use of more effective services. Such interventions are more likely to succeed in bringing about better clinical outcomes.

Close to 850 integrated delivery systems (IDSs) for health care exist in the United States today. Currently, most systems are considered to be in an evolving state of integration as they attempt to provide a full continuum of services in a user-friendly, one-stop-shopping environment that eliminates costly intermediaries, promotes wellness, and improves health outcomes. Many of the functions of healthcare systems depend on adequate financing. If sustainable financing mechanisms are not put in place, innovative ideas for strengthening the primary healthcare base of healthcare systems will not yield results.

Governance of integrated health systems (IHSs) is the subject of extensive discussion in the literature. Governance determines who exercises control over, and is responsible for, the system and can be a particularly difficult issue within communities, even where there is a high degree of willingness to work together. There are a variety of governance models possible for integrated health systems, ranging from affiliation between agencies based on contractual arrangements, to the corporate model, under which all of the components of the system are centrally owned and controlled. In between these two extremes are a variety of systems, sometimes referred to as "federated models," which involve a degree of shared governance for the IHS while maintaining some corporate autonomy for each partner.

Governance of an IHS can be tailored to fit the wishes of the participants in terms of degree of integration. Some communities may approach the exercise as a means to improve linkages from a patient flow perspective, with each group in the alliance maintaining its individual autonomy. Other communities may wish to take a more assertive approach and develop a corporate entity that would maintain control over its constituent parts. Still others may choose a level of integration somewhere in between. It is also useful to recognize that the governance structure for the system may change over time. The governance of the IHS often evolves and becomes more centralized as the system develops.

Communities must determine whether they need to move to a more centralized system and, if so, assess their readiness to make commitments to increased interdependence. The need for a period of trust building and an airing of mutual expectations is critical before moving on to the development of common governance. Governance may take many forms, and each IHS should create a structure that suits its unique characteristics.

Foster Care

"Early identification of service needs and related interventions for children and youth with intensive mental health needs can be cost-efficient by helping them achieve placement stability and permanence" (Park & Ryan, 2009).

In 1980 Congress passed the first comprehensive federal child protective services act, the Adoption Assistance and Child Welfare Act of 1980 (P.L. 96-272). The act focuses on state economic incentives to substantially decrease the length and number of foster care placements. This act also required specific family reunification services, reflecting the goals of the 1999 White House Conference. However, in 1997, to alleviate many of the defects in the 1980 act, Congress passed the Adoption and Safe Families Act, which shifted the focus from family reunification to expeditious permanency for children in adoptive placements. All state child protection systems adopted the federal guidelines as a requirement for receiving federal subsidies. Thus, because of constitutional and federal statutory requirements, the origin of America's child protection system has led to great uniformity among state programs.

Of the approximately half-million children and adolescents in foster care in the United States, experts estimate that 42–60% of them have emotional and behavioral problems. Children in the foster care systems have high levels of mental health needs and receive inpatient psychiatric care for serious emotional and behavioral problems. The most prevalent health needs of children and teens in foster care are multiple childhood traumas that negatively impact their emotional health. In addition to prior trauma, children in foster care must contend with separation from their family, ongoing losses, and the uncertainty of foster care. Thus children and teens in foster care need timely mental health evaluation and treatment. The mental health professional must be knowledgeable of the impact of emotional trauma on children and teens in general, and specifically for children in foster care. More important, mental health professionals must develop a course of treatment in the context of the child's trauma history, individual strengths, family supports, and permanency plan. One of the leading challenges for the mental health professional assisting a child or teen in foster care is assisting a traumatized child to develop a sense of self-efficacy and build relationships in a forever-changing world.

Child Protective Services

The **Child Protective Services** (CPS) programs function is to ensure that all children are provided with safe, permanent, nurturing families by protecting them from abuse and neglect. With the underlying goal to preserve the family unit where possible, CPS also helps protect children from intentional physical or mental injury, sexual abuse, exploitation, or neglect by a person responsible for the child's health or welfare.

In the United States, in 1655, criminal court cases involving child abuse occurred. In 1692, states and municipalities identified care for abused and neglected children as the responsibility of local government and private institutions. In 1696 England first used the legal principle of *parens patriae*, which gave the royal crown care of "charities, infants, idiots, and lunatics returned to the chancery." This principal of *parens patriae* has been identified as the statutory basis for U.S. governmental intervention in families' child-rearing practices.

In the late 1800s, private child protection agencies designed after existing animal protection organizations were developed to investigate reports of child maltreatment and present cases in court and advocate for child welfare legislation. In 1912, the Federal Children's Bureau was established to manage federal child welfare efforts, including services related to child maltreatment. In 1958 amendments to the Social Security Act mandated that states fund child protection efforts. By the mid-1960s, in response to public concern that resulted from article, 49 U.S. states passed child abuse reporting laws. In 1974 efforts by the states resulted in the passage of the federal Child Abuse Prevention and Treatment Act (CAPTA) (P.L. 93-247), providing federal funding for wide-ranging federal and state child maltreatment research and services. This act was amended several times and was most recently amended and reauthorized on June 25, 2003, by the Keeping Children and Families Safe Act of 2003 (P.L. 108-36). Additionally, CAPTA identifies the federal role in supporting research, evaluation, technical assistance, and data-collection activities; establishes the Office on Child Abuse and Neglect; and mandates the National Clearinghouse on Child Abuse and Neglect Information. CAPTA also sets forth a minimum definition of child abuse and neglect.

Child protective services is the name that many states of the United States use; however, some states use other names, to reflect more family-centered (as opposed to child-centered) practices, such as Department of Children & Family Services (DCFS). CPS is also known by the name of Department of Social Services (DSS) or simply "Social Services." The Child Abuse Prevention and Treatment Act (P.L. 93-247) is a law under CPS that provides federal funding to states in support of prevention, assessment, investigation, prosecution, and treatment activities and also provides grants to public agencies and nonprofit organizations for demonstration programs and projects. One key federal legislation addressing child abuse and neglect is the Child Abuse Prevention and Treatment Act originally enacted in 1974 (P.L. 93-247).

Disaster Management

People who are dealing with the consequences of a disaster have normal reactions as they struggle with the disruption and loss caused by the disaster. Often they do not see themselves as needing mental health services and most likely will not seek mental health assistance. The effects of a disaster like Hurricane Katrina or the Loma Prieta earthquake, a terrorist attack like 9/11, or other public health emergencies can be long lasting, and the resulting trauma can occur in those not directly affected by the disaster. As victims of these natural and human disasters struggle to begin recovery and rebuild their lives, the immediate priorities might be access to water, food, shelter, medical care, and security.

For those affected by some disasters like hurricanes, mass murders and fires, however, the mental health effects can be deep and may linger for weeks, months, or years.

An individual who lives through such an event experiences feelings of sadness, hopelessness, anxiety, and depression. Depending on the individual, these feelings can vary in intensity and duration. Moreover, individuals that witness these events on television, the Internet, or read about them in the newspaper might also experience signs of depression, fear, and anxiety. In addition, the rescue workers, emergency medical personnel, and disaster recovery experts engaged in search-and-rescue operations are mentally impacted by a disaster.

Because victims of a disaster might not seek mental health assistance, community outreach may be necessary to seek out and provide mental health services to individuals who may be affected by a disaster. The Federal Emergency Management Agency (FEMA), established in 1979, ensures that victims of presidentially declared disasters receive immediate short-term crisis counseling, as well as ongoing support for emotional recovery. CMHS collaborates with FEMA to train state mental health staff to develop crisis counseling training and preparedness efforts in their states. In addition to FEMA, historically, the Red Cross emphasized an organized system of relief and recovery; however, they now provide mental health services for survivors of tragic accidents and for family members seeking the status of their loved ones.

ROLE OF THE COMMUNITY MENTAL HEALTH PROFESSIONAL

Recent government reports calling for the healthcare field to strengthen its focus on the importance of mental health and recent advances in understanding the prevention and treatment of mental disorders create exciting opportunities for community mental health professionals. Community mental health professionals can provide comprehensive patient-centered mental health care to individuals, groups, and families across the lifespan. Today, the role of community mental health professional can include research, clinical leadership, education, consultation, clinical practice, outreach, and prevention and case management. In areas of the country where the public health department is the primary provider for mental health care for both inpatient and outpatient services, the training of the community mental health professional can play a pivotal role key role in the transformation of mental health services on a local, state, and national level.

In addition, the role of community mental health professionals involves a full range of primary and community mental health care. Focus is placed on biopsychosocial assessment, diagnosis, and management, including medication management, of patients with a mental illness group facilitator in person or via a telehealth treatment modality. Professionals also serve as advocates, develop funding priorities and support policy changes and services. All roles include a practice with a defined patient population (such as adults, elders, or children and adolescents) and work in a variety of settings, including the following:

- Inpatient psychiatry
- Case management
- Emergency and urgent psychiatry
- Outpatient mental health services
- Psychiatric consult-liaison services
- Chronic care management
- Community social support programs

CHAPTER SUMMARY

Community mental health professionals play an integral role in the delivery of health care to these individuals who must interface with local, state, and federal healthcare delivery systems. The Department of Mental Health and Substance Abuse provides leadership and guidance for the achievement of two broad objectives: (1) closing the gap between what is needed and what is currently available to reduce the burden of mental disorders, and (2) promoting mental health.

The implementation of guidelines recommended in the president's Freedom Commission report focuses on forging strategic partnerships and direction to local and state mental health systems to eliminate stigma, enhance capacity, and increase access to timely and accurate information that promotes learning, self-monitoring, and accountability. Healthcare providers will rely on up-to date knowledge to provide the best possible cost-effective care. The highest quality of care and information will be available to clients and families regardless of race, gender, ethnicity, language, age, or place of residence. This chapter described the current forms of mental health service organization found on a local, state, and national level. The current status of service organization was reviewed and recommendations were made for organizing mental health services, based on an optimal mix of a variety of services. The main recommendations are to integrate mental health services, develop an early detection of mental illness, and improve the mental health care delivery system; develop formal and informal community mental health services; and promote and implement community-based alternatives. Finally, the role of the community mental health professional was discussed. Responsibilities include developing many innovative roles to respond to the need for accessible and high-quality mental health services provided in a community setting. For instance, they may work as specialists in settings such as jail health services, high-risk pregnancy clinics, schools, substance abuse centers and recovery programs, or trauma services, or serve as case managers for the severely mentally ill.

REVIEW

1. Discuss the five most costly mental health conditions in the United States.
2. Explain the major changes in the mental health system starting in 1960.
3. Describe the mental health services both public and private, referred to as the *de facto mental health service system*.
4. The charge to the President's New Freedom Commission on Mental Health was to undertake an in-depth review of the public/private mental health system and make recommendations on steps to achieve an effective mental health system in the United States. List recommendations then determine if the goals and objectives have been met.
5. Many persons with mental illness fall into the criminal justice system. Discuss the relationship of mental illness and the criminal justice system.
6. Discuss how health information technology shows promise for improving mental health care delivery.
7. Review the Federal Child Protective Services Act and the Adoption Assistance and Child Welfare Act of 1980.
8. Review the goals and objectives of the Federal Emergency Management Agency (FEMA).

ACTIVITIES

1. Compare the local and state mental health services where you live with those presented in the chapter. What are the differences and similarities?
2. Interview a local, state, or national politician to determine if mental health funding is a priority in your city, county, or state.
3. Write a two-page paper discussing the goals and qualities of a transformed mental health system.
4. Discuss the role or potential roles of the advanced community mental health professional in the mental health system.

REFERENCES AND FURTHER READINGS

American College of Mental Health Administrators. (1997). *Final report of Santa Fe Summit '97. Preserving quality and value in the managed care equation*. Pittsburgh, PA: Author.

American Managed Behavioral Healthcare Association. (1995). *Performance measures for managed behavioral healthcare programs (PERMS 1)*. Washington, DC: AMBHA Quality Improvement and Clinical Services Committee.

American Psychiatric Association. (1994). *Diagnostic and statistical manual of mental disorders* (4th ed.). Washington, DC: Author.

Babigian, H. M., Cole, R. E., Brown, S. W., & Lehman, A. F. (1993). Methods for evaluating the Monroe Livingston capitation system. *Hospital and Community Psychiatry*, *42*(9), 913–919.

Bartsch, D., & Shern, D. (1990). Screening CMHC outpatients for physical illness. *Hospital and Community Psychiatry*, *41*(6), 35–38.

Beigel, A. (1982). Community mental health centers: A look ahead. *Hospital and Community Psychiatry*, *33*(9), 741–745.

Bickman, L., Guthrie, P. R., Foster, E. M., Lambert, E. W., Summerfelt, W. T., Breda, C., & Heflinger, C. A. (1995). *Evaluating managed mental health services: The Fort Bragg experiment*. New York: Plenum.

Bickman, L., Noser, K., & Summerfelt, W. T. (1999). Long term effects of a system of care on children and adolescents. *Journal of Behavioral Health Services and Research*, *26*(2), 185–202.

Bickman, L., & Salzer, M. S. (1997). Quality of mental health care. *Evaluation Review*, *21*, 285–291.

Bickman, L., Summerfelt, W. T., & Noser, K. (1997). Comparative outcomes of emotionally disturbed children and adolescents in a system of services and usual care. *Psychiatric Services*, *48*(12), 1543–1548.

Bureau of the Census. (1996). *Health insurance coverage: 1996. Table A: Health insurance coverage status and type of coverage*: Washington, DC: Author. Retrieved from: http://www.census.gov/hhes/hlthins/cover96/c96taba.html

Centers for Disease Control and Prevention [CDC]. (2000, June 9). Youth risk behavior surveillance—United States, 1999. *MMWR*, *49*(SS-5).

Centers for Disease Control and Prevention [CDC]. (2000). School health policies and programs study (SHPPS). Retrieved from www.cdc.gov/nccdphp/dash/shpps/http://www.cdc.gov/Healthyyouth/shpps/2006/factsheets/pdf/FS_Trends_SHPPS2006.pdf

Centers for Disease Control and Prevention [CDC]. (2002, April 21). Biological and chemical terrorism: Strategic plan for preparedness and response. *MMWR*, *49*(RR04):1–14.

CMHS Uniform Reporting System (2004).

Cradock-O'Leary, J., Young, A. S., Yano, E. M., Wang, M., & Lee, M. L. (2002). Use of general medical services by VA patients with psychiatric disorders. *Psychiatric Services*, *53*, 874–878.

Flaherty, L. T., Garrison, E. G., Waxman, R., Uris, P. F., Keys, S. G., Glass-Siegel, M., & Weist, M. D. (1998). Optimizing the roles of school mental health professionals. *Journal of School Health*, *68*, 420–424.

Glantz, A. (2008). U.S. Insurers told to cover mental health equally. *OneWorld*. Retrieved from http://us.oneworld.net/places/yemen/-/article/357889-insurers-required-cover-mental-health-equally.

Goldman, H., Frank, R., & McGuire, T. (1994). Mental health care. In E. Ginzberg (Ed.), *Critical issues in U.S. health reform* (pp. 73–92). Boulder, CO: Westview.

Goldman, W. (1997). *Goal focused treatment planning and outcomes*. Minneapolis, MN: United Behavioral Health.

Goldman, W., McCulloch, J., & Sturm, R. (1998). Costs and use of mental health services before and after managed care. *Health Affairs (Millwood)*, *17*, 40–52.

Grob, G. N. (1991). *From asylum to community: Mental health policy in modern America*. Princeton, NJ: Princeton University Press.

Gruttadaro, D. (2005). Consumer and family driven care in a transformed mental health delivery system. *NAMI Advocate*, *3*(1), 12–13.

Hadley, T. R., Schinnar, A., & Rothbard, A. (1991). Managed care in the public sector. In S. Feldman (Ed.), *Managed care*. New York: Thomas.

Hall, L. L., Graf, A. C., Fitzpatrick, M. J., Lane, T., & Birkel, R. C. (2003). *Shattered lives: Results of a national survey of NAMI members living with mental illnesses and their families*. TRIAD Report. Arlington, VA: NAMI.

Institute of Medicine. (1997). *Managing managed care: Quality improvement in behavioral health* (Vols. 1 and 2). Washington, DC: National Academy Press.

Joint Commission on Mental Illness and Health. (1961). *Action for mental health: Final report*. New York: Basic Books.

Kann, L., Brener, N. D., & Wechsler, H. (2007). Overview and summary: School Health Policies and Programs Study 2006. *J Sch Health*, 77, 385–397.

Kessler, R. C., Heeringa, S., Lakoma, M. D., Petukhova, M., Rupp, A. E., Schoenbaum, M., . . . Zaslavsky, A. M. (2008). Individual-level and societal effects of mental disorders on earnings in the United States: Results from the national comorbidity survey replication. *American Journal of Psychiatry*, *165*(6), 703–711.

Konrad, E. L. (1996). A multidimensional framework for conceptualizing human services integration initiatives. *New Directions for Evaluation*, *69*(5), 5–19.

McGuire, T. G., & Fairbank, A. (1988). Patterns of mental health utilization over time in a fee-for-service population. *American Journal of Public Health*, *78*(2), 134–136.

The Metropolitan Medical Response System (MMRS), the National Disaster Medical System (NDMS), and the budget authority for the Strategic National Stockpile (SNS) were transferred to DHS from HHS in P.L. 107-296, the Homeland Security Act. The SNS has since been transferred back to HHS, and the MMRS has been transferred to the Office of State and Local Government Coordination and Preparedness (OSLGCP) in DHS.

Morrissey, J. P., Fagan, J. A., & Cocozza, J. J. (2009). New models of collaboration between criminal justice and mental health systems. *American Journal of Psychiatry*, *166*(11), 1211–1214.

Morrissey, J. P., & Ridgely, M. S. (1994). Evaluating the Robert Wood Johnson Foundation program on chronic mental illness. *Milbank Quarterly*, *72*(1), 37–47.

Moteff, J. D. *Critical infrastructures: Background, policy, and implementation*. CRS Report RL30153 Institute of Medicine Report.

National Advisory Mental Health Council. (1998). *Parity in financing mental health services: Managed care effects on cost, access and quality: An interim report to Congress by the National Advisory Mental Health Council*. Bethesda, MD: Department of Health and Human Services, National Institutes of Health, National Institute of Mental Health.

National Alliance for the Mentally Ill. (1999). *State mental illness parity laws*. Arlington, VA: Author.

National Association of County and City Health Officials [NACCHO]. (1991, October). *Local public health agency infrastructure: A chartbook*. Retrieved from http://www.naccho.org/pubs/detail.cfm?id;eq169. Hereafter cited as NACCHO Chartbook.

National Association of State Mental Health Program Directors Research Institute, Inc. (2003). *Position statement on the president's New Freedom Commission on Mental Health*. Alexandria, VA: Author.

National Association of State Mental Health Program Directors Research Institute, Inc. (2004). *Cultural competency: Measurement as a strategy for moving knowledge into practice in state mental health systems: Final report*. Alexandria, VA: Author.

National Association of State Mental Health Program Directors Research Institute, Inc. (2005). *Funding sources and expenditures of state mental health agencies: Fiscal year 2003*. Alexandria, VA: Author.

National Committee for Quality Assurance. (1997). *Health Plan Employer Data and Information Set 3.0 (HEDIS 3.0)*. Washington, DC: Author.

Park, J. M., & Ryan, J. P. (2009) Placement and permanency outcomes for children in out-of-home care by prior inpatient mental health treatment. *Research on Social Work Practice*, 19, 42–51.

Policy Leadership Cadre for Mental Health in Schools. (2001). *Mental health in schools: Guidelines, models, resources, and policy considerations*. Department of Psychology, University of California, Los Angeles. P. L. 110-343.

President's Advisory Commission on Consumer Protection and Quality in the Health Care Industry. (1997). *Final report to the president: Quality first: Better health care for all Americans*. Washington, DC: Author.

President's Commission on Mental Health (1978). Executive Order 11973. February 17, 1977. Washington, DC: Author.

President's New Freedom Commission on Mental Health. (2003). *Achieving the promise: Transforming mental health care in America. Final report*. DDHS Pub. No. SMA-03-3932. Rockville, MD: U.S. Department of Health and Human Services.

Regier, D., Goldberg, I., & Taube, C. (1978). The de facto U.S. mental health services system: A public health perspective. *Archives of General Psychiatry*, *35*, 685–693.

Regier, D. A., Narrow, W., Rae, D. S., Manderscheid, R. W., Locke, B. Z., & Goodwin, F. K. (1993). The de facto US mental and addictive disorders service system. Epidemiologic Catchment Area prospective 1-year prevalence rates of disorders and services. *Archives of General Psychiatry*, *50*, 85–94.

Ridgely, M. S., Morrissey, J. P., Paulson, R. I., Goldman, H. H., & Calloway, M. O. (1998). Characteristics and activities of case managers in the RWJ Foundation program on chronic mental illness. *Psychiatric Services*, *47*(7), 737–743.

Rothbard, A. B. (1999). Managed mental health care for seriously mental ill populations. *Current Opinion in Psychiatry*, *12*, 211–216.

Rothbard, A. B., Hadley, T. R., Schinnar, A. P., Morgan D., & Whitehill, B. (1989). Philadelphia's capitation plan for mental health services. *Hospital and Community Psychiatry*, *40*, 356–358.

Rupp, A., Gause, E., & Regier, D. A. (1998). Research policy implications of cost-of-illness studies for mental disorders. *British Journal of Psychiatry Supplement*, *173*(36), 19–25.

Salzer, M. S., & Bickman, L. (1997). Delivering effective children's services in the community: Reconsidering the benefits of system interventions. *Applied and Preventive Psychology*, *6*(1), 1–13.

Salzer, M. S., Kamis-Gould, E., & Hadley, T. (2001). Current research on mental health systems integration: Implications and future directions. In L. J. Kiser, P. M. Lefkowitz, & L. L. Kennedy (Eds.), *The integrated behavioral health continuum: Models and processes of service delivery* (pp. 235–256). Washington, DC: American Psychiatric Press.

Schlesinger, M. (1986). On the limits of expanding health care reform: Chronic care in prepaid settings. *Milbank Quarterly*, *64*(2), 189–215.

Snow, D., & Newton, P. (1976). Task, social structure and social process in the community mental health center movement. *American Psychologist*, *31*, 582–594.

Soni, A. (2009, July). *The five most costly conditions, 1996 and 2006: Estimates for the U.S. civilian noninstitutionalized population*. Statistical Brief 248. Rockville, MD: Agency for Healthcare Research and Quality. Retrieved from http://www.meps.ahrq.gov/mepsweb/data_files/publications/st248/stat248.pdf

Stuart, M. E., & Weinrich, M. (1998). Beyond managing Medicaid costs: Restructuring care. *Milbank Quarterly*, *76*(2), 251–280.

Sturm, R., McCulloch, J., & Goldman, W. (1999). *Mental health and substance abuse parity: A case study of Ohio's state employee program* (Working Paper No. 128). Los Angeles: UCLA/RAND Center on Managed Care for Psychiatric Disorders.

Sturm, R., & Sherbourne, C. D. (1999). *Are barriers to mental health and substance abuse care still rising*? Manuscript submitted for publication.

Substance Abuse and Mental Health Services Administration. (1998). *State profiles on public sector managed behavioral health care and other reforms*. Rockville, MD: Author.

Substance Abuse and Mental Health Services Administration. (1999). *Background report: Effects of the mental health parity act of 1996*. Rockville, MD: Author.

U.S. Department of Health and Human Services [DHHS]. (1999). *Mental health: A report of the surgeon general—executive summary*. Rockville, MD: U.S. Department of Health and Human Services, Substance Abuse and Mental Health Services Administration, Center for Mental Health Services, National Institutes of Health, National Institute of Mental Health, Retrieved from http://www.surgeongeneral.gov/library/mentalhealth/home.html

U.S. Department of Health and Human Services [DHHS]. (2006). Public Health Functions Project. Retrieved from http://www.health.gov/phfunctions/

U.S. Department of Health and Human Services [DHHS]; Center of Mental Health Services (CMHS); Uniform Reporting System. (2004). Retrieved from http://mentalhealth.samhsa.gov/cmhs/MentalHealthStatistics/. Note: U.S. Department of Health and Human Services: Center for Mental Health Services, Substance Abuse and Mental Health Services Administration. Retrieved from http://mentalhealth.samhsa.gov/publications/allpubs/CA-0014/default.asp

Weist, M.D., Lowie, J. A., Flaherty, L. T., & Pruitt, D. (2001). Collaboration among the education, mental health, and public health systems to promote youth mental health. *Psychiatric Services*, *52*, 1348–1351.

Wells, K. B. (1999). The design of partners in care: Evaluating the cost-effectiveness of improving care for depression in primary care. *Social Psychiatry and Psychiatric Epidemiology*, *34*, 20–29.

World Health Organization. (2005). *Mental health atlas*. Geneva, Switzerland: Author.

Zuvekas, S. H., Banthin, J. S., & Selden, T. M. (1998). Mental health parity: What are the gaps in coverage? *Journal of Mental Health Policy and Economics*, *1*, 135–146.

UNIT III Mental Health Across the Lifespan

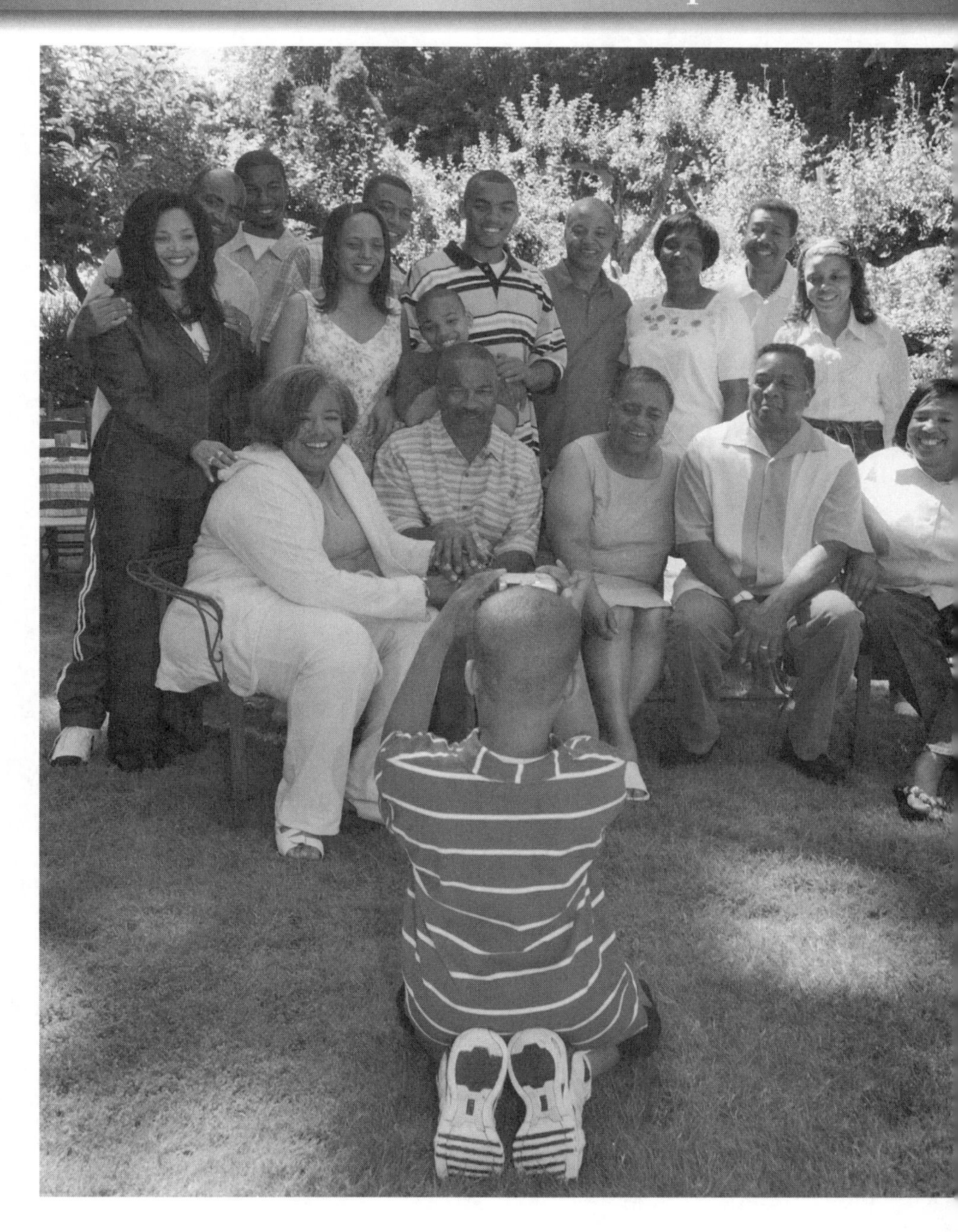

CHAPTER 6

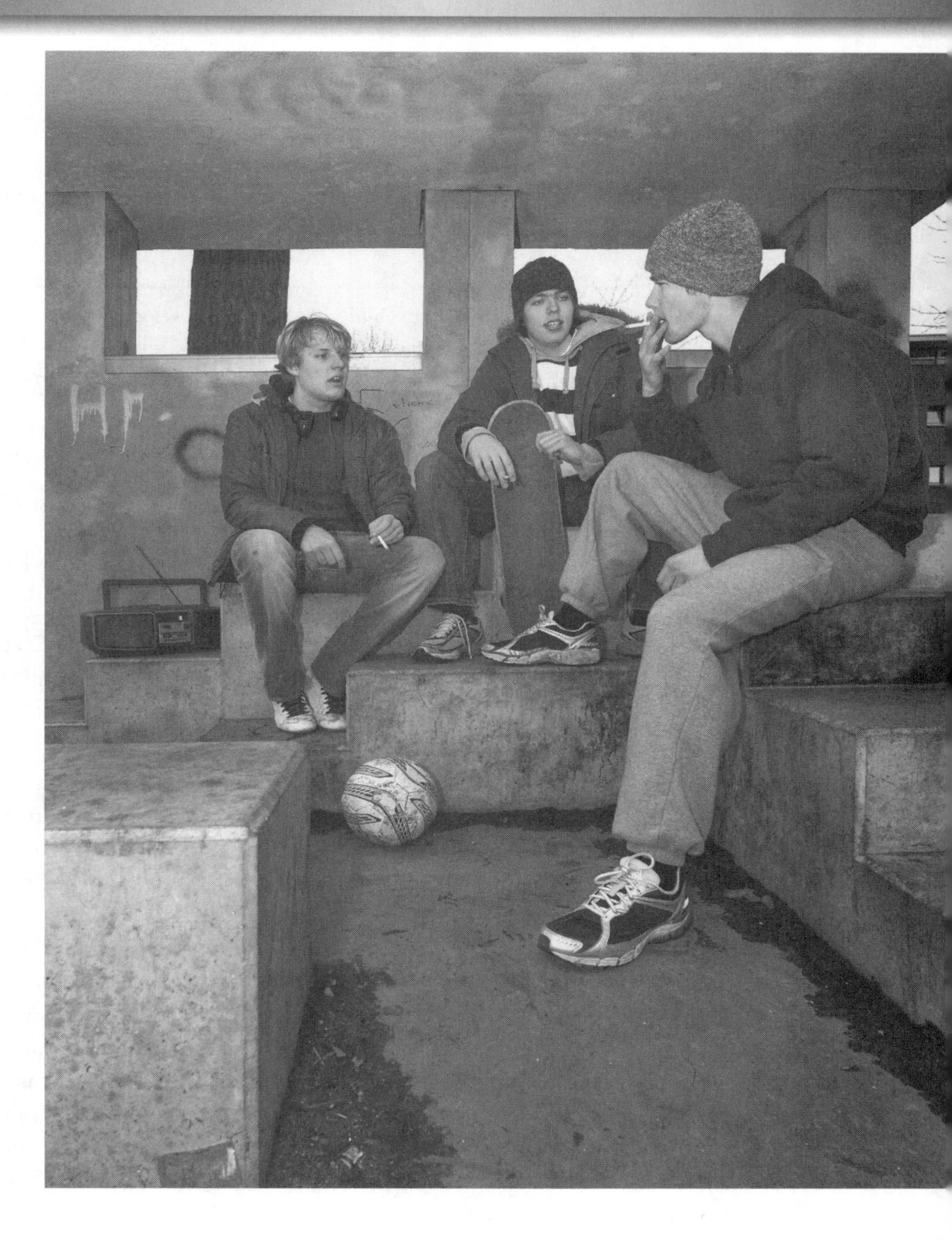

Children, Adolescents, and Mental Health

CHAPTER OBJECTIVES

1. Explain at least four theories related to child and adolescent development.
2. Describe contributing factors to mental health problems among children and adolescents.
3. Describe the challenges associated with diagnosing mental illness among children and adolescents.
4. Explain several common mental health problems among children and adolescents and the related symptoms.

KEY TERMS

- Anxiety disorders
- Attachment theory
- Attention deficient hyperactivity disorder (ADHD)
- Autism
- Bipolar disorder
- Disruptive disorders
- Dysthymic disorder
- Eating disorders
- Pervasive developmental disorder
- Posttraumatic stress disorder (PTSD)
- Reactive attachment disorder (RAD)
- Temperament
- Tourette syndrome

"Mental health in childhood and adolescence is defined by the achievement of expected developmental cognitive, social, and emotional milestones and by secure attachments, satisfying social relationships, and effective coping skills" (U.S. Department of Health and Human Resources [DHHS], 1999). Mentally healthy children and adolescents enjoy a positive quality of life; function well at home, in school, and in their communities; and they are free of disabling symptoms of psychopathology (Hoagwood, Jensen, Petti, & Burns, 1996). Children and adolescence is a time of growth, development, and change and has strong and direct implications for the mental health of an adult. The optimal development of children is considered vital to society, so it is important to understand their social, cognitive, emotional, and educational development. Because about 1 in 10 children in the United States suffer from mental illness and fewer than 1 in 5 receive treatment (Kneisel & Trigoboff, 2009), mental health among this age group is a principal concern.

The developmental process, defined by periods of transition and reorganization, is the focus of much research on this age group. The studies seek to understand and predict the influences that keep children and adolescents mentally healthy and assist with maintaining this health into adulthood. These studies also seek to identify risk and protective factors and understand why children and adolescents who are exposed to the same risk factors have different outcomes. Embedded in this is research on prevention and treatment of mental illness. In these studies, it is essential to consider the children's environment. Children and adolescents must be seen in the context of their social environments such as home and school. These environments can powerfully shape one's development, and they have bidirectional influences.

Treating mental illness among these age groups has unique challenges. This is because the criteria used for adult mental disorders can be difficult to apply to children and adolescents when the signs and symptoms of mental disorders for adults also are characteristics of normal development in children and adolescents. For example, a temper tantrum or an invisible friend could be an expected behavior in a young child, but it is not appropriate in an adult. There is a time in development where it does become apparent that the behavior is not a part of normal development.

Children and adolescents are developing and changing rapidly, which is another reason why treatment can be challenging. Also, disorders in some youth may come and go, and some afflicted children improve as development unfolds, perhaps as a result of healthy influences (DHHS, 1999). Because of the development process, it is important not to characterize the disorder as permanent or unchangeable because the environmental influences and maturity may redirect the child into a healthier state. At the same time, it is essential to not take action and risk the child's not being treated and the condition becoming more severe. As you can see, the science of mental health in childhood and adolescence is complex.

In this chapter we describe the normal development process of children and adolescents and the challenges related to diagnosis and treatment of mental illness among this age group. Also explained are the common mental health problems that children and adolescents experience and the related symptoms.

NORMAL DEVELOPMENT

Development is the lifelong process of growth, maturation, and change that occurs at the fastest pace during childhood and adolescence. An appreciation of normal development is crucial to understanding mental health in children and adolescents and the risks they face in maintaining mental health. Distortions in the process of development may lead to mental disorders. This section focuses on the normal development of children, including progression of their cognitive, social, and temperament attributes.

THEORIES OF DEVELOPMENT

There are numerous theories of development, and we touch on a couple of them. The reason for including these theories of normal development in this chapter is that they provide a foundation on which to understand and identify abnormal development and insight into how children grow into healthy adults. We have broken this section into the stage and nonstage theories.

Stage Theories of Development

The stage theories introduced the concept of thinking about human development and seeing it as a continuous process of physical and psychological tasks that people experience as they age. The stage theories focus on how people mature and hence move through different stages in life. During these stages adaptations are made to physical changes as well as psychological and social changes and challenges. According to these theories, mental health problems occur when the person fails to achieve milestones and objectives in their developmental process. Although these theories have been criticized as being unscientific because they have rarely been tested empirically and are considered not to be culturally sensitive, there are still important concepts to be learned from them.

Psychosocial Stages of Development

Psychoanalyst Erik Erikson was influenced by Freud and believed that the ego exists from birth. Unlike Freud, he believed that personality continues to develop over the lifespan. Erikson also recognized the influence of external factors on development. He felt the course of development is determined by the interaction of the body (genetic biological programming), mind (psychological), and cultural (ethos) influences. Erikson organized life into eight stages that extend from birth to death. The stages contain sets of opposites and are expressed in terms of functioning as an individual and with family and the broader social environment. According to Erikson the stages related to infants, children, and adolescents are as follows:

Infant: *Trust vs Mistrust*. Needs maximum comfort with minimal uncertainty to trust himself/herself, others, and the environment.
Toddler: *Autonomy vs Shame and Doubt*. Works to master physical environment while maintaining self-esteem.
Preschooler: *Initiative vs Guilt*. Begins to initiate, not imitate, activities; develops conscience and sexual identity.
School-Age Child: *Industry vs Inferiority*. Tries to develop a sense of self-worth by refining skills.

Adolescent: *Identity vs Role Confusion*. Tries integrating many roles (child, sibling, student, athlete, worker) into a self-image under role model and peer pressure. (Springhouse Corporation, 1990)

Each stage builds on the successful completion of earlier stages. The challenges of stages not successfully completed may reappear as problems in the future.

Cognitive Development

Jean Piaget, a Swiss psychologist, based his theory on several decades of observations of children (Inhelder & Piaget, 1958). His theory was about how children gradually acquire the ability to understand the world around them through active engagement with it. Piaget was the first to recognize that infants take an active role in getting to know their world and that infants and children are not miniature versions of adult thought.

Although his theory was a great contribution to the field of human development, there are areas of concern. The principal limitations of Piaget's theories are that they are descriptive rather than explanatory. He neglected variability in development and temperament, and he did not consider the important interplay between a child's intellectual development and his or her social experiences (Bidell & Fischer, 1992). These are the stages of cognitive development, according to Piaget:

1. Sensorimotor (*birth to about age 2*): Infants discover motor and reflex actions. The child learns that he or she is separate from the environment. They master the principle of object permanence, and that people and objects continue to exist even though they may be outside the reach of the child's senses.
2. Preoperational (*2 to 7 years of age*): The child begins to use symbols to represent objects, including language. In this stage the child tends to be egocentric and focused on his or her own point of view.
3. Concrete (*7 to 11 years of age*): The ability to think abstractly and make rational judgments begins. Young children begin to think logically.
4. Formal operations (*11 years and older*): Adolescents are capable of hypothetical and deductive reasoning. They have a greater ability to deal with abstractions and engage in scientific thought.

Emotional Development

Erikson believed that an important component of this infancy and childhood is to develop basic trust in others. Many other psychologists hold the belief that children's early relationships are important in their development of relations later in life.

Children must form relationships with their parents as well as with siblings and peers. Peer relationships change throughout the lifespan, and in the very early years children's social skills are very limited so they spend most of their time playing side by side rather than interacting with others.

As children grow, their abilities to form close relationships become highly dependent on their social skills. This includes emotional development and communications skills, including the ability to interpret and understand nonverbal cues. Stanley and Nancy Greenspan proposed seven stages of healthy emotional development from birth to age 4:

1. "0–3 months: Exhibits growing self-regulation and interest in the world
2. 4–5 months: Engages in relationships
3. 6–9 months: Uses emotions in an interactive, purposeful manner
4. 10–14 months: Uses a series of interactive and emotional gestures to communicate
5. 15–18 months: Uses a series of interactive and emotional gestures to solve problems
6. 19–30 months: Uses ideas to convey feelings, wishes, or intentions
7. 31–42 months: Creates logical bridges between emotions and ideas" (Pearson Assessment and Information, n.d.)

Children who lack such skills tend to be withdrawn, are rejected by other children, do not listen to others, and rarely engage with other children in activities (Dodge et al., 1990). They often exhibit features of oppositional defiant or conduct disorder, such as regular fighting, dominating and pushing others around, or being spiteful (Dodge et al., 1990). These social skills can improve if the child is given the opportunity to interact with others. In recent years, knowledge of the importance of children's acquisition of social skills has led to the development and integration of social skills training components into a number of successful therapeutic interventions.

Non-Stage Theories of Development

Other approaches to understanding normal development were less focused on the stages of development. For example, behavioral theorists, such as Ivan Pavlov and B. F. Skinner, explained behavior in terms of responses (behavior) to stimuli (environment); they were interested in how people learn to behave. Social learning theory, developed by Albert Bandura, contributed the idea of role modeling. Several important clinical tools also came out of behaviorism (e.g., reinforcement and behavior modification) and social learning theory (cognitive-behavioral therapy).

Attachment Theory

Attachment refers to an affection bond between one individual and another. Sometimes it is referred to as dependency. **Attachment theory** provides a framework to help with understanding interpersonal relationships between human beings. Attachment theorists believe the human infant has a need for a secure relationship with adult caregivers that fosters social, emotional, and cognitive skills. Separation distress is one way that children show attachment. The children tend to cry, stop their usual activities, and get upset when separated from a caretaker.

The importance of a child's bonds with caregivers was not fully appreciated until John Bowlby introduced the concept of attachment on the effects of maternal deprivation. He believed that attachment has biological foundations and that without it the human species would not survive because an infant needs to be protected and cared for in order to survive. Bowlby (1969) believed that the pattern of an infant's early attachment to parents would form the basis for all later social relationships. On the basis of his experience with disturbed children, he hypothesized that when the mother was unavailable or only partially available during the first months of the child's life, the attachment process would be interrupted, leaving enduring emotional scars and predisposing a child to behavioral problems.

A mother's bond with her child often starts when she feels fetal movements during pregnancy. Immediately after birth, most, but by no means all, mothers experience a surge of affection that is followed by a feeling that the baby belongs to them. This experience does not occur for all mothers or may be delayed, particularly when she has a drug addiction or encounters postnatal depression. Yet, like all enduring relationships, it seems that the relationship between mother and child develops gradually and strengthens over time. Some infants who experience severe neglect in early life may develop mentally and emotionally without lasting consequences. If the neglected infant or child is adopted by parents who provide sensitive, stable, and enriching care, he or she may recover fully. Unfortunately, however, early neglect often continues. When the child remains subject to deprivation, inadequate or insensitive care, lack of affection, low levels of stimulation, and poor education over long periods of time, later adjustment is likely to be severely compromised. One of the problems in the later development of children who experience early institutionalization or significant neglect is that there may have been no opportunities for the caretakers and the infants to establish strong and mutual attachments in a reciprocating relationship. This can cause problems with social relations later in life related to issues such as coping mechanisms, motivation, feelings of security, resiliency, ability to respond to stress, and language acquisition.

Temperament

Temperament is defined as the inherent relatively consistent traits or dispositions that underlie behavior and determine how people react to the world around them. Anna Freud was the first to describe such variations in characteristics, which were systematically derived from her observations of children orphaned by the ravages of World War II. She noticed that some children were affectionate, some wanted to be close but were too shy to approach adults, and some were difficult because they were easily angered and frustrated (Freud, 1965).

For the most part, temperament is an innate quality of the child, one with which he or she is born. It is somewhat modified (particularly in the early years of life) by his or her experiences and interactions with other people and the environment. Interactions with caregivers can modify the child's temperament. When children have difficult temperaments, they usually have more behavioral problems and cause more strain on the mother and family. It is not always clear whether extremes of temperament should be considered within the spectrum of mental disorder (e.g., shyness or anxiety) or whether certain forms of temperament might predispose a child to the development of certain mental disorders.

Examples of the major characteristics that make up temperament are as follows:

- Activity level: The level of physical activity, motion, restlessness or fidgety behavior that a child demonstrates in daily activities (may affect sleep)
- Approach and withdrawal: The way a child initially responds to a new stimulus (rapid and bold or slow and hesitant)
- Adaptability: The degree of ease or difficulty with which a child adjusts to change or a new situation and how well the youngster can modify his reaction
- Intensity: The energy level with which a child responds to a positive or negative situation
- Mood: The mood, positive or negative, or degree of pleasantness or unfriendliness in a child's words and behaviors
- Attention span: The ability to concentrate or stay with a task, with or without distraction
- Distractibility: The ease with which a child can be distracted from a task by environmental stimuli
- Sensory threshold: The amount of stimulation required for a child to respond (American Academy of Pediatrics, 2007).

The relationship between a child's temperament and parenting style is complicated, and it may be either protective if it is good or a risk factor if it is poor. Researchers have long wondered why some children with very supportive and nurturing homes still have done poorly, whereas some from cold and barren home environments have excelled. Part of the answer is that infants are born with differing levels of resilience in their personalities. Another part of the answer is the "goodness of fit" between the child's individual behavior and the way they are reared (Behavioral-Developmental Initiatives, 2008). Generally the better the "fit," the better the results. Temperament is important in parenting in (1) knowing the proper parenting techniques and how to discipline, and (2) how it affects the parent's view of the child and themselves as parents (Behavioral-Developmental Initiatives, 2008). Both of these dimensions are critical in determining how the parent–child relationship evolves over time. Because parents cannot change or determine the child's temperamental style, parenting needs to be molded around the child's temperament. Parents who try to make the child fit their concept of the so-called perfect child usually end up feeling very frustrated (Behavioral-Developmental Initiatives, 2008). A better approach is to observe and learn about the infant's behavioral style and then change the way the parent reacts to the situation. Temperamental characteristics can be very positive in some situations and challenging in others. Only by sensitizing themselves to the infant's personality can parents learn how to respond to it in a helpful way. Most parents learn this through a period of trial and error, but when conflict continues to increase rather than resolve itself, or when it appears unexpectedly, assistance may be welcome (Behavioral-Developmental Initiatives, 2008).

PROTECTIVE FACTORS AND RISK FACTORS

Neuroscience and behavioral research rather than theories are currently used to determine the cause of mental health and illness. Understanding the factors that make children vulnerable to mental illness is important for several reasons. Delineating the range of risk factors for particular mental disorders helps to understand their etiology, the populations most at risk can be identified, understanding the relative strength of different risk factors allows for the design of appropriate prevention programs for children in different contexts, and resources can be better allocated to intervene so as to maximize their effectiveness (DHHS, 1999).

Protective Factors

It is particularly important to prevent mental disorders and to promote healthy development during childhood because many adult mental disorders have related problems in childhood. Therefore it is obviously beneficial to try to intervene early in children's lives before problems occur and they become more unmanageable if they do become evident. The field of prevention has now developed to the point that reduction of risk, prevention of onset, and early intervention are realistic possibilities. Scientific methodologies in prevention are increasingly sophisticated, and the results from high-quality research trials are as credible as those in other areas of biomedical and psychosocial science. There is a growing recognition and increasing supporting research that shows prevention does work.

Prevention is becoming an increasing priority in many social services areas, including prevention. Policymakers and service providers in health, education, social services, and juvenile justice have become invested in intervening early in children's lives: they have come to appreciate that mental health is inexorably linked with general health, child care, and success in the classroom and inversely related to involvement in the juvenile justice system. It also is perceived that investment in prevention may be cost effective.

Some forms of primary prevention are so familiar that they are no longer thought of as mental health prevention activities when, in fact, they are. For example, vaccination against measles prevents its neurobehavioral complications; safer sex practices and maternal screening prevent newborn infections such as syphilis and human immunodeficiency virus (HIV), which also have neurobehavioral manifestations. Efforts to control alcohol use during pregnancy help prevent fetal alcohol syndrome. All these conditions may produce mental disorders in children.

BOX 6-1 Aggressors, Victims, and Bystanders: Thinking and Acting to Prevent Violence

Aggressors, Victims, and Bystanders (AVB): Thinking and Acting To Prevent Violence is a curriculum designed to prevent violence and inappropriate aggression among middle school youth, particularly those living in environments with high rates of exposure to violence. Based on research demonstrating the role of cognitive patterns in mediating aggressive behavior, AVB addresses the differing roles that individuals typically play in promoting or preventing violence.

The core objectives of AVB are to encourage young people to examine their roles as aggressors, victims, and bystanders; develop and practice problem-solving skills; rethink beliefs that support the use of aggression; and generate new ways of thinking about and responding to conflict in each of these roles. A central feature of the curriculum is its four-step Think-First Model of Conflict Resolution. This model helps students pause and reflect when confronted with a conflict so they can define the situation in ways that lead to effective, positive solutions. The curriculum is presented in 12 45-minute classroom sessions conducted one to three times per week over 4 to 12 weeks. AVB can be taught by health educators, language arts teachers, police officers, school resource/safety officers, or physical education instructors.

Source: SAMHSA. (2009). Aggressors, Victims, and Bystanders: Thinking and Acting To Prevent Violence. Retrieved from http://nrepp.samhsa.gov/programfulldetails.asp?PROGRAM_ID=151. Accessed July 15, 2010.

There are some exemplary interventions that focus on enhancing mental health and primary prevention of behavior problems and mental health disorders. Some examples of prevention programs include Project Head Start, the Carolina Abecedarian Project, the Infant Health and Development Program, Elmira Prenatal/Early Infancy Project, and the Primary Mental Health Project.

Risk Factors

Good evidence now indicates that both biological factors and adverse psychosocial experiences during childhood influence—but do not necessarily cause—the mental disorders of childhood. Adverse experiences may occur at home, at school, or in the community. A stressor or risk factor may have no, little, or a profound impact, depending on individual differences among children and the age at which the child is exposed to it, as well as whether it occurs alone or in association with other risk factors. Although children are influenced by their psychosocial environment, most are inherently resilient and can deal with some degree of adversity. However, some children, possibly those with an inherent biological vulnerability (e.g., genes that convey susceptibility to an illness), are more likely to be harmed by an adverse environment, and there are some environmental adversities, especially those that are long-standing or repeated, that seem likely to induce a mental disorder in all but the hardiest of children.

Risk factors for developing a mental disorder or experiencing problems in social-emotional development include biological and psychosocial factors such as prenatal damage from exposure to alcohol, illegal drugs, and tobacco; low birthweight; difficult temperament or an inherited predisposition to a mental disorder; external risk factors such as poverty, deprivation, abuse, and neglect; unsatisfactory relationships; parental mental health disorder; or exposure to traumatic events.

Biological Influences on Mental Disorders

It appears that the origins of most mental disorders are related to some combination of genetic and environmental factors. There is increasing consensus that biological factors exert especially pronounced influences on several disorders including conduct disorder, **pervasive developmental disorder**, **autism**, depression, and attention deficient disorder. It also is likely that biological factors play a large part in the etiology of social phobia, obsessive-compulsive disorder, **Tourette syndrome**, and others.

Two important points about biological factors should be considered. The first is that biological influences are not necessarily synonymous with those of genetics or inheritance. Biological abnormalities of the central nervous system that influence behavior, thinking, or feeling can be caused by injury, infection, poor nutrition, or exposure to toxins such as lead in the environment. These abnormalities are not inherited. Second, it is incorrect to assume that biological and environmental factors are independent of each other. The reality is that they interact, as discussed in Chapter 2. For example, children with a biologically based behavior may modify their environment. For example, low-birthweight infants who have sustained brain damage may become excessively irritable and change the behavior of caretakers in a way that adversely affects the caretaker's ability to provide good care. Thus it is now well documented that a number of biologic risk factors exert important effects on brain structure and function and increase the likelihood of subsequently developing mental disorders. These well-established factors include intrauterine exposure to alcohol or cigarette smoke, perinatal trauma, environmental exposure to lead, malnutrition of pregnancy, traumatic brain injury, nonspecific forms of mental retardation, and specific chromosomal syndromes.

Psychosocial Risk Factors

Environment factors can endanger a child's mental health. Dysfunctional aspects of family life, such as severe parental discord, a parent with substance abuse problems or criminality, a depressed parent, overcrowding, child neglect or abuse, socioeconomic deprivations (which can cause stress in the parents and contribute to child abuse), exposure to violence, or large family size can predispose to conduct disorders and antisocial personality disorders, and the risk is higher if the child does not have a solid and loving relationship with at least one of the parents.

The quality of the relationship between infants or children and their primary caregiver, as manifested by the security of attachment, has long been felt to be of paramount importance to mental health across the lifespan. In this regard, the relationship between maternal problems and those factors in children that predispose them to form insecure attachments, particularly young infants' and toddlers' security of attachment and temperament style and their impact on the development of mood and conduct disorders, is of great interest to researchers. As discussed previously, the attachment process has been shown to be related to mental health problems such as depression, **attention deficient hyperactivity disorder (ADHD)**, and oppositional defiant disorder.

Effects of Parental Depression

Depressed parents may be withdrawn and lack energy and consequently pay little attention to, or provide inadequate supervision of, their children (Center for Mental Health in Schools, 2008). In contrast, depressed parents may be overly critical and irritable, which can be upsetting to children, demoralize them, and distance them (Center for Mental Health in Schools, 2008). At a more subtle level, parents' distress—being pessimistic, tearful, or threatening suicide—is sometimes seen or heard by the child, thereby inducing anxiety. Depressed parents also may not teach their children how to cope with stress through modeling good stress management and resiliency skills, so the child may not learn how to let go of problems and move forward. Depression also is often associated with marital discord, which may have its own adverse effect on children and adolescents. Conversely, the behavior of the depressed child or teenager may contribute to family stress as much as being a product of it. The poor academic performance, withdrawal from normal peer activities, and lack of energy or motivation of a depressed teenager may lead to intrusive or reprimanding reactions from parents that may further reduce the youngster's self-esteem and optimism.

The consequences of maternal depression vary, but they also can be harmful to the mental health of both the parent and the child. An estimated 9–16% of postpartum women experience postpartum depression (American Psychological Association, 2007). The children may become withdrawn, irritable, or inconsolable; display insecure attachment and behavioral problems; experience problems in cognitive, social, and emotional development; and have a higher risk of anxiety disorders and major depression in childhood and adolescence (American Psychological Association, 2007).

During the toddler stage of development, research shows that the playful interactions of a toddler with a depressed mother are often briefer and more likely to be interrupted (by either the mother or the child) than those with a nondepressed parent (Jameson, Gelfand, Kulcsar, & Teti, 1997). Research has shown that some depressed mothers are less able to provide structure or to modify the behavior of excited toddlers, increasing the risk of out-of-control behavior, the development of a later conduct disorder, or later aggressive dealings with peers (Hay, Zahn-Waxler, Cummings, & Iannotti, 1992; Zahn-Waxler, Iannotti, Cummings, & Denham, 1990). A depressed mother's inability to control a young child's behavior may result in the child failing to learn appropriate skills for settling disputes without reliance on aggression.

Stressful Life Events

Stress is related to numerous mental and physical health problems. In most situations, stress is not related to the individual or the situation; it is related to how the individual frames and defines the event or situation. The correlation between stressful life events and risk for child mental disorders is well documented, but this relationship in children and adolescents is complex. The complexity may be due to individual differences and developmental changes. For example, a child's coping mechanisms, level of resiliency, temperament, and social support all impact how the situation is perceived and the effect that it has in both the short- and long-term time frame.

Childhood Maltreatment

Child abuse is a very widespread problem; in 2006, an estimated 3.6 million children were abused, which equates to a rate of 47.8 per 1000 children in the U.S. and Puerto Rico population (National Center on Child Abuse Prevention Research, 2008). Abuse is associated with problems such as insecure attachment, posttraumatic stress disorder, conduct disorder, ADHD, depression, and social and cognitive functioning.

Peer and Sibling Influences

The influence of maladaptive peers can be very damaging to a child and greatly increases the likelihood of adverse outcomes such as delinquency, particularly if the child comes from a family beset by many stressors (Loeber & Farrington, 1998). Sibling rivalry is a common component of family life and may contribute to family stresses. In stressed or large families, parents have many demands placed on their time and find it difficult to oversee, or place limits on, their young children's behavior. When parental attention is in short supply, young siblings squabbling with each other attract available attention. In such situations, parents rarely comment on good or neutral behavior but do pay attention, even if in a highly critical and negative way, when their children start to fight; as a result, the act of fighting may be inadvertently rewarded. Thus, any attention, whether it be praise or physical punishment, increases the likelihood that the behavior is repeated.

ASSESSMENT AND DIAGNOSIS

As with adults, assessment of the mental function of children has several important goals: to learn the unique functional characteristics of each individual (sometimes called formulation) and to diagnose signs and symptoms that suggest the presence of a mental disorder. Case formulation helps the clinician understand the child in the context of family and community. Diagnosis helps identify children who may have a mental disorder with an expected pattern of distress and limitation, course, and recovery. Both case formulation and diagnosis processes are useful in planning for treatment and supportive care. Both are helpful in developing a treatment plan.

Even with the aid of widely used diagnostic classification systems such as the *DSM*, diagnosis and diagnostic classification present a greater challenge with children than with adults for several reasons. Children are often unable to verbalize thoughts and feelings. Clinicians by necessity become more reliant on parents, teachers, and other professionals, who may be unable to assess these mental processes in children. Children's normal development also presents an ever-changing backdrop that complicates clinical presentation. As previously noted, some behaviors may be quite normal at one age but suggest mental illness at another age. Finally, the criteria for diagnosing most mental disorders in children are derived from those for adults, even though relatively little research attention has been paid to the validity of these criteria in children. Expression, manifestation, and course of a disorder in children might be very different from those in adults. The boundaries between normal and abnormal are less distinct and those between one diagnosis and another are fluid. Thus the field of childhood mental health historically downplayed diagnosis.

Most disorders are diagnosed by their manifestations, that is, by symptoms and signs, as well as functional impairment. A diagnosis is made when the combination and intensity of symptoms and signs meet the criteria for a disorder listed in the *DSM*. However, diagnosis of childhood mental disorders, as noted earlier, is rarely an easy task. Many of the symptoms, such as outbursts of aggression, difficulty in paying attention, fearfulness or shyness, difficulties in understanding language, food fads, or distress of a child when habitual behaviors are interfered with, are normal in young children and may occur sporadically throughout childhood. Well-trained clinicians overcome this problem by determining whether a given symptom is occurring with an unexpected frequency, lasting for an unexpected length of time, or is occurring at an unexpected point in development. Clinicians with less experience may either overdiagnose normal behavior as a disorder or miss a diagnosis by failing to recognize abnormal behavior. Inaccurate diagnoses are more likely in children with mild forms of a disorder. We now turn to discussing the more common mental health problems that children and adolescents encounter, which include ADHD, mood disorders, anxiety disorders, autism, disruptive disorders, substance use disorders in adolescents, and eating disorders.

COMMON DISORDERS AMONG CHILDREN AND ADOLESCENTS

Consideration of developmental principles enhances the understanding of mental illness in children and adolescents. According to these principles, a mental disorder results from the interaction of a child and his or her environment. Thus mental illness often does not lie within the child alone. Within the conceptual framework and language of integrative neuroscience, the mental disorder is an emergent property of the transaction with the environment. Proper assessment of a child's mood, thought, and behaviors demands a simultaneous consideration of nature and nurture, genes and environment, and biology and psychosocial influences. These relationships are reciprocal. The brain shapes behavior, and learning shapes the brain.

Mental disorders must be considered within the context of the family and peers, school, home, and community. Taking the social-cultural environment into consideration is essential to understanding mental disorders in children and adolescents, as it is in adults. Focusing on diagnostic labels alone provides too limited a view of mental disorders in children and adolescents.

Mental disorders with onset in childhood and adolescence include, but are not limited to, anxiety disorders, ADHD, autism and other pervasive developmental disorders, eating disorders, and mood disorders. The more common disorders are discussed in this section. Note that it is not uncommon for a child to have more than one disorder or to have disorders from more than one of these groups. Thus children with pervasive developmental disorders often suffer from ADHD. Children with a conduct disorder are often depressed, and the various anxiety disorders may co-occur with mood disorders. Learning and substance-abuse disorders also may coexist.

Anxiety Disorders

Anxiety disorders are a blanket term covering several different forms of abnormal, pathologic anxieties, fears, and phobias. People with anxiety disorders respond to certain objects or situations with fear and dread, as well as with physical signs of anxiety or nervousness, such as a rapid heartbeat and sweating. An anxiety disorder is diagnosed if the person's response is not appropriate for the situation, if the person cannot control the response, or if the anxiety interferes with normal functioning. This section furnishes brief overviews of several anxiety disorders: separation anxiety disorder, generalized anxiety disorder, social phobia, obsessive-compulsive disorder (OCD), and posttraumatic stress disorder (PTSD).

Separation Anxiety Disorder

Separation anxieties are normal among infants and toddlers; they are not appropriate for older children or adolescents and may represent symptoms of separation anxiety disorder. To reach the diagnostic threshold for this disorder, the anxiety or fear must cause distress or affect functioning and last at least 1 month (American Psychiatric Association, 2000). Children with separation anxiety may cling to their parent and have difficulty falling asleep by themselves at night. When separated, they may fear that their parent will be involved in an accident or taken ill, or in some other way be "lost" to the child forever. Their need to stay close to their parent or home may make it difficult for them to attend school or camp, stay at friends' houses, or be in a room by themselves. Fear of separation can lead to headaches, nausea, or vomiting (American Psychiatric Association, 2000). Separation anxiety is often associated with symptoms of depression such as sadness, withdrawal, apathy, or difficulty in concentrating, and such children often fear that they or a family member might die. Young children experience nightmares or fears at bedtime.

The remission rate with separation anxiety disorder is high. However, there are periods where the illness is more severe and other times when it remits. Sometimes the condition lasts many years or is a precursor to panic disorder with agoraphobia. Older individuals with separation anxiety disorder may have difficulty moving or getting married and may, in turn, worry about separation from their own children and partner.

The cause of separation anxiety disorder is not known, although some risk factors have been identified. Affected children tend to come from families that are very close knit. The disorder might develop after a stress such as death or illness in the family, physical trauma, sexual assault, or a move. The disorder sometimes runs in families, but the precise role of genetic and environmental factors has not been established.

Generalized Anxiety Disorder

Children with generalized anxiety disorder (or overanxious disorder of childhood) worry excessively about all manner of upcoming events and occurrences. They worry unduly about their academic performance or sporting activities, about being on time, or even about natural disasters such as earthquakes. The worry persists even when the child is not being judged and has always performed well in the past. Because of their anxiety, children may be overly conforming, perfectionist, or unsure of themselves. They tend to redo tasks if there are any imperfections. They may experience sleep disturbances, restlessness, irritability, and difficulty concentrating (American Psychiatric Association, 2000).

Social Phobia

Children with social phobia (also called social anxiety disorder) have a persistent fear of being embarrassed in social situations, during a performance, or if they have to speak in class or in public; get into conversation with others; or eat, drink, or write in public. People with social anxiety feel that everyone is watching, staring, and judging them (even though rationally they know this is not true). The socially anxious person does not relax and enjoy themselves in public. In fact, they can never fully relax when other people are around. It always feels like others are evaluating them, being critical of them, or judging them in some way. Because the anxiety is so very painful, it is much easier just to stay away from social situations and avoid other people altogether. Many times people with social anxiety simply must be alone—closeted—with the door closed behind them. Even when they're around familiar people, a person with social anxiety may feel overwhelmed and have the feeling that others are noticing their every movement and critiquing their every thought.

Feelings of anxiety in these situations produce physical reactions: palpitations, tremors, sweating, diarrhea, blushing, muscle tension, and so on. Sometimes a full-blown panic attack ensues; sometimes the reaction is much milder. Adolescents and adults are able to recognize that their fear is unreasonable or excessive, although this recognition does not prevent the fear. Children, however, might not recognize that their reaction is excessive, although they may be afraid that others will notice their anxiety and consider them odd or babyish.

Young children do not articulate their fears, but they may cry, have tantrums, freeze, cling, appear extremely timid in strange social settings, shrink from contact with others, stay on the side during social events, and try to stay close to familiar adults. They may fall behind in school, avoid school completely, or avoid social activities among children their age. The avoidance of the fearful situations or worry preceding the feared event may last for weeks and interfere with the individual's daily routine; social life, including speaking in front of people whom they do not know; job; and school.

Attachment Disorders

Attachment is about relationships. Humans need attachments with others for their psychological and emotional development and for survival. Attachment includes the unique relationship between an infant and his or her parents. If the relationship is close and secure, then the child learns to trust and love. If the relationship is not consistent and is emotionally distant, then the child learns not to trust or care. The quality of this relationship has an impact on the rest of his or her life.

Causes include neglect or impaired caregiving, abuse, or loss of parents. Children may experience the loss of primary caregivers because they are physically separated from them, the parents die, or they are incapable of providing adequate care. Even if alternate caregivers are competent, the removal from primary caregivers can cause serious problems by breaking primary attachments.

Reactive attachment disorder (RAD) begins before the age of 5, according to the *DSM-IV-TR*. Inappropriate social relatedness in most contexts is a key marker. The child has either a persistent failure to initiate or respond in a developmentally appropriate fashion to most social interactions (e.g., avoidance, resistance to comforting) or diffuse attachments as manifested by indiscriminate sociability with marked inability to exhibit appropriate selective attachments (e.g., excessive familiarity with relative strangers or lack of selectivity in choice of attachment figures) (American Psychiatric Association, 2000).

Symptoms of attachment disorders include infants resisting being held or touched. Young children may seem withdrawn and passive (Encyclopedia of Mental Disorders, 2010). They may ignore others or respond to others in odd ways. Some may seem overly familiar with strangers and touch or cling to people they have just met. They often lack empathy, and their behavior may come across to others as needy and strange, unlike the normal friendliness of children (Encyclopedia of Mental Disorders, 2010). Other symptoms of reactive attachment disorder in children can include the following:

- Inability to learn from mistakes (poor cause-and-effect thinking)
- Learning problems or delays in learning
- Impulsive behavior
- Abnormal speech patterns
- Destructive or cruel behavior (Encyclopedia of Mental Disorders, 2010).

Attention Deficit Hyperactivity Disorder

Attention deficit and disruptive behavior disorder is an expression used to describe a set of externalizing negativistic behaviors that co-occur during childhood. The three subgroups of externalizing behaviors are oppositional defiant disorder (ODD), conduct disorder (CD), and ADHD. ODD consists of a pattern of negativistic, hostile, and defiant behavior lasting at least 6 months. Examples of behaviors that fall into this category include often loses temper, argues with adults, actively defies or refuses to comply with adults' requests or rules, and deliberately annoys people. CD can include behavior such as aggression to people or animals, property destruction, theft, and serious violations of rules. As its name implies, ADHD is characterized by two distinct sets of symptoms: inattention and hyperactivity impulsivity. Although these problems usually occur together, one may be present without the other to qualify for a diagnosis (American Psychiatric Association, 2000). Inattention or attention deficit may not become apparent until a child enters the challenging environment of elementary school. Such children then have difficulty paying attention to details and are easily distracted by other events that are occurring at the same time; they find it difficult and unpleasant to finish their schoolwork; they put off anything that requires a sustained mental effort; they are prone to make careless mistakes and are disorganized, losing their school books and assignments; they appear not to listen when spoken to and often fail to follow through on tasks (American Psychiatric Association, 2000).

The symptoms of hyperactivity, which become apparent at a rather young age, include fidgeting, squirming around when seated, and having to get up frequently to walk or run around. They always seem to be "on the go" or constantly in motion. They dash around touching or playing with whatever is in sight, have difficulty playing quietly, and/or talk incessantly. Sitting still at dinner or during a school lesson or story can be a difficult task. They squirm and fidget in their seats or roam around the room, wiggle their feet, not wait their turn, or noisily tap their pencil.

Many of these symptoms occur from time to time in normal children. However, in children with ADHD they occur very frequently and in several settings, at home and at school, or when visiting with friends, and they interfere with the child's functioning. Children suffering from ADHD may perform poorly at school; they may be unpopular with their peers, if other children perceive them as being unusual or a nuisance; and their behavior can present significant challenges for parents, leading some to be overly harsh.

Inattention tends to persist through childhood and adolescence into adulthood, whereas the symptoms of motor hyperactivity and impulsivity tend to diminish with age. Many children with ADHD develop learning difficulties that may not improve with treatment (Mannuzza, Klein, Bessler, Malloy, & LaPadula, 1993).

Even though a great many children with this disorder ultimately adjust, some—especially those with an associated conduct or oppositional-defiant disorder—are more likely to drop out of school and fare more poorly in their later careers than children without ADHD. As they grow older, some teens who have had severe ADHD since middle childhood experience periods of anxiety or depression. Hyperactive behavior is often associated with the development of other disruptive disorders, particularly conduct and oppositional-defiant disorder. The *DSM-IV-TR* (American Psychiatric Association, 2000) criteria for ADHD include:

A. Either (1) or (2):
   1. six (or more) of the following symptoms of inattention have persisted for at least six months to a degree that is maladaptive and inconsistent with developmental level:

      Inattention

      - Often fails to give close attention to details or makes careless mistakes in schoolwork, work, or other activities
      - Often has difficulty sustaining attention in tasks or play activities
      - Often does not seem to listen when spoken to directly
      - Often does not follow through on instructions and fails to finish schoolwork, chores, or duties in the workplace (not due to oppositional behavior or failure to understand instructions)
      - Often has difficulty organizing tasks and activities
      - Often avoids, dislikes, or is reluctant to engage in tasks that require sustained mental effort (such as schoolwork or homework)

  - Often loses things necessary for tasks or activities (e.g., toys, school assignments, pencils, books, or tools)
  - Is often easily distracted by extraneous stimuli
  - Is often forgetful in daily activities

2. Six (or more) of the following symptoms of hyperactivity-impulsivity have persisted for at least six months to a degree that is maladaptive and inconsistent with developmental level:

   Hyperactivity

   - Often fidgets with hands or feet or squirms in seat
   - Often leaves seat in classroom or in other situations in which remaining seated is expected
   - Often runs about or climbs excessively in situations in which it is inappropriate (in adolescents or adults, may be limited to subjective feelings of restlessness)
   - Often has difficulty playing or engaging in leisure activities quietly
   - Is often "on the go" or often acts as if "driven by a motor"
   - Often talks excessively

   Impulsivity

   - Often blurts out answers before questions have been completed
   - Often has difficulty awaiting turn
   - Often interrupts or intrudes on others (e.g., butts into conversations or games)

- Some hyperactive-impulsive or inattentive symptoms that cause impairment were present before age 7 years.
- Some impairment from the symptoms is present in two or more settings (e.g., at school [or work] and at home).
- There must be clear evidence of clinically significant impairment in social, academic, or occupational functioning.
- The symptoms do not occur exclusively during the course of a pervasive developmental disorder, schizophrenia, or other psychotic disorder and are not better accounted for by another mental disorder (e.g., mood disorder, anxiety disorder, dissociative disorder, or a personality disorder).

Eating Disorders

Eating disorders involve extreme emotions, attitudes, and behaviors involving weight and food. Eating disorders often are long-term illnesses that may require long-term treatment. In addition, eating disorders frequently occur with other mental disorders such as depression, substance abuse, and anxiety disorders (National Institute of Mental Health, 2002, cited in DHHS, 2003). The earlier these disorders are diagnosed and treated, the better the chances are for full recovery. They usually arise in adolescence and disproportionately affect females. Research shows that more than 90% of those who have eating disorders are women between 12 and 25 years of age (National Alliance for the Mentally Ill, 2003, cited in DHHS, 2003). However, increasing numbers of older women and men also have these disorders. In addition, hundreds of thousands of boys are affected (U.S. DHHS Office on Women's Health, 2000, cited in DHHS, 2003).

The three main eating disorders are anorexia nervosa, bulimia nervosa, and binge-eating disorder. The symptoms are as follows:

- *Anorexia nervosa*: People develop unusual eating habits such as avoiding food and meals, picking out a few foods and eating them in small amounts, weighing their food, and counting the calories of everything they eat. Also, they may exercise excessively.
- *Bulimia nervosa*: People eat an excessive amount of food in a single episode and almost immediately make themselves vomit or use laxatives or diuretics (water pills) to get rid of the food in their bodies. This behavior often is referred to as the "binge/purge" cycle. Like people with anorexia, people with bulimia have an intense fear of gaining weight.
- *Binge-eating disorder*: People with this recently recognized disorder have frequent episodes of compulsive overeating, but unlike those with bulimia, they do not purge their bodies of food (National Institute of Mental Health, 2002, cited in DHHS, 2003). During these food binges, they often eat alone and very quickly, regardless of whether they feel hungry or full. They often feel shame or guilt over their actions. Unlike anorexia and bulimia, binge-eating disorder occurs almost as often in men as in women (National Eating Disorders Association, 2002, cited in DHHS, 2003).

Mood Disorders

Mood disorders, also called affective disorders, involve persistent feelings of sadness or periods of feeling overly happy, or fluctuations from extreme happiness to extreme sadness. Although many people go through sad or elated moods from time to time, people with mood disorders suffer from severe or prolonged mood states that disrupt their daily functioning.

The following are the most common types of mood disorders experienced by children and adolescents:

- Major depression: A 2-week period of a depressed or irritable mood or a noticeable decrease in interest or pleasure in usual activities, along with other signs of a mood disorder.
- Dysthymia (**dysthymic disorder**): A chronic low-grade depressed or irritable mood for at least 1 year.
- Manic depression (bipolar disorder): At least one episode of a depressed or irritable mood and at least one period of a manic (persistently elevated) mood.
- Mood disorder due to a general medical condition: Many medical illnesses (including cancer, injuries, infections, and chronic medical illnesses) can trigger symptoms of depression.
- Substance-induced mood disorder: Symptoms of depression due to the effects of medication, drug abuse, exposure to toxins, or other forms of treatment (Children's Hospital, Boston, 2007).

Seven to 14% of children experience an episode of major depression before the age of 15, and 20–30% of adult bipolar patients report having their first episode before the age of 20 (Children's Hospital, Boston, 2007).

Major depressive disorder is a serious condition characterized by one or more major depressive episodes. Depressed children are sad, they lose interest in activities that used to please them, and they criticize themselves and feel that others criticize them. They feel unloved, pessimistic, or even hopeless about the future; they think that life is not worth living, and thoughts of suicide may be present. Depressed children and adolescents are often irritable, and their irritability may lead to aggressive behavior. They are indecisive, have problems concentrating, and may lack energy or motivation; have a loss of interest or pleasure; and their normal sleep patterns may be disturbed (American Psychiatric Association, 2000).

Dysthymic disorder is a mood disorder like major depressive disorder, but it has fewer symptoms and is more chronic. Because of its persistent nature, the disorder is especially likely to interfere with normal adjustment. The child or adolescent is depressed for most of the day, on most days, and symptoms continue for several years. Sometimes children are depressed for so long that they do not recognize their mood as out of the ordinary and thus may not complain of feeling depressed. When a combination of major depression and dysthymia occurs, the condition is referred to as double depression.

Bipolar disorder is a mood disorder in which episodes of mania alternate with episodes of depression. Frequently, the condition begins in adolescence. The first manifestation of bipolar illness is usually a depressive episode. The first manic features may not occur for months or even years thereafter, or they may occur either during the first depressive illness or later, after a symptom-free period (Strober, Schmidt-Lackner, Freeman, Bower, Lampert, & DeAntonio, 1995). The clinical problems of mania are very different from those of depression. Adolescents with mania or hypomania feel energetic, confident, and special; they usually have difficulty sleeping but do not tire; and they talk a great deal, often speaking very rapidly or loudly. They may complain that their thoughts are racing. They may do schoolwork quickly and creatively but in a disorganized, chaotic fashion. When manic, adolescents may have exaggerated or even delusional ideas about their capabilities and importance, may become overconfident, and may be fresh and uninhibited with others; they start numerous projects that they do not finish and may engage in reckless or risky behavior, such as fast driving or unsafe sex. Sexual preoccupations are increased and may be associated with promiscuous behavior.

Risk Factors for Suicide and Suicidal Behavior

Because mood disorders such as depression substantially increase the risk of suicide, suicidal behavior is a matter of serious concern for clinicians who deal with the mental health problems of children and adolescents. Of 100,000 adolescents, 2000 to 3000 will have a mood disorder, of which 8 to 10 will commit suicide (Children's Hospital, Boston, 2007). The incidence of suicide attempts reaches a peak during the mid-adolescent years. Although suicide cannot be defined as a mental disorder, the various risk factors—especially the presence of mood disorders—that predispose young people to such behavior are given special emphasis in this section, as is a discussion of the effectiveness of various forms of treatment. Risk factors for suicide include personal issues, such as having a mental disorder and being gay or a lesbian; family issues, such as abuse; and environmental issues, such as having access to firearms.

Stressful life events often lead to suicide or a suicide attempt. As indicated earlier, these stressful life events include getting into trouble at school or with a law enforcement agency, a ruptured relationship with a boyfriend or a girlfriend, or a fight among friends. They are rarely a sufficient cause of suicide, but they can be precipitating factors in young people.

Obsessive-Compulsive Disorder

Obsessive-compulsive disorder (OCD), which is classified in the *DSM-IV-TR* (American Psychiatric Association, 2000) as an anxiety disorder, is characterized by recurrent, time-consuming obsessive or compulsive behaviors that cause distress and/or impairment. Obsessions are intrusive, irrational thoughts—unwanted ideas or impulses that repeatedly well up in a person's mind (National Alliance on Mental Illness [NAMI], 2003). The obsessions may be repetitive intrusive images, thoughts, or impulses. Compulsions are repetitive rituals such as handwashing, counting, checking, hoarding, or arranging. An individual repeats these actions, perhaps feeling momentary relief, but without feeling satisfaction or a sense of completion (NAMI, 2003). People with OCD feel they must perform these compulsive rituals or something bad will happen.

There is a strong familial component to OCD, and there is evidence from twin studies of both genetic susceptibility and environmental influences. If one twin has OCD, the other twin is more likely to have OCD if the children are identical twins rather than fraternal twin pairs. It does not appear that the child is simply imitating the relative's behavior because children who develop OCD tend to have symptoms different from those of relatives with the disease (Leonard, Rapoport, & Swedo, 1997).

A large body of scientific evidence suggests that OCD results from a chemical imbalance in the brain. For years, mental health professionals incorrectly assumed OCD resulted from bad parenting or personality defects. This theory has been disproven over the last 20 years. OCD symptoms are not relieved by psychoanalysis or other forms of "talk therapy," but there is evidence that behavior therapy can be effective, alone or in combination with medication (NAMI, 2003). People with OCD can often say "why" they have obsessive thoughts or why they behave compulsively. But the thoughts and the behavior continue. People whose brains are injured sometimes develop OCD, which suggests it is a physical condition. If a placebo is given to people who are depressed or who experience panic attacks, 40% say they feel better (NAMI, 2003). If a placebo is given to people who experience obsessive-compulsive disorder, only about 2% say they feel better (NAMI, 2003). This also suggests a physical condition. Clinical researchers have implicated certain brain regions in OCD. They have discovered a strong link between OCD and a brain chemical called serotonin, a neurotransmitter that helps nerve cells communicate with each other. Scientists also have observed that people with OCD have increased metabolism (NAMI, 2003).

Posttraumatic Stress Disorder

Annually, more than five million children experience some extreme traumatic event in the United States. These include natural disasters (e.g., tornadoes, floods, hurricanes), motor vehicle accidents, life threatening illness, painful medical procedures, physical and sexual abuse, witnessing domestic or community violence, kidnapping and sudden death of a parent (Perry, 2002). Approximately 3 million children each year are diagnosed with PTSD (Cincinnati Children's Hospital Medical Center, 2007), and more than 40% of the 5 million children exposed to trauma will develop some form of chronic neuropsychiatric problem that can significantly impair their emotional, academic, and social functioning (Perry, 2002). Most of these neuropsychiatric problems are classified as anxiety disorders, with the most common being **posttraumatic stress disorder (PTSD)** (Perry, 2002).

PTSD originates from the maladaptive persistence of appropriate and adaptive responses present during traumatic stress. A child's/adolescent's risk for developing PTSD is often affected by the child's or adolescent's proximity and relationship to the trauma, the severity of the trauma, the duration of the traumatic event, the recurrence of the traumatic event, the resiliency of the child, the coping skills of the child, and the support resources available to the child from the family and community following the event(s) (Cincinnati Children's Hospital Medical Center, 2007). The organ mediating the adaptive—and the maladaptive—responses related to traumatic stress is the human brain. PTSD is a clinical syndrome that may develop following extreme traumatic stress (American Psychiatric Association, 2000). According to the *DSM-IV-TR*, the person must have been exposed to a traumatic event in which both of the following were present: (1) The person experienced, witnessed, or was confronted with an event or events that involved actual or threatened death or serious injury, or a threat to the physical integrity of self or others, and (2) the person's response involved intense fear, helplessness, or horror. The *DSM-IV-TR* notes that in children this may be expressed instead by disorganized or agitated behavior. Signs and symptoms must be present for more than 1 month following the traumatic event and cause clinically significant disturbance in functioning. A child is considered to have acute stress disorder if the duration of symptoms is less than 3 months, chronic for more 3 months or more, and delayed onset when symptoms develop initially 6 months or more after the trauma (American Psychiatric Association, 2000). Children with PTSD may present with a combination of problems. In fact, two children may both meet diagnostic criterion for PTSD but have a very different set of symptoms (Perry, 2002).

Typical signs and symptoms of PTSD include impulsivity, distractibility and attention problems, dysphoria, emotional numbing, social avoidance, dissociation, sleep disturbances, aggressive (often reenactment) play, depression, irritability, avoiding certain places or situations that bring back memories, and problems in school (Cincinnati Children's Hospital Medical Center, 2007; Perry, 2002). Young children with PTSD may suffer from delayed development in areas such as toilet training, motor skills, and language. In most studies examining the development of PTSD following a given traumatic experience, twice as many children suffer from significant posttraumatic signs or symptoms but lack all of the criteria necessary for the diagnosis of

PTSD. In these cases, the clinician may identify trauma-related symptoms as part of another neuropsychiatric syndrome.

There are apparent gender differences in the expression and development of PTSD. Clinical experience and recent studies suggest that females tend to exhibit more internalizing (i.e., anxiety, dysphoria, dissociation, avoidance) and males more externalizing (i.e., impulsivity, aggression, inattention, hyperactivity) posttraumatic symptoms. In epidemiologic studies of PTSD in the general adult population, females have higher rates of PTSD than males.

Autism

Autism spectrum disorders (ASDs) are complex developmental disorders of brain function. Each can affect a child's ability through signs of impaired social interaction, problems with verbal and nonverbal communication, and unusual or severely limited activities and interest. These symptoms typically appear during the first 3 years of life (NAMI, 2008). There is no cure for ASDs, but with appropriate early intervention, a child may improve social development and reduce undesirable behaviors.

ASDs affect an estimated 2 to 6 per 1000 children and are about four times more prevalent among males than females (NAMI, 2008). They do not discriminate against racial, ethnic, or social backgrounds. ASDs affect individuals differently and to varying degrees. The ASDs are autism (the defining disorder of the spectrum), Asperger syndrome, pervasive developmental disorder not otherwise specified (PDD-NOS), Rett syndrome, and childhood disintegrative disorder (CDD). The most severe cases are marked by extremely repetitive, unusual, self-injurious, and aggressive behavior. This behavior may persist over time and prove very difficult to change, posing a tremendous challenge to those who must live with, treat, and teach these individuals. The mildest forms of autism resemble a personality disorder associated with a perceived learning disability.

Children diagnosed with an ASD do not embrace the typical patterns of child development. Some hints of future problems may be apparent from birth, whereas in most cases, signs become evident when a child's communication and social skills lag further behind other children of the same age. Some parents report the change as being sudden, and that their children start to reject people, act strangely, and lose language and social skills they had previously acquired.

ASDs are defined by a definite set of behaviors that can range from very mild to severe. Children with ASDs may fail to respond to their name and often avoid eye contact. They also have difficulty interpreting tone of voice or facial expressions and do not respond to others' emotions or watch other people's faces for cues about appropriate behavior. Many children engage in repetitive movements such as rocking and hair twirling, or in self-injurious behavior such as nail biting or head banging. They tend to speak later than other children and may refer to themselves by name instead of "I" or "me." Some speak in a singsong voice about a narrow range of favorite topics, with little regard for the interests of the person to whom they are speaking (NAMI, 2008).

Children do not outgrow ASDs, but studies show that early diagnosis and intervention lead to significantly improved outcomes. Signs to look for include the following:

- Lack of or delay in spoken language (does not babble, point, or make meaningful gestures by 1 year; does not speak one word by 16 months; does not combine two words by 2 years; does not respond to name; or loses language or social skill)
- Repetitive use of language and/or motor mannerisms (e.g., hand-flapping, twirling objects)
- Little or no eye contact
- Lack of interest in peer relationships
- Lack of spontaneous or make-believe play
- Persistent fixation on parts of objects
- Does not smile (NAMI, 2008).

Symptoms of an ASD do not remain static over a lifetime. About a third of children with an ASD—especially those with severe cognitive impairment and motor deficits—eventually develop epilepsy (NAMI, 2008). In many children, symptoms of an ASD improve with intervention or as the children mature. Some eventually lead normal or near-normal lives. ASDs in adolescence could worsen behavior problems in some children as they may become depressed or increasingly unmanageable. Parents should be aware and ready to adjust treatment to fit their child's changing needs (NAMI, 2008).

Disruptive Disorders

Disruptive disorders, such as oppositional defiant disorder (ODD) and conduct disorder (CD), are characterized by antisocial behavior and, as such, seem to be a collection of behaviors rather than a coherent pattern of mental dysfunction. These behaviors are also frequently found in children who suffer from ADHD, another disruptive disorder. Children who develop the more serious conduct disorders often show signs of these disorders at an earlier age. Although it is common for a very young child to snatch something he or she desires from another child, this kind of behavior may herald a more generally aggressive behavior and be the first sign of an emerging oppositional defiant or conduct disorder if it occurs by the ages of 4 or 5 and later. However, not every oppositional defiant child develops conduct disorder, and the difficult behaviors associated with these conditions often remit.

ODD is diagnosed when a child displays a persistent or consistent pattern of defiance, disobedience, and hostility toward various authority figures including parents, teachers, and other adults. It is characterized by such problem behaviors as persistent fighting and arguing, being touchy or easily annoyed, and deliberately annoying or being spiteful or vindictive to other people. Children with ODD may repeatedly lose their temper, argue with adults, deliberately refuse to comply with requests or rules of adults, blame others for their own mistakes, and be repeatedly angry and resentful. Stubbornness and testing of limits are common.

In preschool boys, high reactivity, difficulty being soothed, and high motor activity may indicate risk for the disorder. Marital discord, disrupted child care with a succession of different caregivers, and inconsistent, unsupervised childrearing may contribute to the condition.

Children or adolescents with CD behave aggressively by fighting, bullying, intimidating, physically assaulting, sexually coercing, and/or being cruel to people or animals. Vandalism with deliberate destruction of property, for example, setting fires or smashing windows, is common, as are theft; truancy; early tobacco, alcohol, and substance use and abuse; and precocious sexual activity. Girls with CD are prone to running away from home and may become involved in prostitution. The behavior interferes with performance at school or work, so that individuals with this disorder rarely perform at the level predicted by their IQ or age. Their relationships with peers and adults are often poor. They have higher injury rates and are prone to school expulsion and problems with the law. Sexually transmitted diseases are common. If they have been removed from home, they may have difficulty staying in an adoptive or foster family or group home, which may further complicate their development.

Substance Use Disorders in Adolescents

There are many reasons for drug use among children and adolescents: drugs in the home (e.g., cigarettes, alcohol, etc.); lack of adult supervision (e.g., parents seldom at home); availability of drugs (e.g., easy access to drugs in the community or at school); peer pressure; divorce (which contributes to less adult supervision); curiosity; change in perception (such that children have no fear or very little fear of the risks of drug use); media influence (television, music); escapism (to get away from pressures); and lack of opportunity to participate in alternative activities (e.g., involvement in school activities, clubs, sports). Research has also shown that children who have significant mood and behavior problems, such as prolonged temper tantrums, excessive aggression, impulsivity or risk taking, have a greater chance of developing substance use problems in adolescence compared to those who do not have these behaviors. In addition, children who have learning disabilities or other academic or behavioral problems during elementary and middle school years also may be at higher risk of early drug or alcohol involvement during adolescence.

Some of the recent trends of drug use among adolescents are promising because they indicate a declining trend, but this does not mean it is not an alarming problem. Some examples of positive trends reported by the National Institute on Drug Abuse (2008) include that from 2007 to 2008, the percentage of 10th graders reporting lifetime, past-year, and past-month use of any illicit drug other than marijuana declined significantly. Lifetime use decreased from 18.2% to 15.9%, past-year use declined from 13.1% to 11.3%, and past-month use decreased from 6.9% to 5.3%. Cigarette smoking continues to fall to the lowest rate in the survey's history. Between 2007 and 2008, declines were observed in lifetime, past-month, and daily cigarette use among 10th graders. These findings are particularly noteworthy because tobacco addiction is one of the leading preventable contributors to many of our nation's health problems. Overall, the use of stimulants declined. Lifetime, past-year, and past-month amphetamine use declined among 10th graders. Crystal methamphetamine ("ice") use continues to decline. Past-year use fell among 12th graders, from 1.6% to 1.1%. Also, past-year crack cocaine use declined from 2007 to 2008 among 12th graders, from 1.9% to 1.6% (National Institute on Drug Abuse, 2008).

Although this is good news, drug use continues to be a large problem among adolescents, and the public efforts to decrease drug use need to continue. Some particular areas of concern are that in 2008, 15.4% of 12th graders reported using a prescription drug nonmedically within the past year. This category includes amphetamines, sedatives/barbiturates, tranquilizers, and opiates other than heroin. Vicodin continues to be abused at unacceptably high levels. Many of the drugs used by 12th graders are prescription drugs or, in the case of cough medicine, are available over the counter (National Institute on Drug Abuse, 2008).

COMMUNITY INTERVENTIONS FOR CHILDREN AND ADOLESCENTS

Throughout this book we discuss interventions. In this section, we briefly describe some interventions and locations that are particular for this age group.

For young children, programs and places such as the Women, Infants, and Children (WIC) Program, preschools, day-care centers, hospitals, and Planned Parenthood are good locales for interventions. Many family planning centers offer services beyond contraception such as nutritional counseling and postpartum care. There also are programs in the community for new mothers and parenting classes.

Many schools have programs for child and adolescent mental health. These can include counseling services, as well as educational programs about emotional intelligence, anger management, drug prevention, violence prevention, and bullying. Some of these programs have been shown to be effective; others have not. For example, the well-known Drug Abuse Resistance Education (DARE) program has been shown to be ineffective and, even worse, sometimes counterproductive. The program is used in nearly 80% of the school districts in the United States, in 54 other countries around the world, and is taught to 36 million students each year, yet it has no effective or a negative effective on drug use (Hanson, 2007). That is the conclusion from the U.S. General Accounting Office, U.S. Surgeon General, National Academy of Sciences, U.S. Department of Education, and many others (Hanson, 2007).

There also are after-school programs for youth. These programs include ones that offer mentors, such Big Brothers; education; and skill building. Girls Incorporated (Girls Inc.) is an example of a successful national organization committed to positive youth development and inspiring all girls to be strong, smart, and bold. Girls Inc. is designed to help girls acquire knowledge, skills, and support systems to avoid substance abuse. The program uses a social-influence and life-skills model of prevention, using a combination of adult leadership and peer reinforcement to develop the ability for girls to identify and respond critically to messages and social pressures that encourage substance abuse. Participation has been shown to be significantly related ($p = 0.10$) to delayed onset of drinking among participants, who reported never having drunk alcohol prior to the program (Harvard Family Research Project, n.d.). Participants who reported having already drunk alcohol prior to the program reported lower incidence of drinking at the post-program periods, although this difference was not statistically significant ($p = 0.12$) (Harvard Family Research Project, n.d.). There also are programs outside of school specially designed for children and parents of children with special needs such as autism.

Although we certainly cannot cover all of the programs for these age groups, many have been shown to be effective. It is essential to look at the evaluation results of such programs.

CHAPTER SUMMARY

Childhood is characterized by periods of transition and reorganization, making it critical to assess the mental health of children and adolescents in the context of familial, social, and cultural expectations about age-appropriate thoughts, emotions, and behavior. The range of what is considered normal is wide; still, children and adolescents can and do develop mental disorders that are more severe than the ups and downs in the usual course of development. Mental disorders and mental health problems appear in families of all social classes and of all backgrounds. No one is immune.

In this chapter, we discussed the challenges of assessing mental health problems among this age group. We explained ideas and theories related to normal development and some of the more common mental health problems found among children and adolescents.

REVIEW

1. Explain the theories of child development.
2. Describe the protective and risk factors for mental health problems among this age group.
3. Explain the challenges of assessing mental health among children and adolescents.
4. List the broad categories of mental health illness among children and adolescents.
5. Name some ways to prevent mental illness among children and adolescents.
6. Describe the symptoms of problems such as ADHD, depression, anxiety disorders, autism, mood disorders, and eating disorders.

ACTIVITY

Obtain a copy of the Youth Risk Behavior Surveillance System (YRBSS) for the state that you live in or have lived in previously. Concentrating on the topics related to mental health, review the data. Write a three-page paper that includes a summary of the mental health status of youth in that state and ideas for community interventions that could reduce or eliminate those problems.

REFERENCES AND FURTHER READINGS

American Academy of Pediatrics. (2007). Parenting Corner Q&A: Temperament. Retrieved from http://www.aap.org/publiced/BK5_Temperament.htm

American Psychiatric Association. (2000). *Diagnostic and statistical manual of mental disorders* (*DSM-IV-TR*). Arlington, VA: Author.

American Psychological Association. (2007). *Postpartum depression* [Fact sheet]. Retrieved from http://www.apa.org/pi/wpo/postpartum.html

Anderson, J. C., & McGee, R. (1994). Comorbidity of depression in children and adolescents. In W. M. Reynolds & H. F. Johnson (Eds.), *Handbook of depression in children and adolescents* (pp. 581–601). New York: Plenum.

Bandura, A. (1977). *Social learning theory*. Englewood Cliffs, NJ: Prentice-Hall.

Behavioral-Developmental Initiatives. (2008). Temperament and parenting. Retrieved from http://www.temperament.com/parenting.html

Bidell, T. R., & Fischer, K. W. (1992). Beyond the stage debate: Action, structure, and variability in Piagetian theory and research. In R. Sternberg & C. Berg (Eds.), *Intellectual development* (pp. 100–141). New York: Cambridge University Press.

Birmaher, B., Ryan, N. D., Williamson, D. E., Brent, D. A., & Kaufman, J. (1996). Childhood and adolescent depression: A review of the past 10 years. Part II. *Journal of the American Academy of Child and Adolescent Psychiatry, 35*, 1575–1583.

Birmaher, B., Ryan, N. D., Williamson, D. E., Brent, D. A., Kaufman, J., Dahl, R. E., . . . Nelson, B. (1996). Childhood and adolescent depression: A review of the past 10 years. Part I. *Journal of the American Academy of Child and Adolescent Psychiatry, 35*, 1427–1439.

Black, B., Leonard, H. L., & Rapoport, J. L. (1997). Specific phobia, panic disorder, social phobia, and selective mutism. In J. M. Weiner (Ed.), *Textbook of child and adolescent psychiatry* (2nd ed., pp. 491–506). Washington, DC: American Academy of Child and Adolescent Psychiatry, American Psychiatric Press.

Bowlby, J. (1969). *Attachment and loss. Vol. 1: Attachment*. London: Hogarth Press.

Center for Mental Health in Schools. (2008). *Affect and mood problems related to school aged youth*. Los Angeles, CA: Author.

Children's Hospital, Boston. (2007). Mood disorders. Retrieved from http://www.childrenshospital.org/az/Site1409/mainpageS1409P0.html

Cincinnati Children's Hospital Medical Center. (2007). Post-traumatic stress disorder. Retrieved from http://www.cincinnatichildrens.org/health/info/mental/diagnose/ptsd.htm

Costello, E. J., Angold, A., Burns, B. J., Stangl, D. K., Tweed, D. L., Erkanli, A., & Worthman, C. M. (1996). The Great Smoky Mountains Study of Youth. Goals, design, methods, and the prevalence of DSM-III-R disorders. *Archives of General Psychiatry, 53*, 1129–1136.

de Wilde, E. J., Kienhorst, I. C., Diekstra, R. F., & Wolters, W. H. (1992). The relationship between adolescent suicidal behavior and life events in childhood and adolescence. *American Journal of Psychiatry, 149*, 45–51.

Dodge, K. A., Bates, J. E., & Pettit, G. S. (1990). Mechanisms in the cycle of violence. *Science, 250*, 1678–1683.

Encyclopedia of Mental Disorders. (2010). Reactive attachment disorder of infancy or early childhood. Retrieved from http://www.minddisorders.com/Py-Z/Reactive-attachment-disorder-of-infancy-or-early-childhood.html

Freud, A. (1965). The concept of the rejecting mother. In *The writings of Anna Freud* (Vol. 4, rev. ed., pp. 586–602). New York: International Universities Press.

Gould, M. S., Fisher, P., Parides, M., Flory, M., & Shaffer, D. (1996). Psychosocial risk factors of child and adolescent completed suicide. *Archives of General Psychiatry, 53*, 1155–1162.

Hanson, D. J. (2007). Drug Abuse Resistance Education: The effectiveness of DARE. Retrieved from http://alcoholfacts.org/DARE.html

Harvard Family Research Project (n.d.). A Profile of the Evaluation of Girls Inc.—Friendly PEERsuasion Program. Retrieved from http://www.hfrp.org/out-of-school-time/ost-database-bibliography/database/girls-inc.-friendly-peersuasion-program

Hay, D. F., Zahn-Waxler, C., Cummings, E. M., & Iannotti, R. J. (1992). Young children's views about conflict with peers: A comparison of the daughters and sons of depressed and well women. *Journal of Child Psychology and Psychiatry, 33*, 669–683.

Hoagwood, K., Jensen, P. S., Petti, T., & Burns, B. J. (1996). Outcomes of mental health care for children and adolescents: I. A comprehensive conceptual model. *Journal of the American Academy of Child and Adolescent Psychiatry*, *35*, 1055–1063.

Inhelder, B., & Piaget, J. (1958). *The growth of logical thinking from childhood to adolescence: An essay on the construction of formal operational structures*. New York: Basic.

Jameson, P. B., Gelfand, D. M., Kulcsar, E., & Teti, D. M. (1997). Mother-toddler interaction patterns associated with maternal depression. *Developmental Psychopathology*, *9*, 537–550.

Jensen, P. S., & Hoagwood, K. (1997). The book of names: DSM-IV in context. *Developmental Psychopathology*, *9*, 231–249.

Johnston, L. D., O'Malley, P. M., & Backman, J. G. (1996). *National survey results on drug use from the Monitoring the Future study, 1975–1995. Vol. I: Secondary school students*. (NIH Pub. No. 97-4139). Rockville, MD: National Institute on Drug Abuse.

Kagan, J., Snidman, N., & Arcus, D. (1998). Childhood derivatives of high and low reactivity in infancy. *Child Development*, *69*, 1483–1493.

Kessler, R. C., Nelson, C. B., McKonagle, K. A., Edlund, M. J., Frank, R. G., & Leaf, P. J. (1996). The epidemiology of co-occurring addictive and mental disorders: Implications for prevention and service utilization. *American Journal of Orthopsychiatry*, *66*, 17–31.

Kneisel, C. R., & Trigoboff, E. (2009). Contemporary psychiatric–mental health nursing. Upper Saddle River, NJ: Pearson Prentice Hall.

Kovacs, M., Obrosky, D. S., Gastonis, C., & Richards, C. (1997). First-episode major depressive and dysthymic disorder in childhood: Clinical and sociodemographic factors in recovery. *Journal of American Academy of Child and Adolescent Psychiatry*, *36*, 777–784.

Leonard, H. L., Rapoport, J. L., & Swedo, S. E. (1997). Obsessive-compulsive disorder. In J. M. Weiner (Ed.), *Textbook of child and adolescent psychiatry* (2nd ed., pp. 481–490). Washington, DC: American Academy of Child and Adolescent Psychiatry, American Psychiatric Press.

Loeber, R., & Farrington, D. P. (Eds.). (1998). *Serious and violent juvenile offenders: Risk factors and successful interventions*. Thousand Oaks, CA: Sage.

Mannuzza, S., Klein, R. G., Bessler, A., Malloy, P., & LaPadula, M. (1993). Adult outcome of hyperactive boys. Educational achievement, occupational rank, and psychiatric status. *Archives of General Psychiatry*, *50*, 565–576.

National Alliance on Mental Illness [NAMI]. (2003). Obsessive-compulsive disorder. Retrieved from http://www.nami.org/Template.cfm?Section=By_Illness&Template=/TaggedPage/TaggedPageDisplay.cfm&TPLID=54&ContentID=23035

National Alliance on Mental Illness [NAMI]. (2008). Autism spectrum disorders Fact Sheet. Retrieved from http://www.nami.org/Content/ContentGroups/Helpline1/Autism_Autism_Spectrum_Disorder_Fact_Sheet.htm

National Center on Child Abuse Prevention Research. (2008). 2006 National Child Maltreatment Statistics. Retrieved from http://member.preventchildabuse.org/site/DocServer/Child_Maltreatment_Fact_Sheet_2005.pdf?docID=221

National Institute of Mental Health. (2008). Attention deficit hyperactivity disorder. Retrieved from http://www.nimh.nih.gov/health/publications/adhd/complete-publication.shtml#pub4

National Institute on Drug Abuse. (2008). NIDA InfoFacts: High school and youth trends. Retrieved from http://www.nida.nih.gov/infofacts/HSYouthtrends.html

Pearson Assessment and Information. (n.d.). Greenspan Social-Emotional Growth Chart. Retrieved from http://www.pearsonassessments.com/HAIWEB/Cultures/en-us/Productdetail.htm?Pid=015-8280-229&Mode=summary

Perry, B. D. (2002). Stress, trauma and post-traumatic stress disorders in children. The Child Trauma Center. Retrieved from http://www.childtrauma.org/CTAMATERIALS/PTSDfn_03_v2.pdf

Pickrel, S. G., & Henggeler, S. W. (1996). Multisystemic therapy for adolescent substance abuse and dependence. *Child and Adolescent Psychiatric Clinics of North America*, *5*, 201–211.

Shaffer, D., Fisher, P., Dulcan, M., Davies, M., Piacentini, J., Schwab-Stone, M., . . . Canino, G. R. D. (1996). The second version of the NIMH Diagnostic Interview Schedule for Children (DISC–2). *Journal of the American Academy of Child and Adolescent Psychiatry*, *35*, 865–877.

Shaffer, D., Gould, M. S., Fisher, P., Trautment, P., Moreau, D., Kleinman, M., & Flory, M. (1996). Psychiatric diagnosis in child and adolescent suicide. *Archives of General Psychiatry*, *53*, 339–348.

Springhouse Corporation. (1990). Erikson's development stages. Retrieved from http://honolulu.hawaii.edu/intranet/committees/FacDevCom/guidebk/teachtip/erikson.htm

Stanton, M. D., & Shadish, W. R. (1997). Outcome, attrition, and family-couples treatment for drug abuse: A meta-analysis and review of the controlled, comparative studies. *Psychological Bulletin*, *122*, 170–191.

Strober, M., Schmidt-Lackner, S., Freeman, R., Bower, S., Lampert, C., & DeAntonio, M. (1995). Recovery and relapse in adolescents with bipolar affective illness: A five-year naturalistic, prospective followup. *Journal of the American Academy of Child and Adolescent Psychiatry*, *34*, 724–731.

U.S. Department of Health and Human Services [DHHS]. (1999). *Mental health: A report of the surgeon general.* Rockville, MD: U.S. Department of Health and Human Services, Substance Abuse and Mental Health Services Administration, Center for Mental Health Services, National Institutes of Health, National Institute of Mental Health. Retrieved from http://www.surgeongeneral.gov/library/mentalhealth/home.html

U.S. Department of Health and Human Services [DHHS]. (2003). Eating disorders. Retrieved from http://mentalhealth.samhsa.gov/publications/allpubs/ken98-0047/default.asp

Weinberg, N. Z., Rahdert, E., Colliver, J. D., & Glantz, M. D. (1998). Adolescent substance abuse: A review of the past 10 years. *Journal of the American Academy of Child and Adolescent Psychiatry*, *37*, 252–261.

Weiner, J. M. (1997). Oppositional defiant disorder. In J. M. Weiner (Ed.), *Textbook of child and adolescent psychiatry* (2nd ed., pp. 459–463). Washington, DC: American Academy of Child and Adolescent Psychiatry, American Psychiatric Press.

Werner, E. E., & Smith, R. S. (1992). *Overcoming the odds: High risk children from birth to adulthood.* New York: Cornell University Press.

Zahn-Waxler, C., Iannotti, R., Cummings, E. M., & Denham, S. (1990). Antecedents of problem behaviors in children of depressed mothers. *Development and Psychopathology*, *2*, 271– 291.

CHAPTER 7

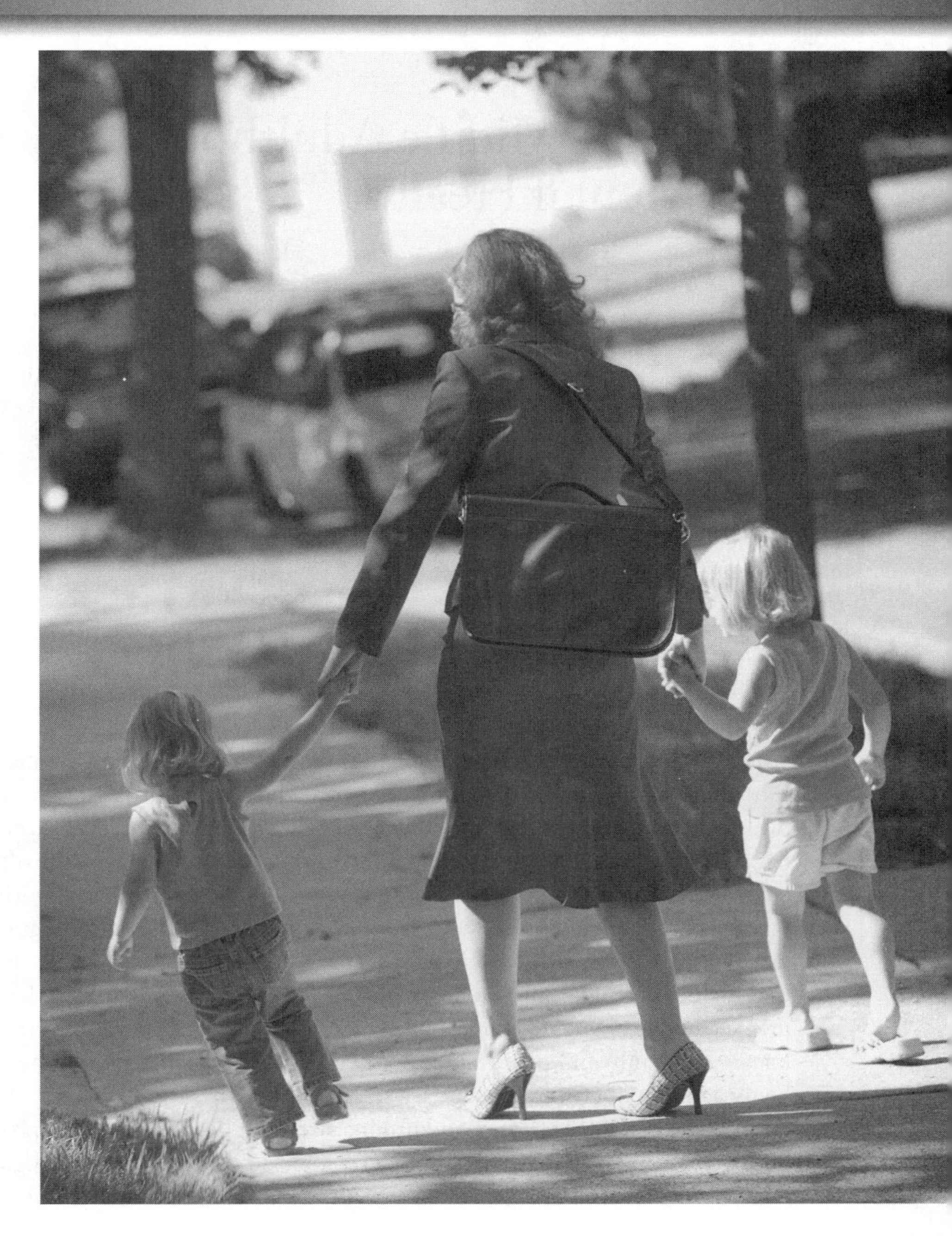

Early and Middle Adulthood and Mental Health

CHAPTER OBJECTIVES

1. Explain the normal development process of adults and midlife crisis.
2. Describe protective and risk factors related to mental health problems among adults.
3. Explain several common mental health problems among adults and the related symptoms.

KEY TERMS

- Agoraphobia
- Anhedonia
- Cyclothymia
- Delirious mania
- Dysphoria
- Dysthymia
- Generalized anxiety disorder
- Jaques's theory
- Midlife crisis
- Neuroticism
- Schizophrenia
- Social phobia
- Sociopathy
- Trichotillomania
- Type A personality

"Mental health in adulthood is characterized by the successful performance of mental function, enabling individuals to cope with adversity and to flourish in their education, vocation, and personal relationships" (U.S. Department of Health and Human Services [DHHS], 1999). Early and middle adulthood are spans of life often filled with change, making it exciting, challenging, adventurous, and stressful. During adulthood one may enter and complete college; begin a career; flourish in intimate, family, community, and professional relationships; start a family; and buy a home. It also is a time that includes changes in intimate relationships; the death of a parent, friend, or family member; divorce and marriage; child rearing; financial difficulties; workload overload; managing family and professional lives; racism and discrimination; health problems; being a victim of criminal assaults; and accidents.

The tremendous changes and productivity that occur during this phase of life may be accompanied by a high amount of stress. It also is a time when biological or genetic factors may be expressed, past events resurface, and personality traits and patterns become attributes that play an important role in personal and professional relationships. Most people manage these stressors successfully, but many people do not, which can lead to mental health problems. The ability to manage these challenges is related to multiple and complex factors.

In this chapter, we discuss normal adult development and factors that protect adults from mental health problems as well as the factors contributing to mental illness. We then describe the common mental health problems that adults experience and their symptoms.

NORMAL DEVELOPMENT

Adult development often looks at how our adult emotional lives are rooted in childhood and infancy. Although this is certainly true, it does not mean that adulthood is only the unconscious reenactment of early childhood conflicts and traumas.

Erikson's Theory

As mentioned in Chapter 6, in the 1950s, psychoanalyst Erik Erikson described the physical, emotional, and psychological stages of development and related specific issues, or developmental work or tasks, of each stage. According to Erikson, there are three phases of adulthood: young, middle, and old age (old age is discussed in Chapter 8). The first two stages are described as follows (Springhouse Corporation, 1990):

1. *Young adulthood*: Intimacy versus Isolation—the person learns to make a personal commitment to another as spouse, parent, or partner.
2. *Middle-aged adulthood*: Generativity versus Stagnation—the adult reaches out beyond their immediate concerns and seeks satisfaction through productivity in career, family, and civic interests.

If these stages are not successfully completed, adults may not create meaningful bonds with others and become preoccupied with themselves. According to Erikson, adults in these stages think about their accomplishments, which can lead to a positive sense of achievement or a negative sense of despair regarding self-worth.

Levinson's Theory

Daniel Levinson also approached understanding adult development from a stage perspective. He saw the primary task of adults as the creation of a structure for life. An individual's life structure is mainly shaped by the social and physical environment, which primarily involves family and work, although other factors such as religion, race, and economic status are often important. This phase of life entails creating new structures and modifying existing ones.

Levinson constructed a framework of stages for males. He identified the stages of a man's adulthood in his theory titled *Seasons of a Man's Life* as follows:

1. *Early adult transition* (17–22): Leave adolescence and family, make preliminary choices for adult life such as entering college or joining the military.
2. *Entering the adult world* (22–28): There is a shift in the center of relationships being family of origin to new adult relationships; makes choices in intimate relationships, friendships, career, values, and lifestyle.
3. *Age 30 transition* (28–33): Changes occur in life structure; people begin to look at their accomplishments in life and realize that time is not infinite.
4. *Settling down* (33–40): Establish a niche in society; makes long-range goals and advances in family and career accomplishments.
5. *Midlife transition* (40–45): Life structure comes into question; usually a time of crisis in the meaning, direction, and value of each person's life; neglected parts of the self (talents, desires, aspirations) seek expression; become more aware of how short life really is.
6. *Entering middle adulthood* (45–50): Choices must be made and a new life structure formed; can be a time of tremendous creative gains or a profound midlife crisis.
7. *Late adulthood* (50+): Spend time reflecting on past achievements and regrets and making peace with one's self and others (including God).

Levinson was working on the stages of transition from women at the time of his death.

Jaques's Theory

Another adult development theorist, Elliott Jaques, emphasized the importance of the midlife crisis in individual development (**Jaques's theory**). He coined the term *midlife crisis*, which declares that the confrontation with personal mortality is the central issue of midlife development. "Midlife crisis" is a phrase used in Western societies. Some cultures may be more sensitive to this phenomenon than others. For example, the Japanese culture is less prone to experience it. Therefore, midlife crisis is likely a cultural construct. This may be due to the fact that some cultures, including Western societies, are more youth focused.

Midlife crisis is the phrase used to describe a period of self-doubt felt by some individuals during the midpoint in their lives. The person begins to become more aware of youth passing and old age coming closer. Sometimes an event can trigger a midlife crisis, such as the death of parents or children leaving home. A midlife crisis can create a desire to change central components of one's life, such as a career shift or a new romantic relationship. Personality type and a history of psychological crisis are believed to predispose some people to a midlife crisis.

Midlife crisis is not always troublesome; it can be a time of renewal. This phase can be a time of internal reflection and a change in priorities and goals. It may be when new hobbies and relationships are formed. Therefore, midlife crisis can be positive. Individuals experiencing a midlife crisis may search for an undefined dream or goal, may feel regret related to goals and dreams that they have not accomplished, may have a need to spend more time with a small core group of people or alone, and/or may have a desire to look and feel youthful.

PROTECTIVE FACTORS AND RISK FACTORS

During any stage of development, certain factors can protect our mental health or put it at risk. Those factors as they relate to adulthood are discussed in this section.

Personality Traits

Personality traits include the qualities of an individual. Personality traits in adults are usually referred to as temperament in infants, children, and adolescents. When we first meet someone, we notice if he or she has a positive outlook, is withdrawn, or is energetic. These traits influence our behavior and health. For example, people who have a **type A personality** are more likely to smoke, consume alcohol, sleep less, drink caffeine, eat less healthy foods, and avoid exercise, as well as have higher stress and irritation levels (Sanderson, 2004). Extraverts tend to have more positive moods, whereas people with higher levels of hostility tend to have more negative moods and are more often uncooperative and aggressive (Sanderson, 2004). Personality traits do tend to stay stable because they are strongly influenced by heredity, yet they are still influenced by our environments and previous experiences (Dombeck & Wells-Moran, 2006).

The various traits and behavioral patterns that epitomize strong mental health do not, of course, exist in isolation: They develop in a social context and impact people's ability to handle psychological and social adversity and stress. In addition, severe or repeated trauma during youth may have enduring effects on neurobiological and psychological development, which can change one's stress response behavior patterns in adulthood (DHHS, 1999). An example of enduring effects has been shown in young adults who experienced severe sexual or physical abuse in childhood. These individuals experience a greatly increased risk of mood, anxiety, and personality disorders throughout adult life.

People's personality traits influence how easy or difficult certain tasks are for them to take on. For instance, it is far easier for an extraverted person to seek social support for a problem than it is for an introverted person to do so. Personality traits are thought to confer either beneficial or detrimental effects on mental health during adulthood, and culture and gender need to be taken into consideration. A brief summary of healthy and maladaptive characteristics follows.

Self-Esteem, Self-Efficacy, and Resilience

Self-esteem refers to a person's beliefs about one's own worth or the extent to which a person values or likes himself or herself. Basically, it is one's favorable or unfavorable attitude toward oneself. Self-esteem also has been conceptualized as buffering the individual from adverse life events. One influential aspect of self-esteem is self-efficacy, which is confidence in one's own abilities to cope with adversity, either independently or by obtaining appropriate assistance from others. Self-efficacy is a major component of the construct known as resilience.

Resilience is the ability to adapt well to stress, adversity, trauma, or tragedy (Mayo Clinic, 2008). It means that, overall, the person can remain stable and maintain healthy levels of psychological and physical functioning in the face of disruption or chaos. If someone has resilience, he or she may experience temporary disruptions in life when faced with challenges. For instance, the person may not sleep as well as usual but is able to continue on with daily tasks, remain generally optimistic about life, and rebound quickly. Resilience is not about toughing it out or living by old clichés, such as "making lemonade out of lemons." It does not mean ignoring feelings of sadness over a loss; nor does it mean the adult always has to be strong and cannot ask others for support. In fact, being willing to reach out to others is a key component of being resilient. Resilience offers protection against developing such conditions as depression, anxiety, or posttraumatic stress disorder (Mayo Clinic, 2008).

Neuroticism

Neuroticism can be defined as an enduring tendency to experience negative emotional states such as fear, shame, anger, anxiety, and guilt. Neurotic individuals respond more poorly to environmental stress and are more likely to interpret ordinary situations as threatening and minor frustrations as hopelessly difficult. A high level of neuroticism is associated with a predisposition toward recognizing the dangerous, harmful, or defeating aspects of a situation and the tendency to respond with worry, anticipatory anxiety, emotionality, pessimism, and dissatisfaction (DHHS, 1999). As a result, individuals who score high on neuroticism are more likely than the average to experience physical symptoms such as headaches and loss of energy as well as emotional issues such as anxiety, anger, guilt, and clinical depression.

Avoidance

Avoidance describes an exaggerated predisposition to withdraw from unusual situations and avoid threatening personal challenges. Closely related to the characteristics of behavioral inhibition or introversion, the trait of avoidance appears to be partly inherited and is associated with shyness, anxiety, and depressive disorders in both childhood and adult life, as well as the subsequent development of substance abuse disorders (Vaughan & Oldham, 1997). People with low levels of harm avoidance are described as healthy extroverts and are characterized by confident, carefree, or outgoing behaviors.

Impulsivity

Impulsivity is a trait associated with people who are inclined to act on impulse rather than thought. People who are overly impulsive seem unable to curb their immediate reactions or think before they act. The inability to delay gratification may be a vulnerability marker for alcoholism, and certain inhibitory-control issues may be specific to antisocial and borderline personality disorders (*Mental Health and Psychiatry News*, 2007). Impulsivity also is linked with physical abuse (both as victim and as a perpetrator), and pathologic conditions such as attention deficit hyperactivity disorder, obsessive-compulsive disorder, and bipolar disorder.

Sociopathy

Sociopathy is a set of traits and behaviors that refers to the predisposition to engage in dishonest, hurtful, unfaithful, and at times dangerous conduct to benefit one's own ends (DHHS, 1999). In its full form, **sociopathy** is referred to as antisocial personality disorder (American Psychiatric Association, 2000). Sociopathy is characterized by a tendency and ability to disregard laws and rules, difficulties reciprocating within empathic and intimate relationships, less internalization of moral standards, and an insensitivity to the needs and rights of others (DHHS, 1999). People scoring high in sociopathy often have problems with aggressiveness and are overrepresented among criminal populations. Although not invariably associated with criminality, sociopathy is associated with problematic, unethical, and morally questionable conduct in the workplace and within social systems.

Additional Personality Traits

Additional personality traits that can affect mental health include social closeness, social potency, being hostile and disagreeable, being conscientious, having an internal locus of control, and being optimistic. As mentioned, these traits do not exist in isolation and they affect other traits. For example, the level of optimism impacts levels of hope.

Biological and Genetic Factors

As mentioned in Chapter 2, genetics can predispose people to certain mental health problems such as depression, anxiety, and insomnia. Symptoms for genetically related mental health problems may manifest themselves during adulthood, but it is important to remember that one single gene has not been found to cause mental health problems. Therefore, personality traits, for example, may protect adults from genetically prone mental illness or they may be risk factors.

Childhood Events

Childhood events can contribute to mental health problems during adulthood. Experiences such as abuse, observing a violent crime, parental mental illnesses, loss of a parent, parental separation or divorce, witnessing domestic violence, being exposed to a natural disaster, or having one or more parents who abuse drugs can certainly be risk factors. It has been found that for people who suffer from schizophrenia (and related disorders), the increased exposure to adverse childhood events is strongly related to psychiatric problems (e.g., suicidal thinking, hospitalizations, distress, and posttraumatic stress disorder), substance abuse, physical health problems (e.g., HIV infection), medical service utilization (e.g., physician visits), and poor social functioning (e.g., homelessness or criminal justice involvement) (Rosenberg, Lu, Mueser, Jankowski, & Cournos, 2007). The higher the degree of impact of traumatic experiences in childhood, the greater the person's vulnerability to stress and mental health problems in adulthood. Childhood experiences such as being raised in a supportive and loving environment can be protective factors.

Stress

During adulthood many positive and negative transitions occur that often lead to stress. As noted previously, assorted traits or personal characteristics have been viewed as factors protective of mental health, including self-esteem, effective coping styles, optimism, and resilience. These and related traits are seen as sources of personal resilience needed to weather the storms of stressful life events.

Stressful life events in adulthood include changes in romantic relationships (including divorce), death of a family member or friend, economic hardship, role conflict, work overload, child rearing, caring for elderly parents and/or in-laws, racism and discrimination, poor physical health, accidental injuries, and intentional assaults on physical safety. Stressful life events in adulthood also may reflect past events. Severe trauma in childhood, including sexual and physical abuse, may persist as a stressor into adulthood or may make the individual more vulnerable to ongoing stresses.

COMMON DISORDERS AMONG ADULTS

Mental disorders are common in adults. An estimated 26.2% of Americans ages 18 and older—about 1 in 4 adults—suffer from a diagnosable mental disorder in a given year (Kessler, Chiu, Demler, & Walters, 2005). When applied to the 2004 U.S. Census residential population estimate for ages 18 and older, this figure translates to 57.7 million people (U.S. Census Bureau Population Estimates by Demographic Characteristics, 2005). Even though mental disorders are widespread in the population, the main burden of illness is concentrated in a much smaller proportion—about 6%, or 1 in 17—who suffer from a serious mental illness (Kessler et al., 2005). In addition, mental disorders are the leading cause of disability in the United States and Canada for ages 15 to 44 (World Health Organization, 2004). Many people suffer from more than one mental disorder at a given time. Nearly half (45%) of those with any mental disorder meet criteria for two or more disorders, with severity strongly related to comorbidity (Kessler et al., 2005).

The social consequences of serious mental disorders—family disruption, loss of employment and housing—can cause great harm. Comprehensive treatment, which includes services that exist outside the formal treatment system, is crucial to reduce or eliminate symptoms, assist recovery, and, to the extent that these efforts are successful, reduce stigma. Consumer self-help programs, family self-help, advocacy, and services for housing and vocational assistance complement and supplement the formal treatment system. Many of these services are operated by consumers, that is, people who use mental health services themselves. The logic behind their leadership in delivery of these services is that consumers are thought to be capable of engaging others with mental disorders, serving as role models, and increasing the sensitivity of service systems to the needs of people with mental disorders (Mowbray et al., 1996).

The three major categories of mental disorders that affect this age group are anxiety and mood disorders and schizophrenia.

BOX 7-1 Coping with Work and Family Stress Evidence-Based Practice

Coping with Work and Family Stress is a workplace preventive intervention designed to teach employees 18 years and older how to deal with stressors at work and at home. The model is derived from Pearlin and Schooler's hierarchy of coping mechanisms as well as Bandura's social learning theory. The 16 90-minute sessions, typically provided weekly to groups of 15 to 20 employees, teach effective methods for reducing risk factors (stressors and avoidance coping) and enhancing protective factors (active coping and social support) through behavior modification (e.g., methods to modify or eliminate sources of stress), information sharing (e.g., didactic presentations, group discussions), and skill development (e.g., learning effective communication and problem-solving skills, expanding use of social network). The curriculum emphasizes the role of stress, coping, and social support in relation to substance use and psychological symptoms. The sessions are led by a facilitator who typically has a master's-level education; is experienced in group dynamics, system theory, and cognitive and other behavior interventions; and is able to manage group process. Facilitator training in the program curriculum is required.

Source: SAMHSA. (2007). Coping With Work and Family Stress. Retrieved from http://nrepp.samhsa.gov/programfulldetails.asp?PROGRAM_ID=142. Accessed July 15, 2010.

Anxiety Disorders

Anxiety disorders are the most prevalent mental disorders in adults, and they affect twice as many women as men. The broad category of anxiety disorders, includes panic disorder, phobias, obsessive-compulsive disorder, posttraumatic stress disorder, and generalized anxiety disorder, among others. The anxiety disorders encompass a group of conditions that share extreme or pathologic anxiety as the principal disturbance of mood or emotional tone. Anxiety, which may be understood as the pathologic counterpart of normal fear, is manifest by disturbances of mood, as well as of thinking, behavior, and physiologic activity. Underlying this heterogeneous group of disorders is a state of heightened arousal or fear in relation to stressful events or feelings. The biological manifestations of anxiety, which are grounded in the fight-or-flight response, include an increased heart rate, sweating, dry mouth, and tensing of muscles as well as numerous other physiologic symptoms. Although the full array of biological causes and correlates of anxiety are not yet understood, numerous effective treatments for anxiety disorders exist now. Treatment draws on an assortment of psychosocial and pharmacologic approaches, administered alone or in combination.

The anxiety disorders include panic disorder (with and without a history of agoraphobia), agoraphobia (with and without a history of panic disorder), generalized anxiety disorder, specific phobia, social phobia, obsessive-compulsive disorder, acute stress disorder, substance-induced anxiety disorder, separation anxiety disorder, posttraumatic stress disorder, and the residual category of anxiety disorder not otherwise specified (American Psychiatric Association, 2000). The disorders tend to be long term, with episodes of reoccurrence and disability.

Panic Attacks and Panic Disorder

A panic attack is a discrete period of intense fear or discomfort associated with numerous somatic and cognitive symptoms (American Psychiatric Association, 2000). These symptoms include palpitations, sweating, trembling, shortness of breath, sensations of choking or smothering, chest pain, nausea or gastrointestinal distress, dizziness or lightheadedness, tingling sensations, chills or blushing, and hot flashes. The attack typically has an abrupt onset, building to maximum intensity within 10 to 15 minutes, and rarely lasts longer than 30 minutes (DHHS, 1999). Most people report a fear of dying, "going crazy," or losing control of emotions or behavior (DHHS, 1999). The experiences generally provoke a strong urge to escape or flee the place where the attack begins and, when associated with chest pain or shortness of breath, frequently results in seeking aid from a hospital emergency department or other type of urgent assistance. Current diagnostic practice specifies that a panic attack must be characterized by at least four of the associated somatic and cognitive symptoms described previously. The panic attack is distinguished from other forms of anxiety by its intensity and its sudden, episodic nature. Panic attacks may be further characterized by the relationship between the onset of the attack and the presence or absence of situational factors. For example, a panic attack may be described as unexpected, situationally bound, or situationally predisposed.

Panic attacks are not always indicative of a mental disorder, and some healthy people experience an isolated panic attack. Panic attacks also are not limited to panic disorder. They commonly occur in the course of social phobia, generalized anxiety disorder, and major depressive disorder (American Psychiatric Association, 2000).

Panic disorder is diagnosed when a person has experienced at least two unexpected panic attacks and develops persistent concern or worry about having further attacks or changes his or her behavior to avoid or minimize such attacks. Although the number and severity of the attacks varies widely, the concern and avoidance behavior are essential features. The diagnosis is inapplicable when the attacks are presumed to be caused by a drug or medication or a general medical disorder such as hyperthyroidism.

Panic disorder is about twice as common among women as men. Age of onset is most common between late adolescence and mid-adult life, with onset relatively uncommon past age 50. There is developmental continuity between the anxiety syndromes of youth, such as separation anxiety disorder. Typically, an early age of onset of panic disorder carries greater risks of comorbidity, chronicity, and impairment.

Agoraphobia

The ancient term *agoraphobia* is translated from Greek as fear of an open marketplace. **Agoraphobia** is a condition where the sufferer becomes anxious in unfamiliar environments or where he or she perceives having little control. Triggers for this anxiety may include crowds, wide open spaces, or traveling (even short distances). This anxiety is often compounded by a fear of social embarrassment because the agoraphobic fears the onset of a panic attack and appearing distraught in public. Most people who present to mental health specialists develop agoraphobia after the onset of panic disorder (American Psychiatric Association, 1998). Thus the formal diagnosis of panic disorder with agoraphobia was established. However, for people who do not meet full criteria for panic disorder, the formal diagnosis of agoraphobia without history of panic disorder is used (American Psychiatric Association, 2000).

Agoraphobia occurs about two times more often in women than men. The gender difference may be attributable to social-cultural factors that encourage, or permit, the greater expression of avoidant coping strategies by women, although other explanations are possible.

Specific Phobias

These common conditions are characterized by marked fear of specific objects or situations that is excessive or unreasonable (American Psychiatric Association, 2000). Exposure to the object of the phobia, either in real life or via imagination or video, invariably elicits intense anxiety, which may include a situationally bound panic attack. Adults generally recognize that this intense fear is irrational. Nevertheless, they typically avoid the phobic stimulus or endure exposure with great difficulty. The most common specific phobias include the following feared stimuli or situations: animals (especially snakes, rodents, birds, and dogs); insects (especially spiders, bees, and hornets); heights; elevators; flying; automobile driving; water; storms; and blood or injections.

The prevalence rates for specific phobias would be higher if less rigorous diagnostic requirements for avoidance or functional impairment were employed. Typically, the specific phobias begin in childhood, although there is a second peak of onset in the middle 20s of adulthood (American Psychiatric Association, 2000). Most phobias persist for years or even decades, and relatively few remit spontaneously or without treatment.

The specific phobias generally do not result from exposure to a single traumatic event (e.g., being bitten by a dog or nearly drowning). Some phobias are learned from family members and social situations. Spontaneous, unexpected panic attacks also appear to play a role in the development of a specific phobia, although the particular pattern of avoidance is much more focal and circumscribed.

Social Phobia

Social phobia, also known as social anxiety disorder, describes people with marked and persistent anxiety in social situations, including performances and public speaking (Ballenger et al., 1998). The critical element of the fearfulness is the possibility of embarrassment or ridicule. Like specific phobias, the fear is recognized by adults as excessive or unreasonable, but the dreaded social situation is avoided or is tolerated with great discomfort. Many people with social phobia are preoccupied with concerns that others will see their anxiety symptoms (e.g., trembling, sweating, or blushing); or notice their halting or rapid speech; or judge them to be weak, stupid, or crazy. Fears of fainting, losing control of bowel or bladder function, or having one's mind go blank also are common (DHHS, 1999). Social phobias generally are associated with significant anticipatory anxiety for days or weeks before the dreaded event, which in turn may further handicap performance and heighten embarrassment.

The prevalence of social phobia is rather low, although the lower figure probably better captures the number of people who experience significant impairment and distress. Social phobia is more common in women. Personality traits such as shyness are attributed to the onset of social phobias for many people with the disorder. A stressful event such as public humiliation may provoke an intensification of difficulties. Once the disorder is established, complete remissions are uncommon without treatment. More commonly, the severity of symptoms and impairments tends to fluctuate in relation to vocational demands and the stability of social relationships.

Generalized Anxiety Disorder

Generalized anxiety disorder is defined by a protracted period (lasting 6 or more months) of anxiety and worry, accompanied by multiple associated symptoms (American Psychiatric Association, 2000). These symptoms include muscle tension, easy fatigability, poor concentration, insomnia, and irritability (DHHS, 1999). In *DSM-IV-TR* (American Psychiatric Association, 2000) an essential feature of generalized anxiety disorder is that the anxiety and worry cannot be attributable to the more focal distress of panic disorder, social phobia, obsessive-compulsive disorder, or other conditions. Rather, as implied by the name, the excessive worries often pertain to many areas, including work, relationships, finances, the well-being of one's family, potential misfortunes, and impending deadlines.

Generalized anxiety disorder is more common in women than men. The disorder typically runs a fluctuating course with periods of increased symptoms usually associated with life stress or impending difficulties. There does not appear to be a specific familial association for general anxiety disorder.

Obsessive-Compulsive Disorder

Obsessions are recurrent, intrusive thoughts, impulses, or images that are perceived as inappropriate, grotesque, or forbidden (American Psychiatric Association, 2000). The obsessions, which elicit anxiety and marked distress, are termed ego alien or ego dystonic because their content is quite unlike the thoughts that the person usually has (DHHS, 1999). Obsessions are perceived as uncontrollable, and the sufferer often fears that he or she will lose control and act on such thoughts or impulses. Common themes include contamination with germs or body fluids, doubts (i.e., the worry that something important has been overlooked or that the sufferer has unknowingly inflicted harm on someone), order or symmetry, or loss of control of violent or sexual impulses.

Compulsions are repetitive behaviors or mental acts that reduce the anxiety that accompanies an obsession or prevent some dreaded event from happening (American Psychiatric Association, 2000). Compulsions include both overt behaviors, such as handwashing or checking, and mental acts including counting or praying. Compulsive rituals often take up long periods of time, even hours, to complete, and they can lead to physical problems. For example, repeated handwashing, intended to remedy anxiety about contamination, is a common cause of contact dermatitis.

Obsessive-compulsive disorder typically begins in adolescence to young adult life. For most, the course is fluctuating and, like generalized anxiety disorder, symptom exacerbations are usually associated with life stress. Common comorbidities include major depressive disorder and other anxiety disorders.

Obsessive-compulsive disorder has a clear familial pattern and somewhat greater familial specificity than most other anxiety disorders. Furthermore, there is an increased risk of obsessive-compulsive disorder among first-degree relatives with Tourette's disorder (DHHS, 1999). Other mental disorders that may fall within the spectrum of obsessive-compulsive disorder include **trichotillomania** (compulsive hair pulling), compulsive shoplifting, body dysmorphic disorder (compulsive and obsessive behavior centering around a preoccupation with one's appearance), gambling, and sexual behavior disorders (Hollander, 1996). The latter conditions vary because the compulsive behaviors are less ritualistic and yield some outcomes that are pleasurable or gratifying.

Acute and Posttraumatic Stress Disorders

Acute stress disorder refers to the anxiety and behavioral disturbances that develop within the first month after exposure to an extreme trauma. Generally, the symptoms of an acute stress disorder begin during or shortly following the trauma. Such extreme traumatic events include rape or other severe physical assault, near-death experiences in accidents, witnessing a murder, and combat. The symptom of dissociation, which reflects a perceived detachment of the mind from the emotional state or even the body, is a critical feature. Dissociation also is characterized by a sense of the world as a dreamlike or unreal place and may be accompanied by poor memory of the specific events, which in severe form is known as dissociative amnesia. Other features of an acute stress disorder include symptoms of generalized anxiety and hyperarousal, avoidance of situations or stimuli that elicit memories of the trauma, and persistent, intrusive recollections of the event via flashbacks, dreams, or recurrent thoughts or visual images.

If the symptoms and behavioral disturbances of the acute stress disorder persist for more than 1 month, and if these features are associated with functional impairment or significant distress to the sufferer, the diagnosis is changed to posttraumatic stress disorder. Posttraumatic stress disorder is further defined in *DSM-IV-TR* (American Psychiatric Association, 2000) as having three subforms: acute (less than 3 months duration), chronic (3 or more months duration), and delayed onset (symptoms began at least 6 months after exposure to the trauma).

By virtue of the more sustained nature of posttraumatic stress disorder (relative to acute stress disorder), a number of changes, including decreased self-esteem, loss of sustained beliefs about people or society, hopelessness, a sense of being permanently damaged, and difficulties in previously established relationships are typically observed (DHHS, 1999). Substance abuse often develops, especially involving alcohol, marijuana, and sedative-hypnotic drugs.

Mood Disorders

Mood disorders are a cluster of mental disorders. The most recognized are being depression or mania. Mood disorders are outside the bounds of normal fluctuations from sadness to elation. They have potentially severe consequences for morbidity and mortality. Mood disorders take a monumental toll in human suffering, lost productivity, and suicide, and when unrecognized, they can result in unnecessary healthcare use. Major depression and bipolar disorder are the most familiar mood disorders, but there are others including **cyclothymia** (alternating manic and depressive states that, although lasting 6 months or more in duration, do not meet criteria for bipolar disorder) and dysthymia (a chronic, milder form of depression). The causes of mood disorders are not fully known. They may be triggered by stressful life events and enduring stressful social conditions (e.g., poverty and discrimination). With the exception of bipolar disorder, they are twice as common in women as men (DHHS, 1999). One subtype of mood disorder, seasonal affective disorder, entails episodes of depression, which occur usually during the darker months (the late fall and winter) and are more common in women than in men. Many psychosocial and genetic factors interact to dictate the appearance and persistence of mood disorders.

Mood disorders, disability and suffering are not limited to the patient. Spouses, significant others, children, parents, siblings, coworkers, and friends experience frustration, guilt, anger, financial hardship, and, on occasion, physical abuse in their attempts to assuage or cope with the depressed person's suffering. Depression also has a negative impact on the economy because of the healthcare costs and loss of productivity. In the workplace, depression is a leading cause of absenteeism and diminished productivity. Although only a minority seek professional help to relieve a mood disorder, depressed people are significantly more likely than others to visit a physician for some other reason. Depression-related visits to physicians thus account for a large portion of healthcare expenditures. Suicide is the most dreaded complication of major depressive disorders. In the United States, men complete suicide four times as often as women do; women attempt suicide four times as frequently as men do.

People have been plagued by disorders of mood for at least as long as they have been able to record their experiences. One of the earliest terms for depression, "melancholy," literally meaning "black bile," dates back to Hippocrates (DHHS, 1999). Since ancient times, dysphoric states outside the range of normal sadness or grief have been recognized, but only within the past 40 years or so have researchers had the means to study the changes in cognition and brain functioning that are associated with severe depressive states.

At some time or another, virtually all adult human beings experience a tragic or unexpected loss, romantic heartbreak, or a serious setback and times of profound sadness, grief, or distress. Indeed, something is awry if the usual expressions of sadness do not accompany such situations so common to the human condition—death of a loved one, severe illness, prolonged disability, loss of employment or social status, or a child's difficulties, for example.

What is now called major depressive disorder, however, differs both quantitatively and qualitatively from normal sadness or grief. Normal states of **dysphoria** (a negative or aversive mood state) are typically less pervasive and generally run a more time-limited course. Moreover, some of the symptoms of severe depression, such as **anhedonia** (the inability to experience pleasure), hopelessness, and loss of mood reactivity (the ability to feel a mood uplift in response to something positive) only rarely accompany normal sadness. Suicidal thoughts and psychotic symptoms such as delusions or hallucinations virtually always signify a pathologic state.

Many other symptoms commonly associated with depression are experienced during times of stress or bereavement. Among them are sleep disturbances, changes in appetite, poor concentration, and ruminations on sad thoughts and feelings. When a person suffering such distress seeks help, the diagnostician's task is to differentiate the normal from the pathologic and, when appropriate, to recommend treatment.

Mood disorders are sometimes caused by general medical conditions or medications. Classic examples include the depressive syndromes associated with dominant hemispheric strokes, hypothyroidism, Cushing disease, and pancreatic cancer (American Psychiatric Association, 2000). Antihypertensives and oral contraceptives are two examples of medications associated with depression. Transient depressive syndromes also are common during withdrawal from alcohol and various other drugs of abuse.

A challenge to diagnosticians is to balance their search for relatively uncommon disorders with their sensitivity to aspects of the medical history or review of symptoms that might have etiologic significance (DHHS, 1999). For example, the onset of a depressive episode a few weeks or months after the patient has begun taking a new blood pressure medication should raise the healthcare provider's suspicion. Cultural influences on the manifestation and diagnosis of depression also are important for the diagnostician to identify (American Psychiatric Association, 2000). As mentioned in Chapter 3, somatization is especially prevalent in individuals from ethnic minority backgrounds.

Major Depressive Disorder

Major depression, also known as unipolar depression, is a serious medical illness affecting 15 million American adults, or approximately 5–8% of the adult population in a given year (National Alliance on Mental Illness [NAMI, 2008]). Unlike normal emotional experiences of sadness, loss, or passing mood states, major depression is persistent and can significantly interfere with an individual's thoughts, behavior, mood, activity, and physical health. Among all medical illnesses, major depression is the leading cause of disability in the United States and many other developed countries (NAMI, 2008).

Depression occurs twice as frequently in women as in men, for reasons that are not fully understood. More than half of those who experience a single episode of depression continue to have episodes that occur as frequently as once or even twice a year (NAMI, 2008). Without treatment, the frequency of depressive illness as well as the severity of symptoms tends to increase over time. Left untreated, depression can lead to suicide.

With regard to symptoms, the onset of the first episode of major depression may not be obvious if it is gradual or mild. The symptoms of major depression characteristically represent a significant change from how a person functioned before the illness. The symptoms of depression include:

- Persistently sad or irritable mood
- Pronounced changes in sleep, appetite, and energy
- Difficulty thinking, concentrating, and remembering
- Physical slowing or agitation
- Lack of interest in or pleasure from activities that were once enjoyed
- Feelings of guilt, worthlessness, hopelessness, and emptiness
- Recurrent thoughts of death or suicide
- Persistent physical symptoms that do not respond to treatment, such as headaches, digestive disorders, and chronic pain (NAMI, 2008)

When several of these symptoms of depressive illness occur at the same time, last longer than 2 weeks, and interfere with ordinary functioning, professional treatment is needed.

There is no single cause of major depression. Psychological, biological, and environmental factors may all contribute to its development. Whatever the specific causes of depression, scientific research has firmly established that major depression is a biological medical illness.

Norepinephrine, serotonin, and dopamine are three neurotransmitters (chemical messengers that transmit electrical signals between brain cells) thought to be involved with major depression. Scientists believe that if there is a chemical imbalance in these neurotransmitters, clinical states of depression result. Antidepressant medications work by increasing the availability of neurotransmitters or by changing the sensitivity of the receptors for these chemical messengers.

Scientists also have found evidence of a genetic predisposition to major depression. There is an increased risk for developing depression when there is a family history of the illness. Not everyone with a genetic predisposition develops depression, but some people probably have a biological makeup that leaves them particularly vulnerable to developing depression. Life events, such as the death of a loved one, a major loss or change, chronic stress, and alcohol and drug abuse, may trigger episodes of depression. Some illnesses such as heart disease and cancer and some medications also may trigger depressive episodes. It is also important to note that many depressive episodes occur spontaneously and are not triggered by a life crisis, physical illness, or other risks.

Dysthymia

Dysthymia is a serious, chronic, and disabling disorder that shares many symptoms with other forms of clinical depression. It is generally experienced as a less severe but more chronic form of major depression. Specifically, dysthymia is characterized by depressed mood experienced most of the time for at least 2 years, along with at least two of the following symptoms: insomnia or excessive sleep, low energy or fatigue, low self-esteem, poor appetite or overeating, poor concentration or indecisiveness, and feelings of hopelessness (*Psychology Today*, 2008b). The more severe symptoms that mark major depression, including anhedonia (inability to feel pleasure), psychomotor symptoms (particularly lethargy or agitation), and thoughts of death or suicide, are often absent in dysthymia (*Psychology Today*, 2008b).

Bipolar Disorder

Bipolar disorder is a recurrent mood disorder featuring one or more episodes of mania or mixed episodes of mania and depression. Bipolar disorder is distinct from major depressive disorder by virtue of a history of manic or hypomanic (milder and not psychotic) episodes. Other differences concern the nature of depression in bipolar disorder. Its depressive episodes are typically associated with an earlier age at onset and a higher familial prevalence (American Psychiatric Association, 2000).

Mania is derived from a French word that literally means "crazed" or "frenzied." The mood disturbance can range from pure euphoria or elation to irritability. Thought content is usually grandiose but also can be paranoid. Grandiosity usually takes the form both of overvalued ideas (e.g., "I am the smartest man in the world") and of frank delusions (e.g., "I have radio transmitters implanted in my head and the government is listening to my thoughts."). Auditory and visual hallucinations complicate more severe episodes. Speed of thought increases and ideas typically race through the manic person's consciousness.

Nevertheless, distractibility and poor concentration commonly impair implementation. Judgment also can be severely compromised; spending sprees, offensive or disinhibited behavior, and promiscuity or other objectively reckless behaviors are commonplace. Subjective energy, libido, and activity typically increase, but a perceived reduced need for sleep can sap physical reserves. Sleep deprivation also can exacerbate cognitive difficulties and contribute to development of a confused state known as **delirious mania**. If the manic patient is delirious, paranoid, or catatonic (motor abnormalities such as immobility or excessive motor activity), the behavior is difficult to distinguish from that of a schizophrenic patient.

Cyclothymia

Cyclothymia, a mild form of bipolar disorder, is characterized by mood swings from mild or moderate depression to hypomania. Hypomania involves periods of elevated mood, euphoria, and excitement but does not disconnect a person from reality (*Psychology Today*, 2008a). A person with cyclothymia experiences symptoms of hypomania but no full-blown manic episodes. Hypomania may feel good to the person who experiences it and may lead to enhanced functioning and productivity (*Psychology Today*, 2008a). Thus even when family and friends learn to recognize the mood swings as possible bipolar disorder, the person may deny that a problem exists. Without proper treatment, however, hypomania can become severe mania or can turn into depression (*Psychology Today*, 2008a).

Signs and symptoms of mania (or a manic episode), which are similar to those of cyclothymia (or a hypomanic episode), include:

- Increased energy, restlessness, and activity
- Excessively "high," overly good, euphoric mood
- Extreme irritability
- Racing thoughts and speech, jumping from one idea to another
- Distractibility, cannot concentrate well
- Need little sleep
- Unrealistic beliefs in one's abilities and powers
- Poor judgment
- Spending sprees
- A lasting period of behavior that is different from usual
- Increased sexual drive
- Abuse of drugs, particularly cocaine, sleeping medications, and alcohol
- Provocative, intrusive, or aggressive behavior
- Denial that anything is wrong (*Psychology Today*, 2008a)

Schizophrenia

Our understanding of **schizophrenia** has evolved since its symptoms were first catalogued by German psychiatrist Emil Kraepelin in the late 19th century. Even though the cause of this disorder remains elusive, its frightening symptoms and biological correlates have come to be quite well defined. Schizophrenia is neither split personality nor multiple personality. Furthermore, people with schizophrenia are not perpetually incoherent or psychotic (American Psychiatric Association, 2000).

Schizophrenia affects a small percentage of the population, yet its severity and persistence reverberate throughout the mental health service system. The course of illness in schizophrenia is quite variable, with most people having periods of exacerbation and remission. Schizophrenia had once been thought to have a uniformly downhill course, but other research shows that many individuals with schizophrenia significantly improve, and more than half recover. Although the causes of schizophrenia are not fully known, experts now agree that schizophrenia develops as a result of interplay between biological predisposition (e.g., inheriting certain genes) and the person's environment. New pharmacologic treatments are at least as effective as past pharmacologic treatments, with fewer troubling side effects.

Schizophrenia is characterized by profound disruption in cognition and emotion, affecting language, thought, perception, affect, and sense of self. The array of symptoms, although wide ranging, frequently includes psychotic manifestations such as hearing internal voices, experiencing other sensations not connected to an obvious source (hallucinations), assigning unusual significance or meaning to normal events, or holding fixed false personal beliefs (delusions). No single symptom is definitive for diagnosis; rather, the diagnosis encompasses a pattern of signs and symptoms, in conjunction with impaired occupational or social functioning (American Psychiatric Association, 2000).

Symptoms are typically divided into positive and negative symptoms because of their impact on diagnosis and treatment. Positive symptoms are those that appear to reflect an excess or distortion of normal functions. The diagnosis of schizophrenia, according to *DSM-IV-TR*, requires at least 1-month duration of two or more positive symptoms, unless hallucinations or delusions are especially bizarre, in which case one alone suffices for diagnosis (DHHS, 1999). Negative symptoms are those that appear to reflect diminished, or loss of, normal functions. These often persist in the lives of people with schizophrenia during periods of low (or absent) positive symptoms. Negative symptoms are difficult to evaluate because they are not as grossly abnormal as positives ones and may be caused by a variety of other factors as well (e.g., as an adaptation to a delusion of being persecuted).

Diagnosis is complicated by early treatment of schizophrenia's positive symptoms. Antipsychotic medications, particularly the traditional ones, often produce side effects that closely resemble the negative symptoms of affective flattening and lack of motivation. In addition, other negative symptoms are sometimes present in schizophrenia but not often enough to satisfy diagnostic criteria (American Psychiatric Association, 2000): loss of usual interests or pleasures; disturbances of sleep and eating; dysphoric mood (depressed, anxious, irritable, or angry mood); and difficulty concentrating or focusing attention (DHHS, 1999).

More than a disease of hallucinations and delusions, many people with schizophrenia also have deficits in cognitive functions, such as memory, learning, and attention. These cognitive problems vary from person to person and can change over time.

Cultural variation is an important consideration in relation to schizophrenia. On first consideration, symptoms like hallucinations, delusions, and bizarre behavior seem easily defined and clearly pathologic. However, what is considered delusional in one culture may be accepted as normal in another. For example, among members of some cultural groups, visions or voices of religious figures are part of normal religious experience. In many communities, seeing or being visited by a recently deceased person are not unusual among family members. Therefore, labeling an experience as pathologic or a psychiatric symptom can be a subtle process for the clinician with a different cultural or ethnic background from the patient; indeed, cultural variations and nuances may occur within the diverse subpopulations of a single racial, ethnic, or cultural group. Often, however, clinicians' training, skills, and views tend to reflect their own social and cultural influences.

No description of symptoms can adequately convey a person's experience of schizophrenia or other serious mental illness. Two individuals with very different internal experiences and outward presentations may be diagnosed with schizophrenia if both meet the diagnostic criteria. Also, people with the disorder can have symptoms that vary. This considerable variation has led to the naming of several subtypes of schizophrenia, depending on what symptoms are most prominent. Currently these are seen as variations within a single disorder. Similarly, the diagnosis is often difficult because other mental disorders share some common features. Diagnosis depends on the details of how people behave and what they report during an evaluation, the diagnostician, and variations in the illness over time. Therefore, many people receive more than one diagnostic label over the course of their involvement with mental health services. Refining the definition of schizophrenia and other serious mental illnesses to account for these individual and cultural variations remains a challenge to researchers and clinicians.

Studying the course of schizophrenia and other serious mental illnesses is difficult because of the changing nature of diagnosis, treatment, and social norms. Overall, research indicates that schizophrenia's course varies considerably from person to person and for each person over time.

The outlook for people with schizophrenia has improved over the last 25 years. Although no totally effective therapy has yet been devised, it is important to remember that many people with the illness improve enough to lead independent, satisfying lives. As we learn more about the causes and treatments of schizophrenia, we should be able to help more patients achieve successful outcomes. Studies that have followed people with schizophrenia for long periods, from the first episode to old age, reveal that a wide range of outcomes is possible. However, the current state of knowledge does not allow for a sufficiently accurate prediction of long-term outcome. Although progress has been made toward better understanding and treatment of schizophrenia, continued investigation is urgently needed. Schizophrenia does not follow a single pathway. Rather, like other mental and somatic disorders, course and recovery are determined by a constellation of biological, psychological, and sociocultural factors. That different degrees of recovery are attainable has offered hope to patients and families.

COMMUNITY INTERVENTIONS FOR ADULTS

Adult programs provide a range of services. Some common places they are offered is at the workplace, hospital, community site, place of worship, and colleges and universities. These programs focus on mental health issues such as stress management, drug rehabilitation, housing and job training for the homeless, and respite care. Outpatient individual and group programs exist as well as inpatient programs.

Support groups are growing. These exist online and in the community. The topics are broad and include examples such as drug dependence, anger management, suicide prevention, divorce, grieving, parenting, and for specific diseases such as depression. An example of a successful program is the U.S. Air Force Suicide Prevention Program (AFSPP). This population-oriented program is geared toward reducing the risk of suicide. A cohort of active-duty U.S. Air Force personnel exposed to the intervention between 1997 and 2002 was compared to a cohort not exposed between 1990 and 1996. The intervention cohort experienced a 33% relative risk reduction compared to the control cohort ($p < 0.001$). The intervention cohort also experienced relative risk reductions for homicide (51%; $p = 0.05$), accidental death (18%; $p = 0.05$), severe family violence (54%; $p < 0.0001$), and moderate family violence (30%; $p < 0.0001$) when compared to the control cohort (Substance Abuse and Mental Health Services Administration [SAMHSA], 2006). A well-known program is Alcoholics Anonymous (AA). The effectiveness of this program has been difficult to measure because of the anonymity of its members and because many members attend meetings in various locations.

CHAPTER SUMMARY

As individuals move into adulthood, developmental goals focus on productivity and intimacy, including pursuit of education, work, leisure, creativity, and personal relationships. Good mental health enables individuals to cope with adversity while pursuing these goals. Untreated, mental disorders can lead to lost productivity, unsuccessful relationships, and significant distress and dysfunction. Mental illness in adults can have a significant and continuing effect on children in their care.

Stressful life events or the manifestation of mental illness can disrupt the balance adults seek in life and result in distress and dysfunction. Severe or life-threatening trauma experienced either in childhood or adulthood can further provoke emotional and behavioral reactions that jeopardize mental health.

In this chapter, we discussed how personality traits affect mental health. Anxiety, mood disorders, and schizophrenia are particular problems in this age group. Anxiety and depression contribute to the high rates of suicide in this population. Schizophrenia is the most persistently disabling condition, especially for young adults, in spite of recovery of function by some individuals in mid to late life.

REVIEW

1. What are some contributing factors to mental illness among adults?
2. What are some personality traits that can contribute to mental illness among adults?
3. What are some personality traits that can protect adults from mental illness?
4. What are the common mental health illnesses that adults encounter?
5. Describe the symptoms of these common mental illnesses.

ACTIVITY

Obtain a copy of the health statistics for your college or university through the National College Health Assessment or student health center. Review the data related to mental health, and write a three-page paper on the status of the problem, the factors related to the cause of the problem, and what could be done to reduce or eliminate the problem.

REFERENCES AND FURTHER READINGS

American Psychiatric Association. (1998). Practice guidelines for the treatment of patients with panic disorder. *American Journal of Psychiatry*, *155*(Suppl. 12), 1–34.

American Psychiatric Association. (2000). *Diagnostic and Statistical Manual of Mental Disorders* (*DSM-IV-TR*). Arlington, VA: Author.

Ballenger, J. C., Davidson, J. R., Lecrubier, Y., Nutt, D. J., Bobes, J., Beidel, D. C., . . . Westenberg, H. G. (1998). Consensus statement on social anxiety disorder from the International Consensus Group on Depression and Anxiety. *Journal of Clinical Psychiatry*, *59*(Suppl. 17), 54–60.

Dombeck, M., & Wells-Moran, J. (2006). Personality trait theory. Retrieved from http://www.mentalhelp.net/poc/view_doc.php?type=doc&id=9715&cn=353

Hollander, E. (1996). Obsessive-compulsive disorder-related disorders: The role of selective serotonergic reuptake inhibitors. *International Clinical Psychopharmacology*, *11*(Suppl. 5), 75–87.

Kessler, R. C, Chiu W. T., Demler O., & Walters E. E. (2005). Prevalence, severity, and comorbidity of twelve-month DSM-IV disorders in the National Comorbidity Survey Replication (NCS-R). *Archives of General Psychiatry, 62*(6), 617–627.

Mayo Clinic. (2008). Resilience: Build skills to endure hardship. Retrieved from http://www.mayoclinic.com/health/resilience/MH00078

Mental Health and Psychiatry News. (2007). Impulsivity may especially vex alcoholics with antisocial and borderline personality disorders. Retrieved from http://www.health.am/psy/more/impulsivity-may-especially-vex-alcoholics/

Mowbray, C. T., Moxley, D. P., Thrasher, S., Bybee, D., McCrohan, N., Harris, S., & Clover, G. (1996). Consumers as community support providers: Issues created by role innovation. *Community Mental Health Journal, 32*, 47–67.

National Alliance on Mental Illness [NAMI]. (2008). Major depression. Retrieved from http://www.nami.org/Template.cfm?Section=By_Illness&template=/ContentManagement/ContentDisplay.cfm&ContentID=7725

Psychology Today. (2008a). Cyclothymia. Retrieved from http://www.psychologytoday.com/conditions/cyclothemia.html

Psychology Today. (2008b). Dysthymia. Retrieved from http://www.psychologytoday.com/conditions/dysthymia.html

Rosenberg, S. D., Lu, W., Mueser, K. T., Jankowski, M. K., & Cournos, F. (2007). Correlates of adverse childhood events among adults with schizophrenia spectrum disorders. *Psychiatry Services, 58*, 245–253, February 2007. doi: 10.1176/appi.ps.58.2.245. Retrieved from http://psychservices.psychiatryonline.org/cgi/content/abstract/58/2/245

Sanderson, C. A. (2004). *Health psychology*. Hoboken, NJ: Wiley.

Springhouse Corporation. (1990). Erikson's development stages. Retrieved from http://honolulu.hawaii.edu/intranet/committees/FacDevCom/guidebk/teachtip/erikson.htm

Substance Abuse and Mental Health Services Administration [SAMHSA]. (2006). SAMSHA's national registry of evidence-based programs and practices. United States Air Force Suicide Prevention Program. Retrieved from http://nrepp.samhsa.gov/listofprograms.asp?textsearch=Search+specific+word+or+phrase&ShowHide=1&Sort=1&A5=5&S7=7

U.S. Census Bureau Population Estimates by Demographic Characteristics. (2005). Table 2: Annual estimates of the population by selected age groups and sex for the United States: April 1, 2000 to July 1, 2004 (NC-EST2004-02). Source: Population Division, U.S. Census Bureau. Release Date: June 9, 2005. Retrieved from http://www.census.gov/popest/national/asrh/

U.S. Department of Health and Human Services. (1999). *Mental health: A report of the surgeon general*. Rockville, MD: U.S. Department of Health and Human Services, Substance Abuse and Mental Health Services Administration, Center for Mental Health Services, National Institutes of Health, National Institute of Mental Health. Retrieved from http://www.surgeongeneral.gov/library/mentalhealth/home.html

Vaughan, S. C., & Oldham, J. M. (1997). Behavioral and adaptive functioning. In A. Tasman, J. Kay, & J. A. Lieberman (Eds.), *Psychiatry* (Vol. 1, pp. 549–562). Philadelphia: Saunders.

World Health Organization. (2004). The World Health report 2004: Changing history, Annex Table 3: Burden of disease in DALYs by cause, sex, and mortality stratum in WHO regions, estimates for 2002. Geneva, Switzerland: Author.

CHAPTER 8

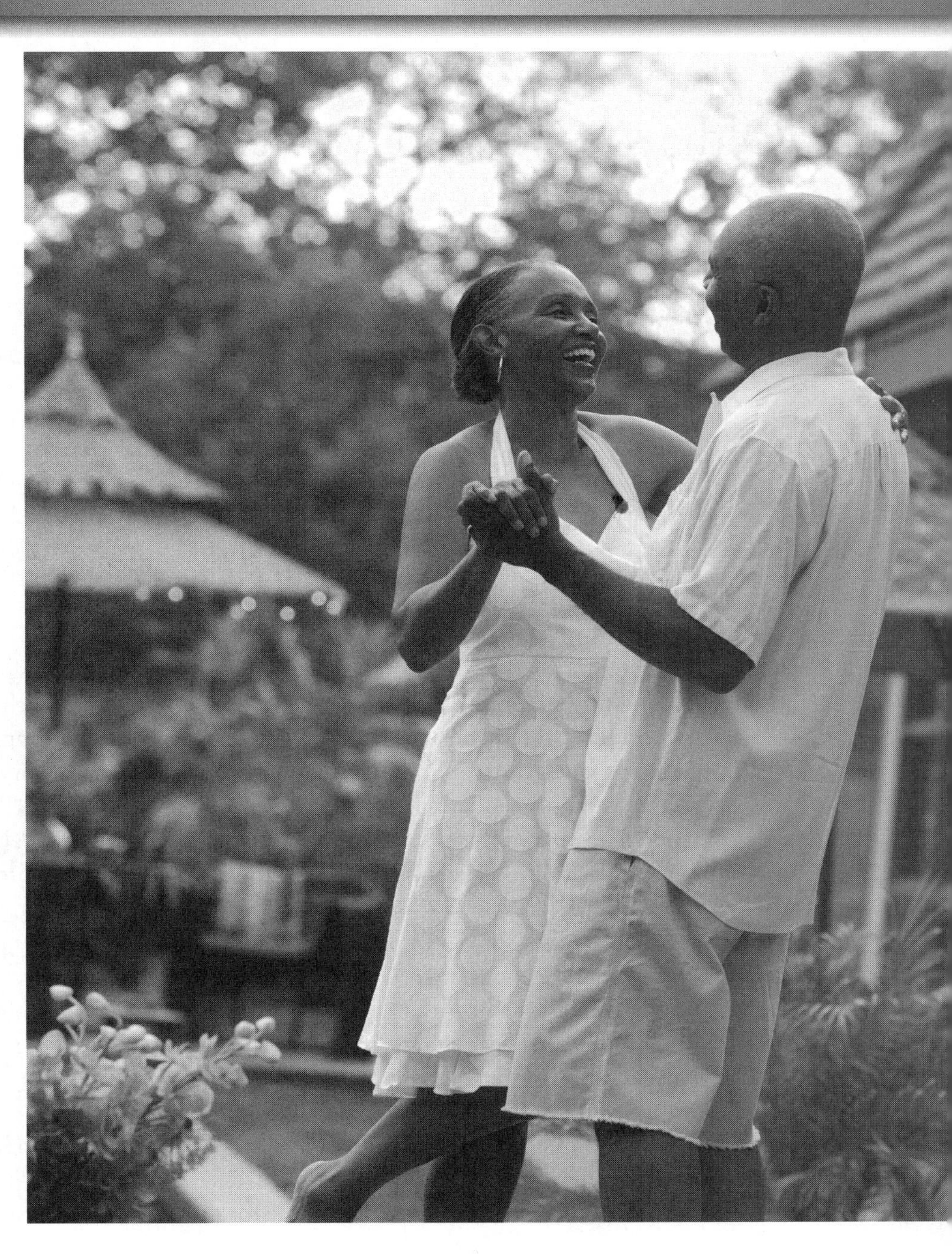

Older Adults and Mental Health

CHAPTER OBJECTIVES

1. Describe the normal milestones of the aging process.
2. Describe the challenges associated with diagnosing and treating mental illness among older adults.
3. Describe contributing factors to mental health problems among older adults.
4. Explain several common mental health problems among older adults and the related symptoms.

KEY TERMS

- Alzheimer's disease
- Crystallized intelligence
- Delirium
- Dementia
- Fluid intelligence
- Normal aging
- Polypharmacy

People are living longer, and the number of older adults is growing at an unprecedented rate. This has caused a growing need and interest in research related to the health of the elderly. Public health efforts to develop, evaluate, and implement mental health programs have led to an increase in the amount of information available about mental health among the elderly.

One model postulates that successful aging is contingent on three elements: avoiding disease and disability, sustaining high cognitive and physical function, and engaging with life (Rowe & Kahn, 1997). The last element encompasses the maintenance of interpersonal relationships and productive activities, as defined by paid or unpaid activities that generate goods or services of economic value. The three major elements are considered to act in concert, for none is deemed sufficient by itself for successful aging. This model broadens the reach of health promotion in aging to entail more than just disease prevention.

Many myths surround the elderly, and although the idea that most elders are incapacitated and immobile is incorrect, elders do have high risk factors for mental illness. The risk factors include having multiple general medical conditions, taking multiple medications, limited and/or fixed income to pay for prevention services and treatment, and psychosocial stressors such as bereavement or isolation. It is estimated that 20% of people age 55 years or older experience some type of mental health concern (American Association for Geriatric Psychiatry, 2004). The most common conditions include anxiety, severe cognitive impairment, and mood disorders (American Association for Geriatric Psychiatry, 2004). These issues often play a role in suicide. Older men have the highest rate of suicide of any age group (Centers for Disease Control and Prevention [CDC], 2009). Suicide rates for men are highest among those aged 75 and older (rate: 35.7 per 100,000) compared to an overall rate of 10.95 per 100,000 for all ages (CDC, 2009).

Treating mental health problems among people in this age group can be challenging because they can be affected by general medical conditions, take multiple medications, have limited finances, and/or are affected by changes in cognitive capacities. Late-life mental disorders also can pose difficulties for family members who assist in caretaking tasks for their loved ones. These issues are a concern, and they highlight the need for preventive interventions. The goal of such prevention strategies may be to limit disability or to postpone or even eliminate the need to institutionalize an ill person.

In this chapter, we explain the normal developmental milestones of aging and methods that older people can use to adapt to the changes that occur during this period of life. The chapter then focuses on mental disorders in older people and the related symptoms and the various risk factors that may complicate the course or outcome of treatment.

NORMAL DEVELOPMENT

According to Erikson, the older adulthood stage of life, Integrity versus Despair, is a time when the person reviews life accomplishments, deals with loss, and prepares for death (Springhouse Corporation, 1990). Erikson saw the period beginning at age 65 years as highly variable. Ideally, individuals at this stage witness the flowering of seeds planted earlier in the prior seven stages of development. When they achieve a sense of integrity in life, they garner pride from their children, students, other significant people in their lives, and past accomplishments. With contentment comes a greater tolerance and acceptance of the decline that naturally accompanies the aging process. Failure to achieve a satisfying degree of ego integrity can be accompanied by despair.

Older adulthood is a time often perceived as a stage of life when capacities and opportunities decline rather than expand. Although it is true that with aging comes certain changes in mental functioning, it also is true that the changes are less extreme than the stereotype leads people to believe. Society's view of getting old has not always kept up with the reality of older Americans' health or the fact that although many people older than 65 years experience some limitations, they learn to live with them and lead happy and productive lives. That being said, it is important to note that an estimated 80% of older adults do have at least one chronic condition, and 50% have at least two (CDC, 2007). Although some disability is the result of more general losses of physiological functions with aging (normal aging), extreme disability in older persons, including that which stems from mental disorders, is not an inevitable part of aging.

Although approximately 1 of 5 people 55 years and older experiences mental disorders that are not part of normal aging, mental disorders in older adults are believed to be underreported (American Association for Geriatric Psychiatry, 2004). It is estimated that only half of older adults who acknowledge mental health problems receive treatment from any healthcare provider (American Association for Geriatric Psychiatry, 2004). Unrecognized or untreated mental health problems such as depression, Alzheimer's disease, alcohol and drug misuse and abuse, anxiety, and late-life schizophrenia can be severely impairing, even fatal. Therefore, it is important that we continue to learn new strategies for preventing and managing mental health among the older population.

But what is normal aging? **Normal aging** is sometimes used to refer to changes attributed to aging itself and refers to the common complex of diseases and impairments that occur in many elderly people. Research that has helped differentiate mental disorders from normal aging has been one of the more important achievements of recent decades in the field of geriatric health. The following paragraphs describe the changes in mental functions that are related to age and part of the normal aging process.

Cognitive Capacity with Aging

Cognition refers to mental capacities such as intellect, language, learning, and memory that are used for remembering, thinking, and perceiving events. With age one's cognitive capacity diminishes, yet important functions are spared. The changes occur at different rates among older adults and are related to genetic and lifestyle factors. Lifestyle choices have a more powerful impact than genetics do on how well the body ages. This indicates that heredity does not solely determine how well one ages and that people are capable of influencing their aging process.

A vast amount of research has investigated changes in cognitive function with aging. Most studies show that, in general, cognitive abilities are at their peak when people are in their 30s and 40s, and they stay at that level until the late 50s or early 60s, at which point they begin to decline, but to only a small degree (American Federation for Aging Research, 2001). The effects of cognitive changes are not usually noticed until the 70s and beyond (American Federation for Aging Research, 2001).

Only certain cognitive abilities decline, and others may improve. These are some of the abilities that tend to change:

- Fluid and crystallized intelligence. Intelligence is commonly categorized into fluid and crystallized intelligence. **Fluid intelligence** (also called native mental ability) is the information-processing system and refers to the ability to think and reason. It includes the speed with which information can be analyzed, and also includes attention and memory capacity. **Crystallized intelligence** is accumulated information and vocabulary acquired from school and everyday life. It also encompasses the application of skills and knowledge to solving problems. Many studies have shown that fluid intelligence is more likely to decline with age than crystallized intelligence. In fact, crystallized intelligence may continue to improve with age. Many people continue to gain expertise and skills in particular areas throughout life (American Federation for Aging Research, 2001).
- Attention. If we do not pay attention to information then it is not taken in, and attention requires the ability to focus on information and to decide whether and how much to process it further. It is possible to pay attention to only a limited amount of information at any one time. Changes in attentional ability have been reported with older age. Some researchers have found that many older adults have increasing difficulty distinguishing between relevant and irrelevant information, so they find it difficult to focus only on the relevant information. This can cause them to be distracted by the irrelevant information and slow down the speed of performing a mental task, compromising accuracy (American Federation for Aging Research, 2001).
- Processing speed. Mental processing and reaction time become slower with age. This slowing of information processing speed actually begins in young adulthood (the late 20s). By the time people are past 60 or older (depending on the individual), they generally take longer to perform mental tasks than when they were younger (American Federation for Aging Research, 2001).
- Memory. There are different types of memory, and not all of them are affected by age. Memory difficulties are usually small and vary widely from person to person, making generalizations difficult. It is widely believed that working memory is most affected by age. Working memory is where conscious mental processing occurs and requires that information be manipulated or transformed in order to be retained. We all have limits on how much we can keep in working memory at one time. As people get older, complex mental tasks can become

more difficult if they require too much information to be held in memory in order to process it. Word retrieval also may become more difficult. The reasons for this are not known. One theory suggests that this also is due to slowed processing speed, and as people age there is more information stored to sort through (American Federation for Aging Research, 2001).

Memory complaints are common in older people; however, subjective memory complaints do not correspond with actual performance. When people forget when they are older they tend to worry more about it than when they forget at younger ages. Fewer than 1 in 5 people over age 65 experiences moderate to severe memory impairment (Population Reference Bureau, 2007). Among those 85 and older, the rate is higher but still less than 50% (Population Reference Bureau, 2007). Sometimes memory problems can be related to other factors such as depression and problems with attention. Somatic symptoms can cause cognitive problems. For example, hypothyroidism can cause dementia, and medications can cause delirium. Dementia and delirium are often confused, so we want to point out the differences here. **Delirium** has a sudden onset, causes fluctuations in mental function, and is usually reversible. When it occurs it is a medical emergency. **Dementia** occurs over a long period of time, progresses slowly, and is usually irreversible. Also, the two disorders affect mental function differently. Delirium affects mainly attention. Dementia affects mainly memory.

Change, Human Potential, and Creativity

Older adults are capable of changing in positive ways later in life, contradictory to the phrase, "You cannot teach an old dog new tricks." Older adults have the ability to be flexible in their attitudes and behavior and can learn and grow intellectually and emotionally. During the later years people have more time to devote to emotional and intellectual growth as external demands on their time may decrease. Also, because we are living longer, there is much more time between retirement and death. In the United States in the late 20th century, late-life expectancy approached another 20 years at the age of 65. In other words, average longevity from age 65 today approaches what had been the average longevity from birth some 2000 years ago. This leaves ample time to embark on new social, psychological, educational, and recreational pathways, as long as the individual retains good health and material resources.

Retirement often is viewed as the most important life event prior to death. Retirement is an event that some people welcome and embrace; others do not have a positive experience with it. Retirement's liberating qualities can provide the person with the opportunity to explore new interests, activities, and relationships.

Cohen (1995) proposed that with increased longevity and health, particularly for people with adequate resources, aging is characterized by two human potential phases.

These phases, which emphasize the positive aspects of the final stages of the life cycle, are termed *Retirement/Liberation* and *Summing Up/Swan Song*.

In the Retirement/Liberation phase, new feelings of freedom, courage, and confidence are experienced. Others do not do well in retirement, particularly if they are in poor health or experience a decline in their standard of living. Having more time and an increased sense of freedom can be liberating and the springboard for creativity in later life. Creative achievement by older people can change the course of an individual, family, community, or culture.

In the late-life Summing Up/Swan Song phase, there is a tendency to appraise one's life, work, ideas, and discoveries and to share them with family or society. The summing up stage can entail giving back to people for receiving so much during their lifetime (U.S. Department of Health and Human Services [DHHS], 1999). There is a tendency to reminisce and elaborate stories during this phase of life. The final part of this phase, referred to as the swan song, denotes the last act or final creative work of a person before retirement or death.

There is much misunderstanding about thoughts of death in later life. Depression, serious loss, and terminal illness trigger the sense of mortality, regardless of age. Most older adults do not fear death. Actually, the fear of death appears to peak in middle age. Periodic thoughts of death—not in the form of dread or angst—do occur, but these are usually associated with the death of a friend or family member. When actual dread of death does occur, it should not be dismissed as accompanying aging but rather as a signal of underlying distress (e.g., depression). This is particularly important in light of the high risk of suicide among depressed older adults.

Coping with Loss and Bereavement

Many older adults experience loss with aging—loss of social status and self-esteem, loss of physical capacities, and death of friends and loved ones. When faced with loss, some older people have the ability to adapt and even thrive. Those experiencing loss may be able to move in a positive direction, either on their own, with the benefit of informal support from family and friends, or with formal support from mental health professionals.

The life and work of William Carlos Williams are illustrative. Williams was a great poet as well as a respected physician. In his 60s, he suffered a stroke that prevented him from practicing medicine. The stroke did not affect his intellectual abilities, but he became so severely depressed that he needed psychiatric hospitalization. Nonetheless, Williams, with the help of treatment for a year, surmounted the depression and for the next 10 years wrote luminous poetry, including the Pulitzer Prize winner *Pictures from Brueghel*, which was published when he was 79. In his later life, Williams wrote about "old age that adds as it takes away." What Williams and his poetry epitomize is that age can be the catalyst for tapping into creative potential (Cohen, 1998).

In 2003, 44% of women and 14% of men 65 and older were widowed (DHHS, 2004). Bereavement is a natural response to death of a loved one. Its features include feelings of sadness, anxiety, anger, and guilt as well as agitation, insomnia, and loss of appetite. This constellation of symptoms, although overlapping somewhat with major depression, does not by itself constitute a mental disorder. Only when symptoms persist for 2 months and longer after the loss does the *DSM-IV-TR* permit a diagnosis of either adjustment disorder or major depressive disorder. Even though bereavement of less than 2 months' duration is not considered a mental disorder, it still warrants clinical attention (American Psychiatric Association, 2000). The justification for clinical attention is that bereavement, as a highly stressful event, increases the probability of, and may cause or exacerbate, mental and somatic disorders.

Bereavement is an important and well-established risk factor for depression. Without treatment, such depression tends to persist, become chronic, and lead to further disability and physical health problems, such as a weakened immune system or headaches. There are interventions that can help prevent the depression from becoming chronic, such as participation in counseling and self-help groups.

Unlike other major adverse life events, recent bereavement is an exclusion criterion for the diagnosis of major depressive disorder in the *DSM-IV-TR*. The rationale is that symptoms of major depression may be confused with symptoms of grief among newly bereaved individuals. In a review of grief course patterns, Bonanno and Kaltman (2001) found that in the first year of bereavement, most people demonstrate four types of disrupted functioning: cognitive disorganization, dysphoria (a negative emotional state), health deficits, and disruptions in both social and occupational functioning. In the group of cognitive changes, they include difficulty in accepting the loss, a sense of loss of part of oneself, uncertainty about the future, and a search for meaning. In most bereaved persons, these four domains of disrupted functioning are common in the first few months of bereavement and generally decline during the first year.

The dynamics around loss in later life need greater clarification. One pivotal question is why some, in confronting loss with aging, succumb to depression and suicide—which, as noted earlier, has its highest frequency after age 65—while others respond with new adaptive strategies. Research on health promotion also needs to identify ways to prevent adverse reactions and to promote positive responses to loss in later life. Meanwhile, despite cultural attitudes that older persons can handle bereavement by themselves or with support from family and friends, it is imperative that those who are unable to cope be encouraged to access mental health services. Bereavement is not a mental disorder, but if unattended to, it has serious mental health and other health consequences.

BOX 8-1 Program of All-Inclusive Care for the Elderly

The Program of All-Inclusive Care for the Elderly (PACE) features a comprehensive and seamless service delivery system and integrated Medicare and Medicaid financing. Eligible individuals are age 55 years or older and meet the clinical criteria to be admitted to a nursing home but choose to remain in the community. An array of coordinated services is provided to support PACE participants to prevent the need for nursing home admission. An interdisciplinary team, consisting of professional and paraprofessional staff, assesses participants' needs; develops care plans; and delivers or arranges for all services (including acute care and, when necessary, nursing facility services), either directly or through contracts. PACE programs provide social and medical services, primarily in an adult day health center setting referred to as the "PACE center," and supplement this care with in-home and referral services in accordance with the participants' needs. Each participant can receive all Medicare- and Medicaid-covered services, as well as other care determined necessary by the interdisciplinary team.

Source: SAMHSA. (2007). Program of All-Inclusive Care for the Elderly (PACE). Retrieved from http://nrepp.samhsa.gov/programfulldetails.asp?PROGRAM_ID=117. Accessed July 15, 2010.

PROTECTIVE FACTORS AND RISK FACTORS

Prevention in mental health has been seen until recently as an area limited to childhood and adolescence. Now there is mounting awareness of the value of prevention in the older population. The body of published literature is not as extensive as that for diagnosis or treatment, but investigators are beginning to shape new approaches to prevention. Yet because prevention research is driven, in part, by refined understanding of disease etiology—and etiology research itself continues to be rife with uncertainty—prevention advances are expected to lag behind those in etiology.

Prevention ideally occurs early in life and throughout life through lifestyles such as exercise, eating a well-balanced diet, timely health screenings, and so on. But that it not to say that prevention is not valuable when people get older. Progress in our understanding of etiology, risk factors, pathogenesis, and the course of mental disorders stimulates and channels the development of prevention interventions. For example, one approach to preventing depression is through grief counseling for widows and widowers. Participation in self-help groups may assist with coping in a healthy manner. Depression can lead to suicide, and this awareness has prompted the development of suicide prevention strategies expressly for primary care. Depression and suicide prevention strategies also are important for nursing home residents.

Prevention models can be applied to older individuals in many ways, provided a broad view of prevention is used (DHHS, 1999). Such a broad view entails interventions for reducing the risk of developing, exacerbating, or experiencing the consequences of a mental disorder. Prevention can occur at the three levels: primary (e.g., exercise), secondary (grief counseling and health screenings), and tertiary (hospitalization). Consequently, this section covers treatment-related prevention, prevention of excess disability, and premature institutionalization. However, many of the research advances noted in this section have yet to be translated into practice.

Treatment-Related Prevention

Prevention of relapse or recurrence of the underlying mental disorder is important for improving the mental health of older patients with mental disorders. Prevention of medication side effects and adverse reactions also is an important goal of treatment-related prevention efforts in older adults. Comorbidity and the associated polypharmacy for multiple conditions are characteristic of older patients. For example, certain medications may cause instability, which can lead to falls, which is a particular concern among older adults.

Prevention of Excess Disability

Prevention efforts in older mentally ill populations also target avoidance of excessive disability. The concept of excess disability refers to the observation that many older patients, particularly those with Alzheimer's disease and other severe and persistent mental disorders, are more functionally impaired than would be expected according to the stage or severity of their disorder. Medical, psychosocial, and environmental factors all contribute to excess disability. For example, depression is a risk factor for patients with Alzheimer's disease. The fast pace of modern life, with its emphasis on independence, also contributes to excess disability by making it more difficult for older adults with impairments to function autonomously. Attention to depression, anxiety, and other mental disorders may reduce the functional limitations associated with concomitant mental and somatic impairments. Many studies have demonstrated that attention to these factors and aggressive intervention, where appropriate, maximize function (DHHS, 1999).

Prevention of Premature Institutionalization

Another important goal of prevention efforts in older adults is prevention of premature institutionalization. Although institutional care is needed for many older patients who suffer from severe and persistent mental disorders, delay of institutional placement until absolutely necessary generally is what patients and family caregivers prefer. It also has significant public health impact in terms of reducing costs.

ASSESSMENT AND DIAGNOSIS

Assessment and diagnosis of late-life mental disorders are especially challenging by virtue of several distinctive characteristics of older adults. First, the clinical presentation of older adults with mental disorders may be different from that of other adults, making detection of treatable illness more difficult. For example, many older individuals present with somatic complaints and experience symptoms of depression and anxiety that do not meet the full criteria for depressive or anxiety disorders. The consequences of these subsyndromal conditions (exhibiting symptoms that are not severe enough for diagnosis as a clinically recognized syndrome) may be just as deleterious as the syndromes themselves. Failure to detect individuals who truly have treatable mental disorders represents a serious public health problem just as misdiagnosis can be.

Detection of mental disorders in older adults is complicated further by high comorbidity with other medical disorders. The symptoms of somatic disorders may mimic or mask psychopathology, making diagnosis more taxing. Also, older adults tend not to report psychological problems for reasons such as stigmas or embarrassment.

Primary care providers carry much of the burden for diagnosis of mental disorders in older adults, and, unfortunately, the rates at which they recognize and properly identify disorders often are low. Most patients with depression who are treated by primary care physicians do not receive care consistent with quality standards (Nauert, 2007).

The large unmet need for treatment of mental disorders reflects patient barriers (e.g., preference for primary care, tendency to emphasize somatic problems, reluctance to disclose psychological symptoms), provider barriers (e.g., lack of awareness of the manifestations of mental disorders, complexity of treatment, and reluctance to inform patients of a diagnosis), and mental health delivery system barriers (e.g., reimbursement policies).

Stereotypes about normal aging also can make diagnosis and assessment of mental disorders in late life challenging. For example, many people believe that senility is normal and therefore may delay seeking care for relatives with dementing illnesses. Similarly, patients and their families may believe that depression and hopelessness are natural conditions of older age, especially with prolonged bereavement.

Cognitive decline, both normal and pathologic, can be a barrier to effective identification and assessment of mental illness in late life. Obtaining an accurate history, which may need to be taken from family members, is important for diagnosis of most disorders and especially for distinguishing between somatic and mental disorders. Normal decline in short-term memory and especially the severe impairments in memory seen in dementing illnesses hamper attempts to obtain good patient histories.

Similarly, cognitive deficits are prominent features of many disorders of late life that make diagnosis of psychiatric disorders more difficult.

While somatic illness can mask psychopathology, elder abuse can be missed by attributing the symptoms to mental deterioration. Elder abuse may appear to be symptoms of dementia, depression, or signs of the elderly person's frailty—or caregivers may explain them that way. In fact, many of the signs and symptoms of elder abuse do overlap with symptoms of mental deterioration, but that does not mean community mental health professionals should dismiss them on the caregiver's say so. As many as 1 in 7 seniors nationwide falls victim to some type of elder abuse—usually at the hands of a family member (State Bar of California, 2009). The abuse can be financial, physical, or psychological. And the consequences can be deadly. Statistics suggest that abused and exploited seniors die sooner than other seniors their age. But in spite of such devastating consequences, most elder abuse goes unreported.

OVERVIEW OF TREATMENT

Treatment of mental disorders in older adults encompasses pharmacologic interventions and psychosocial interventions. Although the pharmacological and psychosocial interventions used to treat mental health problems and specific disorders may be identical for older and younger adults, characteristics unique to older adults may be important considerations in treatment selection.

Pharmacological Treatment

The special considerations in selecting appropriate medications for older people include physiological changes due to aging; increased vulnerability to side effects, the impact of polypharmacy; interactions with other comorbid disorders; and barriers to adherence. All are discussed in the following paragraphs.

The aging process leads to numerous changes in physiology, resulting in altered blood levels of certain medications, prolonged pharmacologic effects, and greater risk for many side effects. Changes may occur in how medications are metabolized. For example, as individuals age, the liver shrinks in size, blood flow to the liver decreases, and enzymes (in the liver) that break down medications decline. Another factor is the decrease in body fluid, which can lead to drugs becoming more highly concentrated, possibly exaggerating the medication's effect.

Because of these pharmacokinetic changes (what the body does to the drug) and pharmacodynamic changes (what a drug does to the body) as people age, it is often recommended that clinicians start low and go slow when prescribing new psychoactive medications for older adults. In other words, efficacy is greatest and side effects are minimized when initial doses are small and the rate of increase is slow. Nevertheless, the medication should generally be titrated to the regular adult dose to obtain the full benefit. The potential pitfall is that because of slower titration and the concomitant need for more frequent medical visits, there is less likelihood of older adults receiving an adequate dose and course of medication.

Increased Risk of Side Effects

The same concerns for psychiatric medications pertain to medications for older adults in general in terms of side effects. Of all the problems older adults face in taking medication, drug interactions are probably the most dangerous. When two or more drugs are mixed in the body, they may interact with each other and produce uncomfortable or even dangerous side effects. This is especially a problem for older adults because they are much more likely to take more than one drug. The more common side effects to psychiatric medications include weight gain, sexual problems, restlessness, irritability, tiredness, drowsiness, hyperactivity, clouded thinking, and memory problems (Hege, 2008).

Polypharmacy

In addition to the effects of aging on how medications are metabolized and the increased risk of side effects, older individuals with mental disorders also are more likely than other adults to be medicated with multiple compounds, both prescription and nonprescription. The annual average number of prescriptions per older adult grew from 19.6 in 1992 to 28.5 in 2000, an increase of 45% (American College of Clinical Pharmacy, 2005). By 2010, the annual average number of prescriptions per older adult is projected to grow to 38.5, an increase of 10 prescriptions or 35% per older adult from 2000 (American College of Clinical Pharmacy, 2005). **Polypharmacy** greatly complicates effective treatment of mental disorders in older adults. Specifically, drug–drug interactions are of concern, both in terms of increasing side effects and decreasing efficacy of one or both compounds.

Treatment Adherence

Adherence with the treatment regimen also is a special concern in older adults, especially in those with moderate or severe cognitive deficits. Physical problems, such as impaired vision, make it likely that instructions may be misread or that one medicine may be mistaken for another. Cognitive impairment also may make it difficult for patients to remember whether or not they have taken their medication. When nonadherence does occur, it may be less easily detected, more serious, less easily resolved, mistaken for symptoms of a new disease, or even falsely labeled as old-age symptomatology. Accordingly, greater emphasis and attention must be placed on adherence by older patients.

Medication nonadherence takes different forms in older adults, that is, overuse and abuse, forgetting, and alteration of schedules and doses. The most common type of deliberate nonadherence among older adults may be the underuse of the prescribed drug, mainly because of side effects and cost considerations. Other reasons include not understanding the need for taking the medication, having to take too many medications, poor relationship with their provider, and not understanding how to take the medication. Better adherence may be achieved by giving simple instructions and by asking specific questions to make sure that the patient understands directions.

Psychosocial Interventions

Several types of psychosocial interventions have proven effective in older patients with mental disorders, but the research is more limited than that on pharmacologic interventions. Both types are frequently used in combination.

Common intervention approaches include cognitive or behavioral training, physical activity training, peer support for dealing with specific stressors, education, and counseling or psychotherapy that is provided in an individual or group setting (Aging Healthy, 2008). Educational interventions are perhaps the most general approach, in that individuals can be educated about a multitude of issues, such as how to manage medications, how to cope with grief, and how to modify their home to make it more accessible. Other approaches include preventive health screening, special packaging of medications, pet therapy, music therapy, light therapy, intergenerational programs, adult day care, and cognitive training (Aging Healthy, 2008). It is becoming more common to target older adults both directly and indirectly through changes in their environment or to target multiple entities within a single intervention (e.g., the older adult, informal or formal caregivers, and the physician) (Aging Healthy, 2008). Important synergies are likely to be achieved by such simultaneous targeting of multiple individuals with intervention strategies that focus both on the pragmatic and psychological aspects of a given health-related problem.

Psychosocial interventions may be preferred for some older patients, especially those who are unable to tolerate, or prefer not to take, medication or who do not have a strong social support system. The benefits of psychosocial interventions are likely to assume greater prominence as a result of population demographics. As the number of older people grows, progressively more older people in need of mental health treatment—especially the very old—are expected to be suffering from greater levels of comorbidity or dealing with the stresses associated with disability. Psychosocial interventions can help relieve the symptoms of a variety of mental disorders and related problems and can play more diverse roles. They can help strengthen coping mechanisms, encourage (and monitor) patients' adherence with medications, and promote healthy behavior (Klausner & Alexopoulos, 1999).

New approaches to service delivery are being designed to realize the benefits of established psychosocial interventions. Many older people are not comfortable with traditional mental health settings, partially as a result of stigma. In fact, many older people prefer to receive treatment for mental disorders by their primary care physicians. Because older people show willingness to accept psychosocial interventions in the primary care setting, new models are striving to integrate into the primary care setting the delivery of specialty mental health services.

COMMON DISORDERS AMONG OLDER ADULTS

Although many older adults adapt to the aging process and change in their lives successfully, the number of older adults with mental illnesses is expected to double in the next 30 years. Mental illnesses have a significant impact on the health and functioning of older people and are associated with increased healthcare use and higher costs. Older adults account for a high percentage of suicide deaths and are at risk of developing both depression and alcohol dependence for perhaps the first time in their lives. In this section we discuss the more common disorders among older adults, which include depression, Alzheimer's disease, anxiety disorders, schizophrenia, and substance abuse.

Depression

Depression in older adults causes distress and suffering and can lead to impairments in physical, mental, and social functioning. Despite being associated with excess morbidity and mortality, depression often goes undiagnosed and untreated. Part of the problem is that depression in older people is hard to disentangle from the many other disorders that affect this age group, and its symptom profile is somewhat different from that in other adults. Another reason is that older people tend not to report psychological problems as often as they do physical ailments. Depressive symptoms are far more common than full-fledged major depression, which is why it is important to note that depression can be major or minor.

Diagnosis of Major and Minor Depression

The term *major depression* refers to conditions with a major depressive episode, such as major depressive disorder, bipolar disorder, and related conditions. Major depressive disorder is characterized by one or more episodes that include the following symptoms: depressed mood, loss of interest or pleasure in activities, significant weight loss or gain, sleep disturbance, psychomotor agitation or retardation, fatigue, feelings of worthlessness, loss of concentration, and recurrent thoughts of death or suicide. Major depressive disorder cannot be diagnosed if symptoms last for less than 2 months after bereavement, among other exclusionary factors (American Psychiatric Association, 2000).

Most older patients with symptoms of depression do not meet the full criteria for major depression. The new diagnostic entity of minor depression has been proposed to characterize some of these patients. Minor depression, a subsyndromal form of depression, is not yet recognized as an official disorder, and *DSM-IV-TR* proposes further research on it. Although the diagnosis of minor depression is not yet standardized, the research criteria proposed in *DSM-IV-TR* are the same as those for major depression, but a diagnosis would require fewer symptoms (with at least two depressive symptoms present for 2 weeks) and less impairment.

Minor depression is a common disorder that may impair a person's functioning and quality of life and is a serious risk factor for major depression. Minor depression, in fact, is not thought to be a single syndrome but rather a heterogeneous group of syndromes that may signify either an early or residual form of major depression, a chronic, although mild, form of depression that does not present with a full array of symptoms at any one time, and it may not be in response to a particular event or stressor. Because depression is more difficult to assess and detect in older adults, research is needed on what clinical features might help identify older adults at increased risk for sustained depressive symptoms and suicide.

Barriers to Diagnosis and Treatment

There are many barriers to the diagnosis of depression in late life. They include:

- Concurrent medical illness
- Medication side effects
- Impaired communication skills in the elderly
- Multiple somatic complaints
- Lack of time in the clinical examination

Some of these barriers reflect the nature of the disorder. Depression occurs in a complex medical and psychosocial context. In the elderly, the signs and symptoms of major depression are frequently attributed to normal aging, atherosclerosis, Alzheimer's disease, or any of a host of other age-associated afflictions. Psychosocial antecedents such as loss, combined with decrements in physical health and sensory impairment, also can divert attention from clinical depression. The consequences of underdiagnosis of this subset of patients can be severe.

Another barrier to diagnosis is that it can and frequently does amplify physical symptoms, distracting patients' and providers' attention from the underlying depression; and many older patients may deny psychological symptoms of depression or refuse to accept the diagnosis because of stigma.

Provider-related factors also appear to play a role in the underdetection of depression and suicide risk. Providers may be reluctant to inform older patients of a diagnosis of depression, owing to uncertainty about diagnosis, reluctance to stigmatize, uncertainty about optimal treatment, concern about medication interactions or lack of access to psychiatric care, and continuing concern about the effectiveness and cost effectiveness of treatment intervention (Unutzer, Katon, Sullivan, & Miranda, 1997).

Societal stereotypes about aging also can hamper efforts to identify and diagnose depression in late life. Many people believe that depression in response to the loss of a loved one, increased physical limitations, or changing societal role is an inevitable part of aging. Even physicians appear to hold such stereotyped views. Suicidal thoughts are sometimes considered a normal facet of old age. These mistaken beliefs can lead to underreporting of symptoms by patients and lack of effort on the part of family members to seek care for patients.

Finally, the healthcare system itself is increasingly restricting the time spent in patient care, forcing mental health concerns to compete with comorbid general medical conditions. Primary care physicians have limited time to spend with patients, which is particularly critical because primary care settings deliver most of the mental health treatment for depressed older adults. Consequently, recognition and management of late-life depression is an important responsibility for the primary care clinician. Given the inseparability of mental and general health in later life particularly, this trend of not having the time to address depression with older patients is worrisome.

Consequences of Depression

The most serious consequence of depression in later life—especially untreated or inadequately treated depression—is increased mortality from either suicide or somatic illness. Older persons (65 years and above) have the highest suicide rates of any age group. White men largely account for the high suicide rate among older people. Because national statistics are unlikely to include more veiled forms of suicide, such as nursing home residents who stop eating, estimates are probably conservative.

Depression is one of the most common conditions associated with suicide in older adults (Conwell, 2001). As stated previously, it is a widely underrecognized and undertreated medical illness. In fact, several studies have found that many older adults who die by suicide—up to 75%—have visited a primary care physician within a month of their suicide (Conwell, 2001). These findings point to the urgency of improving detection and treatment of depression as a means of reducing suicide risk among older persons.

Alzheimer's Disease

Alzheimer's disease is a disorder of pivotal importance to older adults. Every 71 seconds, someone in America develops Alzheimer's disease (Alzheimer's Association, 2008). An estimated 5.2 million Americans of all ages had Alzheimer's disease in 2008 (Alzheimer's Association, 2008). More women than men have Alzheimer's and other dementias, primarily because women live longer, on average, than men, and their longer life expectancy increases the time during which they could develop Alzheimer's or other dementias. The prevalence of Alzheimer's and other dementias also differs for people with fewer versus more years of education and for African Americans compared to whites (Alzheimer's Association, 2008).

Alzheimer's disease is one of the most feared mental disorders because of its gradual, yet relentless, attack on memory. Memory loss, however, is not the only impairment. Symptoms extend to other cognitive deficits in language, object recognition, and executive functioning. Behavioral symptoms—such as psychosis, agitation, depression, and wandering—are common and impose tremendous strain on caregivers. Diagnosis is challenging because of the lack of biological markers, insidious onset, and need to exclude other causes of dementia. The cause of Alzheimer's is unknown, but a genetic factor in Alzheimer's disease that develops after age 65 is apolipoprotein E-e4 (APOE-e4). *APOE e4* is one of three common forms of the *APOE* gene, which provides the blueprint for a protein that carries cholesterol in the bloodstream. Everyone inherits one form of the *APOE* gene from each of his or her parents. Those who inherit one *APOE e4* gene have increased risk of developing Alzheimer's disease (Alzheimer's Association, 2008). Those who inherit two *APOE e4* genes have an even higher risk, but there is still no certainty that they will develop Alzheimer's (Alzheimer's Association, 2008).

This section covers Alzheimer's disease because it is the most prevalent form of dementia and the cause of 60–80% of cases of dementia (Alzheimer's Association, 2008). However, many of the issues raised also pertain to other forms of dementia, such as multiinfarct dementia, dementia of Parkinson's disease, dementia of Huntington's disease, dementia of Pick's disease, frontal lobe dementia, and others.

Assessment and Diagnosis of Alzheimer's Disease: Mild Cognitive Impairment

Declines in cognitive functioning have been identified both as part of the normal process of aging and as an indicator of Alzheimer's disease. Mild cognitive impairment (MCI) characterizes those individuals who have a memory problem but do not meet the generally accepted criteria for Alzheimer's disease such as those issued by the National Institute of Neurological and Communicative Disorders and Stroke–Alzheimer's Disease and Related Disorders Association or *DSM-IV*. MCI is important because it is known that a certain percentage of patients will convert to Alzheimer's disease over a period of time. Thus, if such individuals could be identified reliably, treatments could be given that would delay or prevent the progression to diagnosed Alzheimer's disease.

The diagnosis of Alzheimer's disease depends on the identification of the characteristic clinical features and on the exclusion of other common causes of dementia. The other causes of dementia that must be ruled out include conditions such as cerebrovascular disease, Parkinson's disease, Huntington's disease, brain tumor, systemic conditions (e.g., hypothyroidism, vitamin B_{12} or folic acid deficiency, niacin deficiency, HIV infection), and substance-induced conditions. The diagnosis of Alzheimer's disease requires the presence of memory impairment and another cognitive deficit, such as language disturbance or disturbance in executive functioning. The diagnosis also calls for impairments in social and occupational functioning that represent a significant functional decline (American Psychiatric Association, 2000). Definite Alzheimer's disease can only be diagnosed pathologically through biopsy or at autopsy.

A further challenge in the identification of Alzheimer's disease is the widespread societal view of senility as a natural developmental stage. Early symptoms of cognitive decline may be excused away or ignored by family members and the patient, making early detection and treatment difficult. The clinical diagnosis of Alzheimer's disease relies on an accurate history of the patient's symptoms and rate of decline. Such information is often impossible to obtain from the patient due to the prominence of memory dysfunction. Family members or other informants are usually helpful, but their ability to provide useful information sometimes is hampered by denial or lack of knowledge about signs and symptoms of the disorder.

With diagnosis so challenging, Alzheimer's disease and other dementias are currently underrecognized, especially in primary care settings, where most older patients seek care. The reasons for primary care provider difficulty with diagnosis are speculated to include lack of knowledge or skills, misdiagnosis of depression as dementia, lack of time, and lack of adequate referrals to specialty mental health care.

The urgency of addressing obstacles to recognition and accurate diagnosis is underscored by promising studies that point to the pronounced clinical advantages of early detection. Therapies that slow the progression of Alzheimer's disease or improve existing symptoms are likely to be most effective if given early in the clinical course. Recognition of early Alzheimer's disease, in addition to facilitating pharmacotherapy, has a variety of other benefits that improve the plight of patients and their families. Direct benefits to patients include improved diagnosis of other potentially reversible causes of dementia, such as hypothyroidism, and identification of sources of Alzheimer's disease's excess disability such as depression and anxiety that can be targeted with nonpharmacologic interventions. Family members benefit from early detection by having more time to adjust and plan for the future and by having the opportunity for greater patient input into decisions regarding advanced directives while the patient is still at a mild stage of the illness (Cummings & Jeste, 1999).

Behavioral Symptoms

Alzheimer's disease is associated with a range of symptoms evident in cognition and other behaviors; these include, most notably, psychosis, depression, delusions, hallucinations, depression, agitation, and wandering. Other behavioral symptoms of Alzheimer's disease include insomnia; incontinence; catastrophic verbal, emotional, or physical outbursts; sexual disorders; and weight loss. Behavioral symptoms, however, are not required for diagnosis. Although behavioral symptoms have received less attention than cognitive symptoms, they have serious ramifications: patient and caregiver distress, premature institutionalization, and significant compromise of the quality of life of patients and their families (Kaufer et al., 1998). Alzheimer's disease can contribute to abuse by caregivers, particularly when the patient has behavioral symptoms.

Course

Patients with Alzheimer's disease experience a gradual decline in functioning throughout the course of their illness. Memory dysfunction is not only the most prominent deficit in dementia but also is the most likely presenting symptom. Deficits in language and executive functioning, although common in the disorder, tend to manifest later in its course (Locascio, Growdon, & Corkin, 1995). Depression is prevalent in the early stages of dementia and appears to recede with functional decline (Locascio et al., 1995). Although this may reflect decreasing awareness of depression by the patient, it also could reflect inadequate detection of depression by health professionals. The duration of illness, from onset of symptoms to death, averages 8 to 10 years (American Psychiatric Association, 2000).

Anxiety Disorders

Research on the course and treatment of anxiety in older adults lags behind that of other mental conditions, such as depression and Alzheimer's. Until a few years ago, anxiety disorders were believed to decline with age. But now experts are beginning to recognize that aging and anxiety are not mutually exclusive. Anxiety is as common in the old as in the young, although how and when it appears is distinctly different in older adults. As many as 20% of older adults have excessive anxiety (Glicksman, n.d.). It is believed to be more common than depression in late life. Seniors may find it harder to make changes or deal with stress than when they were younger. They may fear losing their independence and worry about their health, finances, or becoming a burden to their children (Glicksman, n.d.). Some dwell on death after the passing of a spouse or friend.

Anxiety disorders in the older adult population are real and treatable, just as they are in younger people. Another commonality between old and young is the high incidence of depression with anxiety. Depression and anxiety go together in the elderly, as they do in the young, with almost half of those with major depression also meeting the criteria for anxiety and about a quarter of those with anxiety meeting criteria for major depression (Anxiety Disorders Association of America, n.d.). As with younger persons, being a woman and having less formal education are risk factors for anxiety in older adults (Anxiety Disorders Association of America, n.d.).

Most older adults with an anxiety disorder had one when they were younger. What brings out the anxiety are the stresses and vulnerabilities unique to the aging process: chronic physical problems, cognitive impairment, and significant emotional losses.

Late-life anxiety disorders have been underestimated for several reasons, according to experts. For example, older patients are less likely to report psychiatric symptoms and more likely to emphasize their physical complaints, and some major epidemiologic studies have excluded generalized anxiety disorder, one of the most prevalent anxiety disorders in older adults (Anxiety Disorders Association of America, n.d.).

In addition, some disorders that have received less study in older adults may become more important in the near future. For example, military troops who served in the wars such as the Vietnam and Gulf wars; rescue workers involved in the aftermath of disasters like the terrorist attacks on New York City and Washington, D.C.; survivors of the Oklahoma City bombing; survivors of accidents, rape, physical and sexual abuse, and other crimes; immigrants fleeing violence in their countries; survivors of the 1989 California earthquake, the 1997 North and South Dakota floods, and hurricanes Katrina, Hugo, and Andrew; and people who witness traumatic events are among those at risk for developing posttraumatic stress disorder (PTSD). As affected patients age, there is a continuing need for services. In addition, research has shown that PTSD can manifest for the first time long after the traumatic event, and it can develop at any age. Posttraumatic stress is often associated with depression, panic and anxiety disorders, and alcohol and other substance abuse.

Schizophrenia

Although schizophrenia is commonly thought of as an illness of young adulthood, it can both extend into and first appear in later life. Diagnostic criteria for schizophrenia are the same across the lifespan, and *DSM-IV-TR* places no restrictions on age of onset for a diagnosis to be made. Positive symptoms include delusions, hallucinations, disorganized speech, disorganized or catatonic behavior, as well as negative symptoms such as affective flattening, the inability to speak, or avolition (lack of initiative or motivation). Symptoms must cause significant social or occupational dysfunction, must not be accompanied by prominent mood symptoms, and must not be uniquely associated with substance use.

Late-Onset Schizophrenia

Most of the previous research interest in schizophrenia focused on younger adults. With the aging of the general population, there is now an increase in the attention being given to older schizophrenic patients, including those with a late onset of the disorder (Jeste, Paulsen, & Harris, 2000). The literature in this area is still very limited, however, and is also laden with a number of methodological problems (Jeste et al., 2000).

There has been no general agreement on the definition of late-onset schizophrenia (LOS). Some studies chose 40 years of age as the cutoff, whereas others defined late onset as onset after 45, 60, or 65 years of age (Jeste et al., 2000). Furthermore, it is often difficult to determine the age of onset of schizophrenia, especially in older subjects. Elderly patients may not remember and significant others may have died, making confirmation of the patient's history difficult. The presence of premorbid paranoid or schizoid personality traits may further confuse the issue, and older patients with psychotic symptoms may be thought to have organic mental syndromes, mood disorders, or simple sensory deficits (Jeste et al., 2000). The earlier versions of the *Diagnostic and Statistical Manuals* (*DSMs*) did not have an upper age limit for the diagnosis of schizophrenia. It was not until the *DSM-III* that it was stipulated the onset of symptoms for schizophrenia had to be before age 45. Subsequently, the *DSM-III-R* allowed an onset of schizophrenic symptoms after age 45, and it used the term LOS for these individuals (Jeste et al., 2000). The *DSM-IV* and *DSM-IV-TR* do not specify an upper age limit; nor do they include a separate categorization of LOS.

Late-onset psychotic disorders may be fundamentally similar to their early-onset counterparts in the underlying neurobiologic predisposition (Jeste et al., 2000). Certain specific protective factors, however, may prevent an earlier breakdown, whereas other aging-related precipitants may be responsible for the onset of symptoms during later life. Specificity of neurobiologic substrates for different types of late-onset psychoses is yet to be established (Jeste et al., 2000).

Alcohol and Substance Use Disorders

Substance abuse, particularly of alcohol and prescription drugs, among adults 60 and older is one of the fastest-growing health problems facing the country and has been deemed an invisible epidemic. Estimates suggest that the number of substance dependent and abusing adults 50 years and older will climb from approximately 1.7 million in 2001 to 4.4 million by 2020 (Substance Abuse and Mental Health Services Administration, Office of Applied Studies, 2007). This pattern of growth is echoed in admissions to substance abuse treatment, where adult admissions 50 years or older increased from 143,900 to 184,400 (from 8% to 10% of all admissions) between 2001 and 2005 (Substance Abuse and Mental Health Services Administration, Office of Applied Studies, 2007). Yet, even as the number of older adults suffering from these disorders climbs, the situation remains underestimated, underidentified, underdiagnosed, and undertreated. Consequently, treatment for substance abuse may soon need to adapt to address the needs of this growing population.

Substance misuse and abuse for older adults can occur in many forms. It includes the use of drugs that can change mood, such as alcohol, tranquilizers, or illegal drugs. Substance misuse also includes risky drinking or unsafe use of medications. Any substance misuse or abuse can cause serious health problems and problems with family and friends, money, and the law. Medication, both prescription and over-the-counter misuse, is a particular concern with older adults.

Getting older causes bodily changes that can make the person respond differently to alcohol and medications. These changes mean there are differences between the way older adults and younger adults' bodies can handle alcohol. For example, the same amount of alcohol or number of drinks that had hardly any effect before may make an older person feel drunk. This means that as people get older, they can feel the effects with less alcohol (increased sensitivity), and they cannot drink as much as they used to (decreased tolerance to alcohol). Also, alcohol is processed by the body (metabolized) more slowly in older bodies, so blood alcohol levels are higher for a longer amount of time after drinking. This may mean increased danger of accidents, falls, and injuries for older adults even many hours after they drink alcohol.

Older people are more likely to have at least one chronic illness. Many chronic illnesses can make people more likely to have bad reactions to alcohol. Drinking problems also can be more hidden among older people because they are more likely to drink at home, do not have to show up at work the day after drinking, drive less after drinking, and may see friends or other people less frequently.

People 65 years and older take more prescription and over-the-counter medications than any other age group in the United States. Prescription drug misuse and abuse is common among older adults because more drugs are prescribed to them and also because getting older makes the body more likely to feel the effects of drugs (just like with alcohol). Many older adults have problems because some medications do not combine well with other medications. Drinking alcohol with some medications also causes problems for many older adults.

Some prescription and over-the-counter medications can often cause bad side effects that make thinking and regular daily activities more difficult. Older adults can have more adverse drug effects such as excessive daytime sleepiness, problems remembering information or paying attention, slower physical reactions, dizziness, and problems with moving normally. Sometimes drugs can cause memory problems, such as not knowing exactly where you are or what day it is (disorientation) or "acting crazy" (delirium). Sometimes, this is thought to be Alzheimer's disease, even though it is a problem with medications.

COMMUNITY INTERVENTIONS FOR OLDER ADULTS

Programs for older adults often take place in places of worship, senior centers, adult day-care centers, nursing homes, hospitals, medical clinics, retirement communities, and community centers. The programs can include topics such as grieving, medication management, stress management, coping with change, depression, and support groups related to specific disease such as Alzheimer's. As the population grows older, there is an increasing need for such community programs. These programs assist with the particular problem as well as provide a social outlet for seniors. Some seniors are homebound or face transportation issues, so home-based programs such as Program to Encourage Active, Rewarding Lives for Seniors (PEARLS) can be invaluable.

PEARLS is an intervention for people 60 years and older who have minor depression or dysthymia and are receiving home-based social services from community services agencies. The program is designed to reduce symptoms of depression and improve health-related quality of life. PEARLS provides eight 50-minute sessions with a trained social service worker in the client's home over 19 weeks. Counselors use three depression management techniques: (1) problem-solving treatment, in which clients are taught to recognize depressive symptoms, define problems that may contribute to depression, and devise steps to solve these problems; (2) social and physical activity planning; and (3) planning to participate in pleasant events (Substance Abuse and Mental Health Services Administration [SAMHSA], 2007). Counselors encourage participants to use existing community services and attend local events. Symptoms of depression were measured using the Hopkins Symptoms Checklist 20 (HSCL-20), a self-report instrument used for the diagnosis of major depression in adult primary care patients (SAMHSA, 2007). At 12 months, compared with the usual care group, patients receiving the PEARLS intervention were more likely to have at least a 50% reduction in symptoms of depression (43% versus 15%; $p < 0.001$) and to achieve complete remission from depression (36% versus 12%; $p = 0.002$) (SAMHSA, 2007).

CHAPTER SUMMARY

Important life tasks remain for individuals as they age. Older individuals continue to learn and contribute to society, in spite of physiologic changes due to aging and increasing health problems. Continued intellectual, social, and physical activities throughout the life cycle are important for the maintenance of mental health in late life. Stressful life events, such as declining health and/or the loss of mates, family members, or friends, often increase with age. However, persistent bereavement or serious depression is not normal and should be treated. Normal aging is not characterized by mental or cognitive disorders. Mental or substance use disorders that present alone or co-occur should be recognized and treated as illnesses. Disability due to mental illness in individuals older than 65 years will become a major public health problem in the near future because of demographic changes. In particular, dementia, depression, and schizophrenia, among other conditions, will all present special problems in this age group.

In this chapter, we discussed what is normal aging and that mental health disorders among older adults are sometimes attributed to the aging process in error. We discussed some of the contributing factors to mental health problems during this stage of life and the common problems.

REVIEW

1. What are some contributing factors to mental illness among older adults?
2. What are some challenges related to diagnosing mental health problems in older adults?
3. What are the common mental health illnesses that older adults encounter?
4. Describe the symptoms of these common mental illnesses.

ACTIVITY

Interview a retired person older than 65 years. Ask the person about how he or she feels about getting older and retirement. Inquire about their greatest needs, fears, and joys at this stage of life.

REFERENCES AND FURTHER READINGS

Aging Healthy. (2008). Psychosocial-behavioral interventions. Retrieved from http://medicine.jrank.org/pages/937/Interventions-Psychosocial-Behavioral.html

Alzheimer's Association. (2008). *2008 Alzheimer's Disease Facts and Figures*, *4*(2).

American Association for Geriatric Psychiatry. (2004). Geriatrics and mental health—the facts. Retrieved from http://www.aagpgpa.org/prof/facts_mh.asp

American College of Clinical Pharmacy. (2005). Pharmacy practice, research, education, and advocacy for older adults. Retrieved from http://www.accp.com/docs/positions/whitePapers/phco.2005.25.10.pdf

American Federation for Aging Research. (2001). Neurobiology of Aging Information Center. Retrieved from http://www.healthandage.com/html/min/afar/content/other6.htm

American Psychiatric Association. (2000). *Diagnostic and Statistical Manual of Mental Disorders (DSM-IV-TR)*. Arlington, VA: Author.

Anxiety Disorders Association of America. (n.d.). Anxiety disorders in older adults. Retrieved from http://www.adaa.org/GettingHelp/AnxietyDisordersinOlderAdults.asp

Bonanno, G.A., & Kaltman, S. (2001). The varieties of grief experience. *Clinical Psychology Review*, *21*, 705–734.

Centers for Disease Control and Prevention [CDC]. (2007, April). *Healthy aging: Preserving function and improving quality of life among older Americans*. Retrieved from http://www.cdc.gov/nccdphp/publications/aag/pdf/healthy_aging.pdf

Centers for Disease Control and Prevention [CDC]. (2009). Suicide. Retrieved from http://www.cdc.gov/violenceprevention/pdf/Suicide-DataSheet-a.pdf

Cohen, G. D. (1995). Human potential phases in the second half of life: Mental health theory development. *American Journal of Geriatric Psychiatry*, 3, 1–5.

Cohen, G. D. (1998). Creativity and aging: Ramifications for research, practice, and policy. *Geriatrics*, *53*(Suppl. 1), S4–S8.

Conwell, Y. (2001). Suicide in later life: a review and recommendations for prevention. *Suicide and Life Threatening Behavior*, 31(Suppl), 32–47.

Cummings, J., & Jeste, D. (1999). Alzheimer's disease and its management in the year 2010. *Psychiatric Services*, *50*, 1173–1177.

Glicksman, E. (n.d.). Anxiety in older adults. Retrieved from http://www.healthatoz.com/healthatoz/Atoz/common/standard/transform.jsp?requestURI=/healthatoz/Atoz/hc/sen/well/anxsen.jsp

Hege, D. (2008). Psychiatric medication side effects. Retrieved from http://www.eveningpsychiatrist.com/side-effects.htm

Jeste, D. V., Paulsen, J. S., and Harris, M. J. (2000). Late-onset schizophrenia and other related psychoses. Retrieved from http://www.acnp.org/g4/GN401000138/Default.htm

Kaufer, D. I., Cummings, J. L., Christine, D., Bray, T., Castellon, S., Masterman, D., . . . DeKosky, S. T. (1998). Assessing the impact of neuropsychiatric symptoms in Alzheimer's disease: The Neuropsychiatric Inventory Caregiver Distress Scale. *Journal of the American Geriatrics Society, 46*, 210–215.

Klausner, E. J., & Alexopolous, G. S. (1999, September). The future of psychosocial treatments for the elderly. *Psychiatric Research*, 50, 1198–1204.

Locascio, J. J., Growdon, J. H., & Corkin, S. (1995). Cognitive test performance in detecting, staging, and tracking Alzheimer's disease. *Archives of Neurology*, *52*, 1087–1099.

Nauert, R. (2007, September 5). PsychCentral. Primary care for depression may be substandard. Retrieved from http://www.psychcentral.com/news/2007/09/05/primary-care-for-depression-may-be-substandard

Population Reference Bureau. (2007). Today's research on aging. Retrieved from http://66.218.69.11/search/cache?ei=UTF-8&p=memory+older+age&fr=slv1-mdp&u=www.prb.org/pdf07/TodaysResearchAging5.pdf&w=memory+memories+older+old+age+aged+ages&d=ZV34hUfiSAgl&icp=1&.intl=us

Rowe, J. W., & Kahn, R. L. (1997). Successful aging. *Gerontologist*, *37*, 433–440.

Springhouse Corporation. (1990). Erikson's development stages. Retrieved from http://honolulu.hawaii.edu/intranet/committees/FacDevCom/guidebk/teachtip/erikson.htm

State Bar of California. (2009). Elder abuse. Retrieved from http://www.calbar.ca.gov/state/calbar/calbar_generic.jsp?cid=10581&id=24443

Substance Abuse and Mental Health Services Administration, Office of Applied Studies. (2007, November 8). *The DASIS Report: Older Adults in Substance Abuse Treatment: 2005*. Rockville, MD: Author.

Substance Abuse and Mental Health Services Administration [SAMHSA]. (2007). SAMHSA's National Registry of evidence-based programs and practices. Program to Encourage Active, Rewarding Lives for Seniors (PEARLS). Retrieved from http://nrepp.samhsa.gov/programfulldetails.asp?PROGRAM_ID=107

University of New South Wales. (2006, June 23). Brain function and negative thinking linked to late-onset depression. *ScienceDaily*. Retrieved from http://www.sciencedaily.com/releases/2006/06/060623100203.htm

Unutzer, J., Katon, W., Sullivan, M., & Miranda, J. (1997, November 6). *The effectiveness of treatments for depressed older adults in primary care*. Paper presented at Exploring Opportunities to Advance Mental Health Care for an Aging Population, meeting sponsored by the John A. Hartford Foundation, Rockville, MD.

U.S. Department of Health and Human Services [DHHS]. (1999). *Mental Health: A Report of the Surgeon General—Executive Summary*. Rockville, MD: U.S. Department of Health and Human Services, Substance Abuse and Mental Health Services Administration, Center for Mental Health Services, National Institutes of Health, National Institute of Mental Health. Retrieved from http://www.surgeongeneral.gov/library/mentalhealth/home.html

U.S. Department of Health and Human Services [DHHS]. (2004). A profile of older Americans: 2004. Retrieved from http://www.aoa.gov/prof/Statistics/profile/2004/2004profile.pdf

UNIT IV Community Mental Health

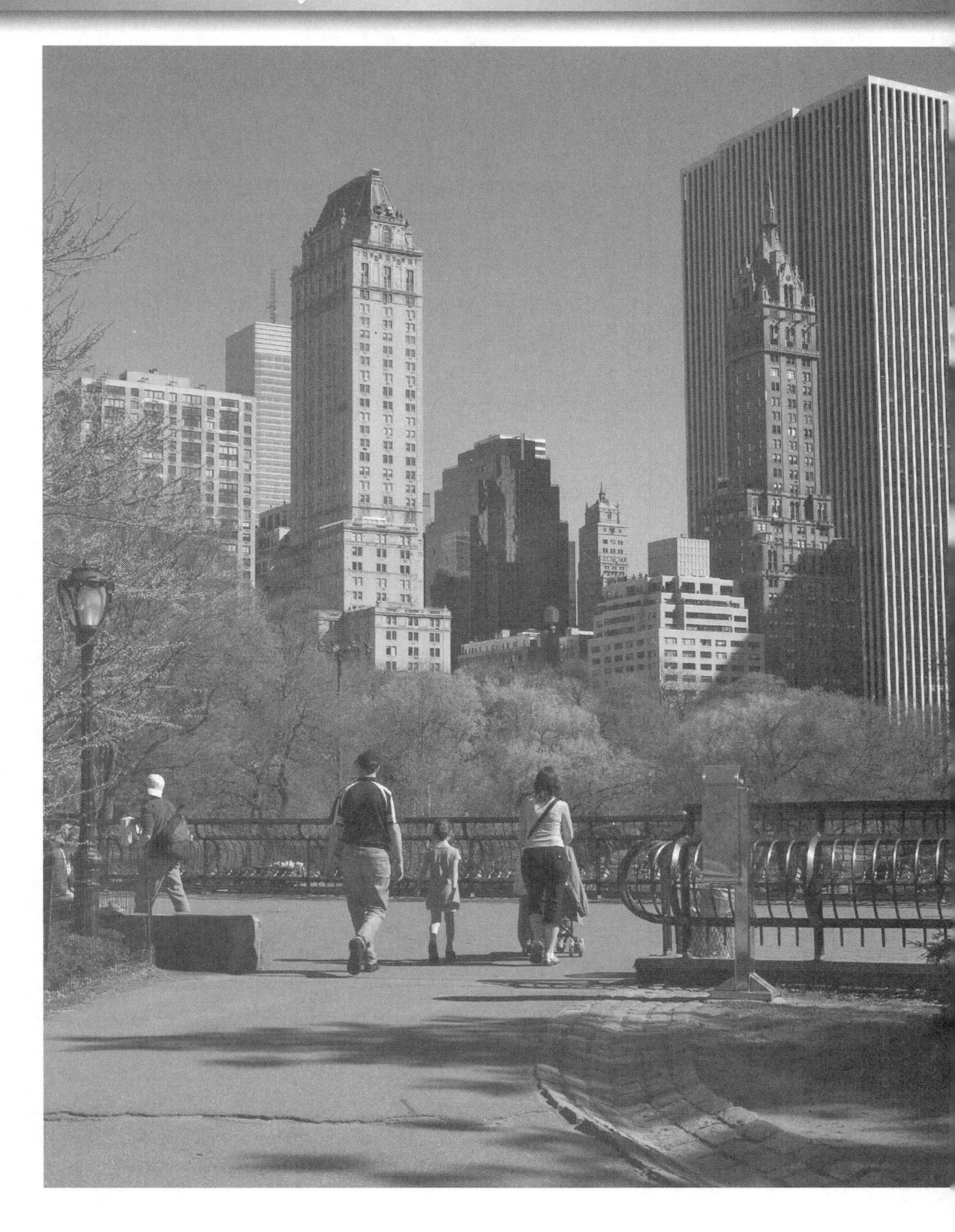

CHAPTER 9

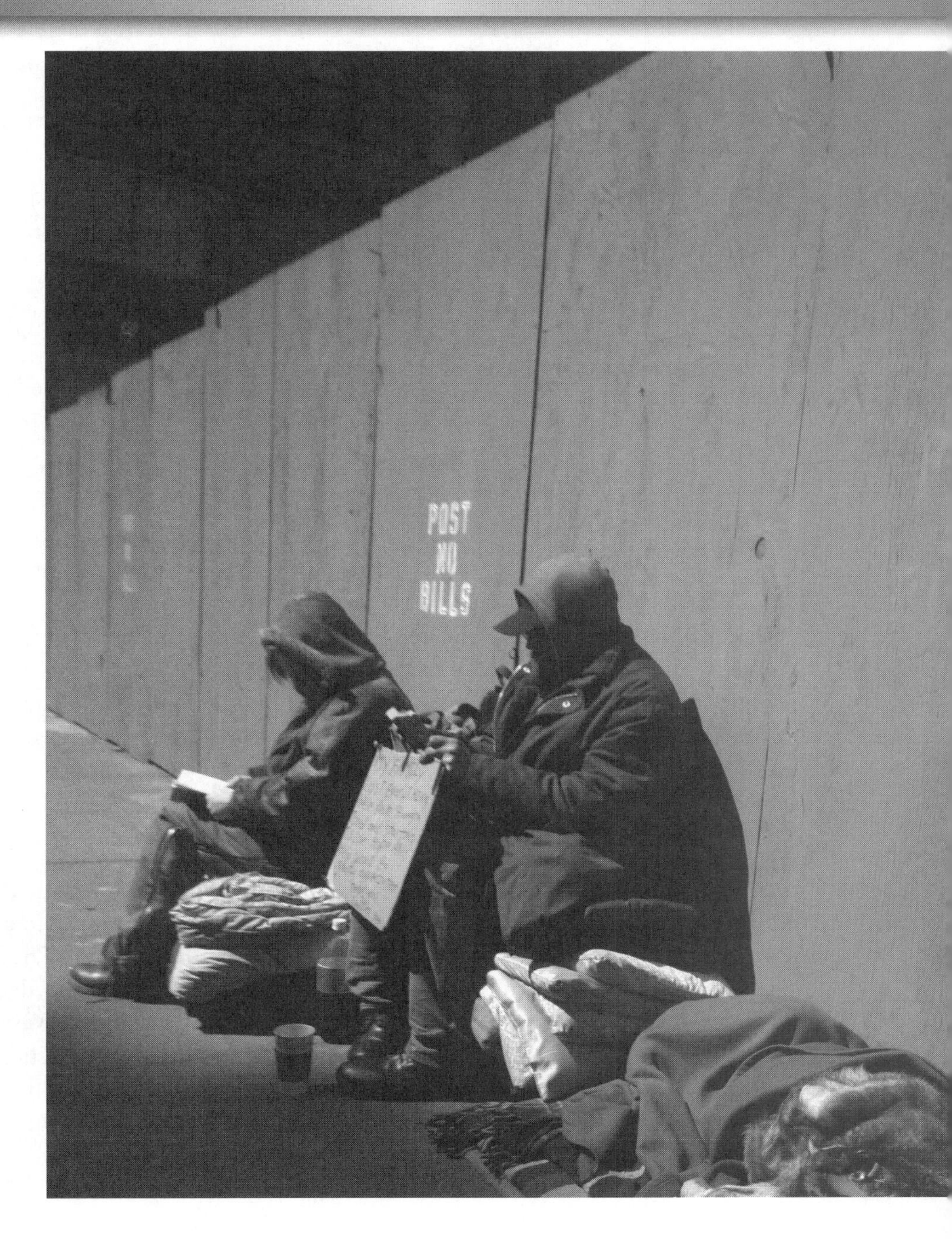

Community Mental Health Problems: Environment

CHAPTER OBJECTIVES

1. Discuss the effects of poverty, discrimination, and homelessness on mental health.
2. Explain how noise can lead to mental illness.
3. Discuss the effects of road rage on mental health.
4. Analyze the role of mental health professionals working with the homeless.
5. Analyze the link between poverty and mental illness.

KEY TERMS

- Discrimination
- Chronically homeless
- Homelessness
- Poverty
- Racism

This chapter examines community health problems that are common among the mentally ill and identifies how psychosocial factors such as discrimination, poverty, and environmental factors like noise, litter, and road rage contribute to mental health problems. The chapter begins with a discussion about poverty and ends with a review of the impact of homelessness and the severely mentally ill.

POVERTY

People living in **poverty** lack financial resources to maintain basic living standards, have fewer educational and employment opportunities, are exposed to adverse living environments, and are less able to access good quality health care. These factors put them at a higher risk of developing mental disorders. People who develop mental disorders who are poor are more likely to descend further into poverty because of increased healthcare costs, decreased productivity, and lost opportunities for employment. When mental health services are available, people are more likely to recover, find employment and provide for themselves and their families, and facilitate the conditions necessary to escape poverty.

Mental health and development are mutually reinforcing. A number of factors like nutrition, education, housing, respect for human rights, empowerment status, work status, social capital, access to health care, livelihood, and coping strategies, among others, mediate this interrelationship. This mutual interaction linking mental health and development can work positively, with good mental health facilitating the active and successful involvement of individuals and communities in development, and negatively, with poor mental health increasing the risk of descending into a vicious cycle of poverty and adverse social and health outcomes. **Figure 9-1** depicts the cycles and factors linking mental health and development and mental ill health and poverty.

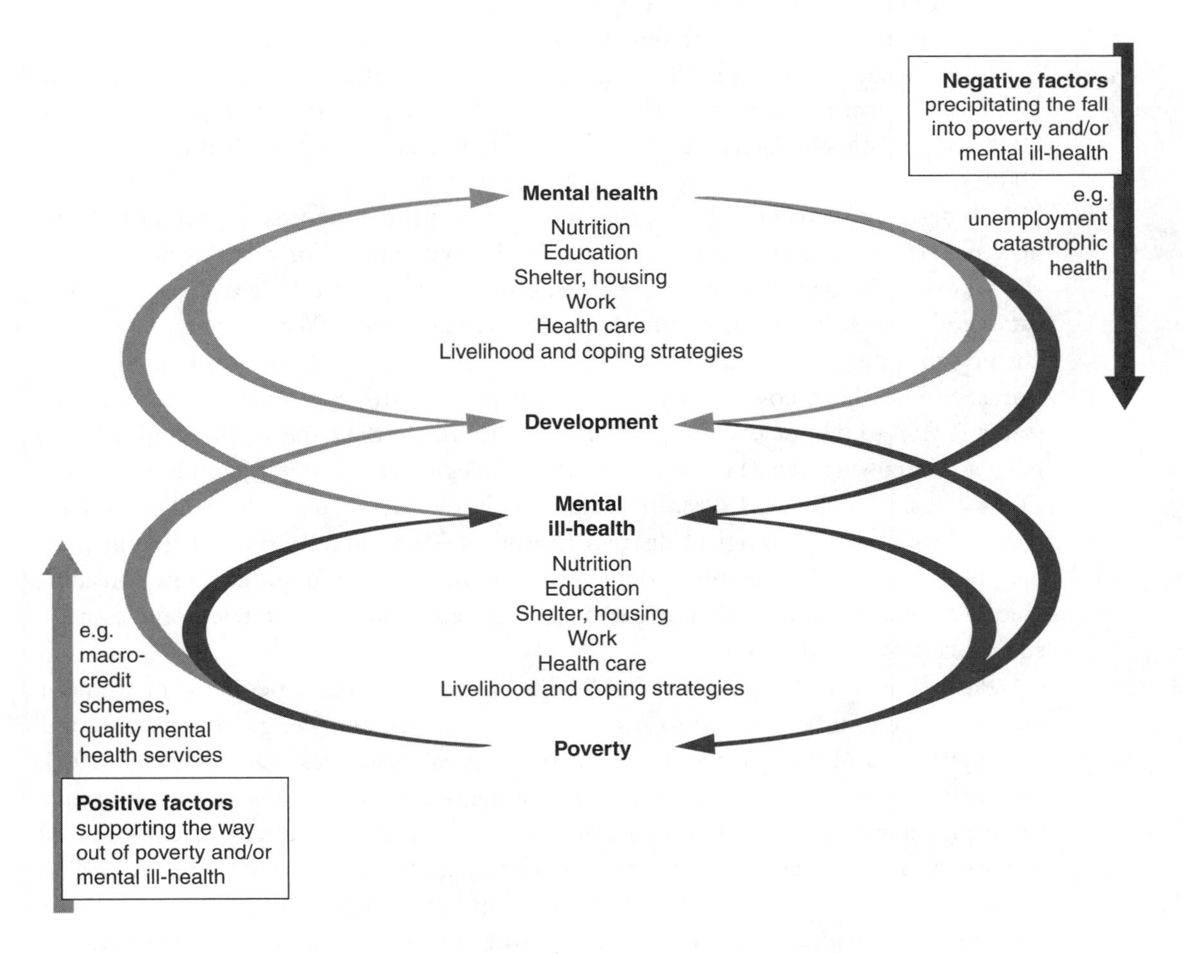

FIGURE 9-1 The Cycles and Factors Linking Mental Health and Development and Mental Ill Health and Poverty

Source: The WHO MIND Project: Mental Improvement for Nations Development Department of Mental Health and Substance Abuse (WHO, 2007).

Poverty, Marginal Neighborhoods, and Community Violence

The overall rate of poverty in the United States varies by race, family, age, and gender. Because of the recent economic downturn, the poverty rate increased between 2007 and 2008. The official poverty rate in 2008 was 13.2%, up from 12.5% in 2007 (DeNavas-Walt, Proctor & Smith, 2009).

This increase in poverty was the first statistically significant annual increase in the poverty rate reported since 2004. At that time, the poverty rate increased from 12.5% in 2003 to 12.7%. In 2008, an alarming 39.8 million people were in poverty, up from 37.3 million in 2007 (DeNavas-Walt, Proctor, & Smith, 2009). Subsequently, in 2008, the poverty rate increased for non-Hispanic whites (8.6% in 2008—up from 8.2% in 2007), Asians (11.8% in 2008—up from 10.2% in 2007), and Hispanics (23.2% in 2008—up from 21.5% in 2007) (DeNavas-Walt et al., 2009). The poverty rate in 2008 was statistically unchanged for African Americans (24.7%) (DeNavas-Walt et al., 2009).

To design effective outreach programs targeting the poor, it is important to know how poverty is related to poorer mental health outcomes. For decades, it has been shown that individuals living in poverty, regardless of race or ethnicity, have the poorest overall health status and health outcomes (Krieger, 1993; Yen & Syme, 1999). According to Adler and colleagues (1994), poverty also is linked to poorer mental health status. Studies have consistently shown that people with the lowest socioeconomic status (SES) are about two to three times more likely than those with high SES to have a mental disorder (Holzer et al., 1986; Kregier et al., 1993; Muntaner, Eaton, Diala, Kessler, & Sorlie, 1998). Individuals with low SES also are more likely to have higher levels of psychological distress (Eaton & Muntaner, 1999) and live in poor neighborhoods. Poor neighborhoods have few resources and suffer from considerable distress and disadvantage in terms of high unemployment rates, homelessness, substance abuse, and crime.

Poverty is linked to poor mental health in two ways. First, people who are poor are more likely to be exposed to stressful social environments (e.g., violence and unemployment) and have access to social or material resources (Dohrenwend, 1973; McLeod & Kessler, 1990). Second, having a mental disorder, such as schizophrenia, can have a negative impact on individual functioning and productivity, which can lead to poverty. Thus poverty is a consequence of mental illness (Dohrenwend et al., 1992). Both explanations provide a robust relationship between poverty and mental illness because the individual might not be able to work or maintain a job (U.S. Department of Health and Human Services [DHHS], 1999). Individuals living in poverty experience increased levels of mental illness, and the experience of racism also has been linked to acts of violence and poor mental health (discussed in the next section).

DISCRIMINATION

America has always struggled with issues related to race, ethnicity, and immigration. Since its inception, the histories of each racial and ethnic minority group can attest to long periods of legalized discrimination or more subtle forms of discrimination (Takaki, 1993). African Americans for example, were forcibly brought to the United States as slaves. The Indian Removal Act of 1830 forced Native Americans off their land and onto reservations in remote areas of the country. These remote areas lacked natural resources and economic opportunities. In 1882 the Chinese Exclusion Act barred immigration from China to the United States and denied citizenship to Chinese Americans until the law was repealed in 1952. Discrimination also was prominent toward Japanese Americans. Over 100,000 Japanese Americans were unconstitutionally incarcerated during World War II, yet none were ever shown to be disloyal. Many Hispanic/Latino Americans, Puerto Ricans, and Pacific Islanders became U.S. citizens through conquest, not choice.

Racism and **discrimination** are terms defining the beliefs, attitudes, and practices that defame individuals or groups because of the color of their skin, gender, age, ethnic or religious group affiliation. Racism and discrimination also have been documented in the administration of medical care. For example, fewer diagnostic and treatment procedures are provided to African Americans versus whites (Shiefer, Escarce, & Schulman, 2000). Additionally, racism and discrimination take forms from daily insults to more severe events, like hate crimes and other acts of violence (Krieger, Sidney, & Coakley, 1999). Institutions or individuals, acting intentionally or unintentionally, can perpetrate racism and discrimination.

Individuals from diverse backgrounds who report experiences with racism and discrimination define these experiences to be stressful (Clark, Anderson, Clark, & Williams, 1999). As race relates to discrimination, Williams (2000) found in a national study of minority groups that African Americans and Hispanic Americans reported experiencing higher overall levels of global stress than whites. The differences were shown in two specific types of stress: financial stress and stress from racial bias. Asian Americans also reported higher overall levels of stress and higher levels of stress from racial bias; however, they did not report financial stress. Hughes and Thomas (1998) linked the experience of racism to poorer mental and physical health. They found that racial inequalities might be the primary cause of differences in reported quality of life between African Americans and whites. Experiences of racism have also been linked to hypertension among African Americans (Krieger & Sidney, 1996; Krieger et al., 1999). Studies also show that African Americans found perceived discrimination to be associated with psychological distress, lower well-being, self-reported ill health, and number of days confined to bed (Ren, Amick, & Williams, 1999).

A national telephone survey, conducted in 1999, looked at two types of racism, their prevalence, and how they may affect mental health (Kessler et al., 1999). The first type of racism was termed "major discrimination" in reference to dramatic events like being "hassled by police" or "fired from a job." This form of discrimination was reported with a lifetime prevalence of 50% among African Americans, in contrast to 31% among whites (Kessler et al., 1999). Major discrimination was associated with psychological distress and major depression in both groups. The second form of discrimination is called "day-to-day perceived discrimination." It was reported more by African Americans (25%) than whites (3%) (Kessler et al., 1999). Day-to-day perceived discrimination was correlated to the development of distress and diagnoses of generalized anxiety and depression in African Americans and whites. The magnitude of the association between these two forms of discrimination and poorer mental health was similar to other commonly studied stressful life events, such as death of a loved one, divorce, or job loss.

There are few studies about the influence of racism on mental illness among racial and ethnic minorities. Perceived discrimination, however, was linked to symptoms of depression in a large sample of 5000 Asian, Latin American, and Caribbean children of immigrants (Rumbaut, 1994). Studies have also found that perceived discrimination was highly related to depressive symptoms among adults of Mexican origin (Finch, Kolody, &Vega, 2000) and among Asians (Yip, Gee, & Takeuchi, 2008).

In summary, racism and discrimination are stressful events that adversely affect health and mental health, and they place minorities at risk for mental disorders such as depression and anxiety (Clark et al., 1999). It has been found that racism may jeopardize the mental health of minorities in three general ways:

1. Racial stereotypes and negative images, when internalized, denigrate individuals' self-worth and negatively affect their psychosocial well-being and functioning.
2. Racism and discrimination by societal institutions have occurred in diverse populations, especially in people with lower socioeconomic status and poorer living conditions, for which poverty, crime, and violence are persistent stressors that can negatively affect mental stability.
3. Racism and discrimination are stressful events leading to psychological distress and physiological changes affecting mental stability (Williams & Williams-Morris, 2000).

ENVIRONMENTAL STRESSORS

Since 2000, environmental health was been considered one of the 22 objectives for the federal government's *Healthy People* initiative. *Healthy People 2020* objectives are presented in **Box 9-1**. As we all witness and cope with smoggy afternoons with poor

BOX 9-1 Proposed *Healthy People 2020* Objectives

ENVIRONMENTAL HEALTH

Objectives Retained as Is from *Healthy People 2010*

5: Reduce the proportion of occupied housing units that have moderate or severe physical problems.

Data Source: American Housing Survey, U.S. Department of Commerce, Bureau of the Census.
Action: Retained *Healthy People 2010* objective 8-23.

Objectives Retained But Modified from *Healthy People 2010*

13: Eliminate elevated blood lead levels in children.

Data Source: National Health and Nutrition Examination Survey (NHANES), CDC, NCHS.
Action: Retained but modified *Healthy People 2010* objective 8-11.

14: Minimize the risks to human health and the environment posed by hazardous sites.

Data Source: Comprehensive Environmental Response and Cleanup Liability Information System (CERCLIS), EPA.
Action: Retained but modified *Healthy People 2010* objective 8-12a.

15: Reduce the amount of toxic pollutants released into the environment.

Data Source: U.S. National Toxics Release Inventory (TRI), EPA.
Action: Retained but modified *Healthy People 2010* objective 8-14.

16: Reduce indoor allergen levels.

a. Reduce indoor allergen levels—cockroach
b. Reduce indoor allergen levels—mouse

Data Source: American Healthy Homes Survey, HUD.
Action: Retained but modified *Healthy People 2010* objective 8-16.

17: Increase the proportion of persons living in homes at risk that have an operating radon mitigation system.

Data Source: Annual estimates of homes with an operating mitigation system developed from annual data provided by radon vent fan manufacturers as reported to EPA, Indoor Environments Division.
Action: Retained but modified *Healthy People 2010* objective 8-18.

19: Increase the proportion of the Nation's elementary, middle, and high schools that have official school policies and engage in practices that promote a healthy and safe physical school environment:

a. Have an indoor air quality management program.
b. Have a plan for how to address mold problems.
c. Have a plan for how to use, label, store, and dispose of hazardous materials.
d. Reduce exposure to pesticides by using spot treatments and baiting rather than widespread application of pesticide.
e. Reduce exposure to pesticides by marking areas to be treated with pesticides.

(continued)

(Continued)

f. Reduce exposure to pesticides by informing students and staff prior to application of the pesticide.
g. Inspect drinking water outlets for lead.
h. Inspect drinking water outlets for bacteria.
i. Inspect drinking water outlets for coliforms.

Data Source: School Health Policies and Programs Study (SHPPS), CDC.

20: Increase the proportion of persons living in pre-1978 housing that has been tested for the presence of lead-based paint hazards.

a. Increase the proportion of pre-1978 housing that has been tested for the presence of lead-based paint.
b. Increase the proportion of pre-1978 housing that has been tested for the levels of lead in dust.
c. Increase the proportion of pre-1978 housing that has been tested for the levels of lead in soil.

Data Source: National Health Interview Survey, CDC, NCHS.
Action: Retained but modified *Healthy People 2010* objective 8-22.

21: Reduce exposure to selected environmental chemicals in the population, as measured by blood and urine concentrations of the substances or their metabolites.

Metals

a. Arsenic
b. Cadmium
c. Lead
d. Mercury, children aged 1 to 5 years.
e. Mercury, females aged 16 to 49 years.

Organochlorine pesticides

f. Chlordane (Oxychlordane)
g. DDT (DDE)
h. beta-hexacyclochlorohexane or beta-HCH

Non-persistent insecticides

i. Paranitrophenol (methyl parathion and parathions)
j. 3,4,6-trichloro-2-pyridinol (chlorpyrifos)
k. 3-phenoxybenzoic acid

Persistent industrial chemicals: Polychlorinated biphenyls (PCBs)

l. PCB 153, representative of nondioxin-like PCBs
m. PCB 126, representative of dioxin-like PCBs

Persistent industrial chemicals: Dioxins

n. 1,2,3,6,7,8-hexachlorodibenzo-p-dioxin, representative of the dioxin class

Potential endocrine disruptors

o. Bisphenol A
p. Perchlorate
q. Mono-n-butyl phthalate

Flame retardants: polybrominated diphenyl ethers (BDEs)

r. BDE 47, (2,2′,4,4′-tetrabromodiphenyl ether)

Data Sources: National Report on Human Exposure to Environmental Chemicals; National Health and Nutrition Examination Survey, NCHS, CDC.
Action: Retained but modified *Healthy People 2010* objectives 8-24 and 8-25.

22: Increase the number of Territories, Tribes, States, and the District of Columbia that monitor diseases or conditions that can be caused by exposure to environmental hazards.

a. Lead poisoning
b. Pesticide poisoning
c. Mercury poisoning
d. Arsenic poisoning
e. Cadmium poisoning
f. Acute chemical poisoning
g. Carbon monoxide poisoning

Data Source: Council of State and Territorial Epidemiologists State Reportable Conditions Data Inventory.
Action: Retained but modified *Healthy People 2010* objective 8-27.

Objectives New to *Healthy People 2020*

20–24: Decrease the number of U.S. homes that are found to have lead-based paint or related hazards.

a. Decrease the number of U.S. homes that have lead-based paint.
b. Decrease the number of U.S. homes that have paint-lead hazards.
c. Decrease the number of U.S. homes that have dust-lead hazards.
d. Decrease the number of U.S. homes that have soil-lead hazards.

Data Source: American Healthy Homes Survey, HUD.
Action: New to *Healthy People 2020*.

25: (Developmental) Decrease the number of new schools sited within 500 feet of a freeway or other busy traffic corridors.

Potential Data Source: GRASP/ATSDR geocoded data from Homeland Security Information Program.
Action: New to *Healthy People 2020*.

26: Increase the development and use of comprehensive municipal heat wave response plans addressing high-risk populations in cities with historic or projected excessive heat events.

Data Sources: National Climatic Data Center (NCDC), NWS; FEMA; public health departments.

Objectives Archived from *Healthy People 2010*

http://www.healthypeople.gov/hp2020/Objectives/files/Draft2009Objectives.pdf

Source: U.S. Department of Health & Human Services, Healthy People 2020 Objectives. http://www.healthypeople.gov/hp2020/Objectives/files/Draft2009Objectives.pdf. Accessed August 25, 2010.

air quality and toxic pollutants released in our oceans and food supply, it is crucial for individuals working with the mentally ill to be aware of underlying factors and risks of environmental toxins that might cause mental illness.

Public health research recognizes the environment as a primary determinant of health (Pope, Snyder, & Mood, 1995). This section briefly discusses the impact of the environment on mental health and the role of mental health professionals in detecting environmental health hazards and in developing and implementing health promotion and treatment programs targeting environmental stressors. Community mental health professionals must be prepared to address the effect the environment plays on the mentally ill and how to treat, prevent, and advocate for better environmental health both from an individual and a global point of view. Many mentally ill persons may live in blighted, rat-infested, single-occupancy hotels, many without running water, with mold and lead-painted walls. In addition, severely mentally ill persons often sleep on flattened cardboard boxes outside, under freeway entrances, and in cold and damp environments. Environmental problems have been a major public health problem for years, recently increasing in severity and frequency. However, private industries and individuals have become more aware of the environmental hazards that we have caused on earth, and more agencies and individuals are focusing on saving the environment by going green.

There has been some convincing data linking environmental factors to schizophrenia that might lead to mental illness. For example, birth in an urban city was linked to schizophrenia in the 1930s by Robert E. Lee Faris and H. Warren Dunham. In their classic study, they found high rates of schizophrenia among children born in inner-city Chicago. These findings have since been replicated numerous times in several countries, and it is believed that children born in urban areas are 50% more likely to be diagnosed with schizophrenia. Other environmental risk factors vary widely and include being born in winter and spring, maternal psychological stress during pregnancy, and obstetric complications. Research led by Brown and colleagues described in the August 2004 issue of the *Archives of General Psychiatry* showed that exposure to influenza in utero also can increase the risk of schizophrenia. Brown has also demonstrated that inflammatory cytokines such as interleukin 8 are expressed at higher levels in the serum of mothers whose children later became schizophrenic. Brown and colleagues (2004) report that high exposures to infectious agents may be more common in inner cities or during colder months when the population is more likely to be sick. In addition, studies have linked schizophrenia and prenatal exposure to a number of microbial infections, including those caused by rubella, toxoplasmosis, and influenza (Brown et al., 2004).

McClellan, Susser, and King (2006) are focusing their efforts on the possibility that schizophrenia can be triggered during pregnancy by maternal starvation. They have centered their research on two historical cohorts: a World War II–era famine in the western Netherlands caused by a Nazi blockade, and the Chinese famine that occurred from 1959 to 1961, precipitated by Mao Zedong's disastrous Great Leap Forward policy. Evidence from both cohorts suggests that maternal famine can double the risk of schizophrenia among offspring (McClellan et al., 2006).

In 1970, the U.S. Environmental Protection Agency (EPA) was formed and given the primary responsibility to control pollution and deal with threats to life and the environment. Although the EPA has regulations and a variety of programs in place to protect the environment, some environmental hazards have reached critical levels, poising a threat to the health status of individuals, our cities, and our nation. Polluting the air affects breathing, life, and health. Hazardous substances enter the environment and are transmitted to people in four ways:

1. Direct exposure to the source, such as lead in paint, mold, insecticides, and the sun.
2. Direct discharge into the air or water, for example exhaust from automobiles and oil spills in the water.
3. Inadequate landfills that result in runoff, leaching hazardous waste into groundwater or through the food chain.
4. Chemical waste buried with toxins like cyanide, heavy metals, and other toxins getting into surface water, groundwater, and soil. **Table 9-1** shows the effects on mental health of some common environmental toxins.

Life depends on food and water. However, for a person who is mentally ill, homeless, or living in an area without water, the circumstances might lead to dehydration, poor adherence with medications, body lice, and poor self-esteem. These individuals also might become ill because of drinking contaminated water or drinking water and consuming food from trash cans and dumpsters, which can lead to neurologic problems and death from high amounts of mold from old food and contaminated water. Moreover, according to a report from MSNBC on May 18, 2008, research conducted in the United States and Canada show that children exposed to pesticides used on foods that children frequently eat, including frozen blueberries, fresh strawberries, and celery, might lead to a diagnosis of attention deficit hyperactivity disorder (ADHD). According to the report, children with high levels of pesticide residue in their urine, particularly from widely used types of insecticide such as malathion, were more likely to have ADHD, a behavior disorder that often disrupts school and social life.

TABLE 9-1 Effects of Toxins on Mental Health

Toxin	Effect on Mental Health
Lead	Lead is a dangerous environmental contaminant known to interfere with learning and brain development. Lead exposure has a wide-ranging effect on children's behavior and development. It has been linked to low IQ and disruptive classroom behavior.
Mercury	Mercury exposure can impair children's memory, attention, and language abilities and interfere with fine motor and visual spatial skills.
Lindane	Lindane was available as recently as 2003 as a prescription medicine to eliminate head lice and was associated with symptoms such as dizziness, headaches, and convulsions.
Polychlorinated biphenyls (PCBs)	Polychlorinated biphenyls (PCBs), some of which are a form of dioxin, for example, have been banned in the United States for years but are still found in the environment. Researchers have found evidence that children exposed in the womb to low levels of PCBs grow up with poor reading comprehension, low IQs, and memory problems.
Endocrine disruptors	Endocrine disruptors are chemicals that can interfere with the human hormonal system, particularly the thyroid gland. During pregnancy, the hormones released by the thyroid are vital for normal development of the fetus's brain.
Plasticizers	Plasticizers are just now coming onto the radar screen as possible sources of health problems. One of them, bisphenol A, is found in pacifiers, baby bottles, and dental sealant used to prevent cavities in children. It's also found in many adult consumer products, according to Elise Miller, MEd, executive director of the nonprofit Institute for Children's Environmental Health and national coordinator of the Learning and Developmental Disabilities Initiative. "We all have bisphenol A in our bodies now," she says. Research on bisphenol A has shown it can affect both the reproductive and neurologic system, and it appears to accumulate at higher concentrations around the fetus—in the umbilical cord and amniotic fluid—than in the mother's blood.
Cyanide	Cyanide is released from natural substances in some foods and in certain plants such as cassava. Cyanide is contained in cigarette smoke and the combustion products of synthetic materials such as plastics. Combustion products are substances given off when things burn. If accidentally ingested (swallowed), chemicals found in acetonitrile-based products that are used to remove artificial nails can produce cyanide. Long-term health effects of exposure to cyanide may lead to heart and brain damage.

In addition, in recent years, more and more people can be seen pushing grocery carts overflowing with glass bottles, aluminum cans, and other recyclable materials for hours down urban streets to recycling locations, which are filled with dirt and grime. Persons who collect cans and bottles from dumpsters and trash cans might be homeless and suffer from mental illness. Daily pushing can lead to blisters and sore hands as well as swollen and painful feet from maneuvering the overloaded carts. Other areas of environmental concern for the mentally ill are secondhand smoke, litter, rats, and vermin like roaches that lead to problems such as asthma, rashes, skin irritations, and delusions.

NOISE

Although no one would say that noise by itself brings on mental illness, there is evidence that noise-related stress can aggravate existing emotional disorders. Research points to higher rates of admission to psychiatric hospitals among people living close to airports, and studies of several industries show that prolonged noise exposure may lead to a larger number of psychological problems among workers.

Noise as a health hazard is based on the level, frequency, and length of exposure. Depending on these factors, noise reaction falls into the categories of annoyance, disruption of activity, loss of hearing, and physical or mental deterioration (Hanlon & Pickett, 1984). The magnitude or level of noise is measured in decibels (dB). The dynamic range of the ear, or the difference between the loudest and the faintest sound, is about 120 dB (Bruce, 1985) as depicted in **Figure 9-2**. The danger level of noise leading to hearing loss for most people is 80 dB, and the current standard for workplace exposure is 90 dB averaged over 8 hours. The United States Environmental Protection Agency (EPA) defines 75 dB as a longtime-range goal for workplace exposure (EPA, 1978). The dB scale is based on powers of 10. Each increase in 10 dB is equivalent to multiplying the intensity by 10.

Of the many health problems related to noise, hearing loss is the most observable and measurable health problem documented by health professionals. Noise might be a complicating factor in heart problems and other diseases for individuals with poor health and causes aggravation and irritability in healthy persons. Moreover, noise may lead to serious outcomes for individuals that suffer mental illness and affects us throughout our lives.

Although the EPA report document regarding noise and health written in 1978 is somewhat outdated, the document is still very valuable today. The EPA report indicates that noise affects the unborn child of women who are exposed to industrial and environmental noise. Infants and children exposed to high noise levels may experience

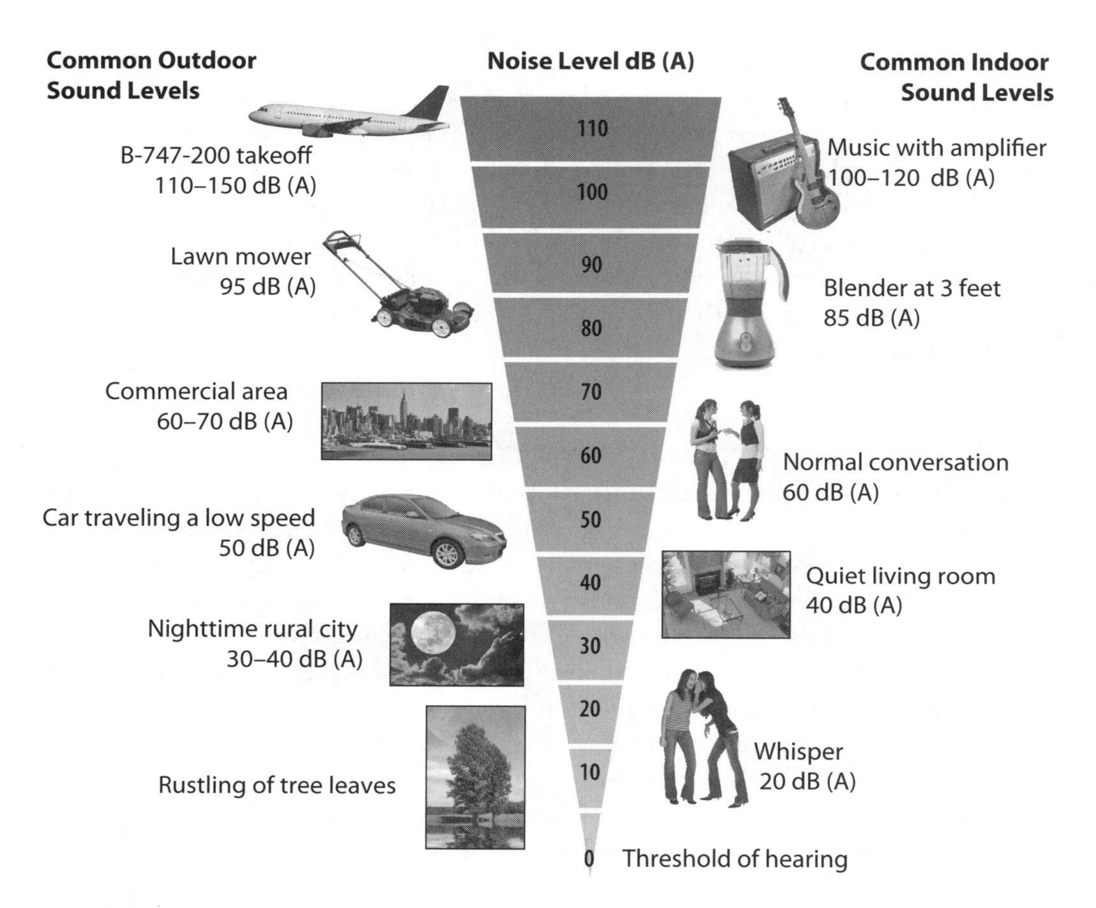

FIGURE 9-2 Sound Levels

learning difficulties and suffer poorer health (EPA, 1978; Evans & Marcynyszyn, 2004). Research also shows that children playing in noisy environments like school play areas and homes may have learning difficulties (EPA, 1978). Overexposure to noise can lead to problems with language development and reading ability. Because they are just learning, children have more difficulty understanding language in the presence of noise than adults do. Consequently, if children learn to speak and listen in a noisy environment, they may have difficulty developing essential skills such as distinguishing the sounds of speech. For example, in an area with high noise levels, a child may confuse the sound of "v" in "very" with the "b" in "berry" and may not learn to tell them apart. Another symptom of this problem is the tendency to distort speech by dropping parts of words, especially their endings (EPA, 1978).

Noise also can have an impact on the quality and quantity of sleep. Sleep is a restorative part of life, and a good night's sleep is crucial to good health. Everyday experience with loud noise suggests that noise interferes with our sleep in a number of ways: difficulty falling asleep, frequently waking up, and noise can cause shifts from deeper to lighter stages of sleep. If noise hindrance with sleep becomes a chronic problem, it may have an impact on the mental and physical well-being of an individual's health. Human response to noise before and during sleep varies among age groups. The elderly and the sick are particularly sensitive to disruptive noise. Compared to young people, an elderly person is more easily awakened by noise and, once awake, has more difficulty returning to sleep. As a group, the elderly require special protection from noises that interfere with their sleep.

Younger age groups seem to be less affected by noise at bedtime and while asleep. However, the adjustment to noise may be the result of failing to remember having awakened during the night (EPA, 1978). Sleep researchers have observed that their subjects often forget and underestimate the number of times they awaken during sleep. It may be that loud noises during the night continue to wake or rouse us when we sleep; as we become familiar with the sounds, however, we return to sleep more rapidly. Factors other than age can influence our sleep. Studies suggest that the more frequent the noise the less likely a sleeper will respond (Botteldooren, De Coensel, Berglund, Nilsson, & Lercher, 2008). Certain kinds of noises can cause almost predictable responses, however. A mother may wake immediately at the sound of a crying baby, but she may tune out louder traffic noise outside (EPA, 1978).

Noise interferes with our sleep by waking us or changing the depth of our sleep. It makes demands on our bodies to constantly adapt. Television news accounts report incidents that point to noise as a trigger of extreme behavior. For instance, a night clerical worker upset about noise outside his apartment shot one of the boys causing the disturbance after he had shouted at them, to no avail, to "Stop the noise." Sanitation workers have been assaulted, construction workers threatened, and motorboat operators shot at because of the noise they produce. Some people cope with loud noise by directing their anger and frustration inward, blaming themselves for being upset and suffering in silence. Others resort to denial of the problem, consider they are tough and pretend that the noise does not bother them. Others deal with noise in a more direct manner. They take sleeping pills, wear earplugs, keep their windows closed, rearrange their sleeping quarters, and spend less time outdoors (EPA, 1978; Stansfeld et al., 2005).

These ways of contending with noise are not likely to eliminate the noise or the underlying annoyance. People who cannot cope with noise typically direct their anger and frustration at others and become more argumentative and moody, although not necessarily violent. Reports from individuals about their worksites suggest that noise increases tension between workers and their supervisors, resulting in grievances against the employer.

Dozens of studies on noise have identified the effects of noise on workers as an important cause of physical and psychological stress, and stress has been directly linked with many common health problems (Cohen, 1981). Thus noise can be associated with disabilities and diseases, including heart disease, high blood pressure, headaches, fatigue, and irritability. However, most Americans are unaware that noise poses such significant dangers to their health and welfare. The reasons for this lack of awareness are clear. Noise is one of many environmental causes of stress and cannot easily be identified as the source of a particular physical or mental health symptom. Another reason is that biomedical and behavioral research is just beginning to assess the effects of noise on the physical and mental well-being of an individual exposed to excessive noise (EPA, 1978).

ROAD RAGE

In recent years, crowded freeway conditions, environmental factors, and a lack of patience have led to yet another concern regarding the mental well-being of individuals in our society. Road rage, also known as road violence, is the name for deliberately dangerous and/or violent behavior under the influence of heightened violent emotion such as anger and frustration involving an automobile in use. Road rage can involve one driver deliberately hitting another driver's vehicle with his or her own and/or firing a weapon at it. Other characteristics of road rage include hitting the person or vehicle with an object other than with a vehicle.

Getting out of one's vehicle and banging on the other driver's vehicle, knocking on the windows, and yelling insults at another driver are also forms of road rage. A variety of events, circumstances, and environments can lead to road rage. The three main categories defining road rage are the environment, instructive responses, and territorial defensiveness. Environmental conditions are the main factors associated with road rage. These conditions can consist of traffic congestion, another's dangerous driving habits, the weather (heat, humidity, etc.), noise levels, and time constraints. Intrusive responses are actions of retaliation to get back at another person for their careless driving, whereas territorial defensiveness is the act of defending one's personal space (the car) in response to another individual's driving. Road rage is a relatively serious act and also seen as a violation of property rights and an endangerment of personal security (Joint, 1995).

Half of drivers who are subjected to aggressive driving behavior on the road also respond with aggression, leading to a more serious confrontation (Connell & Joint,

1996). A survey conducted by Response Insurance Studies in 1995 show 50% of victims who get the finger or are cut off or tailgated respond by honking their horn, yelling, cutting off the driver, giving the finger or tailgating, and using other obscene gestures as well. The study revealed that 34% of drivers honked their horn, 27% yelled, 19% gave the finger back, 17% flashed their headlights, and 7% imitated the initial aggressive behavior (Connell & Joint, 1996). Two percent of the respondents verbalized they would try to run the person off the road if they had the opportunity (Connell & Joint, 1996).

Men are more likely than women to become aggressive, and drivers 18 to 24 years of age are more likely to become agressive than are drivers 65 and older (Connell & Joint, 1996). Drivers with children are more likely to respond aggressively than those without children, and all cell phone users are more aggressive and prone to road rage (Connell & Joint, 1996).

Connell and Joint (1996) offer the following advice for reducing stress and fatigue on the road:

- Before starting a trip, know how to get to the destination and have an alternate route in mind.
- Think about the timing of the journey.
- Service your vehicle and carry out routine checks (tire pressure, oil, water, etc.) regularly.
- Carry spare items (bulbs, fan belt, emergency sign for the windshield, etc.). Also, make sure the windshield is clean, particularly before a long trip. Peering through a dirty windshield is a common source of stress and fatigue when driving. Also, have a window cloth, de-icer, and sunglasses accessible.
- Be comfortable before starting out. Adjust the seat and mirrors, and make sure the seat belt and head restraint are correctly positioned.
- Take trips in stages and never remain behind the wheel of a car for more than three hours without a break. Do not cover more than 300 miles a day, and, on a long trip, be careful on the second day of driving. This is when most people tend to be vulnerable to fatigue.
- Make sure to get out of the car and stretch. Eat a light snack but avoid heavy meals, particularly at lunchtime. Avoid eating in noisy, crowded places.
- Relax before driving. Take time to concentrate on the task at hand, and forget about other problems while driving.
- Anticipate situations that are likely to lead to stress and be tolerant of other road users' errors. If the traffic is congested, try to accept there is little that can be done to prevent the delay.

- Take remedial action before stress and fatigue take over.
- Learn to spot the warning signs of stress and develop positive coping strategies, such as listening to the radio or a CD (many people listen to audiobooks).
- Open the windows to increase ventilation and consciously breathe in the air slowly.
- Do not grip the steering wheel too hard because it will tense arm and neck muscles, leading to fatigue symptoms such as headaches.
- If full images of recent events or conversations are repeatedly replaying in your mind, make a conscious effort to slow them down until they become softer and more distant.

HOMELESSNESS

Homelessness among the mentally ill is increasingly becoming a community health problem in urban areas across the United States. The homeless problem is large and diverse. Different definitions of homelessness are used in different contexts. As it is generally defined, **homelessness** is experienced by a person who "lacks a fixed, regular, and adequate night-time residence." An estimated 842,000 adults and children are homeless in any given week, with that number growing to as many as 3.5 million over the course of a year. People who are among the homeless have lost their jobs, are elderly, are families that may have been evicted, and are physically and/or mentally disabled (Substance Abuse and Mental Health Services Administration [SAMHSA], 1996). According to SAMHSA, approximately half (44%) of homeless people work at least part time; their monthly income averages only $367, compared to a median monthly income of $2840 for U.S. households (SAMHSA, 1996). Those who have disabilities and are unable to work find it nearly impossible to secure affordable housing in virtually every major housing market in the country.

Most homeless persons are unaccompanied adults. Sixty-six percent are single adults, and three quarters of them are men (SAMHSA, 1996). Because of their mental status, many mentally ill homeless people are unable to obtain access to supportive housing, jobs, and/or other treatment services, which can lead to anger and abusive behaviors. About 40% of homeless men are veterans, although veterans make up only 34% of the general adult male population. More important, the number of homeless families continues to grow. Among racial and ethnic minorities, African Americans represent approximately 40% of the homeless population compared to 11% of the general population; Hispanics, 11% compared to 9% of the general population; and 8% are Native Americans compared to 1% of the general population (SAMHSA, 1996).

Homelessness continues to be largely an urban phenomenon: Seventy-one percent are in central cities like San Francisco, Los Angeles, Chicago, and New York. Twenty-one percent are in suburbs, whereas only 9% of homeless individuals live in rural areas (Burt, Aron, Valente, & Iwen, 1999). People who are homeless frequently have health problems: Thirty-eight percent report alcohol use problems. Twenty-six percent of individuals who are homeless report other drug use problems, 39% report some form of mental illness, and between 20% and 25% meet the criteria for a diagnosis of a serious mental illness. Subsequently, 66% report substance use and/or mental health problems, and 3% report having HIV/AIDS. Having a medical problem creates another concern for healthcare professionals. Thus it is important to note that 26% of homeless individuals have acute health problems such as tuberculosis, pneumonia, or sexually transmitted diseases. And 46% of homeless individuals report they have chronic health conditions such as high blood pressure, diabetes, or cancer (SAMHSA, 1996).

People who are homeless also share other common characteristics: 23% are veterans (compared to 13% of the general population), 25% were physically or sexually abused as children, and 27% were in foster care or institutions as children. Twenty-one percent of the homeless population report they were homeless as children; 54% were incarcerated at some point in their lives (SAMHSA, 1996). Finally, the National Coalition for Homelessness estimates that on any given night, 200,000 veterans are homeless. Many homeless veterans suffer severe mental illness. Individuals who are seriously mentally ill and are homeless often have symptoms that are active. If untreated, the symptoms can make it difficult for them to meet basic needs like obtaining food, shelter, and safety. As a matter of fact, many of the health needs of the homeless mentally ill are related to the constant need to find food and shelter. Additionally, many homeless people have problems with their feet due to constant walking and hypothermia due to exposure to cold.

SERIOUS MENTAL ILLNESSES AND THE HOMELESS

Many homeless mentally ill individuals have a dual diagnosis of serious mental illness and substance abuse. Individuals with a dual diagnosis have greater difficulty being homeless than others. They are homeless more often, for longer periods than other homeless populations, and many have been on the streets for years. Moreover, most people with serious mental illnesses who are homeless have had prior contact with the mental health system, either as an inpatient or as outpatient (SAMHSA, 1996). Experiences with the mental health system for these individuals is not always positive; the person may have been hospitalized involuntarily or given treatment services or medications that they feel did not benefit them. The symptoms of severe mental illness are often combined with hygiene problems associated with homelessness; if untreated they can result in many physical health problems such as respiratory infections, dermatologic problems, and risk of exposure to HIV, bug infestations, and tuberculosis (O'Connell et al., 2005).

The social support and family networks of homeless severe mentally ill individuals are usually broken. Homeless individuals who have a family, children, or elderly parents often have lost regular contact with them or are no longer able to connect with the family or serve as a primary caregiver. Homeless individuals without family contact are twice as likely as other homeless people to be arrested or jailed, mostly for misdemeanors. Homeless severe mentally ill individuals are often good candidates for diversion programs that enable them to go from jail to more appropriate treatment, support, and housing programs (Greenwood et al., 2005).

Chronic Homelessness

According to the definition of the Department of Housing and Urban Development (HUD), a person who is **chronically homeless** is an unaccompanied homeless individual with a disabling condition (e.g., substance abuse, serious mental illness, developmental disability, or chronic physical illness) who has been continuously homeless either for a year or more or has had at least four episodes of homelessness in the past 3 years. To be considered chronically homeless, a person must have been sleeping in a place not meant for human habitation and/or in an emergency homeless shelter.

Prevention

To address the problems of homelessness among people with serious mental illnesses, a comprehensive approach to care must be implemented. Discharge planning that helps people who are leaving institutions to access housing, mental health, and other community services and resources can prevent homelessness during such transitions. Planning to prevent homelessness must begin upon admission into an institution, is ready to be implemented upon discharge, and involves consumer input. Providing short-term intensive support services immediately after discharge from hospitals, shelters, or jails has proven effective in further preventing recurrent homelessness during the transition back into the community (SAMHSA, 1996).

Ending Homelessness for People with Serious Mental Illnesses

Research has provided much information about what services and practices are effective in ending homelessness for people with serious mental illnesses. Key findings show that outreach, whether in shelters or on the street, is effective. Given the opportunity, most homeless people with serious mental illnesses are willing to accept treatment and services voluntarily. It is important that mental health professionals provide consistent outreach and introduce services at the client's pace. A key to success is to engage the mentally ill to accept treatment and case management services. A consistent, caring personal relationship is required to engage people who are homeless in treatment. Integrated mental health and substance abuse treatment provided by multidisciplinary treatment teams can also improve mental health, residential stability, and overall functioning in the community. Regular assertive outreach, lower caseloads, and a multidisciplinary approach is a formula that leads to positive treatment and housing outcomes (Rosenheck et al., 1998).

Supportive Services

Supportive housing has also proven to be effective in achieving residential stability, improving mental health, and reducing the costs of homelessness to the community (Greenwood et al., 2005). Many homeless people with serious mental illnesses prefer supported housing and can move directly from homelessness to independent housing with intensive support and attention.

CHAPTER SUMMARY

For the past 30 years, *Healthy People* has provided guidelines to healthcare providers aimed at motivating healthcare providers to design interventions that will improve the health of all Americans. During this time, they have tracked a comprehensive set of national 10-year health promotion and disease prevention objectives aimed at improving the health and mental well-being of all Americans. Environmental toxins, noise, and litter constitute health hazards both physically and mentally for the individual and for community. Prevention of environmental toxins, domestic violence, and noise are goals for prevention in *Healthy People 2020*. It is important that community mental health professionals monitor reports and serve as catalysts for problems that impact the environment and the mental health status of the people they serve. Equally important, community mental health professionals must be able to assess, design, and implement appropriate interventions for persons with mental illness as well as serve as advocates to influence legislation and health policies that affect the environment, poverty, and homelessness.

REVIEW

1. Describe the number of people living in poverty in the United States.
2. List and explain the mutually reinforcing factors of mental health and development.
3. Discuss the history of racism in America and how race influences mental health.
4. Discuss the environmental hazards that pose a threat to the health status of individual lives, our cities, and our nation.
5. Define how the term *homelessness* is used in different contexts.

ACTIVITIES

1. Read the local newspaper or search the Internet to determine information about environmental hazards that are common to persons who are mentally ill.
2. Review police reports regarding the number of road rage incidents that occur in your community. Design a community-based program to address road rage.
3. Identify persons in your community who work with the homeless population. Ask them to identify gaps in services. How would you address these gaps?
4. How would you advocate for noise reduction in your community?

REFERENCES AND FURTHER READINGS

Adler, N. E., Boyce, T., Chesney, M. A., Cohen, S., Folkman, S., Kahn, R. L., & Syme, S. L. (1994). Socioeconomic status and health: The challenge of the gradient. *American Psychologist*, *49*, 15–24.

Bell, C. C. (1996). Pimping the African-American community. *Psychiatric Services*, *47*, 1025.

Botteldooren, D., De Coensel, B., Berglund, B., Nilsson, M. E., & Lercher, P. (2008). Modeling the role of attention in the assessment of environmental noise annoyance. In: Proceedings of the 9th International Congress on Noise as a Public Health Problem (ICBEN) 2008, Foxwoods, CT.

Brown, A., Begg, M., Gravenstein, S., Schaefer, C., Wyatt, R., Bresnahan, M., . . . Susser, E. (2004). Serologic evidence of prenatal influenza in the etiology of schizophrenia *Archives in General Psychiatry*, 61,774–780.

Bruce, R. D. (1985). Noise pollution. In L. L. Jarvis (Ed.), *Community health nursing: Keeping the public healthy* (2nd ed., pp. 847–867). Philadelphia: F. A. Davis.

Burt, L., Aron, D., Valente, L., & Iwen, B. (1999). *Homelessness: Programs and the people they serve.* Findings of the National Survey of Homeless Assistance Providers and Clients. Urban Institute. Retrieved from http://www.urban.org/UploadedPDF/homelessness.pdf

Centers for Disease Control and Prevention. (n.d.). Families. Retrieved from http://www.cdc.gov/mmwr

Centers for Disease Control and Prevention. (n.d.). National Institute for Occupational Safety and Health (NIOSH): Retrieved from http://www.cdc.gov/niosh/npg/

Clark, R., Anderson, N. B., Clark, V. R., & Williams, D. R. (1999). Racism as a stressor for African Americans. A biopsychosocial model. *American Psychologist*, *54*, 805–816.

Cohen, S. (1981). Sound effects on behavior. *Psychology Today*, *15*, 38–46.

Connell, D., & Joint, M. (1996). *Driver aggression*. Road Safety Unit Group Policy.

Cooper-Patrick, L., Gallo, J. J., Gonzales, J. J., Vu, H. T., Powe, N. R., Nelson, C., & Ford, D. E (1999). Race, gender, and partnership in the patient–physician relationship. *Journal of the American Medical Association*, *282*, 583–589.

Cooper-Patrick, L., Gallo, J. J., Powe, N. R., Steinwachs, D. M., Eaton, W. W., & Ford, D. E. (1999). Mental health service utilization by African Americans and whites: The Baltimore Epidemiologic Catchment Area follow-up. *Medical Care*, *37*, 1034–1045.

Cooper-Patrick, L., Powe, N. R., Jenckes, M. W., Gonzales, J. J., Levine, D. M., & Ford, D. E. (1997). Identification of patient attitudes and preferences regarding treatment of depression. *Journal of General Internal Medicine*, *12*, 431–438.

Cross, T. L., Bazron, B. J., Dennis, K. W., & Isaacs, M. R. (1989). *Towards a culturally competent system of care*. Washington, DC: CAASP Technical Assistance Center.

DeNavas-Wait, C., Proctor B. D., Smith J. C. (September 2009). U.S. Census Bureau. Income, poverty and health insurance coverage in the United States: 2008. Retrieved from: http://www.census.gov/prod/2009pubs/p60-236.pdf

Dohrenwend, B. P. (1973). Social status and stressful life events. *Journal of Personality and Social Psychology*, *28*, 225–235.

Dohrenwend, B. P., Levav, I., Shrout, P. E., Schwartz, S., Naveh, G., Link, B. G., . . . Stueve, A. (1992). Socioeconomic status and psychiatric disorders: The causation–selection issue. *Science*, *255*, 946–952.

Eaton, W. W., & Muntaner, C. (1999). Socioeconomic stratification and mental disorder. In A. V. Horwitz & T. K. Scheid (Eds.), *A handbook for the study of mental health: Social contexts, theories, and systems* (pp. 259–283). New York: Cambridge University Press.

Evans, G., & Marcynyszyn, L. A. (2004). Environmental justice, cumulative environmental risk, and health among low- and middle-income children in upstate New York. *American Journal of Public Health*, *94*, 1942–1944.

Faris, R. E. L., & Dunham, W. (1939). *Mental disorders in urban areas* [print]: *An ecological study of schizophrenia and other psychoses*. Chicago: University of Chicago Press.

Finch, B. K., Kolody, B., & Vega, W. A. (2000). Perceived discrimination and depression among Mexican-origin adults in California. *Journal of Health and Social Behavior*, *41*(3), 295–313.

Finkelhor, D. (1979). *Sexually victimized children*. New York: Free Press.

Greenwood, R. M., Schaefer-McDaniel, N. J., Winkel, G., & Tsemberis, S. J. (2005). Decreasing psychiatric symptoms by increasing choice in services for adults with histories of homelessness. *American Journal of Community Psychology*, *36*(3/4), 223–238.

Hanlon, G., & Pickett, J. (1984). *Public Health Administration and Practice*. New York: Times Mirror/Mosby.

Herbers, J. (1986). *The new heartland: America's flight beyond the suburbs and how it is changing our future*. New York: Times Books.

Holzer, C., Shea, B., Swanson, J., Leaf, P., Myers, J., George, L., . . . Bednarski, P. (1986). The increased risk for specific psychiatric disorders among persons of low socioeconomic status. *American Journal of Social Psychiatry*, *6*, 259–271.

Hughes, M., & Thomas, M. E. (1998). The continuing significance of race revisited: A study of race, class and quality of life in America, 1972–1996. *American Sociological Review*, *63*, 785–795.

Joint, M. (1995). *Road rage*. The Automobile Association Group Public Policy Road Safety Unit. Retrieved from: www.aaafoundation.org/resources/index.cfm?button=agdrtext#Driver%20 Aggression

Kessler, R. C., Berglund, P. A., Zhao, S., Leaf, P. J., Kouzis, A. C., Bruce, M. L., . . . Schneier, M. (1996). The 12-month prevalence and correlates of serious mental illness (SMI). In R. W. Manderscheid & M. A. Sonnenschein (Eds.), *Mental health*, *United States* (Pub. No. [SMA] 96–3098). Rockville, MD: Center for Mental Health Services.

Kessler, R. C., Mickelson, K. D., & Williams, D. R. (1999). The prevalence, distribution, and mental health correlates of perceived discrimination in the United States. *Journal of Health and Social Behavior*, *40*, 208–230.

Krieger, N. (1993). Epidemiologic theory and societal patterns of disease. *Epidemiology*, *4*, 276–278.

Krieger, N. (2000). Refiguring "race": Epidemiology, racialized biology, and biological expressions of race relations. *International Journal of Health Services*, *30*, 211–216.

Krieger, N., & Sidney, S. (1996). Racial discrimination and blood pressure: The CARDIA study of young black and white adults. *American Journal of Public Health*, *86*, 1370–1378.

Krieger, N., Sidney, S., & Coakley, E. (1999). Racial discrimination and skin color in the CARDIA study: Implications for public health research. *American Journal of Public Health*, *88*, 1308–1313.

Lachs, M. S., Williams, C. S., O'Brien, S., Pillemer, K. A., & Charlson, M. E. (1998). The mortality of elder mistreatment. *Journal of the American Medical Association*, *280*, 428–432.

Lohr, J. M., DeMaio, C., & McGlynn, F. D. (2003). Specific and nonspecific treatment factors in the experimental analysis of behavioral treatment efficacy. *Behavior Modification*, *27*, 322–367.

McClellan, J., Susser, E., & King, M. C. (2006). Maternal famine, de novo mutations, and schizophrenia. *Journal of the American Medical Association*, *296*, 582–584.

McLeod, J. D., & Kessler, R. C. (1990). Socioeconomic status differences in vulnerability to undesirable life events. *Journal of Health and Social Behavior*, *31*, 162–172.

Muntaner, C., Eaton, W. W., Diala, C., Kessler, R. C., & Sorlie, P. D. (1998). Social class, assets, organizational control and the prevalence of common groups of psychiatric disorders. *Social Science and Medicine*, *47*, 2043–2053.

National Institutes of Health. (2000). *Strategic research plan to reduce and ultimately eliminate health disparities, fiscal years 2002–2006*. Retrieved from: http://www.ncmhd.nih.gov/our_programs/strategic/pubs/VolumeI_031003EDrev.pdf

Noh, S., Beiser, M., Kaspar, V., Hou, F., & Rummens, J. (1999). Perceived racial discrimination, depression and coping: A study of Southeast Asian refugees in Canada. *Journal of Health and Social Behavior*, *40*, 193–207.

O'Connell, J. J., Mattison, S., Judge, C. M., Allen, H. J., & Koh, H. K. (2005). A public health approach to reducing morbidity and mortality among homeless people in Boston. *Journal of Public Health Management and Practice*, *11*(4), 311–116.

Orzech, D. (2007). Chemical kids—environmental toxins and child development. *Social Work Today*, 7(2), 37.

Pope, A. M., Snyder, M. A., & Mood, L. H. (1995). *Nursing, health, & the environment: Strengthening the relationship to improve the public's health*. Institute of Medicine. Washington, DC: National Academy Press.

Ren, X. S., Amick, B., & Williams, D. R. (1999). Racial/ethnic disparities in health: The interplay between discrimination and socioeconomic status. *Ethnicity & Disease*, *9*, 151–165.

Rosenheck, R., Morrissey, J., Lam, J., Calloway, M., Johnsen, M., Goldman, H., . . . Teague, G. (1998). Service system integration, access to services, and housing outcomes in a program for homeless persons with severe mental illness. *American Journal of Public Health*, *88*(11), 1610–1615.

Rumbaut, R. G. (1994). The crucible within: Ethnic identity, self-esteem, and segmented assimilation among children of immigrants. *International Migration Review*, *28*, 748–794.

Shiefer, S. E., Escarce, J. J., & Schulman, K. A. (2000). Race and sex differences in the management of coronary artery disease. *American Heart Journal*, *139*, 848–857.

Snowden, L. R., & Cheung, F. K. (1990). Use of inpatient mental health services by members of ethnic minority groups. *American Psychologist*, *45*, 347–355.

Stansfeld, S. A., Berglund, B., Clark, C., Lopez-Barrio, I., Fischer, P., Öhrström, E., . . . Berry, B. F., RANCH study team. (2005). Aircraft and road traffic noise and children's cognition and health: a cross-national study. *Lancet*, *365*, 1942–1949.

Substance Abuse and Mental Health Services Administration [SAMHSA]. (1996). SAMHSA's. Homelessness Provision of Mental Health and Substance Abuse Services. Retrieved from http://mentalhealth.samhsa.gov/publications/allpubs/homelessness/

Takaki, R. (1993). *A different mirror: A history of multicultural America*. Boston: Little, Brown.

United States Environmental Protection Agency. (1978). *Noise: A Health Problem*. Office of Noise Abatement and Control, Washington, DC: Author.

U.S. Department of Health and Human Services. (1999). *Mental Health: A Report of the Surgeon General*. U.S. Department of Health and Human Services, Substance Abuse and Mental Health Services Administration, Center for Mental Health Services, National Institutes of Health, National Institute of Mental Health, Rockville, MD: Author.

Williams, D. R. (1996). Race/ethnicity and socioeconomic status: Measurement and methodological issues. *International Journal of Health Services*, *26*, 483–505.

Williams, D. R. (2000). Race, stress, and mental health. In C. Hogue, M. Hargraves, & K. Scott-Collins (Eds.), *Minority health in America* (pp. 209–243). Baltimore: Johns Hopkins University Press.

Williams, D. R., & Williams-Morris, R. (2000). Racism and mental health: The African American experience. *Ethnicity and Health*, *5*, 243–268.

Williams, D. R., Yu, Y., Jackson, J. S., & Anderson, N.B. (1997). Racial differences in physical and mental health: Socio-economic status, stress and discrimination. *Journal of Health Psychology*, *2*, 335–351.

Williams, J. W., Jr., Rost, K., Dietrich, A. J., Ciotti, M. C., Zyzanski, S. J., & Cornell, J. (1999). Primary care physicians' approach to depressive disorders: Effects of physician specialty and practice structure. *Archives of Family Medicine*, *8*, 58–67.

World Health Organization. (1973). *Report of the International Pilot Study on Schizophrenia*. Geneva, Switzerland: Author.

World Health Organization. (1992). *International statistical classification of diseases and related health problems* (10th revision; ICD–10). Geneva: Author.

World Health Organization. (2007). Breaking the vicious cycle between mental health and poverty. Retrieved from http://www.who.int/mental_health/policy/ development/1_Breakingviciouscycle_Infosheet.pdf

Yen, I. H., & Syme, S. L. (1999). The social environment and health: A discussion of the epidemiologic literature. *Annual Review of Public Health*, *20*, 287–308.

Yip, T., Gee, F., & Takeuchi, D. T. (2008). Racial discrimination and psychological distress: The impact of ethnic identity and age among immigrant and United States–born Asian adults. *Developmental Psychology*, *44*(3), 787–800.

CHAPTER 10

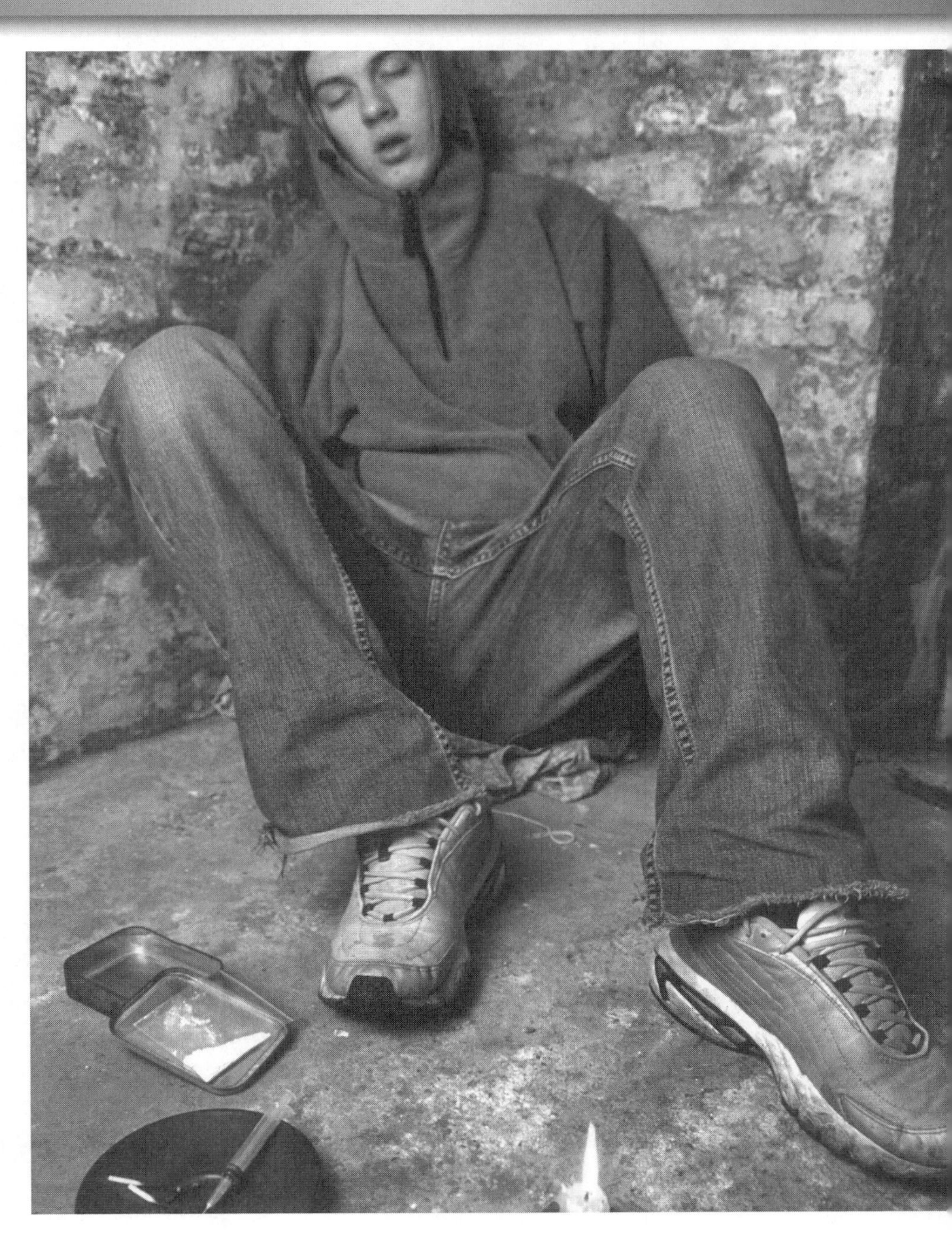

Community Mental Health Problems: Substance Abuse

CHAPTER OBJECTIVES

1. Differentiate between the terms *substance abuse*, *addiction*, *tolerance*, and *dependence*.
2. Explain the scope of the problem of alcohol and substance abuse on mental health.
3. Analyze the role of mental health professionals in working with substance abusers.
4. Examine the differences between drug categories of stimulants, marijuana, club drugs, heroin, anabolic steroids, and inhalants.
5. Define how community health professionals can assist with nicotine/smoking cessation.

KEY TERMS

- Abstinence
- Addiction
- Alcohol abuse
- Alcohol dependence
- Anabolic
- Androgenic
- Blood alcohol content/concentration (BAC)
- Detoxification
- Drug addiction
- Drug dependence
- Glutamate
- Inhalants
- Late-onset alcoholism
- Steroids
- Substance abuse
- Tolerance
- Withdrawal

This chapter examines substance abuse as a public health problem, how substance abuse impacts mental health, and the ways that community mental healthcare providers can help individuals recognize the signs and symptoms of substance abuse. There are several forms of morbidity and mortality linked to substance abuse, coupled with mental health diagnoses. Substance abuse can lead to homicide, domestic violence, family violence, intimate partner violence, school violence, as well as gang violence. These destructive community mental health problems are discussed. Additionally, substance abuse can lead to accidents, low birthweight infants, chronic diseases like cancer, cardiovascular disease, and lung disease as well as death.

Community mental health providers frequently encounter individuals and families who have both substance abuse and mental health problems. To provide the appropriate level of care, community mental health providers must understand potential mental health problems that might affect the community, the individual, and the family. Moreover, community mental health providers must understand ways in which drug and alcohol abuse affect the individual mentally and physically as well as the burdens that substance abuse imposes on society as a whole. Finally, community mental health providers must become aware of the appropriate treatment and therapeutic modalities to implement for individuals who are both mentally ill and substance abusers. This chapter focuses on the extent of substance abuse in our society, defines the most common drug types abused, how they are used, and the physical impact on the body and the current treatment modalities for each drug group. The chapter ends with a discussion about the role of the community mental health provider in substance abuse prevention and treatment.

DRUG/SUBSTANCE ABUSE

Drug abuse, the frequent use of medications in a nonmedical manner, plays a role in many major social problems, such as drugged driving, violence, and stress as well as domestic, intimate partner, and child abuse. Drug abuse can lead to homelessness, crime, and missed work or problems with keeping a job. It harms unborn babies and destroys families. There are several different types of treatment for drug abuse. But the best treatment is to prevent drug abuse in the first place. It is unknown why individuals become addicted to drugs or how drugs change the brain to foster compulsive drug abuse. In addition, many health professionals mistakenly view drug abuse and addiction as strictly a social problem and may characterize those who take drugs as morally weak. A common belief is that drug abusers can just stop taking drugs if they are willing to change their behavior. The complexity of drug addiction is often underestimated. **Drug addiction** is a disease that impacts the brain, and therefore stopping is not just a matter of willpower. Through scientific advances, we now know more about the mechanism of action of drugs in the brain. We have learned that drug addiction can be successfully treated and more about how to assist people to stop abusing drugs and resume their productive lives.

Drug abuse and addiction are a major burden to society. Estimates of the costs of substance abuse in the United States, including health, crime-related costs, and losses in work productivity, exceed half a trillion dollars annually. The cost of substance abuse includes approximately $181 billion for illicit drugs (Office of National Drug

Control Policy, 2004), $168 billion for tobacco (Centers for Disease Control and Prevention [CDC], 2005), and $185 billion for alcohol (Harwood, 2000). These numbers, however, do not completely describe the breadth and depth of the detrimental public health and safety consequences, which include family breakdown, loss of employment, failure in school, domestic violence, child abuse, and other crimes.

UNDERSTANDING DRUG ABUSE

Many terms describe alcohol, tobacco, and drug use. The terms *drug use* and *drug abuse* have limited use because the terms have been narrowed by governmental agencies as well as the general public to include only illegal drugs. Over-the-counter drugs, prescriptions, and legal recreational drugs are not included in these definitions. The term *substance abuse* increases the scope of drug abuse to include alcohol, tobacco, legal drugs, and food. **Substance abuse** is the use of any substance that impairs a person's social or economic well-being and jeopardizes a person's health. *Drug dependence* and *drug addiction* are often used interchangeably. However, the phrases are not the same. **Drug dependence** occurs when there is a psychological change in the central nervous system caused by frequent abuse of drugs and to prevent **withdrawal** symptoms. Addiction is a chronic, often relapsing brain disease that causes compulsive drug-seeking behavior and use despite harmful consequences to the individual who is addicted to drugs and to those in his or her presence. Drug addiction is considered a brain disease because overuse of drugs leads to structural and functional changes in the brain. For most people the initial decision to take drugs is voluntary; over time, however, changes in the brain caused by repeated drug abuse can affect a person's self-control and ability to make sound decisions; additionally the brain sends intense impulses to the individual to take drugs.

These changes in the brain are challenging for a person who is addicted to drugs and trying to stop. Treatments are available to help people counteract addiction's powerful effects and regain control. Combining addiction treatment medications with behavioral therapy ensures success for most patients. Treatment approaches tailored to each patient's drug abuse patterns and any co-occurring medical, psychiatric, and social problems can lead to sustained recovery and a life without drug abuse.

Similar to other *chronic, relapsing* diseases such as diabetes, asthma, or heart disease, drug addiction can be managed successfully. Like other chronic diseases, adhering to the therapeutic regimen is difficult; thus it is not uncommon for a person diagnosed with substance abuse to relapse and begin abusing drugs again. Relapse, however, does not signal failure. Instead a relapse indicates that treatment should be reinstated, adjusted, or that an alternative treatment regimen is needed to help the individual regain control and recover.

THE IMPACT OF DRUGS ON THE BRAIN

Drugs are chemicals that enter into the brain's communication system and disrupt the way nerve cells normally send, receive, and process information. There are two ways that drugs enter into the communication system: (1) by imitating the brain's natural chemical messengers, and/or (2) by overstimulating the "reward circuit" of the brain.

The chemical structure of drugs such as marijuana and heroin have a similar structure to chemical messengers, called *neurotransmitters*, which are naturally produced by the brain. Because of this similarity, these drugs are able to "deceive" the brain's receptors and activate nerve cells to send abnormal messages. Other drugs, like cocaine or methamphetamine, can cause the nerve cells to release large amounts of natural neurotransmitters or prevent the normal recycling of these brain chemicals needed to shut off the signal between neurons. This disruption produces a message that disrupts normal communication patterns. Nearly all drugs, directly or indirectly, target the brain's reward system by inundating the circuit with dopamine. *Dopamine* is a neurotransmitter present in regions of the brain that control movement, emotion, motivation, and feelings of pleasure. The increased stimulation of the communication system normally responds to natural behaviors linked to survival such as eating and spending time with loved ones, and it produces euphoric effects in response to the drugs. This reaction produces a pattern that "leads" people to repeat the behavior of abusing drugs.

As a person continues to abuse drugs, the brain adapts to the overwhelming rush of dopamine by producing less dopamine or by reducing the number of dopamine receptors in the reward circuit. As a result, dopamine's impact on the reward circuit is lessened, reducing the abuser's ability to enjoy the drugs and the things that previously brought pleasure. This decrease compels those addicted to drugs to keep abusing drugs in an attempt to bring their dopamine function back to normal. At this point of substance abuse, the abuse might require larger amounts of the drug to achieve the dopamine high, an effect known as **tolerance**.

Long-term substance abuse causes changes in other brain chemical systems and circuits as well. **Glutamate** is a neurotransmitter that influences the reward circuit and the ability to learn. When the optimal concentration of glutamate is altered by drug abuse, the brain attempts to compensate, which can impair cognitive function. Drug abuse facilitates nonconscious (conditioned) learning, which leads the user to experience uncontrollable cravings when they see a place or person they associate with the drug experience. This learned behavior occurs even when the drug is not available. Imaging studies of the brain among drug-addicted individuals show changes in areas of the brain that are critical to judgment, decision making, learning, and memory, as well as behavior control. These changes together drive an abuser to seek drugs compulsively despite adverse consequences of addiction.

UNDERSTANDING THE ADDICTION PROCESS

No single factor can predict if a person will become addicted to drugs. Risk factors associated with addiction are influenced by a person's biology, social environment, and age or stage of development. The more risk factors an individual has, the greater the chance that taking drugs can lead to addiction. For example:

- *Biology*: The genetic makeup of a person in combination with environmental influences account for addiction vulnerability. Additionally, gender, ethnicity, and the presence of other mental disorders may influence risk for developing drug abuse and addiction.
- *Environment*: The environment of a person has many different influences on developing substance abuse. Examples include family history of substance abuse, socioeconomic status, and quality of life. Factors such as peer pressure, physical and sexual abuse, stress, and parental involvement also can influence the risk of developing drug abuse and addiction.
- *Development*: Addiction is influenced by both genetic and environmental factors and a person's developmental stage in life. For example, adolescents are at high risk of becoming addicted to drugs because of peer pressure and poor judgment and decision-making skills. In addition, adolescents are prone to risk-taking behaviors, including trying new things like abusive drugs. The phenomenon known as **late-onset alcoholism** is when the alcohol problem began after age 60. Many people with late-onset **alcohol abuse** show that alcohol consumption may not be consistent across time; for example, some people may increase their consumption of alcohol as a response to age-related stresses such as the loss of employment or the loss of a loved one.

ALCOHOLISM

Alcohol, one of the oldest and most frequently used drugs in the world, is a central nervous system (CNS) depressant. According to the Substance Abuse and Mental Health Services Administration (SAMHSA), Office of Applied Studies. 2009 report, *Exposure to Substance Use Prevention Messages and Substance Use among Adolescents between 2002 to 2007*, approximately 48.3% of Americans youth 12 years or older reported being current drinkers of alcohol in a 2001 survey. It is estimated that more than 109 million people drink alcohol, an increase from 2000 of 5 million, and that 46.6% of people 12 years or older reported drinking alcohol in the past 30 days (SAMHSA, 2009). Alcoholism, also known as **alcohol dependence**, is a disease that includes four symptoms:

- *Craving*
  - A strong need, or compulsion, to drink
  - Loss of control
  - The inability to limit one's drinking on any given occasion
- *Physical dependence*
  - Withdrawal symptoms such as nausea, sweating, shakiness, and anxiety, occur when alcohol use is stopped after a period of heavy drinking
- *Tolerance*
  - The need to drink greater amounts of alcohol in order to "get high"
- *Loss of control*
  - Craving
  - Loss of control
  - Physical dependence
  - Tolerance

According to the CDC (2008), approximately 79,000 deaths are attributable to excessive alcohol use each year in the United States. This makes excessive alcohol use the third leading lifestyle-related cause of death for the nation (Mokdad, Marks, Stroup, & Gerberding, 2004). In 2005, there were more than 1.6 million alcohol-related hospitalizations (Chen & Yi, 2008) and over 4 million emergency department visits (McCaig & Burt, 2005) for alcohol-related conditions.

The Standard Measure of Alcohol

A standard drink in the United States is a drink that contains 0.6 oz (13.7 g or 1.2 tablespoons) of pure alcohol. Generally, this amount of pure alcohol is found in 12 oz of regular beer or a wine cooler, 8 oz of malt liquor, 5 oz of wine, and 1.5 oz of 80-proof distilled spirits or liquor (e.g., gin, rum, vodka, whiskey).

Definitions of Patterns of Drinking Alcohol

- **Binge drinking**
  - For women, four or more drinks during a single occasion
  - For men, five or more drinks during a single occasion
- **Heavy drinking**
  - For women, an average of more than one drink per day
  - For men, more than two drinks per day on average
- **Excessive drinking**
  - Includes heavy drinking, binge drinking, or both

Most people who binge-drink are not alcoholics or alcohol dependent (Dawson, Grant, & Li, 2005). The U.S. Department of Agriculture and U.S. Department of Health and Human Services (2005) recommends that people drink alcoholic beverages in moderation, which is defined as no more than one drink per day for women and no more than two drinks per day for men. However, some individuals should not drink any alcohol, including those who are pregnant or trying to become pregnant, individuals taking prescription or over-the-counter medications that may cause harmful reactions when mixed with alcohol, and individuals younger than 21 years of age. It is also important that individuals recovering from alcoholism or those who are unable to control the amount they drink; suffering from a medical condition that may be worsened by alcohol; driving; planning to drive; or participating in activities requiring skill, coordination, and alertness should not drink.

Immediate Health Risks

Excessive alcohol use has immediate effects that increase the risk of many harmful health conditions. These immediate effects are most often the result of binge drinking and include the following:

- Unintentional injuries, including traffic injuries, falls, drowning, burns, and unintentional firearm injuries.
- Violence, including intimate partner violence and child maltreatment—offenders are frequently reported to be under the influence of alcohol.
- Child maltreatment and neglect.
- Risky sexual behaviors including unprotected sex, sex with multiple partners, and increased risk of sexual assault, resulting in unintended pregnancy or sexually transmitted diseases.
- Miscarriage and stillbirth among pregnant women, and a combination of physical and mental birth defects among children that last throughout life.
- Alcohol poisoning, a medical emergency that results from high **blood alcohol content/concentration (BAC)**. Blood alcohol content is determined by the concentration of alcohol in a person's blood. BAC is most commonly used as a metric of intoxication for legal or medical purposes. It is usually measured in terms of mass per volume but can also be measured in terms of mass per mass. A normal range of BAC is 0.01–0.029. A BAC of 0.030 or more can suppress the CNS and can cause loss of consciousness, low blood pressure and body temperature, coma, respiratory depression, or death.

Long-Term Health Risks

Over time, excessive alcohol use can lead to the development of chronic diseases, neurologic impairments, and social problems. These include but are not limited to the following:

- Neurologic problems, including dementia, stroke, and neuropathy.
- Cardiovascular problems, including myocardial infarction, cardiomyopathy, atrial fibrillation, and hypertension.
- Psychiatric problems, including depression, anxiety, and suicide.
- Social problems, including unemployment, lost productivity, and family problems.
- Cancer, including cancer of the mouth, throat, esophagus, liver, colon, and breast. In general, the risk of cancer increases with increasing amounts of alcohol.
- Liver disease, including alcoholic hepatitis and cirrhosis, which is among the 15 leading causes of all deaths in the United States (National Center for Health Statistics. Health, United States, 2009). Alcohol abuse in persons with hepatitis C virus causes poor liver function and interference with the medications used to treat hepatitis. Other gastrointestinal problems associated with alcohol abuse include pancreatitis and gastritis.

STIMULANTS

Stimulants are commonly used by people who are looking to become more alert or energetic. Common stimulants include amphetamines, nicotine, cocaine, and caffeine. Additionally, stimulants on the street, commonly called "uppers" or "speed," are abused to increase alertness and physical activity.

Amphetamines

Methamphetamine (meth) is a very addictive stimulant drug. It can be smoked, injected, inhaled, or taken by mouth. It has many street names, such as speed, meth, and chalk. Meth hydrochloride, the crystal form inhaled by smoking, is referred to as chalk, crystal, glass, ice, meth, speed, and tina, and includes benzidine, methedrine, Dexedrine, methamphetamine, and MDMA (methylenedioxymethamphetamine).

Meth affects the brain and can create feelings of pleasure, increase energy, and elevate mood. Abusers quickly become addicted to meth, requiring higher doses more often. Adverse health effects include irregular heartbeat, increased blood pressure, and a variety of psychological problems. Long-term effects may include severe mental disorders, memory loss, and severe dental problems. Most of the meth abused in the United States comes from foreign or domestic superlabs, although it can also be made in small illegal laboratories and private homes, where its production endangers the people in the labs, neighbors, and the environment. Meth is a white, odorless, bitter-tasting crystalline powder that easily dissolves in water or alcohol and is taken orally, intranasally (snorting the powder), intravenously, or by smoking.

The Effect of Methamphetamine on the Brain

Meth increases the release of very high levels of dopamine, which is found in the brain. Dopamine has an impact on motivation, the experience of pleasure, and motor function. Chronic meth abuse changes how the brain functions. Noninvasive human brain imaging studies have shown alterations in the activity of the dopamine system that are associated with reduced motor performance and impaired verbal learning (Volkow et al., 2001). Studies in chronic meth abusers show severe structural and functional changes in areas of the brain associated with emotion and memory (Thompson et al., 2004), which may account for many of the emotional and cognitive problems observed in chronic meth abusers.

Other Adverse Effects of Methamphetamine on Health

Taking the smallest amounts of meth can result in increased wakefulness, increased physical activity, decreased appetite, increased respiration, rapid heart rate, irregular heartbeat, increased blood pressure, and hyperthermia. Long-term meth abuse leads to several harmful consequences, including extreme weight loss, severe dental problems, anxiety, confusion, insomnia, mood disturbances, and violent behavior. Chronic meth abusers also exhibit a number of psychotic symptoms, such as paranoia, visual and auditory hallucinations, and delusions (e.g., the sensation of insects creeping under the skin). The transmission of HIV and hepatitis B and C are also a major concern among meth abusers. Especially among abusers who inject the drug, HIV and other infectious diseases can be spread through contaminated needles, syringes, and other injection equipment that is used by more than one person. The intoxicating effects of meth, regardless of how it is taken, can also alter judgment and lead people to engage in unsafe behaviors. Meth abuse may also worsen the progression of HIV and its consequences. Studies of meth abusers who are HIV positive indicate that the HIV causes greater neuronal injury and cognitive impairment compared with HIV-positive people who do not use the drug (Chang, Ernst, Speck, & Grob, 2005).

Treatment Options

Currently, the most effective treatments are behavioral. For example, the Matrix Model, a comprehensive behavioral treatment approach that combines behavioral therapy, family education, individual counseling, 12-Step support, drug testing, and encouragement for non-drug-related activities has been effective in reducing meth abuse (Rawson et al., 2004). Contingency management interventions have proven to be an effective substance abuse treatment modality. Contingency management provides tangible incentives in exchange for engaging in treatment and maintaining **abstinence** and has also been shown to be effective (Roll et al., 2006). There are no medications at this time approved to treat meth addiction.

The Magnitude of Methamphetamine Abuse

Survey results from the Monitoring the Future Survey (2007), as shown in **Table 10-1**, indicate that 1.8% of 8th graders, 2.8% of 10th graders, and 3.0% of 12th graders have tried meth. In addition, 0.6% of 8th graders, 0.4% of 10th graders, and 0.6% of 12th graders were current (past-month) meth abusers in 2007. Decreases in past-year abuse of meth were seen for 8th (from 1.8% to 1.1%) and 12th graders (from 2.5% to 1.7%) from 2006 to 2007.

According to the 2006 National Survey on Drug Use and Health (NSDUH), there were an estimated 731,000 current users of meth aged 12 or older (0.3% of the population). Of the 259,000 people who used meth for the first time in 2006, the mean age at first use was 22.2 years, which is up considerably from the mean age of 18.6 years in 2005 (NSDUH, 2006). From 2005 to 2006, lifetime meth abuse increased among those 26 and older, particularly among those 26 to 34 years of age.

TABLE 10-1 Methamphetamine Prevalence of Abuse per 2007 Monitoring the Future Survey

	8th Grade	10th Grade	12th Grade
Lifetime (%)	1.8	2.8	3.0
Past Year (%)	1.1	1.6	1.7
Past Month (%)	0.6	0.4	0.6

Source: Johnston, L. D., O'Malley, P. M., Bachman, J. G., & Schulenberg, J. E. (2008). Monitoring the Future national results on adolescent drug use: Overview of key findings, 2007 (NIH Publication No. 08-6418). Bethesda, MD: National Institute on Drug Abuse.

Rates of past-year meth use among persons aged 12 years or older were the highest in the western United States (1.6%), followed by the South (0.7%), Midwest (0.5%), and Northeast (0.3%) regions of the country (NSDUH, 2007).

ANABOLIC STEROIDS

Anabolic steroids are also called anabolic-androgenic steroid and performance-enhancing drugs. Types of anabolic steroids include anadrol, Anavar, Dianabol, Deca-Durabolin, and designer steroids used by professional athletes.

Anabolic-androgenic steroids (AAS) are manufactured substances related to male sex hormones (e.g., testosterone). **Anabolic** refers to muscle building, and **androgenic** refers to increased male sexual characteristics. **Steroids** refers to the class of drugs. These drugs can be legally prescribed to treat conditions resulting from steroid hormone deficiency, such as delayed puberty, but also body wasting in patients with AIDS and other diseases that result in loss of lean muscle mass. Bodybuilders and athletes often use anabolic steroids to build muscles and improve athletic performance; however, using AAS for this purpose is not legal or safe. Abuse of anabolic steroids has been linked with many health problems.

How AAS Are Abused

Some people, both athletes and nonathletes, abuse AAS in an attempt to enhance performance and/or improve physical appearance. AAS are taken orally or injected, typically in cycles of weeks or months interrupted by shorter resting periods (this is referred to as "cycling"). In addition, users often combine several different types of steroids, a practice referred to as "stacking," to get an immediate effect of AAS.

How AAS Affect the Brain

The immediate effects of AAS in the brain are mediated by their binding to androgen and estrogen receptors, which can then shuttle into the cell nucleus to influence patterns of gene expression. Because of this, the acute effects of AAS in the brain are substantially different from those of other drugs of abuse. The most important difference is that AAS are not euphorigenic, meaning they do not trigger rapid increases in the neurotransmitter dopamine, which are responsible for the high that often drives substance abuse behaviors. However, long-term use of AAS can eventually have an impact on the same brain pathways and chemicals—such as dopamine, serotonin, and opioid systems—that are affected by drugs of abuse. The combined effect of the complex direct and indirect actions of AAS can affect mood and behavior in significant ways. For the individual with mental illness, these changes in the mood can have a major impact on the behavior of a person in crisis or not adhering to their therapeutic regimen.

AAS and Mental Health

Taken together, the preclinical, clinical, and anecdotal reports suggest that steroids may contribute to psychiatric dysfunction. Research shows that abuse of anabolic steroids may lead to aggression and other adverse effects (Pope, Kouri, & Hudson, 2000). For example, many users report feeling good about themselves while on anabolic steroids, but extreme mood swings can also occur, including manic-like symptoms that could lead to violence (Pope & Katz, 1998). Researchers have also observed that users may suffer from paranoid jealousy, extreme irritability, delusions, and impaired judgment stemming from feelings of invincibility.

Addictive Potential

Animal studies have shown that AAS are reinforcing; that is, animals self-administer AAS when given the opportunity, just as they do with other addictive drugs (Arnedo, Salvador, Martinez-Sanchi, & Gonzalez-Bono, 2000). This property is more difficult to demonstrate in humans, but the potential for AAS abusers to become addicted is consistent with their continued abuse despite physical problems and negative effects on social relations (Brower, 2002). Several hours and dollars are spent obtaining AAS drugs, which is another indication of addiction. Individuals who abuse steroids can experience withdrawal symptoms when they stop taking AAS, such as mood swings, fatigue, and restlessness, loss of appetite, insomnia, reduced sex drive, and steroid cravings, all of which may contribute to the need for continued abuse. One of the most dangerous withdrawal symptoms of AAS is depression; when persistent, depression can lead to attempts of suicide.

Research also indicates that some users might turn to other drugs to alleviate of the negative side effects of AAS. For example, a study of 227 men admitted in 1999 to a private treatment center for dependence on heroin or other opioids found that 9.3% had abused AAS before trying other illicit drugs. Eighty-six percent of this sample indicated that they used opioids to counteract insomnia and irritability resulting from the steroids (Arvary & Pope, 2000).

Other Adverse Effects of AAS on Health

Steroid abuse can lead to serious and even irreversible health problems. The most common and dangerous problems include liver damage, jaundice (yellowish pigmentation of skin, tissues, and body fluids), fluid retention, high blood pressure, increases in low-density lipoproteins (LDL; bad cholesterol), and decreases in high-density lipoproteins (HDL; good cholesterol). Other reported effects of AAS are renal failure, severe acne, and trembling. In addition, there are some gender- and age-specific adverse effects as follows:

- Men: Shrinking of the testicles, reduced sperm count, infertility, baldness, development of breasts, increased risk for prostate cancer
- Women: Growth of facial hair, male-pattern baldness, changes in or cessation of the menstrual cycle, enlargement of the clitoris, deepened voice
- Adolescents: Stunted growth due to premature skeletal maturation and accelerated puberty changes; adolescents risk not reaching their expected height if they take AAS before the typical adolescent growth spurt

In addition, people who inject AAS are at risk of contracting or transmitting HIV/AIDS or hepatitis, which causes serious damage to the liver.

Treatment Options

There has been very little research on the treatment for AAS abuse. Current knowledge derives largely from the experiences of a small number of physicians who have worked with patients undergoing steroid withdrawal. Supportive therapy combined with education about possible withdrawal symptoms from AAS is an effective treatment method. Occasionally, medications are used to restore the balance of the hormonal system after the system has been interrupted by steroid abuse. If symptoms are severe or prolonged, medications related to the symptom are used, or the person might require hospitalization.

The Magnitude of AAS Abuse: Monitoring the Future

Steroid use among 8th-, 10th-, and 12th-grade boys and girls remained unchanged from 2006 to 2007 as illustrated in **Table 10-2**; however, significant reductions were noted since 2001 for lifetime and past-year use among all grades, and for past-month use among 8th and 10th graders. Among high school seniors in 2007, past-year steroid use was reported by 2.3% of boys versus 0.6% of girls.

TABLE 10-2 Anabolic Steroid Use by Students per 2007 Monitoring the Future Survey			
	8th Grade	**10th Grade**	**12th Grade**
Lifetime (%)	1.5	1.8	2.2
Past Year (%)	0.8	1.1	1.4
Past Month (%)	0.4	0.5	1.0

Source: Johnston, L. D., O'Malley, P. M., Bachman, J. G., & Schulenberg, J. E. (2008). Monitoring the Future national results on adolescent drug use: Overview of key findings, 2007 (NIH Publication No. 08-6418). Bethesda, MD: National Institute on Drug Abuse.

CLUB DRUGS

The term *club drug* refers to a wide variety of dangerous drugs. These drugs are often used by young adults at all-night dance parties known as raves or trance scenes, night clubs, and bars. They include methylenedioxymethamphetamine (MDMA), also known as ecstasy, XTC, X, adam, clarity, and lover's speed; gamma-hydroxybutyrate (GHB), also known as grievous bodily harm, G, liquid ecstasy, and Georgia home boy; ketamine, also known as special K, K, vitamin K, cat valium; Rohypnol, also known as roofies, rophies, roche, forget-me pill; methamphetamine, also known as speed, ice, chalk, meth, crystal, crank, fire, glass; lysergic acid diethylamide (LSD), also known as acid, boomers, yellow sunshines, thizz, and E pills.

Club drugs are a pharmacologically heterogeneous group of psychoactive compounds that have become more common in recent years. Sometimes people use them to commit sexual assaults. Club drugs can cause serious health problems, even death, especially when taken in combination with alcohol.

GHB (Xyrem) is a CNS depressant that was approved by the Food and Drug Administration (FDA) in 2002 for use in the treatment of narcolepsy (a sleep disorder). This approval came with severe restrictions, including the requirement for a patient registry monitored by the FDA. GHB is also a metabolite of the inhibitory neurotransmitter gamma-amino butyric acid (GABA); thus it is found naturally in the brain but at concentrations much lower than doses that are abused. *Rohypnol* (flunitrazepam) started appearing in the United States in the early 1990s. It is a benzodiazepine (chemically similar to valium or Xanax), but it is not approved for medical use in this country, and its importation is banned. *Ketamine* is a dissocialized anesthetic, mostly used in veterinary practice.

How Club Drugs Are Abused

Raves and trance events are generally night-long dances, often held in warehouses. Many people who attend raves and trances do not use club drugs, but those who do may be attracted to their generally low cost and the intoxicating highs that are said to deepen the rave or trance experience. Rohypnol is usually taken orally, although there are reports that it can be ground up and snorted. GHB and Rohypnol have both been used to facilitate date rape (also known as "drug rape," "acquaintance rape," or "drug-assisted" assault). Club drugs can be colorless, tasteless, and odorless, and they can be added to beverages and ingested unbeknownst to the victim. When mixed with alcohol, Rohypnol can incapacitate victims and prevent them from resisting sexual assault. GHB also has anabolic effects (it stimulates protein synthesis) and has been sought by bodybuilders to aid in fat reduction and muscle building. Ketamine is usually snorted or injected intramuscularly.

How Club Drugs Affect the Brain

GHB acts on at least two sites in the brain: the GABA-B receptor and a specific GHB binding site. At high doses, GHB's sedative effects may result in sleep, coma, or death. Rohypnol, like other benzodiazepines, acts at the GABA-A receptor. It can produce anterograde amnesia, in which individuals may not remember events they experienced while under the influence of the drug. Ketamine is a dissociative anesthetic because it distorts perceptions of sight, sound, and produces feelings of detachment from the environment and self. Ketamine acts on a type of glutamate receptor (NMDA receptor) to produce its effects, similar to those of the drug PCP (Maeng & Zarate, 2007). Low-dose intoxication results in impaired attention, learning ability, and memory. At higher doses, ketamine can cause dreamlike states and hallucinations, and at higher doses still, ketamine can cause delirium and amnesia.

Addictive Potential

Repeated use of GHB may lead to withdrawal effects, including insomnia, anxiety, tremors, and sweating. Severe withdrawal reactions have been reported among patients presenting from an overdose of GHB or related compounds, especially if other drugs or alcohol are involved (Maxwell & Spence, 2005).

Like other benzodiazepines, chronic use of Rohypnol can produce tolerance and dependence. There have been reports of people binging on ketamine, a behavior that is similar to that seen in some cocaine- or amphetamine-dependent individuals. Ketamine users also can develop signs of tolerance and cravings for the drug (Jansen & Darracot-Cankovic, 2001).

Other Adverse Effects Club Drugs Have on Health

Uncertainties about the sources, chemicals, and possible contaminants used to manufacture many club drugs make it extremely difficult to determine toxicity and associated medical consequences. Coma and seizures can occur following use of GHB after the first experience with GHB. Combined use with other drugs such as alcohol can result in nausea and breathing difficulties. GHB and two of its precursors, gamma butyrolactone (GBL) (Smith, Larive, & Romanelli, 2004) and butanediol (BD), have been involved in poisonings, overdoses, date rapes, and deaths. Rohypnol may be lethal when mixed with alcohol and/or other CNS depressants. Ketamine in high doses can cause impaired motor function, high blood pressure, and potentially fatal respiratory problems.

Treatment Options

There is very little information in the scientific literature about the treatment for persons who abuse or are dependent on club drugs. There are no GHB detection tests for use in emergency departments, and many clinicians are unfamiliar with the drug; thus many GHB incidents likely go undetected. According to case reports, however, patients who abuse GHB appear to present a mixed picture of problems upon admission, yet they have a good response to treatment, which often involves residential services (Maxwell & Spence, 2005).

According to Maxwell and Spence (2005), treatment for Rohypnol follows accepted protocols for benzodiazepine, which may consist of a 3- to 5-day inpatient **detoxification** program, with 24-hour intensive medical monitoring and management of withdrawal symptoms, given that withdrawal from benzodiazepines can be life threatening. Patients with a ketamine overdose are managed through supportive care for acute symptoms, with special attention to cardiac and respiratory functions (Smith et al., 2004).

The Magnitude of Club Drug Abuse: Monitoring the Future Survey

According to results of the 2007 Monitoring the Future (MTF) survey, 0.7% of students in the 8th grade reported past-year use of GHB, as did 0.6% and 0.9% of students in grades 10 and 12, respectively. This is consistent with use reported in 2006. Past-year use of ketamine did not change significantly from 2006 to 2007 and was reported by 1.0% of 8th graders, 0.8% of 10th graders, and 1.3% of 12th graders in 2007. There was no significant change in the illicit use of Rohypnol from 2006 to 2007, according to 2007 MTF results, which report consistently low levels of Rohypnol use since the drug was added to the survey in 1996.

COCAINE

Cocaine is also called blow, C, coke, crack, flake, snow, and rich man's drug. It is a powerfully addictive stimulant drug. The powdered hydrochloride salt form of cocaine can be snorted or dissolved in water and injected intravenously. Crack is the cocaine base that has not been neutralized by an acid to make the hydrochloride salt. This form of cocaine comes in the form of a rock crystal that is smoked in a pipe, cigarette, or cigar. The term *crack* refers to the crackling sound produced by the rock as it is heated.

How Cocaine Is Abused

Three routes of administration are commonly used for cocaine: snorting, injecting, and smoking. Snorting is the process of inhaling cocaine powder through the nose, where it is absorbed into the bloodstream through the nasal tissues. Injecting is the use of a needle to release the drug directly into the bloodstream. Smoking involves inhaling cocaine vapor or smoke into the lungs, where absorption into the bloodstream is as rapid as by injection.

The intensity and duration of cocaine's effects, which include increased energy, reduced fatigue, and reduced mental alertness, depend on the route of the drug administration. The faster cocaine is absorbed into the bloodstream and delivered to the brain, the more intense the high. Injecting or smoking cocaine produces a quicker, stronger high than snorting. But faster absorption usually means shorter duration of action. The high from snorting cocaine may last 15 to 30 minutes, but the high from smoking may last only 5 to 10 minutes. To sustain the high, a cocaine abuser has to administer the drug frequently. For this reason, cocaine is sometimes abused in binges, taken repeatedly within a relatively short period of time, at increasingly high doses.

How Cocaine Affects the Brain

Cocaine is a strong CNS stimulant that increases levels of dopamine, a brain chemical associated with pleasure and movement, in the brain's reward circuit. Certain brain cells, or neurons, use dopamine to communicate. Normally, dopamine is released by a neuron in response to a pleasurable signal (e.g., the smell of good food), and then recycled back into the cell that released it, shutting off the signal between neurons. Cocaine acts by preventing the dopamine from being recycled, causing excessive amounts of dopamine to build up, amplifying the message and ultimately disrupting normal communication. The excess of dopamine is responsible for cocaine's euphoric effects. With repeated use, cocaine can cause long-term changes in the brain's reward system and in other brain systems as well, which may eventually lead to addiction. With repeated use, tolerance to the cocaine high also often develops. Many cocaine abusers report that they seek but fail to achieve as much pleasure as they did from their first exposure. Some users increase their dose in an attempt to intensify and prolong the euphoria, but this can also increase the risk of adverse psychological or physiologic effects.

Adverse Effects of Cocaine on Health

Abusing cocaine has a variety of adverse effects on the body. For example, cocaine constricts blood vessels, dilates pupils, and increases body temperature, heart rate, and blood pressure. It can also cause headaches and gastrointestinal complications such as abdominal pain and nausea. Because cocaine tends to decrease appetite, chronic users can become malnourished as well. Different methods of taking cocaine can produce different adverse effects. Regularly snorting cocaine, for example, can lead to loss of the sense of smell, nosebleeds, problems with swallowing, hoarseness, and a chronically runny nose. Ingesting cocaine can cause severe bowel gangrene as a result of reduced blood flow. Injecting cocaine can bring about severe allergic reactions and increased risk for contracting HIV and other blood-borne diseases. Binge patterns of use may lead to irritability, restlessness, anxiety, and paranoia. Cocaine abusers can suffer a temporary state of full-blown paranoid psychosis, in which they lose touch with reality and experience auditory hallucinations.

Regardless of how or how frequently cocaine is used, a user can experience acute cardiovascular or cerebrovascular emergencies, such as a heart attack or stroke, which may cause sudden death. Cocaine-related deaths are often a result of cardiac arrest or seizure followed by respiratory arrest.

Added Danger: Cocaethylene

When people consume cocaine and alcohol together, they compound the danger each drug poses and unknowingly perform a complex chemical experiment within their bodies. Researchers have found that the human liver combines cocaine and alcohol to produce a third substance, cocaethylene, which intensifies cocaine's euphoric effects. Cocaethylene is associated with a greater risk of sudden death than cocaine alone (Harris, Everhart, Mendelson, & Jones, 2003).

Treatment Options

Behavioral interventions such as cognitive-behavioral therapy have been shown to be effective for decreasing cocaine use and preventing relapse. Treatment must be tailored to the individual patient's needs to optimize outcomes and often involves a combination of treatment, social support, and other services.

Currently, there are no medications for treating cocaine addiction; however, researchers are looking for medications that help alleviate the severe craving experienced by people in treatment for cocaine addiction. In addition, researchers are investigating the use of medications to counteract triggers of relapse, such as stress. Several compounds are currently being investigated for their safety and efficacy, including a vaccine that would sequester cocaine in the bloodstream and prevent it from reaching the brain. To be effective addiction medications must be used as a part of a comprehensive treatment program.

The Magnitude of Cocaine Abuse: Monitoring the Future Survey

According to the 2007 MTF survey, cocaine use among 8th-, 10th-, 12th-grade students as shown in **Tables 10-3** and **10-4** did not show a significant increase; nonetheless, the rates remained at unacceptably high levels: 3.1% of 8th graders, 5.3% of 10th graders, and 7.8% of 12th graders have tried cocaine; 0.9% of 8th graders, 1.3% of 10th graders, and 2.0% of 12th graders were current (past-month) cocaine users.

TABLE 10-3 Use of Cocaine in *Any Form* by Students per 2007 Monitoring the Future Survey

	8th Graders	10th Graders	12th Graders
Lifetime (%)	3.1	5.3	7.8
Past Year (%)	2.0	3.4	5.2
Past Month (%)	0.9	1.3	2.0

Source: Johnston, L. D., O'Malley, P. M., Bachman, J. G., & Schulenberg, J. E. (2008). Monitoring the Future national results on adolescent drug use: Overview of key findings, 2007 (NIH Publication No. 08-6418). Bethesda, MD: National Institute on Drug Abuse.

TABLE 10-4 Crack Cocaine Use by Students

	8th Graders	10th Graders	12th Graders
Lifetime (%)	2.1	2.3	3.2
Past Year (%)	1.3	1.3	1.9
Past Month (%)	0.6	0.5	0.9

Source: Johnston, L. D., O'Malley, P. M., Bachman, J. G., & Schulenberg, J. E. (2008). Monitoring the Future national results on adolescent drug use: Overview of key findings, 2007 (NIH Publication No. 08-6418). Bethesda, MD: National Institute on Drug Abuse.

HEROIN

Heroin is also called H, junk, skag, and smack. It is a synthetic opiate drug that is highly addictive. It is made from morphine, a naturally occurring substance extracted from the seed pod of the Asian opium poppy plant. Heroin usually appears as a white or brown powder or as a black sticky substance known as "black tar heroin." Heroin abuse is a serious problem in the United States. Major health problems from heroin include miscarriages, heart infections, and death from overdose. People who inject the heroin also are at risk for contracting infectious diseases, including HIV/AIDS and hepatitis. Regular use of heroin can lead to tolerance; that is, users need more and more of the drug to have the same effect. At higher doses over time, the body becomes dependent on heroin. If dependent users stop heroin, they have withdrawal symptoms such as restlessness, muscle and bone pain, diarrhea, vomiting, and cold flashes.

How Heroin Is Abused

Heroin can be injected, snorted/sniffed, or smoked—routes of administration that rapidly deliver the drug to the brain. Injecting is the use of a needle to release the drug directly into the bloodstream. Snorting is the process of inhaling heroin powder through the nose, where it is absorbed into the bloodstream through the nasal tissues. Smoking heroin involves inhaling the smoke into the lungs. All three methods of administering heroin can lead to addiction and other severe health problems.

The Effect of Heroin on the Brain

Heroin enters the brain, where it is converted to morphine and binds to receptors known as opioid receptors. These receptors are located in many areas of the brain (and in the body), especially those involved in the perception of pain and in the reward system. Opioid receptors are also located in the brainstem and are important for automatic processes critical to life, such as breathing, blood pressure, and arousal.

After an intravenous injection of heroin, users report feeling a surge of euphoria ("rush") accompanied by dry mouth, a warm flushing of the skin, and a heaviness of the extremities. Following this initial euphoria, the user goes "on the nod," an alternately wakeful and drowsy state. Mental functioning becomes clouded. Users who do not inject the drug may not experience the initial rush, but other effects are the same. With regular heroin use, tolerance develops. The abuser must use more of the heroin to achieve the same intensity. Eventually, chemical changes in the brain can lead to addiction.

What Other Adverse Effects Does Heroin Have on Health?

Heroin abuse is associated with serious health conditions, including fatal overdose, spontaneous abortion, and—particularly in users who inject the drug—infectious diseases, including HIV/AIDS and hepatitis. Chronic users may develop collapsed veins, infection of the heart lining and valves, abscesses, and liver or kidney disease. Pulmonary complications, including various types of pneumonia, may result from the poor health of the abuser, as well as from heroin's depressing effects on respiration. In addition to the effects of the drug itself, street heroin often contains toxic contaminants or additives that can clog the blood vessels leading to the lungs, liver, kidneys, or brain, causing permanent damage to vital organs and death.

Chronic use of heroin leads to physical dependence, a state in which the body has adapted to the presence of the drug. If a dependent user reduces or stops use of the drug abruptly, he or she may experience severe symptoms of withdrawal. These symptoms, which can begin as early as a few hours after the last drug administration, include restlessness, muscle and bone pain, insomnia, diarrhea and vomiting, cold flashes with goose bumps ("cold turkey"), kicking movements ("kicking the habit"), and other symptoms. Users also experience severe craving for the drug during withdrawal, precipitating continued abuse and/or relapse. Major withdrawal symptoms peak between 48 and 72 hours after the last dose and typically subside after about a week; however, some individuals may show persistent withdrawal symptoms for months.

Although heroin withdrawal is considered less dangerous than alcohol or barbiturate withdrawal, sudden withdrawal by heavily dependent users who are in poor health is occasionally fatal. Heroin abuse during pregnancy, together with related factors like poor nutrition and inadequate prenatal care, has been associated with adverse consequences including low birthweight, an important risk factor for later developmental delay. If the mother is regularly abusing the drug, the infant may be born physically dependent on heroin and could suffer from serious medical complications requiring hospitalization.

Treatment Options

A range of treatments exist for heroin addiction, including medications and behavioral therapies. Science has taught us that when medication treatment is integrated with other supportive services, patients are often able to stop using heroin (or other opiates) and return to stable and productive lives. Treatment often begins with medically assisted detoxification from the process of cleaning toxins from the body and withdrawing from the drug safely. Medications such as clonidine and, now, buprenorphine can be used to help minimize symptoms of withdrawal. However, detoxification alone is not treatment and has not been shown to be effective in preventing relapse—it is merely the first step.

Medications to help prevent heroin relapse include:

- *Methadone*, which has been used for more than 30 years to treat heroin addiction, is a synthetic opiate medication that binds to the same receptors as heroin; but when taken orally, as dispensed, it has a gradual onset of action and sustained effects, reducing the desire for other opioid drugs while preventing withdrawal symptoms. Properly prescribed methadone is not intoxicating or sedating, and its effects do not interfere with ordinary daily activities. At the present time, methadone is only available through specialized opiate treatment programs.
- *Buprenorphine* is a more recently approved treatment for heroin addiction (and other opiates). It differs from methadone in having less risk for overdose and withdrawal effects, and importantly, it can be prescribed in the privacy of a doctor's office.
- *Naltrexone* is approved for treating heroin addiction but has not been widely used because of compliance issues. It is an opioid receptor blocker, which has been shown to be effective in highly motivated patients. It should only be used in patients who have already been detoxified in order to prevent severe withdrawal symptoms. Naloxone is a shorter acting opioid receptor blocker, used to treat cases of overdose.

For pregnant heroin abusers, methadone maintenance combined with prenatal care and a comprehensive drug treatment program can improve many of the detrimental maternal and neonatal outcomes associated with untreated heroin abuse. Preliminary evidence suggests that buprenorphine also is a safe and effective treatment during pregnancy, although infants exposed to either methadone or buprenorphine prenatally may require treatment for withdrawal symptoms. For women who do not want or are not able to receive pharmacotherapy for their heroin addiction, detoxification from opiates during pregnancy can be accomplished with medical supervision, although potential risks to the fetus and the likelihood of relapse to heroin use should be considered.

There are many effective behavioral treatments available for heroin addiction in combination with medication. These behavioral treatments can be delivered in residential or outpatient settings. Examples are contingency management, which uses a voucher-based system where patients earn "points" based on negative drug tests, which they can exchange for items that encourage healthy living; and cognitive-behavioral therapy, designed to help modify a patient's expectations and behaviors related to drug abuse, and to increase skills in coping with various life stressors.

Monitoring the Future Survey

According to the 2007 MTF survey on heroin use, as shown in **Table 10-5**, there were no significant changes since 2006 in the proportion of students in the 8th, 10th, and 12th grades reporting lifetime, past-year, and past-month use of heroin overall. Heroin use has been steadily declining since the mid-1990s. Recent peaks in heroin use were observed in 1996 for 8th graders, 1997 to 2000 for 10th graders, and 2000 for 12th graders. Annual prevalence of heroin use in 2007 dropped significantly, by between 38% and 40%, from these recent peak use years for each grade surveyed.

TABLE 10-5 Heroin Use by Students per 2007 Monitoring the Future Survey

	8th Grade	10th Grade	12th Grade
Lifetime (%)	1.3	1.5	1.5
Past Year (%)	0.8	0.8	0.9
Past Month (%)	0.4	0.4	0.4

Source: Johnston, L. D., O'Malley, P. M., Bachman, J. G., & Schulenberg, J. E. (2008). Monitoring the Future national results on adolescent drug use: Overview of key findings, 2007 (NIH Publication No. 08-6418). Bethesda, MD: National Institute on Drug Abuse.

INHALANTS

Inhalant use is also called huffing. Many parents fear that their children will use drugs such as marijuana or LSD; however, they may not realize the dangers of substances in the home. Household products such as glue, hair spray, paint, and lighter fluid are drugs used by kids in search of a quick high. Many young people inhale vapors from inhalants not knowing that serious health problems can result. Parents and kids both need to know the dangers of inhalants. One session of inhalant abuse can disrupt heart rhythms and lower oxygen levels; either of these can cause death. Regular abuse can result in serious harm to the brain, heart, kidneys, and liver.

Inhalants are a diverse group of volatile substances whose chemical vapors can be inhaled to produce psychoactive (mind-altering) effects. Although other abused substances can be inhaled, the term *inhalants* is used to describe substances that are rarely, if ever, taken by any other route of administration. A variety of products common in the home and workplace contain substances that can be inhaled to get high; however, people do not typically think of these products (e.g., spray paint, glue, and cleaning fluids) as drugs because they were never intended to induce intoxicating effects. Yet young children and adolescents can easily obtain these extremely toxic substances and are among those most likely to abuse them. In fact, 8th graders have tried inhalants more than any other illicit drug (Johnston, O'Malley, Bachman, & Schulenberg, 2007). Moreover, a person with hallucinations might mistakenly drink lighter fluid as water and intensify the hallucinations.

Types of Products Abused as Inhalants

Inhalants fall into the following categories:

- Volatile solvents are liquids that vaporize at room temperature. Industrial or household products, including paint thinners or removers, degreasers, dry cleaning fluids, gasoline, lighter fluid, art or office supply solvents, including correction fluids, felt-tip marker fluid, electronic contact cleaners, and glue.
- Aerosol sprays that contain propellants and solvents. Household aerosol propellants in items such as spray paint, hair or deodorant spray, fabric protector spray, aerosol computer cleaning products, and vegetable oil spray.
- Gases found in household or commercial products and those used as medical anesthetics, in household or commercial products including butane lighters and propane tanks, in whipped cream aerosol cans or dispensers (whippets), and refrigerant gases. Medical anesthetics, such as ether, chloroform, halothane, and nitrous oxide ("laughing gas").

- Nitrites, a special class of inhalants that are used primarily as sexual enhancers. Organic nitrites are volatiles that include cyclohexyl, butyl, and amyl nitrites, commonly known as "poppers." Amyl nitrite is still used in certain diagnostic medical procedures. When marketed for illicit use, they are often sold in small brown bottles labeled as "video head cleaner," "room odorizer," "leather cleaner," or "liquid aroma." These various products contain a wide range of chemicals such as toluene (spray paints, rubber cement, gasoline), chlorinated hydrocarbons (dry cleaning chemicals, correction fluids), hexane (glues, gasoline), benzene (gasoline), methylene chloride (varnish removers, paint thinners), butane (cigarette lighter refills, air fresheners), and nitrous oxide (whipped cream dispensers, gas cylinders).

According to the Substance Abuse and Mental Health Services Administration, Office of Applied Studies NSDUH Report, *Inhalant Use Across the Adolescent Years*, adolescents tend to abuse different products at different ages (http://nida.nih.gov/infofacts). Among new users 12 to 15 years of age, the most commonly abused inhalants were glue, shoe polish, spray paints, gasoline, and lighter fluid. Among new users age 16 or 17, the most commonly abused products were nitrous oxide or whippets. Nitrites are the class of inhalants most commonly abused by adults (Wu, Schlenger, & Ringwalt, 2005).

How Inhalants Are Abused

Inhalants can be breathed in through the nose or mouth in a variety of ways, such as sniffing or snorting fumes from a container, spraying aerosols directly into the nose or mouth, or placing an inhalant-soaked rag in the mouth ("huffing"). Users may also inhale fumes from a balloon or a plastic or paper bag that contains an inhalant. The intoxication produced by inhalants usually lasts just a few minutes; therefore, users often try to extend the "high" by continuing to inhale repeatedly over several hours.

The Effect of Inhalants on the Brain

The effects of inhalants are similar to those of alcohol, including slurred speech, lack of coordination, euphoria, and dizziness. Inhalant abusers may also experience lightheadedness, hallucinations, and delusions. With repeated inhalations, many users feel less inhibited and less in control. Some may feel drowsy for several hours and experience a lingering headache. Chemicals found in different types of inhaled products may produce a variety of additional effects, such as confusion, nausea, or vomiting.

By displacing air in the lungs, inhalants deprive the body of oxygen, a condition known as hypoxia. Hypoxia can damage cells throughout the body, but the cells of the brain are especially sensitive to inhalants. The symptoms of brain hypoxia vary according to which regions of the brain are affected. The hippocampus, for example, helps control memory, so someone who repeatedly uses inhalants may lose the ability to learn new things or may have a hard time carrying on simple conversations. Long-term inhalant abuse can also break down myelin, a fatty tissue that surrounds and protects some nerve fibers. Myelin helps nerve fibers carry their messages quickly and efficiently, and when damaged can lead to muscle spasms and tremors or even permanent difficulty with basic actions like walking, bending, and talking.

Although not very common, addiction to inhalants can occur with repeated abuse. Based on the 2006 Treatment Episode Dataset, inhalants were reported as the primary substance abused by less than 0.1% of all individuals admitted to substance abuse treatment (Office of Applied Studies, 2008). However, of those individuals who reported inhalants as their primary, secondary, or tertiary drug of choice, nearly half were adolescents 12 to 17 years of age. This age group represents only 8% of total admissions to treatment (Office of Applied Studies, 2008).

Other Adverse Effects of Inhalants on Health

Lethal Effects

Sniffing highly concentrated amounts of the chemicals in solvents or aerosol sprays can directly induce heart failure and death within minutes of a session of repeated inhalations. This syndrome is known as "sudden sniffing death" and can affect an otherwise healthy young person. Sudden sniffing death is particularly associated with the abuse of butane, propane, and chemicals in aerosols.

High concentrations of inhalants also may cause death from suffocation by displacing oxygen in the lungs, causing the user to lose consciousness and stop breathing. Deliberately inhaling from a paper or plastic bag or in a closed area greatly increases the chances of suffocation. Even when using aerosols or volatile products for their legitimate purposes (e.g., painting, cleaning), it is wise to do so in a well-ventilated room or outdoors.

Harmful Irreversible Effects

- Hearing loss: Spray paints, glues, dewaxers, dry cleaning chemicals, correction fluids

- Peripheral neuropathies or limb spasms: Glues, gasoline, whipped cream dispensers, gas cylinders
- CNS or brain damage: Spray paints, glues, dewaxers;
- Bone marrow damage: Gasoline
- Serious but potentially reversible effects include liver and kidney damage: Correction fluids, dry cleaning fluids, and blood oxygen depletion from varnish removers and paint thinners
- HIV/AIDS: Nitrites are abused to enhance sexual pleasure and performance, and they can be associated with unsafe sexual practices that greatly increase the risk of contracting and spreading infectious diseases such as HIV and hepatitis

The Magnitude of Inhalant Abuse: Monitoring the Future

The MTF survey (2007) reports more 8th graders (15.6%) have tried inhalants in their lifetime than any other illicit drug, including marijuana. Lifetime use (use at least once during a respondent's lifetime) of inhalants was reported by 15.6% of 8th graders, 13.6% of 10th graders, and 10.5% of 12th graders in 2007; 3.9% of 8th graders, 2.5% of 10th graders, and 1.2% of 12th graders were current users of inhalants (had used at least once during the 30 days preceding response to the survey).

MARIJUANA

Marijuana is also called cannabis, ganja, grass, hash, herb, pot, and weed. It is the most commonly abused illegal drug in the United States. Abusing marijuana can result in problems with memory, learning, and social behavior. Longer term, it can lead to problems such as lung cancer and increased risk of infections. It can interfere with family, school, work, and other activities. Scientific studies are under way to test the safety and usefulness of cannabis compounds for treating certain medical conditions. Currently, smoking marijuana is not recommended for the treatment of any disease or condition. The main active chemical in marijuana is delta-9-tetrahydrocannabinol (THC).

How Marijuana Is Abused

Marijuana is usually smoked as a cigarette (joint) or in a pipe. It is also smoked in blunts, which are cigars that have been emptied of tobacco and refilled with marijuana. Because the blunt retains the tobacco leaf used to wrap the cigar, this mode of delivery combines marijuana's active ingredients with nicotine and other harmful chemicals. Marijuana can also be mixed in food or brewed as a tea. As a more concentrated, resinous form, marijuana is called hashish, and as a sticky black liquid, hash oil. Marijuana smoke has a pungent, distinctive, and usually a sweet-and-sour odor.

How Marijuana Affects the Brain

When someone smokes marijuana, THC rapidly passes from the lungs into the bloodstream, which carries the chemical to the brain and other organs throughout the body. THC acts on specific sites in the brain, called cannabinoid receptors, kicking off a series of cellular reactions that ultimately lead to the "high" that users experience when they smoke marijuana. Some brain areas have many cannabinoid receptors; others have few or none. The highest density of cannabinoid receptors are found in the parts of the brain that influence pleasure, memory, thoughts, concentration, sensory and time perception, and coordinated movement (Herkenham et al., 1990).

Not surprisingly, marijuana intoxication can cause distorted perceptions, impaired coordination, difficulty in thinking and problem solving, and problems with learning and memory. Research has shown that marijuana's adverse impact on learning and memory can last for days or weeks after the acute effects of the drug wear off (Pope, Gruber, Hudson, Huestis, & Yurgelun-Todd, 2001). As a result, someone who smokes marijuana every day may be functioning at a suboptimal intellectual level all of the time.

Research on the long-term effects of marijuana abuse indicates some changes in the brain similar to those seen after long-term abuse of other major drugs. For example, cannabinoid withdrawal in chronically exposed animals leads to an increase in the activation of the stress-response system (Rodríguez, de Fonseca, Carrera, Navarro, Koob, & Weiss, 1997) and changes in the activity of nerve cells containing dopamine (Diana, Melis, Muntoni, & Gessa, 1998). Dopamine neurons are involved in the regulation of motivation and reward, which are directly or indirectly affected by all abused drugs.

Addictive Potential

Long-term marijuana abuse can lead to addiction and cause harmful effects on social functioning in the family, school, work, and recreational activities. Long-term marijuana abusers trying to quit report irritability, sleeplessness, decreased appetite, anxiety, and drug craving, all of which make it difficult to quit. These withdrawal symptoms begin approximately 1 day following abstinence, peak at 2 to 3 days, and subside within 1 or 2 weeks following drug cessation (Budney, Vandrey, Hughes, Thostenson, & Bursac, 2008).

Marijuana and Mental Health

A number of studies have shown an association between chronic marijuana use and increased rates of anxiety, depression, suicidal ideation, and schizophrenia. Some of these studies have shown age at first use to be a factor, where early use is a marker of vulnerability to later problems. However, at this time, it not clear whether marijuana use causes mental problems, exacerbates them, or is used in attempt to self-medicate symptoms already in existence. Chronic marijuana use, especially in a very young person, may also be a marker of risk for mental illnesses, including addiction, stemming from genetic or environmental vulnerabilities such as early exposure to stress or violence, which is the strongest evidence in the literature that links marijuana use and schizophrenia and/or related disorders (Moore et al., 2007). High doses of marijuana also can produce an acute psychotic reaction, and research suggests that in vulnerable individuals, marijuana use may be a factor that increases risk for the disease.

Other Adverse Effects of Marijuana on Health

Effects on the Heart

One study found that an abuser's risk of heart attack quadruples in the first hour after smoking marijuana (Mittleman et al., 2001). The researchers suggest that such an outcome might occur from marijuana's effects on blood pressure and heart rate (it increases both) and reduced oxygen-carrying capacity of blood.

Effects on the Lungs

Numerous studies have shown marijuana smoke to contain carcinogens and to be an irritant to the lungs. In fact, marijuana smoke contains 50–70% more carcinogenic hydrocarbons than tobacco smoke. Marijuana users usually inhale more deeply and hold their breath longer than tobacco smokers do, which further increases the lungs' exposure to carcinogenic smoke. Marijuana smokers show dysregulated growth of epithelial cells in their lung tissue, which could lead to cancer (Tashkin, 2005); however, a case-controlled study found no positive associations between marijuana use and lung, upper respiratory, or upper digestive tract cancers (Hashibe et al., 2006). Thus the link between marijuana smoking and these cancers remains unsubstantiated at the time of writing this book.

Nonetheless, marijuana smokers can have many of the same respiratory problems as tobacco smokers, such as daily cough and phlegm production, more frequent acute chest illness, a heightened risk of lung infections, and a greater tendency toward obstructed airways. A study of 450 individuals found that people who smoke marijuana frequently but do not smoke tobacco have more health problems and miss more days of work than nonsmokers (Polen et al., 1993). Many of the extra sick days among the marijuana smokers in the study were for respiratory illnesses.

Effects on Daily Life

Research clearly demonstrates that marijuana has the potential to cause problems in daily life or make a person's existing problems worse. In one study, heavy marijuana abusers reported that the drug impaired several important measures of life achievement including physical and mental health, cognitive abilities, social life, and career status (Gruber, Pope, Hudson, & Yurgelun-Todd, 2003). Several studies associate workers' marijuana smoking with increased absences, tardiness, accidents, workers' compensation claims, and job turnover.

Treatment Options

Behavioral interventions, including cognitive-behavioral therapy and motivational incentives (e.g., providing vouchers for goods or services to patients who remain abstinent) have shown efficacy in treating marijuana dependence. Although no medications are currently available, recent discoveries about the workings of the cannabinoid system offer promise for the development of medications to ease withdrawal, block the intoxicating effects of marijuana, and prevent relapse.

The latest treatment data indicate that in 2006 marijuana was the most common illicit drug of abuse and was responsible for about 16% (289,988) of all admissions to treatment facilities in the United States. Marijuana admissions were primarily male (73.8%), white (51.5%), and young (36.1% were in the 15 to 19 age range). Those in treatment for primary marijuana abuse had begun use at an early age: 56.2% had abused it by age 14 and 92.5% had abused it by age 18.

The Magnitude of Marijuana Abuse

According to the data from the National Survey on Drug Use and Health, in 2006, 14.8 million Americans age 12 or older used marijuana at least once in the month prior to being surveyed; these findings are similar to the 2005 rates. About 6000 people a day in 2006 used marijuana for the first time, approximately 2.2 million Americans. Of these, 63.3% were under age 18.

Monitoring the Future Survey

According to the 2007 MTF survey, marijuana use has been declining since the late 1990s. Between 2000 and 2007, past-year use decreased more than 20% in all three grades combined (8th, 10th, and 12th graders) shown in **Tables 10-6, 10-7**, and **10-8**. Nevertheless, marijuana use remains at high levels, with more than 40% of high school seniors reporting use at least once in their lifetimes.

TABLE 10-6 Percentage of 8th Graders Who Have Used Marijuana per 2007 Monitoring the Future Study

	2001	2002	2003	2004	2005	2006	2007
Lifetime (%)	20.4	19.2	17.5	16.3	16.5	15.7	14.2
Past Year (%)	15.4	14.6	12.8	11.8	12.2	11.7	10.3
Past Month (%)	9.2	8.3	7.5	6.4	6.6	6.5	5.7
Daily (%)	1.3	1.2	1.0	0.8	1.0	1.0	0.8

Source: Johnston, L. D., O'Malley, P. M., Bachman, J. G., & Schulenberg, J. E. (2008). Monitoring the Future national results on adolescent drug use: Overview of key findings, 2007 (NIH Publication No. 08-6418). Bethesda, MD: National Institute on Drug Abuse.

TABLE 10-7 Percentage of 10th Graders Who Have Used Marijuana per 2007 Monitoring the Future Study

	2001	2002	2003	2004	2005	2006	2007
Lifetime (%)	40.1	38.7	36.4	35.1	34.1	31.8	31.0
Past Year (%)	32.7	30.3	28.2	27.5	26.6	25.2	24.6
Past Month (%)	19.8	17.8	17.0	15.9	15.2	14.2	14.2
Daily (%)	4.5	3.9	3.6	3.2	3.1	2.8	2.8

Source: Johnston, L. D., O'Malley, P. M., Bachman, J. G., & Schulenberg, J. E. (2008). Monitoring the Future national results on adolescent drug use: Overview of key findings, 2007 (NIH Publication No. 08-6418). Bethesda, MD: National Institute on Drug Abuse.

TABLE 10-8 Percentage of 12th Graders Who Have Used Marijuana per 2007 Monitoring the Future Study

	2001	2002	2003	2004	2005	2006	2007
Lifetime (%)	19.0	47.8	46.1	45.7	44.8	42.3	41.8
Past Year (%)	37.0	36.2	34.9	34.3	33.6	31.5	31.7
Past Month (%)	22.4	21.5	21.2	19.9	19.8	18.3	18.8
Daily (%)	5.8	6.0	6.0	5.6	5.0	5.0	5.1

Source: Johnston, L. D., O'Malley, P. M., Bachman, J. G., & Schulenberg, J. E. (2008). Monitoring the Future national results on adolescent drug use: Overview of key findings, 2007 (NIH Publication No. 08-6418). Bethesda, MD: National Institute on Drug Abuse.

PRESCRIPTION DRUG ABUSE

Most people take medicines only for the reasons their doctors prescribe them. But an estimated 20% of people in the United States have used prescription drugs such as narcotic painkillers, sedatives, tranquilizers, and stimulants for nonmedical reasons, a practice known as prescription drug abuse. Prescription drug abuse is a serious and growing problem.

The availability of prescription drugs is probably one reason this has become so prevalent. Doctors are prescribing more drugs for more health problems than ever before. Online pharmacies make it easy to get prescription drugs without a prescription, even for youngsters, as depicted in **Table 10-9**.

NICOTINE

Street names for nicotine include smokes, fags, cigs, and cancer sticks. Modes of administration are inhalation, chewing, prescription gum or patch.

According to the 2004 National Survey on Drug Use and Health (2005), an estimated 70.3 million Americans age 12 or older reported current use of tobacco—59.9 million (24.9% of the population) were current cigarette smokers, 13.7 million (5.7%) smoked cigars, 1.8 million (0.8%) smoked pipes, and 7.2 million (3.0%) used smokeless tobacco, confirming that tobacco is one of the most widely abused substances in the United States. Although these numbers are still unacceptably high, they represent a decrease of almost 50% since peak use in 1965 (Giovino et al., 1995).

The 2005 MTF survey of the National Institute of Drug Abuse (NIDA) showed a significant decrease in smoking trends among the nation's youth. The results indicate that about 9% of 8th graders, 15% of 10th graders, and 23% of 12th graders had used cigarettes in the 30 days prior to the survey (NIDA, 2005). Despite cigarette use being at the lowest levels of the survey since a peak in the mid-1990s, the past few years indicate a clear slowing of this decline. And although perceived risk and disapproval of smoking had been on the rise, recent years have shown the rate of change to be dwindling. In fact, current use, perceived risk, and disapproval leveled off among 8th graders in 2005, suggesting that renewed efforts are needed to ensure that teens understand the harmful consequences of smoking.

Moreover, the declining prevalence of cigarette smoking among the general U.S. population is not reflected in patients with mental illnesses. For them, it remains substantially higher, with the incidence of smoking in patients suffering from post-traumatic stress disorder, bipolar disorder, major depression, and other mental illness twofold to fourfold higher than the general population, and smoking incidence among

TABLE 10-9 Prescription Drug Abuse

Substances: Category and Name	Examples of *Commercial* and Street Names	DEA Schedule*/ How Administered**	*Intoxication Effects*/Potential Health Consequences
Depressants			*Reduced pain and anxiety; feeling of well-being; lowered inhibitions; slowed pulse and breathing; lowered blood pressure; poor concentration*/confusion, fatigue; impaired coordination, memory, judgment; respiratory depression and arrest, addiction
Barbiturates	*Amytal, Nembutal, Seconal, Phenobarbital*; barbs, reds, red birds, phennies, tooies, yellows, yellow jackets	II, III, V/injected, swallowed	*Also, for barbiturates—sedation, drowsiness*/depression, unusual excitement, fever, irritability, poor judgment, slurred speech, dizziness
Benzodiazepines (other than flunitrazepam)	*Ativan, Halcion, Librium, Valium, Xanax*; candy, downers, sleeping pills, tranks	IV/swallowed	*For benzodiazepines—sedation, drowsiness*/dizziness
Flunitrazepam***+	*Rohypnol*; forget-me pill, Mexican Valium, R2, Roche, roofies, roofinol, rope, rophies	IV/swallowed, snorted	*For flunitrazepam*—visual and gastrointestinal disturbances, urinary retention, memory loss for the time under the drug's effects
Dissociative Anesthetics			*Increased heart rate and blood pressure, impaired motor function*/memory loss; numbness; nausea/vomiting
Ketamine	*Ketalar SV*; cat Valium, K, Special K, vitamin K	III/injected, snorted, smoked	*Also, for ketamine—at high doses, delirium, depression, respiratory depression and arrest*
Opioids and Morphine Derivatives			*Pain relief, euphoria, drowsiness*/respiratory depression and arrest, nausea, confusion, constipation, sedation, unconsciousness, coma, tolerance, addiction

Codeine	*Empirin with Codeine, Fiorinal with Codeine, Robitussin A-C, Tylenol with Codeine*; Captain Cody, Cody, schoolboy; (with glutethimide) doors & fours, loads, pancakes and syrup	II, III, IV/injected, swallowed	*Also, for codeine—less analgesia, sedation, and respiratory depression than morphine*
Fentanyl	*Actiq, Duragesic, Sublimaze*; Apache, China girl, China white, dance fever, friend, goodfella, jackpot, murder 8, TNT, Tango and Cash	II/injected, smoked, snorted	
Morphine	*Roxanol, Duramorph*; M, Miss Emma, monkey, white stuff	II, III/injected, swallowed, smoked	
Opium	*laudanum, paregoric*; big O, black stuff, block, gum, hop	II, III, V/swallowed, smoked	
Other opioid pain relievers (oxycodone, meperidine, hydromorphone, hydrocodone, propoxyphene)	*Tylox, OxyContin, Percodan, Percocet*; oxy 80s, OxyContin, Oxycet, hillbilly heroin, percs*Demerol, meperidine hydrochloride*; demmies, pain killer*Dilaudid*; juice, dillies*Vicodin, Lortab, Lorcet; Darvon, Darvocet*	II, III, IV/swallowed, injected, suppositories, chewed, crushed, snorted	
Stimulants			*Increased heart rate, blood pressure, metabolism; feelings of exhilaration, energy, increased mental alertness*/rapid or irregular heart beat; reduced appetite, weight loss, heart failure
Amphetamines	*Biphetamine, Dexedrine*; bennies, black beauties, crosses, hearts, LA turnaround, speed, truck drivers, uppers	II/injected, swallowed, smoked, snorted	*Also, for amphetamines—rapid breathing; hallucinations*/tremor, loss of coordination; irritability, anxiousness, restlessness, delirium, panic, paranoia, impulsive behavior, aggressiveness, tolerance, addiction

(continued)

TABLE 10-9 Prescription Drug Abuse (*Continued*)

Substances: Category and Name	Examples of *Commercial* and Street Names	DEA Schedule*/ How Administered**	*Intoxication Effects*/Potential Health Consequences
Stimulants (*Continued*)			
Cocaine	*Cocaine hydrochloride*; blow, bump, C, candy, Charlie, coke, crack, flake, rock, snow, toot	II/injected, smoked, snorted	*For cocaine*—increased temperature/ chest pain, respiratory failure, nausea, abdominal pain, strokes, seizures, headaches, malnutrition
Methamphetamine	*Desoxyn*; chalk, crank, crystal, fire, glass, go fast, ice, meth, speed	II/injected, swallowed, smoked, snorted	*For methamphetamine—aggression, violence, psychotic behavior*/memory loss, cardiac and neurological damage; impaired memory and learning, tolerance, addiction
Methylphenidate	*Ritalin*; JIF, MPH, R-ball, Skippy, the smart drug, vitamin R	II/injected, swallowed, snorted	*For methylphenidate—increase or decrease in blood pressure, psychotic episodes*/ digestive problems, loss of appetite, weight loss
Other Compounds			
Anabolic steroids	*Anadrol, Oxandrin, Durabolin, Depo-Testosterone, Equipoise*; roids, juice	III/injected, swallowed, applied to skin	*No intoxication effects*/hypertension, blood clotting and cholesterol changes, liver cysts and cancer, kidney cancer, hostility and aggression, acne; adolescents, premature stoppage of growth; in males, prostate cancer, reduced sperm production, shrunken testicles, breast enlargement; in females, menstrual irregularities, development of beard and other masculine characteristics

* Schedule I and II drugs have a high potential for abuse. They require greater storage security and have a quota on manufacturing, among other restrictions. Schedule I drugs are available for research only and have no approved medical use; Schedule II drugs are available only by prescription (unrefillable) and require a form for ordering. Schedule III and IV drugs are available by prescription, may have five refills in 6 months, and may be ordered orally. Most Schedule V drugs are available over the counter.

** Taking drugs by injection can increase the risk of infection through needle contamination with staphylococci, HIV, hepatitis, and other organisms. Associated with sexual assaults.

+ Not available by prescription in the United States.

Source: National Institute on Drug Abuse: The Science of Drug Abuse & Addiction, Prescription Drug Abuse. Retrieved from: http://www.nida.nih.gov/DrugPages/PrescripDrugsChart.html. Accessed August 8, 2010.

people with schizophrenia as high as 90% higher than the general population (Lasser et al., 2000).

Tobacco use is the leading preventable cause of death in the United States. The impact of tobacco use in terms of morbidity and mortality costs to society is staggering, as shown in **Figure 10-1**. Economically, more than $75 billion of total U.S. healthcare costs each year is attributable directly to smoking (Surgeon General Report, 2004). However, this cost is well below the total cost to society because it does not include burn care from smoking-related fires, perinatal care for low birthweight infants of mothers who smoke, and medical care costs associated with disease caused by secondhand smoke. In addition to healthcare costs, the costs of lost productivity due to smoking effects are estimated at $82 billion per year, bringing a conservative estimate of the economic burden of smoking to more than $150 billion per year (CDC, 2004; NIDA, 2006).

More than 4000 chemicals are found in the smoke of tobacco products. Of these, nicotine, first identified in the early 1800s, is the primary reinforcing component of tobacco that acts on the brain. Cigarette smoking is the most popular method of using

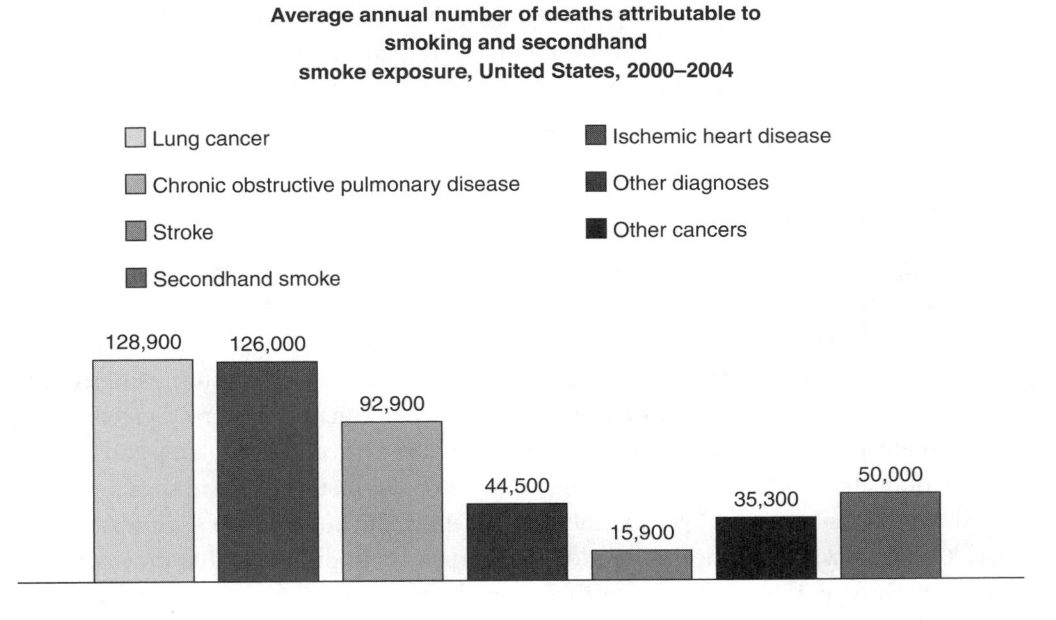

FIGURE 10-1 Average Annual Number of Deaths Attributable to Smoking and Secondhand Smoke Exposure, United States, 2000–2004

Source: CDC, MMWR 2008; 57(45): 1226–1228. "Other diagnoses" or causes include other cardiovascular diseases, perinatal conditions, and residential fires.

tobacco; however, there has also been a recent increase in the sale and consumption of smokeless tobacco products, such as snuff and chewing tobacco. These smokeless products also contain nicotine, as well as many toxic chemicals.

The cigarette is a very efficient and highly engineered drug delivery system. By inhaling tobacco smoke, the average smoker takes in 1 to 2 mg of nicotine per cigarette (Federal Trade Commission, 2000). When tobacco is smoked, nicotine rapidly reaches peak levels in the bloodstream and enters the brain. A typical smoker takes 10 puffs on a cigarette over a period of the 5 minutes that the cigarette is lit. Thus, a person who smokes about 1.5 packs (30 cigarettes) daily gets 300 "hits" of nicotine to the brain each day. In those who typically do not inhale the smoke, such as cigar and pipe smokers and smokeless tobacco users, nicotine is absorbed through the mucosal membranes and reaches peak blood levels and the brain more slowly.

Immediately after exposure to nicotine, there is a "kick" caused in part by the drug's stimulation of the adrenal glands and resulting discharge of epinephrine (adrenaline). The rush of adrenaline stimulates the body and causes a sudden release of glucose, as well as an increase in blood pressure, respiration, and heart rate (Benowitz, 1996). Nicotine also suppresses insulin output from the pancreas, which means that smokers are always slightly hyperglycemic (i.e., they have elevated blood sugar levels; Bornemisza & Suciu, 1980). The calming effect of nicotine reported by many users is usually associated with a decline in withdrawal effects rather than the direct effects of nicotine.

Nicotine Addiction

According to Benowitz (1996), most smokers use tobacco regularly because they are addicted to nicotine (**addiction** is characterized by compulsive drug seeking and use, even in the face of negative health consequences). It is well documented that most smokers identify tobacco use as harmful and express a desire to reduce or stop using it, and nearly 35 million of them want to quit each year. Unfortunately, according to the U.S. Department of Health and Human Services (HHS) Office on Smoking and Health (2000), only about 6% of people who try to quit are successful for more than a month.

Research has shown how nicotine acts on the brain to produce a number of effects. Of primary importance to its addictive nature are findings that nicotine activates reward pathways, the brain circuitry that regulates feelings of pleasure. A key brain chemical involved in mediating the desire to consume drugs is the neurotransmitter dopamine, and research has shown that nicotine increases levels of dopamine in the reward circuits. This reaction is similar to that seen with other drugs of abuse and is thought to underlie the pleasurable sensations experienced by many smokers. Nicotine's pharmacokinetic properties also enhance its abuse potential. Cigarette smoking produces a rapid distribution of nicotine to the brain, with drug levels peaking within 10 seconds of inhalation (Benowitz, 1996). However, the acute effects of nicotine dissipate in a few minutes, as do the associated feelings of reward, which causes the smoker to continue dosing to maintain the drug's pleasurable effects and prevent withdrawal.

Withdrawal

Nicotine withdrawal symptoms include irritability, craving, cognitive and attention deficits, sleep disturbances, and increased appetite. These symptoms may begin within a few hours after the last cigarette, quickly driving people back to tobacco use. Symptoms peak within the first few days of smoking cessation and may subside within a few weeks (Henningfield, 1995). For some people, however, symptoms may persist for months.

Although withdrawal is related to the pharmacologic effects of nicotine, many behavioral factors can also affect the severity of withdrawal symptoms. For some people, the feel, smell, and sight of a cigarette and the ritual of obtaining, handling, lighting, and smoking the cigarette are all associated with the pleasurable effects of smoking and can make withdrawal or craving worse. Although nicotine gum and patches may alleviate the pharmacologic aspects of withdrawal, cravings often persist. Other forms of nicotine replacement, such as inhalers, attempt to address some of these other issues; behavioral therapies can help smokers identify environmental triggers of withdrawal and craving so they can employ strategies to prevent or avoid symptoms and urges to smoke.

CAFFEINE

Caffeine, also known by street names java and joe, is considered the most commonly used psychoactive drug in the world. Approximately 80% of the world's population consumes it daily, and continuous research is being done on its health benefits and consequences. High caffeine drinks like Red Bull, lattes from McDonald's, and iced coffee drinks from Pete's and Starbucks are a growing drug of choice among teens and young adults.

Caffeine is the common name for 1,3,7-trimethylxanthine. When purified, caffeine produces an intensely bitter white powder that provides a distinctive taste in soft drinks. The word "caffeine" came from the German word *kaffee* and the French word *café*, each meaning coffee. After ingesting caffeine, it is completely absorbed within 30 to 45 minutes, and its effects substantially diminish within about 3 hours. It is eventually excreted, so there is no accumulation in the body. Caffeine has been shown to affect mood, stamina, the cerebrovascular system, and gastric and colonic activity.

Sources of Caffeine

Caffeine is naturally found in certain leaves, seeds, and fruits of over 60 plants worldwide. The most common sources in our diet are coffee, tea leaves, cocoa beans, cola, and energy drinks. Caffeine can also be produced synthetically and added to food, beverages, supplements, and medications. Product labels are required to list caffeine in the ingredients but are not required to list the actual amounts of the substance. A low to moderate intake is 130 to 300 mg of caffeine per day; heavy caffeine consumption corresponds to more than 6000 mg/day. It is estimated that the average daily caffeine consumption among Americans is about 280 mg/day; 20–30% consume more than 600 mg daily. Large amounts are usually consumed in residential care facilities, homeless shelters, and care homes for people with individuals with mental illness. Frequently clients in these facilities have open access to drinks such as coffee and tea all day and throughout the evening. The caffeine content of some foods and beverages are listed in **Table 10-10**.

TABLE 10-10 Amount of Caffeine in Food

Coffees	Serving Size	Caffeine (mg)
Coffee, generic brewed	8 oz	133 (range: 102–200) (16 oz = 266)
Starbucks Brewed Coffee (Grande)	16 oz	320
Einstein Bros. regular coffee	16 oz	300
Dunkin' Donuts regular coffee	16 oz	206
Starbucks Vanilla Latte (Grande)	16 oz	150
Coffee, generic instant	8 oz	93 (range: 27–173)
Coffee, generic decaffeinated	8 oz	5 (range: 3–12)
Starbucks Espresso, doppio	2 oz	150
Starbucks Frappuccino Blended Coffee Beverages, average	9.5 oz	115
Starbucks Espresso, solo	1 oz	75

TABLE 10-10 Amount of Caffeine in Food (*Continued*)

Coffees (*Continued*)	**Serving Size**	**Caffeine (mg)**
Einstein Bros. Espresso	1 oz	75
Espresso, generic	1 oz	40 (range: 30–90)
Starbucks Espresso decaffeinated	1 oz	4
Teas	**Serving Size**	**Caffeine (mg)**
Tea, brewed	8 oz	53 (range: 40–120)
Starbucks Tazo Chai Tea Latte (Grande)	16 oz	100
Snapple, Lemon (and diet version)	16 oz	42
Snapple, Peach (and diet version)	16 oz	42
Snapple Raspberry (and diet version)	16 oz	42
Arizona Iced Tea, black	16 oz	32
Nestea	12 oz	26
Snapple, Just Plain Unsweetened	16 oz	18
Arizona Iced Tea, green	16 oz	15
Snapple, Kiwi Teawi	16 oz	10
Soft Drinks	**Serving Size**	**Caffeine (mg)**
FDA official limit for cola and pepper soft drinks	12 oz	71
Vault	12 oz	71 (20 oz = 118)
Jolt Cola	12 oz	72
Mountain Dew MDX, regular or diet	12 oz	71 (20 oz = 118)
Coke Blak	12 oz	69 (20 oz = 115)
Coke Red, regular or diet	12 oz	54 (20 oz = 90)
Mountain Dew, regular or diet	12 oz	54 (20 oz = 90)
Pepsi One	12 oz	54 (20 oz = 90)
Mellow Yellow	12 oz	53
Diet Coke	12 oz	47 (20 oz = 78)
Diet Coke Lime	12 oz	47 (20 oz = 78)
TAB	12 oz	46.5
Pibb Xtra, Diet Mr. Pibb, Pibb Zero	12 oz	41 (20 oz = 68)

(*continued*)

TABLE 10-10 Amount of Caffeine in Food (*Continued*)

Soft Drinks (*Continued*)	**Serving Size**	**Caffeine (mg)**
Dr. Pepper	12 oz	42 (20 oz = 68)
Dr. Pepper diet	12 oz	44 (20 oz = 68)
Pepsi	12 oz	38 (20 oz = 63)
Pepsi Lime, regular or diet	12 oz	38 (20 oz = 63)
Pepsi Vanilla	12 oz	37
Pepsi Twist	12 oz	38 (20 oz = 63)
Pepsi Wild Cherry, regular or diet	12 oz	38 (20 oz = 63)
Diet Pepsi	12 oz	36 (20 oz = 60)
Pepsi Twist, diet	12 oz	36 (20 oz = 60)
Coca-Cola Classic	12 oz	35 (20 oz = 58)
Coke Black Cherry Vanilla, regular or diet	12 oz	35 (20 oz = 58)
Coke C2	12 oz	35 (20 oz = 58)
Coke Cherry, regular or diet	12 oz	35 (20 oz = 58)
Coke Lime	12 oz	35 (20 oz = 58)
Coke Vanilla	12 oz	35 (20 oz = 58)
Coke Zero	12 oz	35 (20 oz = 58)
Barq's Diet Root Beer	12 oz	23 (20 oz = 38)
Barq's Root Beer	12 oz	23 (20 oz = 38)
7-Up, regular or diet	12 oz	0
Fanta, all flavors	12 oz	0
Fresca, all flavors	12 oz	0
Mug Root Beer, regular or diet	12 oz	0
Sierra Mist, regular or free	12 oz	0
Sprite, regular or diet	12 oz	0
Energy Drinks	**Serving Size**	**Caffeine (mg)**
Spike Shooter	8.4 oz	300
Cocaine	8.4 oz	288

TABLE 10-10 Amount of Caffeine in Food (*Continued*)

Energy Drinks (*Continued*)	**Serving Size**	**Caffeine (mg)**
Monster Energy	16 oz	160
Full Throttle	16 oz	144
Rip It, all varieties	8 oz	100
Enviga	12 oz	100
Tab Energy	10.5 oz	95
SoBe No Fear	8 oz	83
Red Bull	8.3 oz	80
Red Bull Sugarfree	8.3 oz	80
Rockstar Energy Drink	8 oz	80
SoBe Adrenaline Rush	8.3 oz	79
Amp	8.4 oz	74
Glaceau Vitamin Water Energy Citrus	20 oz	50
SoBe Essential Energy, Berry or Orange	8 oz	48
Frozen Desserts	**Serving Size**	**Caffeine (mg)**
Ben & Jerry's Coffee Heath Bar Crunch	8 fl. oz	84
Ben & Jerry's Coffee Flavored Ice Cream	8 fl. oz	68
Haagen-Dazs Coffee Ice Cream	8 fl. oz	58
Haagen-Dazs Coffee Light Ice Cream	8 fl. oz	58
Haagen-Dazs Coffee Frozen Yogurt	8 fl. oz	58
Haagen-Dazs Coffee & Almond Crunch Bar	8 fl. oz	58
Starbucks Coffee Ice Cream	8 fl. oz	50–60
Chocolates/Candies/Other	**Serving Size**	**Caffeine (mg)**
Jolt Caffeinated Gum	1 stick	33
Hershey's Special Dark Chocolate Bar	1.45 oz	31
Hershey's Chocolate Bar	1.55 oz	9
Hershey's Kisses	41 g (9 pieces)	9
Hot Cocoa	8 oz	9 (range: 3–13)

(continued)

TABLE 10-10 Amount of Caffeine in Food (*Continued*)

Over-the-Counter Drugs	Serving Size	Caffeine (mg)
NoDoz (Maximum Strength)	1 tablet	200
Vivarin	1 tablet	200
Excedrin (Extra Strength)	2 tablets	130
Anacin (Maximum Strength)	2 tablets	64

Most information was obtained from company Web sites or direct inquiries (as of September 2007).

Serving sizes are based on commonly eaten portions, pharmaceutical instructions, or the amount of the leading-selling container size. For example, beverages sold in 16-oz or 20-oz bottles were counted as one serving.

Source: Adapted from Juliano, L. M., & Griffiths, R. R. (2005). Caffeine. In J. H. Lowinson, P. Ruiz, P., R. B. Millman, & J. G. Langrod (Eds.), *Substance abuse: A comprehensive textbook* (4th ed.; pp. 403–421). Baltimore: Lippincott Williams & Wilkins.

Site of Action

Caffeine absorption occurs within minutes, and brain levels remain stable for 1 hour. Caffeine increases activity in the frontal lobe where working memory is centered and in the anterior cingulum, which controls attention. Caffeine is an adenosine receptor antagonist. Blockage of this receptor results in mental alertness, reduction in cerebral blood flow, and bronchodilation (dilation of the bronchiole tubes).

Withdrawal

Caffeine withdrawal may occur within 24 to 48 hours of stoppage and is marked by headaches, fatigue or drowsiness, anxiety or depression, irritability, muscle tension, and nausea or vomiting.

THE ROLE OF THE COMMUNITY MENTAL HEALTH PROFESSIONAL

Promoting a healthy lifestyle and education about drugs and their use is the first step of preventing drug abuse. Community mental health professionals can help to promote and facilitate support groups and assist with harm reduction education about drug use and their destruction. In addition to helping them understand the consequences of drug abuse on their health, they can also help clients with a dual diagnosis of mental health and substance abuse understand the consequences of drug abuse on their family, community, and society as a whole. Mental health professionals also assist people to learn interventions for stress, fatigue, sleep, and pain management, rather than depending on drugs, which can lead to substance abuse.

A key component to program design, mental health professionals can design community-based programs to keep children away from areas at high risk for drug abuse and provide counseling services for children and families living in abusive homes. Mental health professionals can develop community drug education programs and teach community members the purpose, side effects, and the dangers of drugs when used inappropriately as well as provide case management services and social support for individuals with documented substance abuse problems. Finally, community health professionals must have knowledge about community resources for inpatient, outpatient, and community-based programs to refer individuals to depending on their readiness for change or for signs of withdrawal.

CHAPTER SUMMARY

To assist the substance abuser with the appropriate interventions, community mental health professionals must be able to identify risk factors and assess each individual's mental and physical status as well as the adverse effects of the substance on the individual behaviorally, cognitively, and physically. Once drug abuse dependence, addiction, or signs of withdrawal are identified, the community health professional must help the client understand the appropriate level of treatment and understand when and where to refer the substance abuser and his or her family. Healthcare professionals facilitate emotional support and counseling programs.

The need for community education and prevention is paramount to prevention and to help individuals understand the consequences of smoking and illicit drug use as well as participate in appropriate evidence-based treatment programs. The abuse of a variety of substances poses health problems for all. The abuse of alcohol, drugs, cigarettes, and even coffee constitutes health hazards and social problems. For example, individuals living in mental health facilities, in shelters, or in supervised boarding homes are impacted by secondhand smoke. Prevention of substance and tobacco abuse are goals in the *Healthy People 2020*. Review the *Healthy People 2020* box (**Box 10-1**), which lists the objectives directed at substance and tobacco abuse. Although these objectives are crucial to the prevention of substance abuse, many times funding is eliminated in economic downturns.

BOX 10-1 Proposed *Healthy People 2020* Objectives

SUBSTANCE ABUSE

Objectives Retained as Is from *Healthy People 2010*

1: Reduce cirrhosis deaths.

Data Source: National Vital Statistics System (NVSS), CDC, NCHS.
Action: Retained *Healthy People 2010* objective 26-2.

2: Reduce drug-induced deaths.

Data Source: National Vital Statistics System (NVSS), CDC, NCHS.
Action: Retained *Healthy People 2010* objective 26-3.

3: Reduce drug-related hospital emergency department visits.

Data Source: Drug Abuse Warning Network (DAWN), SAMHSA.
Action: Retained *Healthy People 2010* objective 26-4.

4: Reduce the proportion of adolescents who report that they rode, during the previous 30 days, with a driver who had been drinking alcohol.

Data Source: Youth Risk Behavior Surveillance System (YRBSS), CDC, NCCDPHP.
Action: Retained *Healthy People 2010* objective 26-6.

5: Increase the age and proportion of adolescents who remain alcohol and drug free.

a. Increase in average age of first use among adolescents aged 12 to 17 years: alcohol
b. Increase in average age of first use among adolescents aged 12 to 17 years: marijuana
c. Increase in high school seniors never using substances: alcoholic beverages
d. Increase in high school seniors never using substances: illicit drugs

Data Sources: National Survey on Drug Use and Health (NSDUH), SAMHSA; Monitoring the Future study, NIH.
Action: Retained *Healthy People 2010* objective 26-9.

6: Reduce past-month use of illicit substances.

a. Increase the proportion of adolescents not using alcohol or any illicit drugs during the past 30 days.
b. Reduce the proportion of adolescents reporting use of marijuana during the past 30 days.
c. Reduce the proportion of adults using any illicit drug during the past 30 days.

Data Source: National Survey on Drug Use and Health (NSDUH), SAMHSA.
Action: Retained *Healthy People 2010* objective 26-10.

7: Reduce the proportion of persons engaging in binge drinking of alcoholic beverages.

a. Reduction in students engaging in binge drinking during the past 2 weeks: high school seniors
b. Reduction in students engaging in binge drinking during the past 2 weeks: college students
c. Reduction in adults and adolescents engaging in binge drinking during the past month: adults aged 18 years and older

d. Reduction in adults and adolescents engaging in binge drinking during the past month: adolescents aged 12 to 17 years

Data Sources: Monitoring the Future study, NIH; National Survey on Drug Use and Health (NHDUH), SAMHSA.
Action: Retained *Healthy People 2010* objective 26-11.

8: Reduce average annual alcohol consumption.

Data Source: Epidemiologic Data System, NIH.
Action: Retained *Healthy People 2010* objective 26-12.

9: Reduce steroid use among adolescents.

a. Among 8th graders
b. Among 10th graders
c. Among 12th graders

Data Source: Monitoring the Future Study, NIH.
Action: Retained *Healthy People 2010* objective 26-14.

10: Reduce the proportion of adolescents who use inhalants.

Data Source: National Survey on Drug Use and Health (NSDUH), SAMHSA.
Action: Retained *Healthy People 2010* objective 26-15.

11: Increase the proportion of adolescents who disapprove of substance abuse.

a. Increase in adolescents who disapprove of having one or two alcoholic drinks nearly every day: 8th graders
b. Increase in adolescents who disapprove of having one or two alcoholic drinks nearly every day: 10th graders
c. Increase in adolescents who disapprove of having one or two alcoholic drinks nearly every day: 12th graders
d. Increase in adolescents who disapprove of trying marijuana or hashish once or twice: 8th graders
e. Increase in adolescents who disapprove of trying marijuana or hashish once or twice: 10th graders
f. Increase in adolescents who disapprove of trying marijuana or hashish once or twice: 12th graders

Data Source: Monitoring the Future study, NIH.
Action: Retained *Healthy People 2010* objective 26-16.

12: Increase the proportion of adolescents who perceive great risk associated with substance abuse.

a. Increase in adolescents aged 12 to 17 years perceiving great risk associated with substance abuse: consuming five or more alcoholic drinks at a single occasion once or twice a week
b. Increase in adolescents aged 12 to 17 years perceiving great risk associated with substance abuse: smoking marijuana once per month

(continued)

(Continued)

c. Increase in adolescents aged 12 to 17 years perceiving great risk associated with substance abuse: using cocaine once per month

Data Source: National Survey on Drug Use and Health (NSDUH), SAMHSA.
Action: Retained *Healthy People 2010* objective 26-17.

13: Increase the number of admissions to substance abuse treatment for injection drug use.

Data Source: Treatment Episodes Data Set (TEDS), SAMHSA.
Action: Retained *Healthy People 2010* objective 26-20.

Objectives Retained But Modified from *Healthy People 2010*

14: Increase the proportion of persons who need alcohol and/or illicit drug treatment and received specialty treatment for abuse or dependence in the past year.

a. Illicit drug treatment
b. Alcohol and illicit drug treatment
c. Alcohol abuse or dependence

Data Source: National Survey on Drug Use and Health (NSDUH), SAMHSA.
Action: Retained but modified *Healthy People 2010* objectives 26-18 and 26-21.

15: (Developmental) Increase the proportion of persons who are referred for follow-up care for alcohol problems, drug problems after diagnosis, or treatment for one of these conditions in a hospital emergency department.

Potential Data Source: National Hospital Ambulatory Medical Care Survey (NHAMCS), CDC, NCHS.
Action: Retained but modified *Healthy People 2010* objective 26-22.

Objectives New to *Healthy People 2020*

16: Decrease the proportion of adults who drank excessively in the previous 30 days.

Data Source: National Survey on Drug Use and Health (NSDUH), SAMHSA.
Action: New to *Healthy People 2020*.

17: Increase the number of driving while impaired (DWI) courts in the United States.

Data Source: National Association of Drug Court Professionals (NADCP) database.
Action: New to *Healthy People 2020*.

18: Increase the number of level I and level II trauma centers that implement evidence-based alcohol screening and brief intervention.

Data Source: National Trauma Verification Registry, American College of Surgeons.
Action: New to *Healthy People 2020*.

19: Reduce the past-year nonmedical use of prescription drugs.

a. Pain relievers
b. Tranquilizers
c. Stimulants
d. Sedatives
e. Any psychotherapeutic drug (including any of those noted above)

Data Sources: National Survey on Drug Use and Health (NSDUH), SAMHSA; Monitoring the Future study, NIH.
Action: New to *Healthy People 2020.*

20: Decrease the rate of alcohol-impaired driving (.08;pl blood alcohol content [BAC]) fatalities.

Data Source: Fatality Analysis Reporting System (FARS), DOT.
Action: New to *Healthy People 2020.*

Objectives Archived from *Healthy People 2010*

26-1: Reduce deaths caused by alcohol-related motor vehicle crashes.

HP2010 Data Source: Fatality Analysis Reporting System (FARS), DOT.
Action: Archived due to target being met in 2007.

26-5: (Developmental) Reduce alcohol-related hospital emergency department visits.

HP2010 Potential Data Source: National Hospital Ambulatory Medical Care Survey (NHAMCS), CDC, NCHS.
Action: Archived due to lack of adequate data source.

26-7: (Developmental) Reduce intentional injuries resulting from alcohol and illicit drug-related violence.

HP2010 Potential Data Source: National Crime Victimization Survey (NCBS), DOJ, BJS.
Action: Archived due to lack of adequate data source.

26-8: Reduce the cost of lost productivity in the workplace due to alcohol and drug use.

HP2010 Data Source: Periodic estimates of economic cost of alcohol and drug use, NIH, NIAAA, and NIDA.
Action: Archived due to lack of adequate data source.

26-13: Reduce the proportion of adults who exceed guidelines for low-risk drinking.

HP2010 Data Source: National Epidemiologic Survey on Alcohol and Related Conditions, NIH, NIAAA.
Action: Archived due to lack of adequate data source; issue addressed in new objective SA HP2020-16.

26-19: (Developmental) Increase the proportion of inmates receiving substance abuse treatment in correctional institutions.

HP2010 Potential Data Source: Uniform Facility Data Set Survey of Correctional Facilities, SAMHSA, OAS.
Action: Archived due to lack of adequate data source.

26-23: (Developmental) Increase the number of communities using partnerships or coalition models to conduct comprehensive substance abuse prevention efforts.

HP2010 Potential Data Source: Community Partnerships Data, SAMHSA.
Action: Archived due to lack of adequate data source.

(continued)

(Continued)

26-24: Extend administrative license revocation laws, or programs of equal effectiveness, for persons who drive under the influence of intoxicants.

HP2010 Data Source: DOT, NHTSA.
Action: Archived due to lack of adequate data source.

26-25: Extend legal requirements for maximum blood alcohol concentration (BAC) levels of 0.08 percent for motor vehicle drivers aged 21 years and older.

HP2010 Data Source: DOT, NHTSA.
Action: Archived due to target being met in 2005.

Objectives Archived from *Healthy People 2010*

http://www.healthypeople.gov/hp2020/Objectives/files/Draft2009Objectives.pdf

Source: U.S. Department of Health & Human Services, Healthy People 2020 Objectives. http://www.healthypeople.gov/hp2020/Objectives/files/Draft2009Objectives.pdf. Accessed August 25, 2010.

Community mental health providers are in key positions to detect community problems that might impact individuals who are mentally ill. The effects of substance abuse include several life-threatening conditions and can result in death. Individuals who abuse drugs, smoke cigarettes, or drink coffee often know the consequences of their use, however, they need emotional support and education to help them cope with the life trials leading to drug addiction and the tools necessary to quit when they are ready.

Numerous substance abuse programs are available for assisting individuals with substance abuse. However, it is important that community health providers know what programs and resources are available. The role of the community health provider includes support education, counseling health education, and referral.

REVIEW

1. Discuss the impact of substance abuse on mental health, child abuse, elder abuse, and homelessness.
2. Explain the role of the mental health provider in preventing and treating substance abuse.
3. List and explain the impact of substance abuse on the brain, body, and the cost of society.
4. Define the most commonly abused drugs and substances by teens.
5. Discuss nicotine and caffeine addiction.
6. Explain the withdrawal process.

ACTIVITIES

1. Look at your local community resources; identify agencies that might serve as a referral for substance abuse for the individual and the family.
2. Have the students discuss their personal attitudes toward substance abuse and mental health.
3. Design a community-based program addressing substance abuse.

REFERENCES AND FURTHER READINGS

Advance Data from Vital and Health Statistics. (2005). No. 358. Hyattsville, MD: National Center for Health Statistics.

Alcoholism. (2007). NIAAA Surveillance Report #80, 2007. Retrieved from http://pubs.niaaa.nih.gov Volume I: Secondary school students (NIH Pub. No. 07-6205). Bethesda, MD: National Institute on Drug Abuse.

American Academy of Pediatrics, Committee on Substance Abuse and Committee on Children with Disabilities. (2000). Fetal alcohol syndrome and alcohol-related neurodevelopmental disorders. *Pediatrics, 106*, 358–361.

Arnedo, M. T., Salvador, A., Martinez-Sanchis, S., & Gonzalez-Bono, E. (2000). Rewarding properties of testosterone in intact male mice: A pilot study. *Pharmacology, Biochemistry, and Behavior, 65*, 327–332.

Arvary, D., & Pope, H. G., Jr. (2000). Anabolic-androgenic steroids as a gateway to opioid dependence. *New England Journal of Medicine, 342*, 1532.

Benowitz, N. L. (1996). Pharmacology of nicotine: Addiction and therapeutics. *Annual Review of Pharmacology and Toxicology, 36*, 597–613.

Bor Diana, M., Melis, M., Muntoni, A. L., & Gessa, G. L. (1998). Mesolimbic dopaminergic decline after cannabinoid withdrawal. *Proceedings of the National Academy of Science, USA, 95*(17), 10269–10273.

Bornemisza, P., & Suciu, I. (1980). Effect of cigarette smoking on the blood glucose level in normals and diabetics. *Medicina Interna, 18*, 353–356.

Breslau, N. (1985)Psychiatric comorbidity of smoking and nicotine dependence. *Behavior Genetics, 25*, 95–101.

Brower, K. J. (2002). Anabolic steroid abuse and dependence. *Current Psychiatry Report, 4*(5), 377–387.

Budney, A. J., Vandrey, R. G., Hughes, J. R., Thostenson, J. D., & Bursac, Z. (2008). Comparison of cannabis and tobacco withdrawal: Severity and contribution to relapse. *Journal of Substance Abuse Treatment, 35*(4), 362–368.

Centers for Disease Control and Prevention [CDC]. (2005). Annual Smoking–Attributable Mortality, Years of Potential Life Lost, and Productivity Losses—United States, 1997–2001. *Morbidity and Mortality Weekly Report, 54*(25), 625–628.

Centers for Disease Control and Prevention [CDC]. (2006). Youth risk behavior surveillance—United States, 2005. *Morbidity and Mortality Weekly Report, 55*(No. SS-5).

Centers for Disease Control and Prevention [CDC]. (2008). Alcohol-Related Disease Impact (ARDI). Atlanta, GA: Author. Retrieved from http://www.cdc.gov/alcohol/ardi.htm.

Centers for Disease Control and Prevention [CDC]. (2008). National youth risk behavior survey 1991–2005: Trends in the prevalence of selected risk behaviors. Retrieved from http://www.cdc.gov/HealthyYouth/yrbs/pdf/trends /YRBS_Risk_Behaviors.pdf

Chang, L., Ernst, T., Speck, O., & Grob, C. S. (2005). Additive effects of HIV and chronic methamphetamine use on brain metabolite abnormalities. *American Journal of Psychiatry*, *162*, 361–369.

Chen, C.M., & Yi, H. (2008). *Surveillance Report #84: Trends in Alcohol-Related Morbidity among Short-Stay Community Hospital Discharges, United States, 1977–2006*. Arlington, VA.

Dawson, D. A., Grant, B. F., & Li, T-K. (2005). Quantifying the risks associated with exceeding recommended drinking limits. *Alcoholism, Clinical and Experimental Research*, *29*, 902–908.

Diana, M., Melis, M., Muntoni, A. L., & Gessa, G. L. (1998). Mesolimbic dopaminergic decline after cannabinoid withdrawal. *Proc. Natl. Acad. Sci. U.S.A.*, 95, 10269-10273.

Federal Trade Commission. (2000). *"Tar," nicotine, and carbon monoxide of the smoke of 1294 varieties of domestic cigarettes for the year 1998*. Washington, DC: Author.

Giovino, G. A., Henningfield, J. E., Tomar, S. L., Escobedo, L. G., Slade, G. A., Henningfield, J. E., . . . Slade, J. (1995). Epidemiology of tobacco use and dependence. *Epidemiology Review*, *17*(1), 48–65.

Greenfield, L. A. (1998). Alcohol and crime: An analysis of national data on the prevalence of alcohol involvement in crime. Report prepared for the Assistant Attorney General's National Symposium on Alcohol Abuse and Crime. Washington, DC: U.S. Department of Justice. Retrieved from http://www.ojp.usdoj.gov/bjs/pub/pdf/ac.pdf

Gruber, A. J., Pope, H. G., Hudson, J. I., & Yurgelun-Todd, D. (2003). Attributes of long-term heavy cannabis users: A case-control study. *Psychological Medicine*, *33*(8), 1415–1422.

Harris, D. S., Everhart, T., Mendelson, J., & Jones, R. T. (2003). The pharmacology of cocaethylene in humans following cocaine and ethanol administration. *Drug and Alcohol Dependence*, *72*(2), 169–182.

Harwood, H. (2000). Updating estimates of the economic costs of alcohol abuse in the United States: Estimates, update methods, and data report. Prepared by the Lewin Group for the National Institute on Alcohol Abuse and Alcoholism.

Hashibe, M., Morgenstern, H., Cui, Y., Tashkin, D. P., Zhang, Z. F., Cozen, W., . . . Greenland, S. (2006). Marijuana use and the risk of lung and upper aerodigestive tract cancers: Results of a population-based case-control study. *Cancer Epidemiology, Biomarkers & Prevention*, *15*(10), 1829–1834.

Henningfield, J. E. (1995). Nicotine medications for smoking cessation. *New England Journal of Medicine*, *333*, 1196–1203.

Herkenham, M., Lynn, A., Little, M. D., Johnson, M. R., Melvin, L. S., de Costa, B. R., & Rice, K. C. (1990). Cannabinoid receptor localization in the brain. *Proceedings of the National Academy of Science, USA*, *87*(5), 1932–1936.

Highlights 2006. (2008). National Admissions to Substance Abuse Treatment Services, DASIS Series S-40, DHHS Pub. No. (SMA) 08-4313, Rockville, MD.

Hughes, J. R., Hatsukami, D. K., Mitchell, J. E., & Dahlgren, L. A. (1986). Prevalence of smoking among psychiatric outpatients. *American Journal of Psychiatry*, *143*, 993–997.

Jansen, K. L., & Darracot-Cankovic, R. (2001). The nonmedical use of ketamine, part two: A review of problem use and dependence. *Journal of Psychoactive Drugs*, *33*(2), 151–158.

Johnston, L. D., O'Malley, P. M., Bachman, J. G., & Schulenberg, J. E. (2007). *Monitoring the Future national survey results on drug use, 1975–2006*. Bethesda, MD: National Institute on Drug Abuse.

Johnston, L. D., O'Malley, P. M., Bachman, J. G., & Schulenberg, J. E. (2009). *Monitoring the Future national results on adolescent drug use: Overview of key findings, 2008* (NIH Pub. No. 09-7401). Bethesda, MD: National Institute on Drug Abuse.

Kesmodel, U., Wisborg, K., Olsen, S. F., Henriksen, T. B., & Sechler, N. J. (2002). Moderate alcohol intake in pregnancy and the risk of spontaneous abortion. *Alcohol & Alcoholism*, *37*(1), 87–92.

Lasser, K., Boyd, J. W., Woolhandler, S., Himmelstein, D. U., McCormick, D., & Bor, D. H. (2000). Smoking and mental illness. A population-based prevalence study. *Journal of the American Medical Association*, *284*, 2606–2610.

Maeng, S., & Zarate, C. A., Jr. (2007). The role of glutamate in mood disorders: Results from the ketamine in major depression study and the presumed cellular mechanism underlying its antidepressant effects. *Current Psychiatry Reports*, *9*(6), 467–474.

Maxwell, J. C., & Spence, R. T. (2005). Profiles of club drug users in treatment. *Substance Use and Misuse*, *40*(9–10), 1409–1426.

McCaig, L. F., & Burt, C. W. (2005). National Hospital Ambulatory Medical Care Survey: 2003 emergency department summary (PDF-875K). Advance Data from Vital and Health Statistics; No. 358. Hyattsville, MD: National Center for Health Statistics.

Mittleman, M. A., Lewis, R. A., Maclure, M., Sherwood, J. B., Muller, M. A., Lewis, R. A., . . . Colley, B. G. (2003). Binge drinking in the preconception period and the risk of unintended pregnancy: Implications for women and their children. *Pediatrics*, *11*(5), 1136–1141.

Mokdad, A. H., Marks, J. S., Stroup, D. F., & Gerberding, J. L. (2000). Actual causes of death in the United States. *Journal of the American Medical Association*, *291*(10), 1238–1245.

Moore, T. H., Zammit, S., Lingford-Hughes, A., Barnes, T. R., Jones, P. B., Burke, M., & Lewis, G. (2007). Cannabis use and risk of psychotic or affective mental health outcomes: A systematic review. *Lancet*, *370*(9584), 319–328.

National Center on Addiction and Substance Abuse at Columbia University. (1999). No safe haven: Children of substance-abusing parents. Retrieved from. http://www.casacolumbia.org.

National Institute on Drug Abuse (NIDA). (2006). Research report series on tobacco addiction: NIH Pub. No. 01-4342. Bethesda, MD: NIDA, NIH, DHHS. Publication number 06-4342.

National Center for Health Statistics. Health, United States (2009). With special feature on medical technology. Hyattsville, MD.

Office of National Drug Control Policy. (2004). *The Economic Costs of Drug Abuse in the United States: 1992–2002*. Washington, DC: Executive Office of the President (Pub. No. 207303).

Polen, M. R., Sidney, S., Tekawa, I. S., Sadler, M., Friedman, M. R., Sidney, S., . . . Friedman, G. D. (1993). Health care use by frequent marijuana smokers who do not smoke tobacco. *Western Journal of Medicine*, *158*(6), 596–601.

Pope, H. G., Jr., Gruber, A. J., Hudson, J. I., Huestis, M. A., & Yurgelun-Todd, D. (2001). Neuropsychological performance in long-term cannabis users. *Archives of General Psychiatry*, *58*(10), 909–915.

Pope, H. G., & Katz, D. L. (1998). Affective and psychotic symptoms associated with anabolic steroid use. *American Journal of Psychiatry*, *145*(4), 487–490.

Pope, H. G., Jr., Kouri, E. M., & Hudson, M. D. (2000). Effects of supraphysiologic doses of testosterone on mood and aggression in normal men: A randomized controlled trial. *Archives of General Psychiatry*, *57*(2), 133–140.

Rawson, R. A., Marinelli-Casey, P., Anglin, M. D., Dickow, A., Frazier, Y., Gallagher, C., . . . Zweben, J. (2004). A multi-site comparison of psychosocial approaches for the treatment of a methamphetamine dependence. *Addiction*, *99*, 708–717.

Rodríguez de Fonseca, F., Carrera, M. R. A., Navarro, M., Koob, G. F., & Weiss, F. (1997). Activation of corticotropin-releasing factor in the limbic system during cannabinoid withdrawal. *Science*, *276*(5321), 2050–2054.

Roll, J. M., Petry, N. M., Stitzer, M. L., Brecht, M. L., Peirce, J. M., McCann, M. J., . . . Kellogg, S. (2006). Contingency management for the treatment of methamphetamine use disorders. *American Journal of Psychiatry*, *163*, 1993–1999.

Sherwood, J. B., & Muller, J. E. (2001). Triggering myocardial infarction by marijuana. *Circulation*, *103*(23), 2805–2809.

Smith, G. S., Branas, C. C., & Miller, T. R. (1999). Fatal nontraffic injuries involving alcohol: A metaanalysis. *Annals of Emergency Medicine*, *33*(6), 659–668.

Smith, K. M., Larive, L. L., & Romanelli, F. (2004). Club drugs: Methylenedioxymethamphetamine, flunitrazepam, ketamine hydrochloride, and γ–hydroxybutyrate. *American Journal of Health-System Pharmacy*, *59*(11),1067–1076.

Substance Abuse and Mental Health Services Administration. (2005). Results from the 2004 National Survey on Drug Use and Health: National Findings (Office of Applied Studies, NSDUH Series H-28, DHHS Publication No. SMA 05-4062). Rockville, MD.

Substance Abuse and Mental Health Services Administration. (2007). Results from the 2006 National Survey on Drug Use and Health: National Findings (Office of Applied Studies, NSDUH Series H-32, DHHS Publication No. SMA 07-4293). Rockville, MD.

Substance Abuse and Mental Health Services Administration, Office of Applied Studies. (2008). Treatment Episode Data Set (TEDS). Highlights—2006. National Admissions to Substance Abuse Treatment Services, DASIS Series S-40, DHHS Pub. No. (SMA) 08-4313, Rockville, MD.

Substance Abuse and Mental Health Services Administration, Office of Applied Studies. (2008). The DASIS Report: Adolescent Admissions Reporting Inhalants: 2006. Retrieved from http://www.oas.samhsa.gov

Substance Abuse and Mental Health Services Administration, Office of Applied Studies. (2009). The NSDUH Report: Exposure to Substance Use Prevention Messages and Substance Use among Adolescents: 2002–2007. Rockville, MD.

Tashkin, D. P. (2005). Smoked marijuana as a cause of lung injury. *Monaldi Archives for Chest Disease*, *63*(2), 92–100.

Thompson, P. M., Hayashi, K. M., Simon, S. L., Geaga, J. A., Hong, M. S., Sui, Y., . . . London, E. D. (2004). Structural abnormalities in the brains of human subjects who use methamphetamine. *Journal of Neuroscience*, *24*, 6028–6036.

U.S. Department of Agriculture and U.S. Department of Health and Human Services. (2005). In: *Dietary guidelines for Americans* (pp. 43–46). Washington, DC: U.S. Government Printing Office; 2005. Retrieved from http://www.health.gov/document/html U.S. Department of Health and Human Services/

U.S. Department of Health and Human Services. (2000). *Healthy People 2010* (2nd ed.). With *Understanding and improving health* and *Objectives for improving health* (2 vols.). Washington, DC: Author.

U.S. Department of Health and Human Services. (2000). *Reducing tobacco use: A report of the surgeon general*. Atlanta, GA: U.S. Department of Health and Human Services, Centers for Disease Control and Prevention; National Center for Chronic Disease Prevention and Health Promotion; Office on Smoking and Health.

U.S. Department of Health and Human Services. (2004). *The health consequences of smoking: A report of the surgeon general*. Atlanta, GA: U.S. Department of Health and Human Services; Centers for Disease Control and Prevention; National Center for Chronic Disease Prevention and Health Promotion; Office on Smoking and Health.

U.S. Department of Health and Human Services, National Institutes of Health. (2006). Tobacco Addiction: Research Series. (NIH Pub. No. 06-4342). Retrieved from www.drugabuse.gov/PDF/TobaccoRRS_v16.pdf

Volkow, N. D., Chang, L., Wang, G. J., Fowler, J. S., Leonido-Yee, M., Franceschi, D. . . . Miller, E. N. (2001). Association of dopamine transporter reduction with psychomotor impairment in methamphetamine abusers. *American Journal of Psychiatry, 158*, 377–382.

Wang, G. J., Volkow, N. D., Chang, L., Miller, E., Sedler, M., Hitzemann, R., . . . Fowler, J. S. (2004). Partial recovery of brain metabolism in methamphetamine abusers after protracted abstinence. *American Journal of Psychiatry, 161*, 242–248.

Wechsler, H., Davenport, A., Dowdall, G., Moeykens, B., & Castillo, S. (1994). Health and behavioral consequences of binge drinking in college. *Journal of the American Medical Association, 272*(21), 1672–1677.

Wu, L. T., Schlenger, W. E., & Ringwalt, C. L. (2005). Use of nitrite inhalants ("poppers") among American youth. *Journal of Adolescent Health, 37*, 52–60.

CHAPTER 11

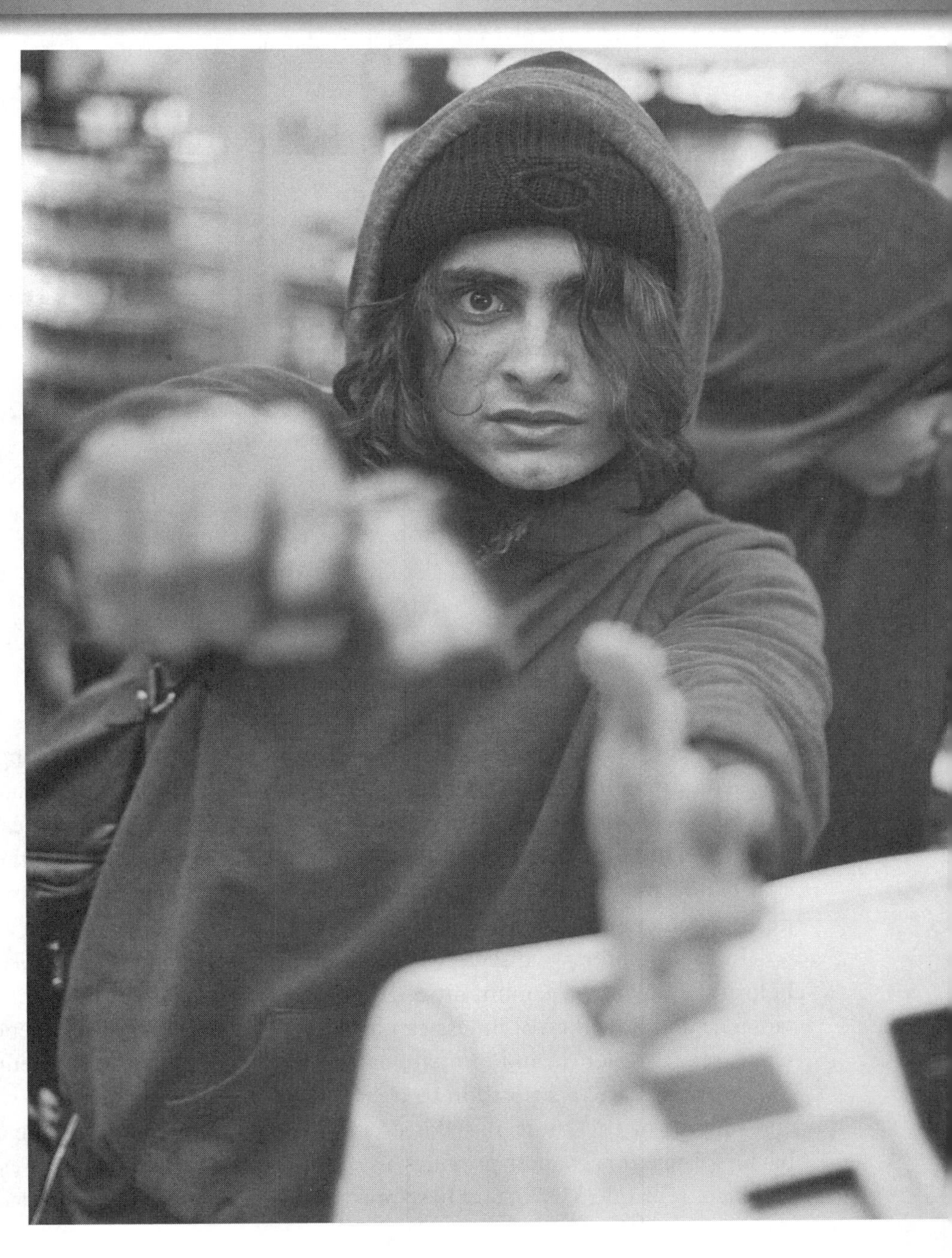

Community Mental Health Problems: Violence

CHAPTER OBJECTIVES

1. Describe the problem of violence in American communities.
2. Examine the predictors of child and elder abuse.
3. Identify the predictors and onset of sexual and intimate partner abuse.
4. Analyze the role of mental health professionals working with survivors of violence.
5. Define interventions to assist victims of violence.

KEY TERMS

- Affective violence
- Assault
- Child abuse
- Child neglect
- Emotional abuse
- Homicide
- Incest
- Munchausen syndrome
- Neglect
- Physical abuse
- Rape
- Suicide bomber

As we celebrate the dawning of the new decade, the joy of its beginning is plagued by frequent announcements of violent acts committed by individuals against themselves and others. In almost every newspaper we read, we discover headlines about college students being murdered or committing suicide or we learn about the escalation of street and hate crimes. This chapter is the third chapter addressing community mental health problems that mental health professionals must be prepared to address.

In this chapter, we discuss ways that community mental health professionals can help individuals and communities recognize the signs and symptoms of abuse and violence and how mental illness can lead to homicide, domestic violence, family violence, sexual violence, and intimate partner violence. Community mental health professionals also are in a position to treat individuals and communities who are abused and support or encourage individuals and the community to engage in alternative behaviors; thus, this chapter provides an overview of interventions addressing domestic violence, referral sources, and best-practice interventions addressing violence.

VIOLENCE AGAINST OTHERS

According to Sigmund Freud (1955), the most powerful obstacle to culture is the innate, independent, and instinctual human tendency toward aggression. Other scholars, however, believe that aggression is a learned behavior and not innate. For example, American children between 2 and 18 years of age spend an average of 6 hours and 32 minutes each day using media (television, commercial or self-recorded video, movies, video games, print, radio, recorded music, computer, and the Internet (Henry J. Kaiser Family Foundation, 1999). A large proportion of this media exposure includes acts of violence that are witnessed or "virtually perpetrated" (in the form of video games) by young people. It has been estimated that by age 18, the average young person will have viewed 200,000 acts of violence on television alone (Clark, 1993; Manganello & Taylor, 2009; Swing, Gentile, Anderson, & Walsh, 2010). This learned behavior and constant exposure to violence can lead to desensitization to violence and lead to senseless acts of violence. Recently, for example, the report of a 15-year-old teenage girl being gang **raped** by 15 boys in Richmond, California, while being watched by several students, captured the headlines of local and national television networks and newspapers. Similarly, displays on YouTube of beatings (www.youtube.com) and senseless hate crimes are more prominent than ever before among teens and the homeless, as reported by Hector Becerra and Richard Winton, *Los Angeles Times* staff writers who covered the story of a homeless man doused in gasoline and set on fire ("Cruel end for a man who asked for little," October 2008). Moreover, people in war-torn developing countries with internal conflict continue to harm and kill others as well as themselves as **suicide bombers** (Dahlberg & Butchart, 2005; Volkan, 1997).

In addition to this exposure to violence, exposure to violent video games and television programs leads to abusive gestures, language, play, and hostility. Hostility appears to be one factor leading to the occurrence of violence among others and oneself. Hostility includes aggressive behavior, anger, and hatred as well as passive gestures such as gossip and neglect. Withholding affection and fair treatment can also lead to hostility. In today's hustle and bustle, people may harbor more feelings that are hostile and use fewer constructive ways to resolve built-up feelings.

Because of our constant exposure to violence and hostile feelings, we fear we will be touched by violence, and we grieve stories about children held captive by sexual predators as well as members of their family. For example, Tracy Dugard was kidnapped and lived for 18 years with a known sex offender, Elizabeth Smart, and numerous nameless girls and boys are kidnapped from their home, neighborhood park, city, state, or country are abused or murdered. We also hear news briefs about sexual predators killed by their former victims, now adults seeking to wash away recurring dreams of sexual abuse they endured when they were a child or students being murdered on college campuses by their friends and ex-lovers. Furthermore, we have witnessed mothers throwing their innocent children in the bay or the bathtub because of mental illness, neglect, and abuse. To understand community violence, it is important for healthcare professionals to understand the salient factors; that is, each person can lash out and hurt himself, herself, or others at any point in time. It is equally important to know that violence is a community health problem, and community health professionals play an integral role in developing and providing the best care and interventions possible. The next section examines the prevalence of violence as a community problem, and it explores how community mental health providers can help individuals, families, and communities cope with violence and abuse.

Extent of the Problem

The prevalence of violence in the American culture is significant, and crime has undergone severe changes. According to the U.S. Department of Justice (2005), a violent crime is committed every 23.1 seconds and a property crime every 3.1 seconds. Subsequently, U.S. residents age 12 and older experienced an estimated 23 million crimes of violence and theft. Even more startling, the violent crime rate was 20.7 victimizations per 1000 persons age 12 or older, and for property crimes it was 146.5 per 1000 households (U.S. Department of Justice, Bureau of Justice Statistics, 2008). Finally, the number of homicides involving African American youth as victims and perpetrators also surged from 2002 to 2007 (Fox & Swatt, 2008). Although the overall murder rates across the United States have been relatively stable, according to a study conducted by researchers at Northeastern University in 2008, the number of African American murder victims rose by more than 31% (Fox & Swatt, 2008). Additionally, the number of murders involving young African American perpetrators rose by 43% over the same period (Fox & Swatt, 2008), noting that guns were the weapon of choice in most of the killings.

Affective violence is the verbal expression of intense anger and emotions such as bullying, taunts, disrespect, alienation, and physical threats. The primary goal of a violent crime is to injure the target. Violent behavior is typically impulsive, in response to interpersonal stress. In contrast, predatory violence includes hate crimes, which are also referred to as bias crimes. Hate crimes are motivated by bias and hatred of minority groups and sexual and gender orientation. Additionally, hate crimes are more common against African Americans and lesbian, bisexual, gay, or transgendered individuals. Another form of violence involves the phenomenon of stalking.

Stalking is a predatory violence viewed on the continuum of delusional and nondelusional behavior. At the delusional end of stalking, the relationship exists only in the mind of the perpetrator, who may have a delusion that a famous person is in love with him or her or that the perpetrator is a famous person. At the nondelusional end of the stalking continuum, a relationship between the victim and the perpetrator exists. The relationship tends to be or has been an interpersonal relationship or contact; in addition, stalkers can be motivated by religious delusions or hallucinations directing them to a particular person. Frequently, a preoccupation with the victim becomes consuming and could lead to the death of the victim and the stalker.

The Internet and other telecommunications technologies are promoting advances in every aspect of society, improving education and health care and facilitating communications among family and friends, whether across the street or around the world. Unfortunately, several attributes of the Internet and telecommunications, its low cost, ease of use, and anonymous nature, make it an attractive medium for fraudulent scams, child sexual exploitation, and increasingly, a new concern known as *cyberstalking*. Online dating sites like date.com and Internet sites like Facebook, Twitter, and MySpace have become sites of concern for individuals using them to find companionship online. As a result, cyberstalking has become a major area of violence that must be understood by community mental health professionals. Cyberstalking refers to the use of the Internet, e-mail, or other electronic communication devices to stalk a person.

Typology of Stalkers

Cyber stalkers are categorized into five types (Mullen, Pathé, Purcell, & Stuart, 1999), classified as follows. The *rejected stalker* has had an intimate relationship with the victim (although occasionally the victim may be a family member or close friend) and views the termination of the relationship as unacceptable. Their behavior is characterized by a mixture of revenge and desire for reconciliation.

Intimacy seekers attempt to bring to fruition a relationship with a person who has engaged their desires and who they may also mistakenly perceive reciprocates that affection.

Incompetent suitors tend to seek to develop relationships, but they fail to abide by the social rules governing courtship. They are usually intellectually limited and/or socially incompetent.

Resentful stalkers harass their victims with the specific intention of causing fear and apprehension out of a desire for retribution for some actual or supposed injury or humiliation.

Predatory stalkers stalk for information-gathering purposes or fantasy rehearsal in preparation for a sexual attack.

Other types of stalkers include:

- Delusional stalkers usually have a history of mental illness, which may include schizophrenia or manic depression. The delusional/schizophrenic stalker may have stopped taking his or her medication and now lives in a fantasy world composed of part reality and part delusion that the person is unable to differentiate. If they're not careful, targets of the delusional stalker are likely to be sucked in to this fantasy world and start to have doubts about their own sanity, especially if the stalker is intelligent and intermittently and seamlessly lucid and "normal."
- Erotomaniac stalkers are also delusional and mentally ill. They believe they are in love with the victim and create an entire relationship in their head.
- Harasser stalkers like to be the center of attention and may have an attention-seeking personality disorder. They may not be stalkers in the strict sense of the word but repeatedly pester anyone (especially anyone who is kind, vulnerable, or inexperienced) who might be persuaded to pay them attention. If they exhibit symptoms of **Munchausen syndrome**, they may select a victim who they stalk by fabricating claims of harassment by this person against themselves.
- Love rats may not be stalkers in the strict sense of the word, but they have many similar characteristics. Love rats surf the Internet with the intention of starting relationships and may have several simultaneous relationships. The targets of a cyberstalker may know little about the person they are talking to (other than what they've convincingly been fed) and be unaware of a trail of other targets past and present.
- Trolls want to be given more credibility than they deserve and to suck people into useless, pointless, never-ending, emotionally draining, ranting discussions full of verbal loops and "word labyrinths," playing people against each other, hurting their feelings, and wasting their time and emotional energy (www.BullyOnline.org).

According to Indianchild.com (2000), another form of stalking is obsession stalking. Obsession stalkers are motivated by sexual harassment and obsession for love, which can begin with an online romance. The online relationship is usually halted by one person in the relationship, and the rejected lover cannot accept it. Obsession stalkers are also usually jealous and possessive people. Death threats via e-mail or through live chat messages are a manifestation of obsession stalking. More important, revenge and hate stalkers often originate from an obsession stalker. Often an argument has gotten out of hand, leading to a hate and revenge relationship. Revenge vendettas are often the result of something that may have been said or done online, which may have offended someone or began with arguments where someone may have been rude to another user. Sometimes, hate cyberstalking occurs for no reason at all. A person might not know why he or she is being targeted, what he or she has done, or who is stalking him or her. The cyberstalker may not even know the victim. Finally, there are the ego and power trip stalkers, who are harassers or stalkers online showing off their skills to themselves and their friends. They do not have any grudges; rather they use the victim to show off their power to their friends or are stalking just for fun and do not have any means to carry out the physical threats they make.

Victims of Cyberstalking

A stalker is someone who wants to be in control and usually picks a victim who is equal to them. This philosophy keeps the victim submissive. The main targets of cyberstalkers are individuals who are "new to the Internet," women, children, and people who might be emotionally unstable. It is easy to pick out a new person online. Most of them do not know the chat room lingo, obvious by their profile information and lack of Internet knowledge. The type of channel or chat room entered may also indicate that a person is new online and using sources like Newbie Chats, Getting Started Tour, and so on. These are traits that stalkers pick up quickly. The U.S. Justice Department estimates there could be hundreds of thousands of victims being stalked. Mostly women are stalked, but men are too. More men than women look for companionship online. If a man is rejected, the rejection may leave him with a hurt ego, and he may seek revenge through stalking.

The lack of knowledge about cyberstalking by mental health professionals and criminal justice officials also means that the harm suffered by victims of cyberstalking might be overlooked. Cyberstalking can involve behaviors that range from posting offensive messages to physical attacks (Bocjj & McFarlane, 2002). Specific risks to a victim of cyberstalking include a loss of personal safety, the loss of a job, sleeplessness, and a change in work or social habits. Bocjj (2003) describes several cases of cyberstalking that have resulted in even more serious outcomes, including murder.

These are the characteristics of the victims of cyberstalking:

- Male or female depending on the age group; in 18- to 32-year-olds, females predominate
- Often involved in a real or imagined romantic or sexual relationship

- May be a member of a targeted minority group or special group (e.g., ethnic, racial, and religious minorities; gays and lesbians; patients with cancer or other serious illnesses; adoptive or birth parents; political or special interest group)

The U.S. Department of Justice and the National Center for Victims of Crime in the United States suggests victims of cyberstalking take the following steps:

- Victims younger than age 18 should tell their parents or another adult they trust about any harassments and/or threats.
- Experts suggest that in cases where the offender is known, victims should send the stalker a clear written warning. Specifically, victims should communicate that the contact is unwanted and ask the perpetrator to cease sending communications of any kind. Victims should do this only once. Then, no matter the response, victims should under no circumstances ever communicate with the stalker again.
- File a complaint with the stalker's Internet service provider, as well as with their own service provider.
- Many Internet service providers offer tools that filter or block communications from specific individuals.
- As soon as individuals suspect they are victims of online harassment or cyberstalking, they should start collecting all evidence and document all contact made by the stalker. Save all e-mail, postings, or other communications in both electronic and hard-copy form. If possible, save all of the header information from e-mails and newsgroup postings. Record the dates and times of any contact with the stalker.
- Victims may also want to start a log of each communication explaining the situation in more detail. Victims may want to document how the harassment is affecting their lives and what steps they have taken to stop the harassment.
- Victims may want to file a report with local law enforcement or contact their local prosecutor's office to see what charges, if any, can be pursued. Victims should save copies of police reports and record all contact with law enforcement officials and the prosecutor's office.
- Victims who are being continually harassed may want to consider changing their e-mail address, Internet service provider, a home phone number, and should examine the possibility of using encryption software or privacy protection programs. Any local computer store can offer a variety of protective software, options, and suggestions. Victims may also want to learn how to use the filtering capabilities of email programs to block e-mails from certain addresses.

- Furthermore, victims should contact online directory listings such as www.four11.com, www.switchboard.com, and www.whowhere.com to request removal from their directory.
- Finally, under no circumstances should victims agree to meet with the perpetrator face-to-face to "work it out" or "talk." No contact should ever be made with the stalker. Meeting a stalker in person can be very dangerous (National Center for Victims of Crime, 1999; 2003).

HOMICIDE

Homicide is the killing of one human being by the act or omission of another. The term applies to all such killings, whether criminal or not. Homicide is considered noncriminal in a number of situations, including deaths as the result of war and putting someone to death by the valid sentence of a court. Killing may also be legally justified or excused, as it is in cases of self-defense or when someone is killed by another person who is attempting to prevent a violent felony. Criminal homicide occurs when a person purposely, knowingly, recklessly, or negligently causes the death of another. Murder and manslaughter are both examples of criminal homicide.

A homicide may be justifiable or excusable by the surrounding circumstances. In such cases, the homicide is not considered a criminal act. A justifiable homicide is a homicide that is commanded or authorized by law. For instance, soldiers in a time of war may be commanded to kill enemy soldiers. Generally, such killings are considered justifiable homicide unless other circumstances suggest they were not necessary or were not within the scope of the soldier's duty. In addition, a public official is justified in carrying out a death sentence because state or federal law commands the execution.

DOMESTIC VIOLENCE

This discussion of domestic violence outlines the problems, causes, symptoms, treatments, prevention, programs, and the role of the mental health professional. The concept of domestic violence is important to community mental health professionals because knowledge of this domestic violence will help steer them to effective prevention programs and interventions. Domestic violence is defined "as any physical or psychological harm experienced by one person from another with whom an intimate relationship is shared" (Ascione & Arkow, 1999, p. 43). Domestic violence is also known as gender violence, interpersonal violence, and domestic abuse. Domestic violence can occur daily and can often be deadly. People from all age ranges, ethnic groups, and financial backgrounds can become victims of domestic violence. According to the Family Violence Prevention Fund, an estimated 960,000 incidents of violence occur against a current or former spouse, boyfriend, or girlfriend per year (Dutton & Golant, 1995). Domestic violence has a vast spectrum of problems and causes, but there are many treatments and prevention programs to aid in the lifelong healing process.

At the 153rd annual meeting in 2000, members of the association discussed the correlation of violence toward treating and preventing violence. Experts at the meeting indicated that many psychiatric diagnoses are seen with domestic violence, including, but not limited to, mood disorders such as depression and bipolar depression; anxiety disorders such as posttraumatic stress disorder (PTSD); personality disorders such as avoidant personality disorder or dependent personality disorder; sexual dysfunction disorders such as sexual aversion disorder and hypoactive sexual disorder; and substance abuse disorders (American Psychiatric Association, 2000). Ehrensaft, Moffitt, and Caspi (2006) found that women involved in abusive relationships had an increased risk of adult psychiatric morbidity; thus, to develop and implement successful programs to decrease domestic violence in our communities, it is important to understand the correlation of depression and the abovementioned behaviors.

Domestic abuse or domestic violence occurs when one person in an intimate relationship tries to dominate and control the other person (Helpguide.org). The abuser uses fear, guilt, shame, and intimidation to wear the victim down and gain complete dominance over them. The abuser may threaten or hurt the victim or those around them. Additionally, the abuse may occur when the abuser has low self-esteem, extreme jealously, difficulties regulating anger and other strong emotions, or feels inferior to the other partner in terms of education or socioeconomic background (Goldsmith, 2006). Attacks are perpetrated in settings that include public streets, places of employment, in the home, military settings, and in places of worship. Economic, cultural, political, and legal factors can lead someone to become violent. Women's economic dependence on men, limited access to cash and credit, limited employment opportunities, and limited education create the economic factors that influence violence.

The abuse that occurs usually is cyclic, meaning the abuser has encountered this type of behavior through family history, the community, or other influences while growing up and is repeating those behaviors. When an abuser is under the influence of a substance such as alcohol or drugs, it increases the likelihood that the abuse will occur because the abuser has limited control over his or her emotions (Helpguide.org). According to Helpguide.org, a cycle of steps occurs when domestic violence takes place:

Step 1: Abuse

The abuse is a power display to show "who is boss." The abuser shows aggressive and abusive behavior.

Step 2: Guilt

The abuser feels guilt over being caught and facing the consequences, not what he has done to the victim.

Step 3: Rationalizing or Excuses

The abuser has deep thoughts of what happened. He makes excuses about what happened or even blames the victim for his aggressive behavior.

Step 4: "Normal" Behavior

The abuser acts as if nothing has happened and does everything in his power to keep the victim in the relationship and to keep control.

Step 5: Fantasy and Planning

The abuser fantasizes about abusing again, thinks of what the victim has done wrong this time and about ways of punishment, and then turns the plan into reality.

Step 6: Setup

The abuser sets up the situation where he can justify abusing again and sets the plan into motion as shown in **Figure 11-1** (Helpguide.org).

The symptoms of domestic violence vary greatly among victims; depression, anxiety, increased risky behaviors, shame, and fear are just some of the many symptoms experienced by a victim. Smoking, alcohol, and drug use are common coping mechanisms for some women. Sleep and appetite may increase or decrease according to how a victim responds to stress. "Stress and anxiety vary considerably among victims" (Morewitz, 2004, p. 74). Stressors eventually manifest physically, and the health status of the victim may decline (Morewitz, 2004). The victim's symptoms are many and can range in severity. The aggressor's symptoms are also very complex and deep rooted. Some of the behaviors identified are denial, shift of blame, a promise to change, and anger or rage. The abuser is as quick to deny that anything happened at all as not to deal with the situation. Shifting the blame to the victim is also very common, making the victim feel as though it was his or her fault. Some aggressors plead with and beg their partners to forgive them because they are going to change. At times anger and rage is seen throughout the episode and is sometimes seen outside of the home (Dutton & Golant, 1995).

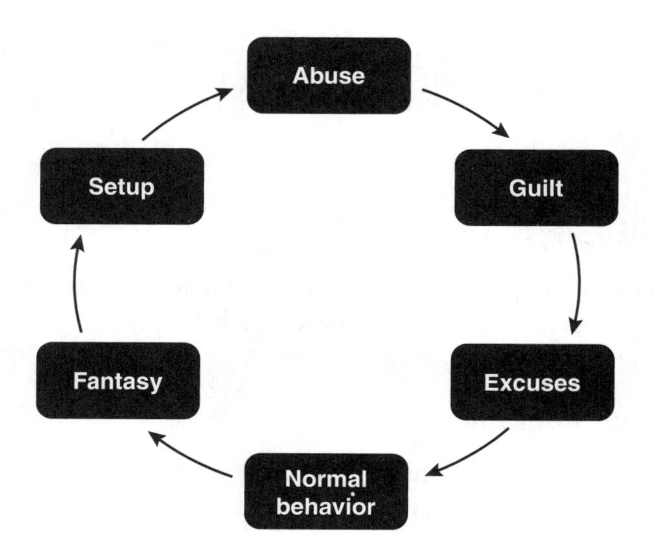

FIGURE 11-1 Cycle of Domestic Violence
Source: Courtesy of Helpguide.org © 2001–2010. All rights reserved. For more articles in this series, visit www.Helpguide.org. Accessed October 6, 2010.

SEXUAL VIOLENCE

Currently sexual violence is one of the most underreported forms of abuse in the United States (Logan & Walker, 2009). Sexual violence (SV) refers to sexual activity where consent is not obtained or freely given. Anyone can be a victim of SV, but most victims are female. The person responsible for the violence is typically male and is usually someone known to the victim. The perpetrator of SV can be a friend, coworker, neighbor, or family member. Sexual abuse committed by a family member is called **incest**. There are many types of SV. Not all include being forced to have sex or include physical contact between the victim and the perpetrator. Examples include sexual harassment, threats, intimidation, peeping, and taking nude photos of a person.

Both the Smith, Farole, and U.S. Department of Justice, Office of Justice Programs, Bureau of Justice Statistics Selected Findings of Female Victims of Violence (2009), and Catalano, Smith, and Snyder (2009) report that in 2008 females age 12 or older experienced about 552,000 nonfatal violent victimizations (rape/sexual **assault**, robbery, or aggravated or simple assault) by an intimate partner (a current or former spouse, boyfriend, or girlfriend) where the consent to have sex is not obtained or freely given. The National Violence Against Women (NVAW) survey sampled 8000 women and 8000 men and found that 1 in 6 women (17%) and 1 in 33 men (3%) reported experiencing an attempted or completed rape at some time in their lives (Tjaden & Thoennes, 1998).

Furthermore, according to the Centers for Disease Control and Prevention Youth Risk Behavior Surveillance (2006), SV is also a significant problem among high school students in the United States: Among high school students surveyed nationwide, approximately 8% reported having been forced to have sex. Females (11%) were more likely than males (4%) to report having been forced to have sex. On a college level, an estimated 20–25% of college women in the United States experience attempted or completed rape during their college career (Fisher, Cullen, & Turner, 2000). As previously noted, however, these numbers might underestimate the problem. Many cases are not reported because victims are afraid to tell the police, friends, or family about the abuse. Also victims think that their stories of abuse will not be believed and they will not be helped by the police. Furthermore, victims are often afraid of the stigma associated with SV and may also keep quiet about it because they have been threatened with further harm if they tell anyone (Basile, Arias, Desai, & Thompson, 2004; Bureau of Justice Statistics, U.S. Department of Justice, 2008).

Health issues associated with SV are serious and can lead to long-term problems. Common health problems include chronic pain, headaches, stomach problems, sexually transmitted diseases, sterilization, HIV/AIDS, sleep and food deprivation, extreme stress, and violence (Rekart, 2005). In addition, rape results in about 32,000 pregnancies each year (Holmes, Resnick, Kilpatrick, & Best, 1996), and SV can have an emotional impact leading the victims to be fearful and anxious (Goldsmith, 2006b). Many victims of SV may replay their attack over and over in their minds, have problems with trust, and become cautious about being inappropriately involved with others. The anger and stress that victims feel about the incident also may lead to eating disorders, depression, and attempted suicide; SV is also linked to negative health behaviors.

The cost of SV was an estimated $5.8 billion in 1995. Updated to 2003 dollars, that is more than $8.3 billion, including $6.2 billion for physical assault, $461 million for stalking, $460 million for rape, and $1.2 billion for lives lost. The Centers for Disease Control and Prevention (CDC) reports that victims of severe domestic violence annually miss 8 million days of paid work—the equivalent of 32,000 full-time jobs— and approximately 5.6 million days of household productivity. This cost includes medical care, mental health services, and lost productivity (e.g., time away from work) (CDC, 2006; Max, Rice, Finkelstein, Bardwell, & Leadbetter, 2004).

More important, according to the 2006 report of the Department of Justice, Bureau of Justice Statistics, homicide trends in the United States, intimate partner violence (IPV) resulted in 1544 deaths in 2004. Of these deaths, 25% were males and 75% were females.

INTIMATE PARTNER VIOLENCE

IPV, also known as domestic violence, not only hurts the women who are being abused but it also affects their overall health, their ability to earn a living, and their children. Although men can suffer from IPV, women are much more likely to be abused by an intimate partner than are men.

The Effect of Intimate Partner Violence on Health

IPV is abuse that occurs between two people in a close relationship. The term *intimate partner* includes current and former spouses and dating partners. IPV exists along a continuum from a single episode of violence to ongoing battering. IPV includes four types of behavior (CDC, 2006):

- *Physical abuse* is when a person hurts or tries to hurt a partner by hitting, kicking, burning, or using other physical force.
- *Sexual abuse* is forcing a partner to take part in a sex act when the partner does not consent.
- *Threats* of physical or sexual abuse include the use of words, gestures, weapons, or other means to communicate the intent to cause harm.
- *Emotional abuse* is threatening a partner or his or her possessions or loved ones, or harming a partner's sense of self-worth. Examples are stalking, name-calling, intimidation, or not letting a partner see friends and family.

Often IPV starts with emotional abuse and can progress to physical or sexual assault. Several types of IPV may occur together, and like SV can affect the health of the victim in many ways. Many victims suffer relatively minor physical injuries like cuts, scratches, bruises, and welts. Others injuries are more serious and can cause long-term disabilities. Serious injuries include broken bones, internal bleeding, and head trauma. Not all injuries are physical. IPV can also cause emotional harm. Victims of IPV often have low self-esteem; they may have a hard time trusting others and succeeding in long-term relationships. In addition to physical injuries, the anger and stress that victims feel may lead to eating disorders and/or depression, and some victims think about or attempt to commit suicide. The longer the IPV occurs, the more serious the effects are on the victim. IPV is also linked to harmful health behaviors. Victims of IPV are more likely to smoke, abuse alcohol, use drugs, and engage in risky sexual activity (Tjaden & Thoennes, 2000).

Assessing Risk for Intimate Partner Violence

Several factors can increase the risk that someone will hurt his or her partner. However, having these risk factors does not always lead to IPV (CDC, 2006).

Risk factors for perpetration (hurting a partner) include but are not limited to the following:

- Using drugs or alcohol, especially drinking heavily
- Seeing or being a victim of violence as a child
- Unemployment that causes feelings of stress

Interventions for Intimate Partner Violence

Traditionally, women's groups have addressed IPV by setting up crisis hotlines and shelters for battered women. Both men and women can work with young people to prevent IPV. They can help change social norms, be role models and mentor youth, and work with others to help end this type of violence. For example, by modeling non-violent relationships, men and women can send the message to young boys and girls that violence is unacceptable.

UNDERSTANDING SEXUAL VIOLENCE

The ultimate goal for preventing SV and IPV is to prevent it before it begins. Prevention efforts at many levels are needed to accomplish this goal. Some examples include:

- Engaging high school students in mentoring programs or other skill-based activities that address healthy sexuality and dating relationships
- Helping parents identify and address social and cultural influences that may promote attitudes and violent behaviors in their kids
- Creating policies at work, at school, and in other places that address sexual harassment
- Developing mass media (e.g., radio, TV, magazine, newspaper) messages that promote norms, or shared beliefs, about healthy sexual relationships

The CDC uses a four-step approach to address public health problems like sexual violence.

Step 1: Define the problem.
Step 2: Identify risk and protective factors.
Step 3: Develop and test prevention strategies.
Step 4: Share the best prevention strategies.

Community mental health care professionals should ask questions about violence in the home, at work, at school, or in a relationship. Assessments should included questions about previous/current abuse, family history of abuse, and if children are being abused. Community mental health providers also can assist victims of abuse in finding a safe place away from the abuser. Some women may be afraid to say they have been abused, but the longer a woman stays in an abusive relationship, the more danger she and her children may endure; more important, abusive behavior often becomes worse over time.

Abuse does not just occur among women and their children. Elder abuse is a concern in today's society because individuals are living longer. Based on the U.S. Census Bureau, Population Projections (2008), on January 1, 2011, as baby boomers begin to celebrate their 65th birthdays, 10,000 people will turn 65 every day—this will continue for 20 years. According to the 2008 projections, by 2050, more than 20% of Americans will be over 65 years of age. Additionally, during the 20th century, the population of Americans age 85 and older grew from 100,000 to 4.2 million. In this age group, known as the oldest old, women outnumber men by 2.6 to 1 (Campion, 1994). The number of people age 100 and older increased 36% between 1990 and 2003, growing from 37,306 to 50,639. Now there are more than 60,000 centenarians (Campion, 1994). According to the Administration on Aging, 2004 A Profile of Older Americans, by 2045, the number of centenarians in the United States is projected to reach 757,000. In addition, as a person ages and becomes frail, many elderly persons are being cared for by their young children, relatives, or a caregiver. In the next section, we discuss the extent of elder abuse in the community, symptoms and prevention of elder abuse, reporting laws, as well as the role of mental health professionals working with abused elderly persons in the community.

ELDER ABUSE

Older people today are more visible, active, and independent than ever before. They are living longer and in better health. However, as the population of older Americans grows, so does the hidden problem of elder abuse, exploitation, and neglect. In a recent national study of Adult Protective Services (APS), there were 253,421 reports of abuse of adults age 60 and older or 832.6 reports for every 100,000 people over the age of 60 (Teaster, Otto, Dugar, Mendiondo, Abner, & Cecil, 2006). The National Elder Abuse Incidence Study (National Center on Elder Abuse, 1998) found that more than 500,000 persons 60 years of age and older were victims of domestic abuse and that an estimated 84% of incidents are not reported to authorities. Findings of their research suggest that elders who have been abused tend to die earlier than those who are not abused, even in the absence of chronic conditions or life-threatening disease.

Like other forms of abuse, elder abuse is a complex problem, and it is easy for people to have misconceptions about it. Many people who hear "elder abuse and neglect" think about older people living in nursing homes or about elderly people who live all alone and never have visitors. Elder abuse is not just a problem of older people who are marginalized or suffered by individuals on the outskirts of life. Elder abuse is prominent in every neighborhood and is endured by both the rich and the poor.

Elder abuse, like other forms of violence, is never an acceptable response to any problem or situation, however stressful. Effective interventions can prevent or stop elder abuse. By increasing awareness among physicians, mental health professionals, home healthcare workers, and others who provide services to the elderly as well as family members, patterns of abuse or neglect can be broken, and both the abused person and the abuser can receive needed help.

Defining Elder Abuse

Elder abuse is defined as the infliction of physical, emotional, or psychological harm to older adults. Elder abuse also can take the appearance of financial exploitation or intentional or unintentional neglect of an older adult by the caregiver. Physical abuse can range from slapping or shoving to severe beatings and restraining with ropes or chains. When a caregiver or other person uses enough force to cause unnecessary pain or injury, even if the reason is to help the older person, the behavior can be regarded as abusive. Physical abuse can include hitting, beating, pushing, kicking, pinching, burning, or biting. It can also include acts against the older person such as over- or undermedicating, depriving the elder of food, or exposing the person to severe weather, deliberately or inadvertently.

Emotional or psychological abuse can range from name-calling or letting somebody have the "silent treatment" to intimidating and threatening an elderly individual. When a person behaves in a way that causes fear, mental anguish, and emotional pain or distress, the behavior can be regarded as abusive. Emotional and psychological abuse can also include insults, threats, treating older people in a childlike way, and isolating them from family, friends, and regular activities, either by force, threats, or through manipulation.

With more elderly people living longer, many of them elect to live at home rather than enter a convalescence hospital or assisted living program. These individuals might require a family care provider or paid caregiver to assist them with activities of daily living in order for them to remain living alone. With the increased use of caregivers comes increased rates of caregiver neglect. Caregiver neglect, another form of elder abuse, can range from withholding appropriate attention from the individual to intentionally failing to meet the physical, social, or emotional needs of the older person. Neglect, in contrast, includes failure to provide food, water, clothing, medications, and assistance with the activities of daily living or failure to help with personal hygiene. If the caregiver has responsibility for paying bills for the older person, neglect also can include failure to pay the bills or to manage the elder person's finances responsibly.

Sexual abuse among the elderly is also a problem elderly persons might face in the community setting. Sexual abuse in the elderly population can range from sexual exhibition to rape. It can include inappropriate touching, photographing the person in suggestive poses, forcing the person to look at pornography, forcing sexual contact with a third party, or any unwanted sexualized behavior. Sexual abuse among the elderly also includes rape, sodomy, or coerced nudity. However sexual abuse is often not reported as a form of elder abuse.

In addition to sexual abuse, financial exploitation is a prominent form of elder abuse. Financial exploitation can range from misuse of an elder's funds to embezzlement. Financial exploitation includes fraud, taking money under false pretenses, forgery, forced property transfers, purchasing expensive items with the older person's money without their knowledge or permission, or denying the older person access to his or her own funds or home. Financial exploitation also includes the improper use of legal guardianship arrangements, powers of attorney, or conservatorships, and it also includes a variety of scams perpetrated by salespeople for health-related services, mortgage companies, and financial managers or friends.

Although elder abuse is commonly perpetrated by others, older adults sometime harm themselves through self-neglect (e.g., not eating, not going to the doctor for needed care) or because of alcohol or drug abuse. One of the most difficult problems family members face is achieving a balance between respecting an older adult's autonomy and intervening before self-neglect becomes dangerous (National Center on Elder Abuse, 1998).

Older adults with signs of dementia may become abusive toward family members or caregivers as part of the disease process. The object of the abuse is often another older adult, for example, a spouse who is caring for the impaired elder. The abuse may take the form of hitting or gripping the caregiver to the extent of causing bruises or creating hazards such as setting furniture on fire. Abuse creates potentially dangerous situations and feelings of worthlessness, and it might isolate the older person from people who can provide them with assistance.

Institutional abuse is another form of elder abuse in our nation. Generally, institutional abuse involves abuse committed by a person who has a legal or contractual obligation to care for the elderly adult in a nursing home, foster home, or other similar residential facility. A federal study conducted by the General Accounting Office in 1998 found that nearly 1 in 3 California nursing homes have been cited for "serious or potentially life-threatening care problems ("California Nursing Homes: Federal and State Oversight Inadequate to Protect Residents in Homes with Serious Care Violations," July 28, 1998). The study was requested by the Senate Special Committee on Aging in response to allegations that 3113 California nursing home residents died in 1993 from malnutrition, dehydration, and other conditions resulting from substandard care. Elder abuse in nursing homes is still prevalent today; for example, an Escondido nursing home repeatedly cited for serious violations and abuse in the past received the highest penalty in California of $100,000 after a resident receiving oxygen caught on fire when he was smoking unsupervised. According to a *San Diego Union-Tribune* article ("Neglected patient burns to death in San Diego nursing home," February, 28, 2008) this violation was the fourth accusation in 3 years made by state officials against Palomar Heights Care Center. In addition, according to the *Chicago Tribune*, December 1, 2009, violent patients and felons with mental disorders and improper care rape, threaten, and kill vulnerable elderly patients. Tribune reporters Gary Marx and David Jackson wrote the story after they learned of a patient at an Aurora, Illinois, nursing home who was killed in a fight with another patient. Illinois is unique among states in relying on nursing homes to house younger adults with mental illness, including several thousand felons. An investigation by the newspaper also documented reports that violent psychiatric patients who were not receiving proper treatment assaulted, raped, and even murdered their elderly and disabled housemates ("Chicago Nursing Homes," 2009).

Symptoms That May Signal Elder Abuse

Many of the symptoms listed here can occur as a result of dementia, chronic disease condition, or medications. The appearance of these symptoms should prompt further investigation to determine the appropriate intervention.

Physical Abuse

Bruises or grip marks around the arms or neck
Rope marks or welts on the wrists and/or ankles
Repeated unexplained injuries
Dismissive attitude or statements about injuries
Refusal to go to the emergency department for repeated injuries

Emotional/Psychological Abuse

Uncommunicative and unresponsive
Unreasonably fearful or suspicious
Lack of interest in social contacts
Chronic physical or psychiatric health problems
Evasiveness

Sexual Abuse

Unexplained vaginal or anal bleeding
Torn or bloody underwear
Bruised breasts
Sexually transmitted diseases

Financial Abuse or Exploitation

Life circumstances do not match with the size of the estate
Large withdrawals from bank accounts, switching accounts, unusual ATM activity
Signatures on checks do not match elder's signature

Neglect

Poor hygiene or disheveled appearance
Sunken eyes or loss of weight
Extreme thirst or hunger
Bedsores

What Causes Elder Abuse

There is no one explanation of what characteristics lead to elder abuse and neglect. Elder abuse is a complex problem that can emerge from several root causes and multiple factors. These factors include but are not limited to family situations, caregiver issues, and cultural issues.

Family Situations and Elder Abuse

Family situations contributing to elder abuse include conflict in the family, a history and pattern of violent interactions within the family, social isolation, or the stresses of one or more family members who care for the older adult and lack knowledge about care and caregiving skills.

Intergenerational and marital violence that persist into old age also are factors leading to elder abuse. In some instances, elder abuse is simply a continuation of abuse that has been occurring in the family for years. If a woman has been abused during a 50-year marriage, she is not likely to report abuse when she is old and in poor health. For example, a woman who has been abused for years may turn her rage on her husband if his health fails (National Elder Abuse Incidence Study, 1998). If there has been a history of violence in the family, an adult child may take the role of an abuser if abused as a child. In this instance, the adult child might abuse the parent by withholding nourishment or by overmedicating the elderly parent. Family stress is another factor that can trigger elder abuse. When a frail or disabled older parent moves into a family member's home, the lifestyle adjustments and accommodations can be staggering. In some instances, the financial burdens of paying for health care for an aging parent or living in overcrowded quarters can lead to stress that can trigger elder abuse. Such a situation can be especially difficult when the adult child has no financial resources other than those of the aging parent. Marital stress between older couples when they must share a home with their adult children can lead to elder abuse. The new living arrangements could cause tension between an adult child and his or her spouse; when problems and stress mount, the potential for abuse or neglect increases.

Finally, social isolation from friends and family can show that a family may be in trouble, and it also can be a risk factor for abuse. Social isolation can be a strategy for keeping abuse a secret or the result of the stresses of caring for a dependent older family member. Social isolation is dangerous because it cuts off family members from outside help and the support they need to cope with the stresses of caregiving. Social isolation also makes it harder for outsiders to see and intervene in a volatile abusive situation or to protect the older person from harm. Additionally, social isolation inhibits the abuser from getting outside help.

Caregiver Issues and Elder Abuse

Personal troubles leading a caregiver to abuse a frail older person include caregiver stress, or burnout, mental or emotional illness, addiction to alcohol or drugs, job loss or other personal crises, financial dependency on the older person, and a tendency to use violence to solve problems. At times, the person being cared for is physically abusive to the caregiver, especially when the older person has Alzheimer's or other forms of dementia.

Caregiver stress is a significant risk factor for abuse and neglect. When caregivers are all of a sudden placed into the position of being responsible for providing daily care for an elder without appropriate training and information about how to balance the needs of the older person with their own needs, they frequently experience intense frustration and anger that can lead to a range of abusive behaviors (National Elder Abuse Incidence Study, 1998). The risk of elder abuse is greater when the caregiver is responsible for an older person who is sick or is physically or mentally incapacitated. Caregivers providing for physically or mentally ill parents often feel trapped and hopeless and are unaware of available resources and assistance. Without skills for managing difficult behaviors, caregivers can find themselves using physical force to cope with the stress of caregiving.

At times the caregiver's own self-image as an "obedient child" may compound the elder abuse by causing the child to feel that the older person deserves and wants only their care, and considering respite or residential care is a betrayal of the older person's trust. Dependency is a contributing factor in elder abuse. When the caregiver is financially dependent on an elderly person, there may be financial exploitation or abuse. Or if the older person is completely dependent on the caregiver, the caregiver may resent the older person, leading to abusive behavior.

Finally, emotional and psychological problems of the caregiver can put the caregiver at risk for abusing an older person in their care. A caregiver who is addicted to drugs or alcohol is more likely to become an abuser than individuals who are not addicted to drugs or alcohol. More important, caregiving can lead to greater use of alcohol, in an attempt to manage stress, and a caregiver with an emotional or personality disorder may be unable to control his or her impulses when feeling angry or resentful of the older person.

Cultural Issues and Elder Abuse

Certain societal attitudes make it easier for abuse to continue without detection or intervention. These factors include the lack of appreciation and respect for older adults and society's belief that what happens in the home is a private "family matter." Certain cultural beliefs and behaviors, such as language barriers, make some situations more difficult to distinguish from abuse or neglect, and it is important, however, not to ignore abuse by attributing the cause to cultural differences or diversity. Understanding cultural diversity and differences will help mental health professionals not to mistake cultural mores and beliefs for abuse or neglect. It is also important for mental health professionals to understand that definitions of what is considered "abuse" vary across diverse cultural and ethnic communities. Lack of respect for the elderly may contribute to violence against older people. When older people are regarded as disposable, society fails to recognize the importance of assuring dignified, supportive, and nonabusive life circumstances for every older person.

The idea that what happens at home is "private" can be a major factor in keeping an older person locked in an abusive situation. Those outside the family who observe or suspect abuse or neglect may fail to intervene because they fear they might misinterpret a private fight. Finally, shame and embarrassment often make it difficult for older persons to reveal abuse because they do not want others to know that such events occur in their family.

Religious or ethical belief systems can also contribute to the mistreatment of family members, especially women. Individuals who participate in religious behaviors that are abusive do not consider the behaviors to be abusive. In some cultures, women's basic rights are not honored, and older women in these cultures may not realize they are being abused. In addition to religious beliefs, cultural values, beliefs, and traditions significantly affect family life. They dictate family members' roles and responsibilities toward one another, how family members relate to one another, how decisions are made within families, how resources are distributed, and how problems are defined. Culture further influences how families cope with stress and determines if and when families will seek help from outsiders. Understanding these factors can significantly increase professionals' effectiveness. Colleagues, coworkers, and clients themselves, as well as members of the community, are valuable resources in understanding the role of culture and abuse. Although it is not possible to achieve an understanding of all the diverse cultures community mental health professionals are likely to encounter, learning what questions to ask is an important first step to understanding abuse from a cultural perspective. Questions include:

- What role do seniors play in the family? In the community?
- Who within the family is expected to provide care to frail members? What happens when they fail to do so?
- Who makes decisions about how family resources are expended? About other aspects of family life?
- Who, within the family, do members turn to in times of conflict or strife? What conduct is considered abusive?
- Is it considered abusive to use an elder's resources for the benefit of other family members? To ignore a family member?
- With immigrant seniors, when did they come to the U.S. and under what circumstances? Did they come alone or with family members?
- Did other family members sponsor them and, if so, what resources did those family members agree to provide?
- What is their legal status?
- What religious beliefs, past experiences, attitudes about social service agencies or law enforcement, or social stigmas may affect community members' decisions to accept or refuse help from outsiders?
- Under what circumstances will families seek help from outsiders?
- To whom will they turn for help (e.g., members of the extended family, respected members of the community, religious leaders, and physicians)?
- What are the trusted sources of information in the community?

- What television and radio stations, shows, and personalities are considered reliable?
- What newspapers and magazines do people read?
- How do persons with limited English speaking or reading skills get their information about resources?

The answers to these questions can provide guidance to mental health professionals working with members of diverse ethnic and cultural communities. These guidelines also will help mental health providers understand expectations and dynamics within families and determine what services will be most appropriate and acceptable. Answers to these questions also will help health professionals identify trusted persons and leaders in the community whom they can call to provide assistance. Additionally, the answer to these questions might provide insight into promising approaches and vehicles for increasing awareness about available elder abuse services (Fulmer, Firpo, Guadagno, Easter, Kahan, & Paris, 2003; Pillemer & Suitor, 1992). Substance abuse has been identified as the most frequently cited risk factor associated with elder abuse and neglect (Bradshaw & Spencer, 1999). It may be the victim and/or the perpetrator who has the substance abuse problem.

Elder Abuse and Substance Abuse

Substance abuse is believed to be a major factor in all types of elder abuse, including physical mistreatment, emotional abuse, financial exploitation, and neglect. It is also a significant factor in self-neglect (Bradshaw & Spencer, 1999).

The following patterns have been observed with respect to perpetrators of elder abuse who abuse drugs or alcohol: They may view older family members, acquaintances, or strangers as easy targets for financial exploitation and seek money to support a drug habit or to provide a source of income if they do not work. Perpetrators often move into an older person's home and use it as a base of operation for drug use or trafficking. Acts of domestic violence also occur more frequently when the perpetrator or abusive partners are under the influence of drugs or alcohol. The relationship between domestic violence and substance abuse, however, is not fully understood. It has been assumed, however, that alcohol and drugs reduce the self-consciousness of the abuser; perpetrators of domestic violence may also use drugs and alcohol to rationalize their behavior. Caregivers who are having difficulty coping with the demands of providing care may use drugs as a coping mechanism.

The following patterns have been observed among victims who abuse drugs or alcohol: They may have impairments related to substance abuse, such as cognitive loss, that reduce their ability to resist or detect coercion or fraud. Physical disabilities associated with substance abuse increase risk by rendering the older person dependent on others for assistance or care and giving caregivers physical access to the older person and his or her home. Caregivers are also likely to have access to an older person's financial resources. Abusive caregivers may encourage or force older people to drink excessively or to use drugs to make them more compliant or easier to care for. Moreover, victims of abuse might use drugs or alcohol as a coping mechanism to relieve anxiety and fear. Seniors who have long-standing alcohol or substance abuse problems are likely to have poor relationships with their families or be estranged entirely. If the older person needs care, their family members may be unwilling to help or may harbor resentments that impede their ability to provide good care. Older persons who self-neglect are more likely to have substance abuse or alcohol problems (Bradshaw & Spencer, 1999).

In addition to the rights and services generally available to all crime victims by statute, legislators at both the federal and state levels have enacted laws that provide special protections and privileges to elderly victims of crime.

Elder Abuse Laws

Frequent accounts of elder abuse in our society led policymakers to pass a series of laws to protect elderly persons from violence. The passage of the federal Older Americans Act (OAA) of 1965 and the creation of the Vulnerable Elder Rights Protection Program in 1992 were instrumental in promoting state laws to address the needs and concerns of the elderly. The Vulnerable Elder Rights Protection Program legislation promoted advocacy efforts through ombudsmen offices; abuse, neglect, and exploitation prevention programs; and legal assistance on behalf of older Americans. It also offered federal funding incentives, which made it possible for states to develop and maintain programs designed to assist the elderly. Most state elder abuse laws are designed after legislation addressing child abuse and neglect. Elder abuse laws often involve both the criminal justice and social services system.

In some states, elder abuse laws are incorporated into assault, battery, domestic violence or sexual assault statutes, and sentencing is enhancement imposed if the victim is over a specified age. For example, the state of Illinois uses a combination approach to prosecute crimes for aggravated battery of an elderly person and for criminal neglect or financial exploitation of an elderly person. In addition, the state includes the age of the victim as a special classification under its aggravated criminal sexual assault and abuse laws.

Mandatory Reporting

One of the earliest legislative trends to assist elderly victims mandated the reporting of elder abuse. Most states require certain classes of professionals to report suspected abuse and neglect. The most common categories of mandatory reporters are medical professionals, healthcare providers, mental health counselors, service providers, and all government agents who are exposed to the elderly. These health professionals must report evidence that leads them to "reasonably believe" that the elderly person in question is the victim of abuse or neglect. A few states have established 24-hour hotlines in an attempt to make reporting of abuse easier and to secure the safety of the victim as quickly as possible. Most statutes establish penalties for those who fail to report, and many also provide immunity from civil suits or prosecution to those who make reports in "good faith." Immunity is provided to individuals reporting elder abuse even if those reports cannot be substantiated, to further encourage reporting of suspected abuse.

According to the National Elder Abuse Incidence Study (1998), although these laws have helped to increase the reporting of elder abuse by 150% from 1986 to 1996, elder abuse is still underreported. Training programs to increase public awareness and better prepare health professions required by law to report elder abuse have been implemented in California, Florida, and Mississippi, in an attempt to further promote reporting mandates.

Investigation and Intervention

Most states empower both social service and law enforcement agencies to investigate reports, intervene, and even remove elderly victims from abusive circumstances. In some jurisdictions, multidisciplinary teams are used to combine the knowledge of health, mental health, social service, legal, and law enforcement professionals to better evaluate the needs of the elderly victimized by abuse. In Colorado, a restraining order may be imposed to prohibit further emotional abuse of an elderly victim.

In an attempt to further improve intervention mechanisms, Tennessee has created an innovative Victimization Prevention Program that is an extension of the Tennessee State University's Center for Aging program (National Elder Abuse Incidence Study, 1998). The program is designed to collect data on the problems of elderly abuse, neglect, and criminal victimization, as well as engage the community in prevention activities through presentations at churches, community centers, schools, and senior centers. In addition, the program conducts workshops for government employees and police, as well as for the elderly and their families, and it implements an advocacy program to assist victims in responding to and recovering from abuse, neglect, and criminal victimization.

Special Provisions for Institutional Abuse

Because of institutional abuse, state officials have been given special authority to investigate reports of abuse in nursing homes and care facilities. The state officials can revoke or deny operating permits to institutions that violate laws or allow their employees to commit offenses against the elderly in their care. Provisions to protect employees who report institutional abuse from retaliation by their employers are also becoming more common. All states and the District of Columbia have established ombudsman programs to receive, investigate, and resolve the grievances of patients residing in long-term care facilities. Finally, the states have established registries of caregivers and medical personnel convicted of elder abuse and required some healthcare personnel to be fingerprinted before starting a position in a healthcare setting. These procedures have been implemented to allow potential employers to conduct a more complete criminal history and background checks on applicants for positions involving care of the elderly. For example, Missouri maintains an employee disqualification list of persons who have misappropriated funds or property of a resident while employed in a long-term care facility.

Special Classification Under General Crime

Special classifications for elderly victims are often included in a state's robbery, assault, battery, murder, and even carjacking statutes. A few states, such as Iowa and Oregon, have chosen to include age as a hate violence characteristic. States are also starting to address telemarketing schemes and consumer fraud crimes that often seem to target vulnerable victims, including the elderly.

In Nevada, an offender who commits a crime against a person over the age of 60 is subject to a prison term twice as long as that normally allowed for the same offense. A Louisiana law mandates that all violent crimes against the elderly be punished by a minimum of 5 years of imprisonment with no opportunity for parole. Georgia imposes an enhanced penalty for unfair or deceptive business practices directed toward the elderly, and other states consider the victim's advanced age to be an aggravating factor to be taken into account when determining a sentence.

Special Trial Provisions

An elderly victim's availability as a witness is often limited due to mobility problems resulting from advanced age and related health concerns. Videotaping depositions is one option available to elderly victims/witnesses who cannot attend court to testify in person. Giving civil and/or criminal cases involving an older victim or witness docket priority is a method that states such as California, Colorado, Nevada, and New York have adopted to address potential time limitations in such cases. In addition, to make court appearances more manageable and less traumatic, services for physically challenged elderly persons, such as personal care attendants and interpreters for the hearing impaired, are provided in certain states.

Compensation and Restitution

All victims of violent crime are allowed to file for compensation to recoup the economic losses they suffer because of such crime. However, many of these programs have created "minimum loss standards" ranging from $100 to $200, precluding claims for lesser amounts. Other compensation programs require victims to absorb the first $100 or $200 of their loss in much the same way as a deductible is paid in conjunction with private insurance policies. Mindful of the economic hardship even a small financial loss might inflict on elderly victims with fixed incomes, many states have waived minimum loss and deductibility provisions in cases where the victim is 65 years of age or older. The specific age does vary from state to state.

Although many programs do not compensate victims for the loss of personal property, most states have created an exception when the property lost is considered essential to elderly crime victims (such as eyeglasses, dentures, hearing aids, or other medical equipment). A few states have compensated homebound victims for the loss of their television or radios.

Restitution laws of some states also contain special provisions for elderly victims. In California, restitution for medical and psychological treatment is mandatory for victims of assault, battery, or assault with a deadly weapon for victims over the age of 65 (Byers & Hendricks, 1993; National Center for Victims of Crime, 1997). Rhode Island mandates restitution for breaking and entering the dwelling of an elderly victim (Byers & Hendricks, 1993; National Center for Victims of Crime, 1997b). The Juvenile Court in Louisiana may distribute unclaimed restitution to elderly victims of other nonviolent crimes for whom restitution has been ordered but not paid (Byers & Hendricks, 1993; National Center for Victims of Crime, 1997b).

Preventing Elder Abuse

In addition to promoting the social attitude that no one regardless of age should be abused, the criteria necessary to decrease elder abuse are included in the following steps:

- Help families understand the needs of respite care.
- Increase the availability of respite care.

- Promote increased social contact and provide social support for families with dependent older adults, and encourage counseling and treatment to cope with personal and family problems that contribute to abuse.

Violence, abuse, and neglect toward elders are signs that the people involved in the abusive act need help—immediately. Education is the cornerstone of preventing elder abuse. Media, newspaper, and journal coverage of abuse in nursing and care homes has made the public knowledgeable about and outraged against abusive treatment in those settings. Because most elderly abuse occurs in the home by family members or caregivers; a concerted effort is needed to educate the public about caregiver stress that might lead to abuse, the magnitude of elderly abuse, and the risk of abuse faced by the elderly as a result of caregiver stress.

Every caregiver needs time alone, free from the worry and responsibility of providing continuous care. Respite care, having someone else care for the elderly for a few hours each week, is essential in reducing caregiver stress, a major contributing factor in elder abuse. Respite care is especially important for caregivers taking care of people suffering from Alzheimer's disease or other forms of dementia or elders who are severely disabled or mentally ill.

Social contact and support can be a benefit to elderly family members as well as caregivers. When a caregiver receives social support, the stress of caring for an elderly person is less likely to reach unmanageable levels. Having other people to talk to is an important part of relieving stress. Families in similar circumstances can unite to share solutions and provide informal respite for each other. Moreover, when there is a large social support group or network, abuse is less likely to go unnoticed. Isolation of elders increases the probability of abuse and may be an important sign that abuse is occurring.

Counseling for behavioral or personal problems in the family can also play a significant role in helping people change lifelong patterns of negative behavior or find solutions to problems emerging from current stresses. If there is a substance abuse problem in the family, treatment is the first step in preventing violence against the older family member. In some instances, it may be in the best interest of the older person to move him or her to a different, safer setting. In some cases, a nursing home, assisted living facility, or boarding home might be more suitable for the elderly than living with children who are not equipped emotionally or physically to handle the responsibility of caring for an elderly parent or relative. Even in situations where it is difficult to tell whether abuse has really occurred, counseling can be helpful in alleviating stress.

Although significant strides have been made in recent years to address the needs and concerns of elderly victims of abuse, there is still much to be done. Public education; mandatory reporting; special training for criminal justice, social services, and mental health professionals; as well as stronger legal penalties for offenders who target the elderly, are just a few of the legislative prevention tools being used by mental health professionals to protect the elderly from abuse. In addition, support groups, education about how to be a caregiver, and respite care are excellent interventions that are available to families to prevent or decrease elder abuse.

CHILD ABUSE

Frederick Douglass commented, "It is far easier to build strong children than to repair broken men." **Child abuse**, also known as child maltreatment, is an intergenerational crisis that continues to increase and devastate a large number of children and teenagers in American society. Many people still narrowly define child abuse as physical abuse, yet anytime someone inflicts harm of any kind on a child, it is a form of child abuse. Although child abuse takes on many forms, it can be categorized under the following areas: **child neglect**, physical and emotional abuse, and sexual abuse, discussed later in this chapter.

Child Abuse as a Social Problem

It may be difficult to grasp why anyone would harm a vulnerable child; however, many child abusers were probably once also abused. According to the National Center for Victims of Crime, a parent or guardian is at greater risk of abusing a child if he or she was abused (ncvc.org), thus contributing to a vicious intergenerational cycle that continues to plague our society as shown in **Figure 11-2**. Despite the large number of abused children in society and the numerous cases of child abuse, little explanation into the biopsychosocial aspects of child mistreatment exists to explain why child mistreatment incidents occur. Although we do not know what leads to child mistreatment, it is important to know that child maltreatment occurs across all socioeconomic, ethnic, and demographic boundaries and remains a serious and widespread public health problem. Although a multitude of articles have been written on child abuse, articles providing insight into the long-term damage of child abuse on the victim are minimal. Children who endure abuse suffer behavioral, cognitive, and social hurdles and require costly medical treatment, counseling for themselves and family members, and possible out-of-home placements such as foster care (Dube et al., 2005; Wang & Holton, 2007).

Child Abuse Statistics in the United States

According to the federal Child Abuse Prevention and Treatment Act, also known as CAPTA, child abuse and neglect is defined as "Any recent act or failure to act on the

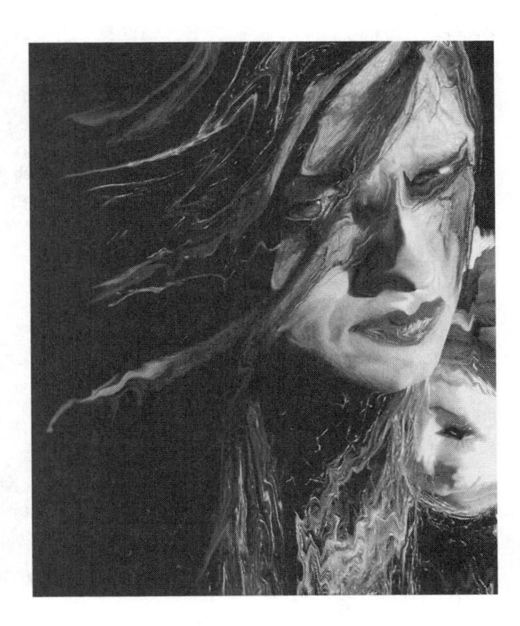

FIGURE 11-2 Regina Lafay, *Inner Child*
Source: Reprinted with permission Regina Lafay.

part of a parent or caretaker which results in death, serious physical or emotional harm, sexual abuse or exploitation; or an act or failure to act which presents an imminent risk of serious harm" (Child Welfare Information Gateway). Even though child abuse in this country is being reported at epidemic levels, the statistics do not truly reflect the actual numbers of abuse cases. Incidences of abuse are underreported for a several reasons, for example, shame, fear, and isolation. The U.S. Department of Health and Human Services (DHHS) Children's Bureau reported the following data on child abuse for 2005: Child Protective Services (CPS) (2006) received 2.9 million referrals alleging child maltreatment. Approximately two-thirds of the referrals were accepted for investigation or assessment. After investigation, CPS agencies determined that 906,000 children were victims of child maltreatment. The national rate of victimization was 12.4 per 1000 children. Over half of the reports of alleged child maltreatment were made by professionals including educators, law enforcement personnel, medical professionals, social service personnel, and child-care staff. The largest proportion of child abuse reports were made by educators at 16.3% of the reports, followed by law enforcement and legal personnel at 16%. Social services professionals made 11.6% of the reports; friends, neighbors, and relatives submitted approximately 43.2% of the reports. Children younger than 3 years suffered the highest rate of victimization, and it was reported that girls were more at risk than boys (DHHS, 2006).

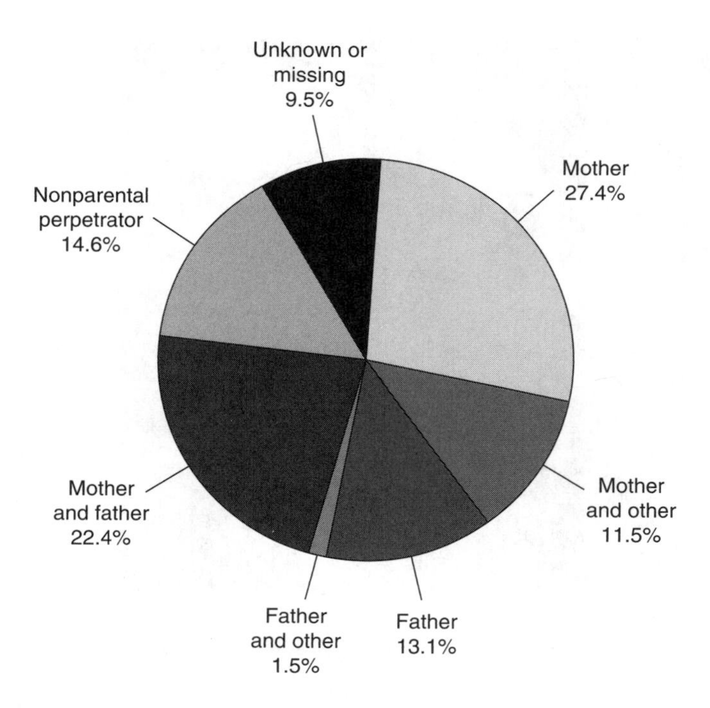

FIGURE 11-3 Perpetrator Relationships of Child Fatalities, 2006
Source: U.S. Department of Health and Human Services, Administration for Children and Families.

The classifications of child abuse are as follows: 60% neglect, 20% physical abuse, 10% sexual abuse, 17% other types of abuse, and 5% emotionally maltreated. Additionally, a child can be a victim of more than one type of child maltreatment. Nearly 76% of perpetrators of sexual abuse were friends or neighbors; 30% were other relatives. Less than 3% of parental perpetrators were associated with sexual abuse. Finally, approximately 15% of child victims were placed in foster care. Nearly 57% of victims and 25% of nonvictims received services as a result of a CPS investigation or assessment. Approximately 80% of perpetrators of child maltreatment were parents, as shown in **Figure 11-3** (DHHS, 2006).

Another important and heartbreaking reality of child abuse is that interventions to help abused children often come too late. The U.S. Department of Health and Human Services estimates there are approximately 1500 fatalities each year as a result of child maltreatment and that more than three quarters of these children are younger than 4 years of age (DHHS, 2005). Moreover, according to Childhelp, a leading national nonprofit organization dedicated to helping victims of child abuse and neglect, the number of deaths caused by abuse is steadily rising, as illustrated in **Figure 11-4**.

Forms of Child Abuse/Maltreatment

Although most states have their own definitions of child abuse and neglect, most recognize the four major types of child maltreatment: neglect, physical, sexual abuse, and emotional abuse.

Neglect is the failure to provide the basic needs of a child. The basic needs of children are broken down into the following categories: physical needs (failure to provide necessary food or shelter or lack of appropriate supervision), medical needs (failure to provide necessary medical or mental health treatment), educational needs (failure to educate a child or attend to special education needs), and emotional needs (not paying attention to a child's emotional needs, failure to provide psychological care, or permitting the child to use alcohol or other drugs). These situations may vary based on differences in cultures, standards of a particular community, and poverty level.

Physical abuse is often what people think of when they hear about child abuse. **Physical abuse** can be defined as an injury or injuries to a child that are intentional. Physical abuse includes physical signs such as welts, burns, bites, strangulation, broken bones, internal injuries, cigarette burns, absorption burns, and/or dry burns. According to the National Committee for the Prevention of Child Abuse, like SV and IPV the longer the abuse persists, the more serious the injuries are to the child and the more difficult it is to eliminate the abusive behavior. Physical abuse is not only physically traumatizing and emotionally devastating for an abused child, but it can also lead to delayed development, learning and motor disorders, mental retardation, and hearing loss.

Sexual abuse is defined as the exploitation of a child for the sexual gratification of another. The sexual contact, abuse, or the use of a child for adult sexual pleasure, even if perpetrated by an individual not considered an adult, is sexual abuse. Sexual abuse may include one or more of the following: obscene language, pornography, exposure in privacy or online, fondling, molesting, oral sex, intercourse, and sodomy. The perpetrators of sexual abuse are usually persons well known to the child, and it is considered the most malicious form of abuse that exists. The long-term effects of sexual abuse can include depression, low self-esteem, to posttraumatic stress disorder, promiscuity, and multiple personality and borderline disorders (Dube et al., 2005; Kilpatrick et al., 2003).

Lastly, the most difficult form of child maltreatment to recognize is emotional abuse. **Emotional abuse** is a behavior that affects a child's emotional development and sense of self-worth. Emotional abuse can include name-calling, ridiculing, humiliation, intensifying a fear, destroying personal property or favorite toys, torture or destruction of a pet, excessive criticism, inappropriate demands, withholding of communications, or routine labeling or belittling. Most victims of emotional abuse are

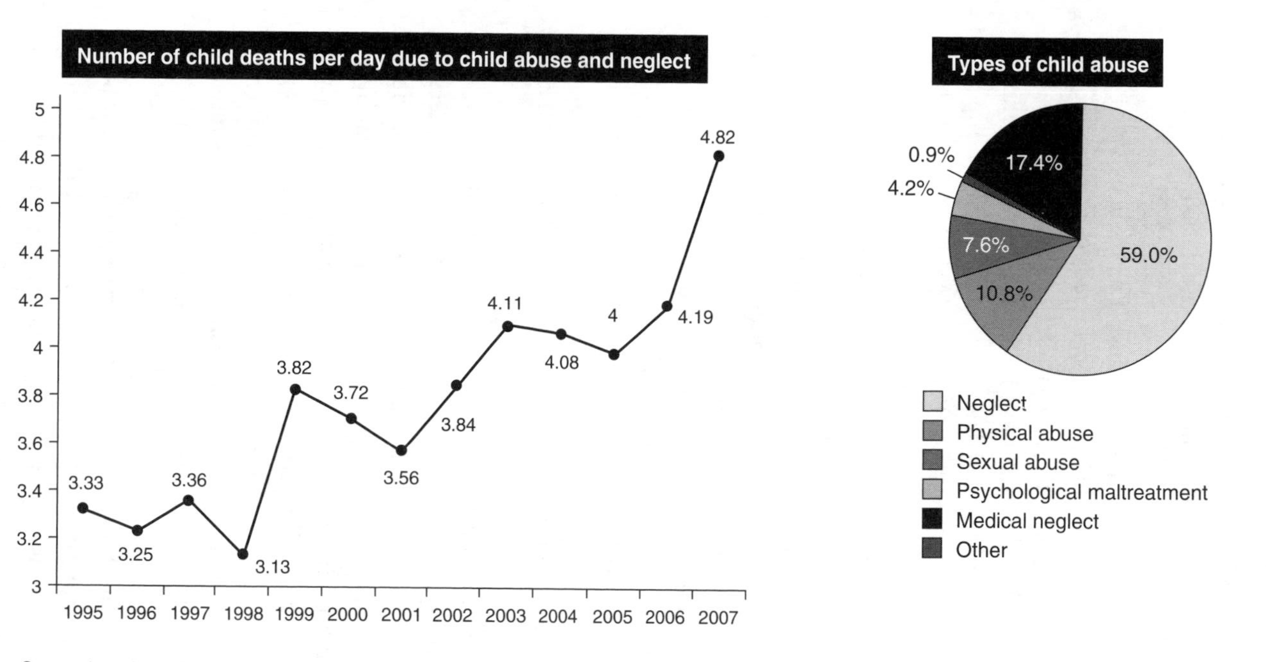

General statistics

- **A report of child abuse is made every ten seconds.**
- Almost **five children die every day** as a result of child abuse.
- More than three out of four are under the age of four.
- It is estimated that between 60–85% of child fatalities due to maltreatment are **not recorded as such on death certificates**.
- 90% of child sexual abuse victims know the perpetrator in some way; 68% are abused by family members.
- Child abuse occurs at every socioeconomic level, across ethnic and cultural lines, within all religions and at all levels of education.
- 31% percent of women in prison in the United States were abused as children.
- Over **60% of people in drug rehabilitation centers report being abused or neglected** as a child.
- About 30% of abused and neglected children **will later abuse their own children**, continuing the horrible cycle of abuse.
- About 80% of 21-year-olds that were abused as children met criteria for **at least one psychological disorder**.
- The estimated annual cost of child abuse and neglect in the United States for 2007 is **$104 billion**.
- Abused children are **25% more likely to experience teen pregnancy**.
- Abused teens are **three times less likely** to practice safe sex, putting them at greater risk.

FIGURE 11-4 Number of Child Deaths Per Day Due to Child Abuse and Neglect: Type of Abuse

Reprinted with permission Childhelp.org.

Sources: Centers of Disease Control and Prevention and The Federal Administration for Children and Families. The CDC publication: http://www.cdc.gov/mmwr

Prevent Child Abuse America: Current Trends in Child Abuse Reporting & Fatalities: The 2000 Fifty State Survey

National Center on Child Abuse Prevention Research: Prevent Child Abuse America; Current Trends in Child Abuse Reporting and Fatalities: The Results of the 1997 Annual Fifty State Survey

Lung, C., & Daro D. (1996). *Current trends in child abuse reporting and fatalities: The results of the 1995 annual fifty state survey*. Chicago: National Committee to Prevent Child Abuse. Retrieved from http://www.childabuse.com/fs9.htm

U.S. Department of Health & Human Services Administration for Children & Families. Child Maltreatment 2003: Summary of Key Findings.

National Clearinghouse on Child Abuse & Neglect Information. Long-Term Consequences of Child Abuse & Neglect 2005.

U.S. Department of Justice

Becker-Weidman, A. Child abuse and neglect study.

National Institute on Drug Abuse 2000 Report.

DePanfilis, D. (2006). Child neglect: A guide for prevention, assessment and intervention. U.S. Department of Health and Human Services.

Long-Term Consequences of Child Abuse and Neglect. Child Welfare Information Gateway. Washington, DC: U.S. Department of Health and Human Services, 2006. Retrieved from http://www.childwelfare.gov/pubs/factsheets/long_term_consequences.cfm

Wang, C-T, & Holton, J. (2007). Total estimated cost of child abuse and neglect in the United States. Prevent Child Abuse America funded by The Pew Charitable Trusts.

U.S. Department of Health & Human Services, Administration on Children Youth & Families. Child Maltreatment 2007. Washington, DC: U.S. Government Printing Office, 2009). Retrieved from http://www.acf.hhs.gov/programs/cb

likely to internalize the abusive message, leading to severe psychological damage and lack of trust. Emotional abuse in children can also lead to abnormal or disrupted attachment development and the victim's blaming him- or herself for the abuse, leading to a learned helplessness, emotional numbing, and passive behavior (Finkelhor, 1979; Finkelhor, Ormrod, Turner, & Hamby, 2005).

Indicators of Child Abuse and Long-Term Effects

No matter what form of abuse a child might experience, he or she will be affected by the abuse in several ways. Although the reactions and coping mechanisms exhibited by abused children vary, many of the coping mechanisms are common. The environment of a violent home can be a traumatic experience for a child. If abused children do not have a good support system they can trust around them, such as family members and friends, they will be less likely to connect with others for help and will attempt to deal with the abuse on their own in silence. Thus it is critical for community mental health professionals to be able to recognize the key indicators of abuse and to intervene on behalf of the child.

Indicators of sexual abuse can include:

- Injury to the genital area
- Pain when sitting or walking
- Sexually suggestive
- Promiscuous behavior or verbalization
- Age-inappropriate knowledge of sexual relations
- Sexual victimization of other children

Indicators of maltreatment can include:

- Malnourishment
- Listlessness or fatigue
- Stealing or begging for food
- Poor personal hygiene
- Torn and/or dirty clothes
- Untreated need for glasses, dental care, or other medical attention
- Frequent absence from or tardiness to school and child inappropriately left unattended or without supervision

Children exposed to abuse throughout their childhood usually suffer long-term effects into adulthood. Abused children physically hurt themselves and do not care about what happens to them (Dube et al., 2005). They often have low self-esteem and feel unimportant or unworthy of love and respect. Behavioral manifestations of abused children include being overly aggressive and taking anger out on people, children, or pets. Subsequently, these children grow up to become abusers of their own children and families and have lack-of-trust issues with people throughout their life (Das, 2006). Abused children are at higher risk of being diagnosed with a psychiatric disorder once they reach adulthood, including anxiety, depression, eating disorders, and suicidal tendencies (Das, 2006). Similarly, victims of abuse may suffer psychological problems such as nightmares and flashbacks, which are both signs of posttraumatic stress disorder (Das, 2006). Lastly, studies show that victims of abuse have a higher likelihood of being involved in criminal activity and violence during their adolescence or adulthood, and they are at higher risk of becoming drug users or drug abusers (Das, 2006).

Treatment

Often victims of child abuse do not know where to get help and usually will not report that they are being abused. Many of them do not know how to define abuse. Thus many states require professionals who work with children to report possible signs of abuse if it becomes apparent. In California, the California Child Abuse and Neglect Reporting Law identifies which professions are required to report and what signs to look for in an abused child. The law also provides procedures on how to report possible abuse, and the law ensures that children are protected from their parents or anyone abusing them. The purpose of the law is not to negatively affect the parents but rather serve as a catalyst to bring about change in the home environment, which in turn may help to lower the risk of abuse.

There is no quick fix for treating an abused child because of the mental and emotional impact of abuse on the health of a child. One method of treatment for child abuse is family therapy. This approach to treatment targets the whole family. The family usually participates in counseling to attempt to resolve the abuse and help the family identify alternative coping mechanisms. If the family does not cooperate with the treatment plan or the abused child is severely traumatized, the child can be admitted into a child abuse treatment program. Private and public programs are available that offer 24-hour care. There are three primary types of programs. Residential care centers are staffed by specialists who monitor a large number of patients. Group homes house a small number of children in a residence-type setting rather than a facility (so it is less restrictive). Therapeutic foster care, which provides for long-term care, is more available in most urban cities. The goals of the facilities are to provide a positive environment and setting to alter the behaviors of the patients.

Prevention

Focusing on prevention is the key to reducing child abuse. Child abuse is linked to unhealthy and unstable family units; thus, counseling as a treatment modality can help parents understand the difference between discipline and punishment, and it can also provide parents with the skills they need to be better parents and with tools to better help them cope with daily stress and demands. According to founders of the SafeState .org Web site, "Parents may be unable to ask for help directly, and child abuse may be their way of calling attention to family problems" (safestate.org).

Another avenue for prevention is through social support and community outreach. Being active in the community can have a tremendous impact on reducing child abuse. Parents who lack social and community support and abuse children are usually socially isolated. An intervention to decrease abuse for parents who are isolated includes providing social as well as group and community activities. Parents often lack the support systems they need that can help them cope with their problems. Providing community involvement, community education, and support programs targeting children and parents can serve as a learning opportunity for parents through observation of positive and healthy family behaviors and outcomes (Bethea, 1999).

Best Practices

In the city of San Francisco, California, an organization called the San Francisco Child Abuse Prevention Center (SFCAPC) is a successful program targeting child abuse. The SFCAPC consist of two organizations: the San Francisco Child Abuse Council, which deals with training professionals who serve children, and the TALK Line Family Support Center, which offers counseling and other direct social services to help children and their families. The program also offers indirect services to promote awareness and prevention of child abuse. The SFCAPC organization trains health professionals and individuals who work with children to recognize signs of abuse, teaches children how to recognize abuse, provides families with assistance, and takes triage calls from families in crisis (sfcapc.org).

The San Francisco Child Abuse Council has three main goals: provide safety education for children at school, train professionals about child abuse detection and reporting, and increase public awareness about child abuse. An important goal of this program is to educate elementary school children about safety habits, for example, traffic safety, abuse awareness, and response to emergencies.

The SFCAPC also operates the TALK Line Family, which focuses on assisting families with child abuse problems and the Parental Stress Line (415-441-KIDS) a

24-hour crisis and counseling line that provides counseling for parents who are in crisis. In addition, there is a drop-in center for parents who prefer to talk to someone in person. Parents who come in for services leave their child in a supervised play area where they are monitored. The center also offers a variety of other helpful services, such as job-search assistance. Approximately a quarter of the parents seen at the center are homeless and/or jobless (sfcapc.org).

Child abuse continues to be an understated and underreported epidemic. It is a devastating phenomenon with long-term residual complications not just for the individual but for society as a whole. Great strides have been made to educate health professionals on how to detect child maltreatment and about reporting laws. Several social programs also exist in the community. The goals and objectives of these programs are to increase awareness of and to educate children as well as adults about child abuse. Child abuse programs also provide counseling for children, parents, and families as a whole. Nevertheless, more work is needed to prevent and protect children from abuse in our society. The consequences of child abuse are not just physical, but mental and psychological as well. The physical injuries can be severe and even fatal; however, the emotional and mental scarring is lifelong, and for some, devastating.

CHAPTER SUMMARY

The prevalence of violence continues to be significant. Moreover, the ways to commit violent acts against individuals, communities, and the world have advanced with the industrialized world. With increasing frequency we read about children, adolescents, and adults playing out the violent images that they see on television or in video games in real time. We hear about suicide bombers across the world sacrificing their bodies for what they believe is a just cause, and all too often, we learn about neglected and abused elderly men and women who live in the community with loved ones in institutions where they thought they could retire in peace. Community mental health professionals are in key positions to detect the risk factors that lead to acts of violence on an individual or community level. Furthermore, community health professionals also are mandated to report child and elder abuse, as well as domestic, sexual, and intimate partner violence, and to provide emotional support to victims of abuse. Thus this chapter provided a summary of elder abuse and mandatory reporting laws.

In addition to knowing the risk factors leading to violence, it is important that community mental health professionals specialize in assessing, designing, and implementing programs that help people change destructive behaviors and protect others from harm. The community mental health professional needs to know what programs and resources are available in the local area, what they charge, eligibility, and what degree of success has been reported. Community mental health professionals are also trained to identify gaps in services and develop evidence-based programs targeting violence.

REVIEW

1. Explain the prevalence and types of violence in America.
2. Describe primary and secondary prevention actions community mental health professionals may take related to violence.
3. Describe the cultural aspects of violence in the United States.
4. Discuss the impact of substance abuse on mental health, child abuse, elder abuse, and homelessness.

ACTIVITIES

1. Review homicide rates in your local newspaper.
2. Look at your local community resources; identify agencies that might serve as a referral for elder abuse, child abuse, and domestic violence for the individual and the family.
3. Have the students discuss their personal attitudes toward and domestic violence.

REFERENCES AND FURTHER READINGS

American Psychiatric Association. (2000). *Diagnostic and statistical manual of mental disorders*: Fourth Edition, Text Revision (4th ed.). Washington, DC: American Psychiatric Association.

Ascione, F. R., & Arkow, P. (1999). *Child abuse, domestic violence, and animal abuse: Linking the circles of compassion for prevention and intervention*. West Lafayette, IN: Purdue University Press.

Attorney General's Office: Crime and Violence Prevention Center. (2007). *California Child Abuse & Neglect Reporting Law*. Retrieved from http://www.safestate.org/

Basile, K.C., Arias, I., Desai, S., & Thompson, M. P. (2004). The differential association of intimate partner physical, sexual, psychological, and stalking violence and post-traumatic stress symptoms in a nationally representative sample of women. *Journal of Traumatic Stress*, *17*, 413–421.

Bethea, L. (1999). Primary prevention of child abuse. American Family Physician, University of South Carolina School of Medicine, Columbia, South Carolina.

Bocjj, P. (2002). Corporate cyber stalking: An Invitation to Build Theory. *First Monday*, 7(11). Retrieved from http://firstmonday.org/ issues/issue7_11/bocij/index.html

Bocjj, P. (2003). Victims of cyber stalking: An exploratory study of harassment perpetrated via the Internet. *First Monday*, *8*(10). Retrieved from http://firstmonday.org/issues/issue8_10/bocij/index.html

Bocjj, P., & McFarlane, L. (2002). Online harassment: Towards a definition of cyber stalking. *Prison Service Journal*, *139*, 31–38.

Bradshaw, D., & Spencer, C. (1999). The role of alcohol in elder abuse cases. In J. Pritchard (Ed.), Elder abuse work: Best practices in Britain and Canada. London: Jessica Kingsley Press.

Bullyonline (n.d.). Retrieved from http://www.bullyoffline.org/related/stalking.htm

Byers, B., & Hendricks, J. E. (1993). *Adult protective services: Research and practice*. Springfield, IL: Thomas Books.

California Courts Self-Help Center. (n.d.). *Can a domestic violence restraining order help me*? Retrieved from http://www.courtinfo.ca.gov

California Department of Public Safety. (n.d.). *Information for victims of domestic violence*. Retrieved from http://www.dps.state.ak.us/

California Nursing Homes. (1998). Federal and State Oversight Inadequate to Protect Residents in Homes with Serious Care Violations, Op. Gen. Accounting Off./T-HEHS98-219.

Campion, E. W. (1994). The oldest old. *New England Journal of Medicine*, *330*(25), 1819–1820.

Catalano, S., Smith, E., and Snyder, H. (2009). Selected Findings Female Victims of Violence. Retrieved from: http://bjs.ojp.usdoj.gov/index.cfm?ty=pbdetail&iid=2020

Centers for Disease Control and Prevention. (2006). Youth risk behavior surveillance—United States, 2005. *Morbidity and Mortality Weekly Report*, *55*(No. SS-5).

"Chicago nursing homes: Slaying of nursing-home resident in nearby motel shows how violence can spill into neighborhoods. Crimes frustrate Uptown and Edgewater, where a cluster of nursing homes admit mentally ill felons," *Chicago Tribune*, December 1, 2009.

Childhelp.org. (2006). *Treatment*. Retrieved from http://www.childhelp.org/about/programs-and-services/residential-treatment-centers

Clark, C. S. (1993). TV violence. *CQ Researcher*, *3*, 265-288.

"Cruel end for a man who asked for little," *LA Times*, October, 2008.

Dahlberg, L., & Butchart, A. (2005). State of the science: violence prevention efforts in developing and developed countries. *International Journal of Injury Control and Safety Promotion*, *12*(2):93–104.

Das, T. (2006). *Long-term consequences of child abuse*. Retrieved from http://www.chakra.org/. Warrick County, Indiana.

Dube, S. R., Anda, R. F., Whitfield, C. L., Brown, D. W., Felitti, V. J., Doug, M., & Giles, W. H. (2005). Long-term consequences of childhood sexual abuse by gender of victim. *American Journal of Preventive Medicine*, *28*, 430–438.

Dutton, D. G., & Golant, S .K. (1995). *The batterer: A psychological profile*. New York: Basic Books.

Ehrensaft, M., Moffitt, T. E., & Caspi, A (2006). Domestic violence is followed by increased risk of psychiatric disorder among women, but not men. *American Journal of Psychiatry*, *163*, 885–892.

Federal Interagency Forum on Aging-Related Statistics. Older Americans 2010: Key Indicators of Well-Being. Federal Interagency Forum on Aging-Related Statistics. Washington, DC: U.S. Government Printing Office. July 2010.

Finkelhor, D. (1979). *Sexually victimized children*. New York: Free Press.

Finkelhor, D., Ormrod, R. K., Turner, H. A., & Hamby, S. L. (2005). The victimization of children and youth: A comprehensive, national survey. *Child Maltreatment*, *10*(1), 5–25.

Fisher, B., Cullen, F., & Turner, M. (2000). *The sexual victimization of college women: Findings from two national level studies*. Washington, DC: National Institute of Justice and Bureau of Justice Statistics.

Fox, J., & Swatt, M. (2008). *The recent surge in homicides involving black males and guns: Time to reinvest in prevention and crime control*. Boston: Northestern University.

Freud, S. (1955). Civilization and its discontents. In J. Strachey (Ed.), *The complete psychological works of Sigmund Freud*. London: Hogarth Press.

Fulmer, T., Firpo, A., Guadagno, L., Easter, T. M., Kahan, F., & Paris, B. (2003). Themes from a grounded theory analysis of elder neglect assessment by experts. *Gerontologist, 43*(5), 745–752.

Goldsmith, T. D. (2006a). Symptoms of domestic violence. Psych Central. Retrieved from http://www.pyschcentral.com

Goldsmith, T. D. (2006b). The physical and emotional injuries of domestic violence. Psych Central. Retrieved from http://www.psychcentral.com

Helpguide.org. (2007). Domestic violence and abuse: Signs and symptoms of abusive relationships. Retrieved from http://www.helpguide.org

Henry J. Kaiser Family Foundation. (1999). *Kids and media at the new millennium: A KaiserFamily Foundation report*. Menlo Park, CA: Henry J. Kaiser Family Foundation.

Holmes, M. M., Resnick, H. S., Kilpatrick, D. G., & Best, C. L. (1996). Rape-related pregnancy: Estimates and descriptive characteristics from a national sample of women. *American Journal of Obstetrics and Gynecology, 175*, 320–325.

Indianchild.com (n.d.). *A parent's guide to Internet Safety: Raising good kids*. Retrieved from www.indianchild.com

Kilpatrick, D. G., Ruggerio, K. J., Acierno, R., Saunders, B. E., Resnick, H. S., & Best, C. L. (2003). Violence and risk of PTSD, major depression, substance abuse/dependence, and comorbidity: Results from the national survey of adolescents. *Journal of Consulting and Clinical Psychology, 71*, 692–700.

Logan, T., & Walker, R. (2009). Partner stalking: Psychological dominance or business as usual? *Trauma, Violence, and Abuse, 10*(3), 247–270.

Long-Term Consequences of Child Abuse and Neglect. (2006). Child Welfare Information Gateway. Washington, DC: U.S. Department of Health and Human Services. Retrieved from http://www.childwelfare.gov/pubs/factsheets/long_term_consequences.cfm

Manganello, J. A., & Taylor, C. A. (2009). Television exposure as a risk factor for aggressive behavior among 3-year-old children. *Archives of Pediatrics and Adolescent Medicine, 163*(11), 1037–1045.

Max, W., Rice, D. P., Finkelstein, E., Bardwell, R.A., & Leadbetter, S.(2004). The economic toll of intimate partner violence against women in the United States. *Violence and Victims, 19*(3), 259–272.

Morewitz, S. J. (2004). *Domestic violence and maternal and child health*. New York: KlewerAcademic/Plenum.

Mullen, P. E., Pathé, M., Purcell, R., & Stuart, G. W. (1999). A study of stalkers. *American Journal of Psychiatry, 156*, 1244–1249.

National Center for Victims of Crime. (1997). Child abuse. Retrieved from http://www.ncvc.org/

National Center for Victims of Crime. (1997). *Elder abuse*. Arlington, VA: Author.

National Center on Elder Abuse. (1998). National Elder Abuse Incidence Study. Final Report. Retrieved from http://www.aoa.gov/AoARoot/AoA_Programs/Elder_Rights/Elder_Abuse/docs/ABuseReport_Full.pdf

National Child Abuse Statistics. (2006). Childhelp: Prevention and treatment of child abuse. Retrieved from http://www.childhelp.org/resources/learning-center/statistics

National Coalition Against Domestic Violence (NCADV). (n.d.). *Domestic violence awareness month*. Retrieved from http://www.ncadv.org/takeaction Domestic Violence AwarenessMonth_134.html

"Neglected Patient Burns To Death In San Diego Nursing Home." (2008). *San Diego Union-Tribune*.

Nemours Foundation. (2008). Stress. Retrieved from http://www.kidshealth.org/teen/your_mind/emotions/stress.html

New Generation. (2007). *Health Center*. Retrieved from www.ucsf.edu

Office of Children and Family Services. (n.d.). Signs of child abuse or maltreatment. Retrieved from http://www.ocfs.state.ny.us/

Pillemer, K. A., & Suitor, J. J. (1992). Violence and violent feelings: What causes them among family caregivers? *The Journals of Gerontology. Series B, Psychological Sciences and Social Sciences*, *47*(4), S165–S172.

Rekart, M. L. (2005). Sex-work harm reduction. *Lancet*, *366*, 2123–2134.

San Francisco Child Abuse Prevention Center. (2005a). Programs: Overview. Retrieved from http://www.sfcapc.org/programs.htm

San Francisco Child Abuse Prevention Center. (2005b). Programs: TALK line. Retrieved from http://www.sfcapc.org/

Smith, E. L., & Farole, Jr., D. J. Bureau of Justice Statistics. (2009). *Profile of Intimate Partner Violence Cases in Large Urban Counties* (NCJ 228193). Washington, DC.

Swing, E. L., Gentile, D. A., Anderson, C. A., and Walsh, D. A. (2010). Television and Video Game Exposure and the Development of Attention Problems. *Pediatrics*. *126*(2): 214–221.

Symptoms of Acute Stress Disorder. (2008). Acute stress disorder symptoms. Retrieved from http://counsellingresource.com/Administration on Aging 2004, A Profile of Older Americans

Teaster, P. B., Otto, J. M., Dugar, T. D., Mendiondo, M. S., Abner, E. L., & Cecil, K. A. (2006). The 2004 survey of state adult protective services: Abuse of adults 60 years of age and older. Report to the National Center on Elder Abuse, Administration on Aging, Washington, D.C.

Tjaden, P., & Thoennes, N. (1998). *Stalking in America*: *Findings from the National Violence Against Women Survey*. Research in Brief. Washington, DC: U.S. Census Bureau. Population Projections, 2008. Retrieved from http://www.census.gov/population/www/projections/2008projections.html

U.S. Center for Mental Health Services. (2000). *Cultural competence standards in managed care mental health services*: *Four underserved/underrepresented racial/ethnic groups*. Rockville, MD: Author.

U.S. Department of Health and Human Services. (1998). *National elder abuse incidence study*. Retrieved from www.aoa.dhhs.gov

U.S. Department of Health and Human Services. (1999). *Mental health*: *A report of the Surgeon General*. Rockville, MD: Author.

U.S. Department of Health and Human Services. (2000). *Healthy People 2010* (2nd ed.). With *Understanding and improving health* and *Objectives for improving health* (2 vols.). Washington, DC: Author.

U.S. Department of Health and Human Services. (2001). *Youth violence*: *A report of the Surgeon General*. Rockville, MD: Author.

U.S. Department of Health and Human Services. (2004). Silence hurts: Alcohol abuse and violence against women. Retrieved from http://www.pathwayscourses

U.S. Department of Health and Human Services, Administration for Children and Families. (2003). Child maltreatment: Summary of key findings.

U.S. Department of Health and Human Services, Administration on Children, Youth, and Families. (2009). Child Maltreatment 2007. Washington, DC: U.S. Government Printing Office. Retrieved from http://www.acf.hhs.gov/programs/cb

U.S. Department of Health and Human Services, Administration on Children, Youth, and Families, Children's Bureau. (2006). *The AFCARS report #13*. Retrieved from http://www.acf.hhs.gov/programs/cb/stats_research/index.htm#afcars

U.S. Department of Justice. (1999, 2003). Cyberstalking: A New Challenge for Law Enforcement and Industry—A Report from the Attorney General to the Vice President. Washington, DC: U.S. Department of Justice, pp. 2, 6. Retrieved from http://www.justice.gov/criminal/cybercrime/cyberstalking.htm#N_1_

U.S. Department of Justice, Bureau of Justice Statistics. (2008). Criminal Victimization, 2007. NCJ 224390. Rockville, MD.

U.S. Department of Justice, Federal Bureau of Investigation. (2005). *FBI Law Enforcement Bulletin, 74*(5). Washington, D.C., 20535-0001.

Understanding and Combating Elder Abuse in Minority Communities. (1997). Proceedings of a 1997 conference sponsored by the National Center on Elder Abuse (NCEA) and funded by the Archstone Foundation. Single copies are available at no cost from the Archstone Foundation.

Volkan, V. D. (1997). *Bloodlines: From Ethnic Pride to Ethnic Terrorism*. New York: Farrar, Straus, and Giroux.

Wang, C-T., & Holton, J. (2007). *Total estimated cost of child abuse and neglect in the United States*. Prevent Child Abuse America, funded by The Pew Charitable Trusts.

Appendix A: Resources: Where to Go for Help

The National Domestic Violence Hotline: 1-800-799-SAFE (7233)

Sexual Violence Prevention: Beginning the Dialogue: www.cdc.gov/ncipc/dvp/SVPrevention.htm

Rape, Abuse and Incest National Network Hotline: www.rainn.org or (800) 656-HOPE

National Sexual Violence Resource Center: www.nsvrc.org

Violence Against Women Network (VAWnet): www.vawnet.org

Men Can Stop Rape: www.mencanstoprape.org

STOP IT NOW!: www.stopitnow.org

National Center on Elder Abuse
1225 Eye Street, NW, Suite 725, Washington, DC 20005; phone: (202) 898-2586; fax: (202) 898-2583; www.elderabusecenter.org
NCEA is a resource for public and private agencies, professionals, service providers, and individuals interested in elder abuse prevention information, training, technical assistance, and research.

Eldercare Locator
Sponsored by the Administration on Aging (AoA). If the address and ZIP code of the older person being abused is known, Eldercare Locator can refer you to the appropriate agency in the area to report the suspected abuse; (800) 677-1116.

Area Agency on Aging
Most states have an information and referral line that can be helpful in locating services for victims or potential perpetrators of elder abuse and neglect. Check your local telephone directory.

Medicaid Fraud Control Units (MFCU)
Each state attorney general's office is required by federal law to have an MFCU that investigates and prosecutes Medicaid provider fraud and patient abuse and neglect in healthcare programs and home health services that participate in Medicaid.

Adult Protective Services
In many states, Adult Protective Services is designated to receive and investigate allegations of elder abuse and neglect. Every state has some agency that holds that responsibility. It may be the Area Agency on Aging, the Division of Aging, the Department of Aging, or the Department of Social Services.

National Domestic Violence Hotline
The hotline provides support counseling for victims of domestic violence and provides links to 2500 local support services for abused women. The hotline operates 24 hours a day, every day of the year; (800) 799-SAFE; TDD (800) 787-3224.

Administration on Aging
330 Independence Avenue, SW, Washington, DC 29201; (202) 245-0641

American Association of Retired Persons
601 E Street, NW, Washington, DC 20049; (202) 434-2277

Commission on Legal Problems of the Elderly
American Bar Association, 1800 M Street, NW, Washington, DC 20036; (202) 331-2297

National Center on Elder Abuse
University of Delaware, 297 Graham Hall, Newark, DE 19716; www.ncea.aoa.gov; phone: (302) 831-3525; fax: (302) 831-4225; e-mail: ncea-info@aoa.hhs.gov

National Committee for the Prevention of Elder Abuse
c/o Institute on Aging, 119 Belmont Street, Worcester, MA 01605; (508) 793-6166

National Council on Aging
409 3rd Street, NW, Second Floor, Washington, DC 20024; (202) 479-6688

National Association of State Units on Aging
1225 I Street, NW, Room 725, Washington, DC 20005; (202) 898-2578

State Attorney General, county/city prosecutor, or county/city law enforcement
Check in the yellow pages of the local phone book under the appropriate section heading of "Local Governments," "County Governments," or "State Government." Detailed information about youth violence: www.cdc.gov/injury.

California Nursing Homes
Federal and State Oversight Inadequate to Protect Residents in Homes with Serious Care Violations, Op. Gen. Accounting Off./T-HEHS98-219 (July 28, 1998).

National Center for Injury Prevention and Control
Resources for learning more about the relationship between substance abuse and elder abuse; (800) CDC-INFO; www.cdc.gov/injury cdcinfo@cdc.gov.

CHAPTER 12

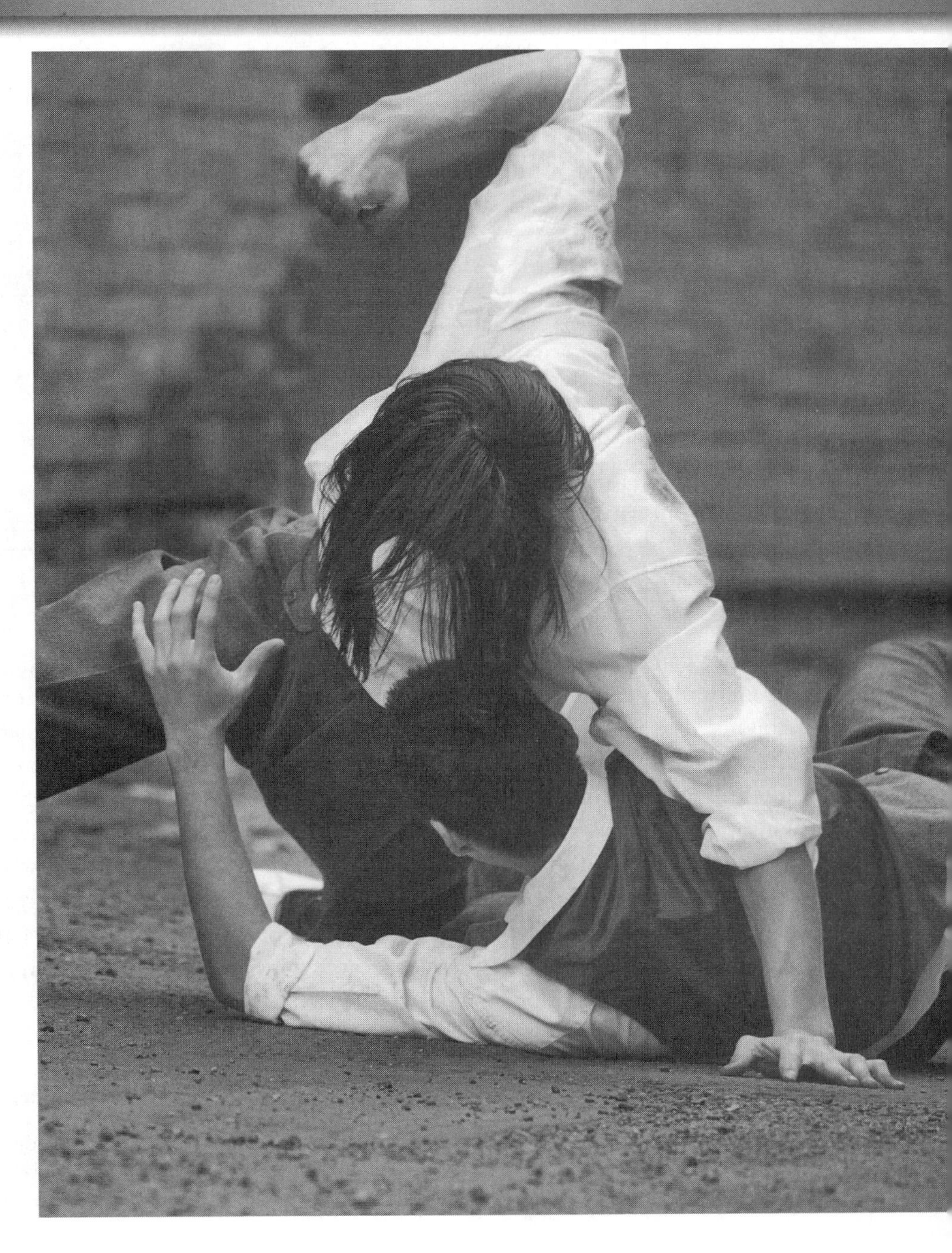

Community Mental Health Problems: Violence Across the Lifespan

CHAPTER OBJECTIVES

1. List the complications caused by physical abuse during pregnancy.
2. Define the characteristics of school violence.
3. Describe the characteristics of gang membership.
4. Discuss the risk factors that perpetrate youth violence.
5. Discuss the role of the mental health professional in preventing violence across the lifespan.
6. Define the best practices to address violence across the lifespan.

KEY TERMS

- Infanticide

Violence can influence every state of life whether in an intimate relationship, school, or community setting. This chapter provides an overview of risk factors that lead to violence. For example, prebirth violence includes battering women during pregnancy, affecting birth outcomes. In infancy, female **infanticide**, the practice of intentionally killing an infant, can occur, as well as physical, sexual, and psychological abuse. Moreover, adolescence presents issues of dating and courtship violence, for example, throwing acid on a girl or a woman to punish her. Adolescents also participate in school violence and homicide. This is the fourth and final chapter addressing common community health problems that community mental health professionals must know about, and it also discusses effective interventions and prevention strategies to address violence across the lifespan.

ABUSE AGAINST PREGNANT WOMEN

Pregnancy is a time of increased risk for abuse. There is more incidence of violence during pregnancy than hypertension, gestational diabetes, or placenta previa, all of which are routinely assessed during the pregnancy. Between 16% and 25% of women report physical and emotional abuse during pregnancy. Pregnant teens and Hispanic women have a higher rate of abuse than other women. Nonpregnant women are usually beaten in the face or chest, whereas pregnant women are beaten in the abdomen. Physical abuse during pregnancy leads to miscarriage, placenta abruption, fetal loss, premature labor, fetal fractures, pelvic fractures, rupture of the uterus, and hemorrhage. Battering during pregnancy is associated with the severity of abuse. Men who beat pregnant women are usually extremely violent and dangerous. Battering during pregnancy is also a risk for homicide of the female partner and unborn child (Sarkar, 2008).

The first prenatal visit is associated with the pattern of abuse. Women who are abused are more likely to delay prenatal care until the third trimester. Furthermore, abused women report the abuser forced them to avoid prenatal care by denying them access to transportation or preventing them from leaving the home. Abuse during pregnancy is often overlooked by healthcare professionals.

ROLE OF THE COMMUNITY MENTAL HEALTH PROVIDER

The goal of domestic violence treatment is to end the abuser's violent and abusive behavior, increase victim safety, hold batterers accountable, and find treatment for the abuser and the abused. Several types of treatment are available for victims. The efforts required to prevent violence can be primary, secondary, or tertiary prevention. The community mental health professional might be involved at all levels of care of abused victims and treatment. In addition, the community health provider might be involved in program development and operation for individuals who are abused as well as for the abuser.

Community-based prevention programs might be designed to address abuse on an individual, group, or family level. The target audience guides program goals and objectives. For example, a prevention program for children might be teaching the core values of human life and appropriate touching. A common therapeutic approach for batterers is anger management, which focuses on the batterer's learning to control his or her anger. The programs are not designed to address the fundamental causes of domestic violence, safety, and accountability issues; thus they can be ineffective.

Another treatment is couple's therapy, which focuses on helping the couples understand one another and designing ways that couples can learn how to get along better. Engaging in couple's therapy requires the acceptance of the idea that both parties are at fault. Couple's therapy allows the batterer to stay focused on criticism of his or her partner rather than dealing with his or her own problems.

Dr. Christopher Eckhardt, a professor at Purdue University and an expert on domestic violence, has released a series of recommendations on how to improve the therapy regimen (*Purdue News*, 2005). He encourages individual therapy for batterers instead of group therapy. He states, "Concerns about sharing personal information in a group setting also may keep some men from talking about personal issues, such as being a victim of abuse themselves." In the past, it was thought that domestic violence was about problematic anger. It is now known to be about the abuser's desire to control a partner using whatever behaviors are necessary. Many abusers are not angry when they use a control tactic. Abusers in treatment often say they used their expression of anger as a way to intimidate and control their partners (Murphy & Eckhardt, 2005). Mental health care professionals who specialize in domestic violence can help abusers find their emotional wounds, which is the first vital step in stopping a person from battering.

A study by the University of Arkansas shows that sorting abusers by categories may be a therapeutic benefit during treatment. They found three distinct subgroups of abusers. The first subgroup, "antisocial," has no regard for authority, ends up in trouble with the law, and gets into frequent fights. The second subgroup, "passive-aggressive/dependent," tends to be reactive and emotional, angry, and depressed. The third group, "nonpathological," shows no antisocial or anger traits; they simply just abuse their spouses (Lohr, DeMaio, & McGlynn, 2003). Determining what type of batterer an individual is will make developing a therapy geared toward their personality easier. Lee, Sebold, and Uken (2003) approach abuse by holding offenders accountable and responsible for building solutions, rather than focusing on their problems and deficits, and they purport therapy should focus on "solution-talk" where clients are assisted in developing useful goals and solution behaviors that are then amplified, supported, and reinforced through a solution-building process.

There are several ways to prevent domestic violence. Increasing the knowledge about domestic violence and the signs of abusive behavior is the key to prevention. Awareness and education campaigns can be provided in school, faith-based organizations, and at community health fairs. A nationwide campaign, Domestic Violence Awareness Month, evolved from the first Day of Unity observed in October 1981 by the National Coalition Against Domestic Violence (NCADV). In October 1994, the NCADV, in conjunction with *Ms. Magazine*, created the "Remember My Name" project, a national registry to increase public awareness about domestic violence deaths. Treatment for victims of domestic violence involves a strong focus on safety in addition to providing therapy, counseling, legal information, shelters, and access to other community resources.

The safety of victims of domestic violence is the primary concern before starting any other treatment. A safety plan should be in place that includes how and when to leave an abuser in addition to where to go. A safety kit should also be kept in a protected place that includes important articles such as clothing, medications, money, copies of important documents, and keys, which can be taken with the victim when he or she decides to leave. Legal options can also be considered, including filing a restraining order or reporting an abuser to the police (Rice, 2007).

Local domestic violence programs are effective in providing confidential assistance, which includes emergency safety services such as shelter and 24-hour crisis hotlines. Domestic violence program advocates are knowledgeable in criminal justice, family court, and social services systems in addition to having useful contacts in other community resources that can be helpful, including housing, education, counseling, alcohol and drug treatments, child care, employment, and medical treatment. Many programs provide safe shelter for victims and their children, legal information, help with filling out protective order paperwork, information on domestic violence, crisis hotlines, transportation, and clothing (California Department of Public Safety, 2007).

After safety has been addressed, psychological treatment may be needed to help victims cope with the emotional consequences of domestic violence. Two of the most common types of treatment for domestic violence are individual and support group counseling. Goals to help victims should include help with identifying the impact abuse has had on their life as well as helping them work toward regaining independence (Rice, 2007). Support groups are especially helpful for victims because many are forced to be isolated from their friends, family, and community. Victims benefit from support groups because they can share their experience with other victims and learn that they are not alone. In addition to support groups, individual counseling is helpful for victims of domestic violence. Counselors offer resources and options but cannot decide what is best for the victim. Instead, victims must decide on what is best for them and are encouraged by the counselor to do what is best for their situation. Additional treatment may be needed for some victims who show symptoms of depression, posttraumatic stress disorder (PTSD), substance abuse, or other disorders often associated with domestic violence (Rice, 2007).

Best Practices

Safe Alternatives to Violent Environments (SAVE) is a nonprofit community-based organization funded by federal, state, and local jurisdictions; private foundations; corporations; and concerned citizens (SAVE, 2007). This organization was founded in

1976, in an effort to reach out to those experiencing family violence. SAVE's mission is to "Provide alternatives to domestic violence through support services, advocacy and education, and to assist domestic violence victims and their families to end the cycle of violence" (SAVE, 2007). The organization is currently located in southern Alameda County, serving mostly the San Francisco Bay Area; however, they offer their services to any city, state, or country.

SAVE's free services are not only a way of treating the victim but they act as a safety net, a means of changing a lifestyle. They provide a variety of services, starting with prevention. Their prevention services include community education, teen dating violence prevention, crisis calls, temporary retraining hours, as well as workplace violence education. The cost of domestic violence to U.S. businesses is between $3 and $5 billion per year in lost productivity, and approximately 94% of U.S. corporate security directors rank domestic violence as a high security challenge at their companies. With these statistics in mind, it is imperative for corporations and businesses to educate their management staff about the impact of domestic violence (SAVE, 2007). Intervention services include a 24-hour crisis hotline, Police Department Advocates medical outreach, emergency shelter, long-term housing, as well as temporary restraining order clinics. Emergency shelters, which offer beds for up to 90 days, may include food, clothing, and transportation. When room at the shelter is not available, the organization provides motel and food vouchers for the individuals (SAVE, 2007). SAVE offers a children's program, with child development groups and counseling for children. In addition, violence and abuse prevention provides training, support groups, individual counseling, and staff to accompany the victim to court for emotional support and assistance through the legal proceedings (SAVE, 2007).

Domestic violence is cyclical and can affect people of all ages, ethnic groups, and financial backgrounds. This violence is not limited to only physical abuse and can include psychological, sexual, and financial abuse. There are numerous symptoms related to violence that vary from individual to individual. The treatment for victims of domestic violence involves a strong focus on safety in addition to providing therapy, counseling, legal information, shelter, and other community resources. However, treatment for abusers is limited, not thoroughly understood, and still underresearched. In 2008, in a CNN television news headline, it was reported that a 14-year-old boy shot and killed a classmate who dressed in girls' clothing and self-identified as transgendered. The shooting took place in February 2008 during class while his teacher and dozens of classmates watched in horror. The bullied transgendered youth was killed because he allegedly told classmates that he was friends with the 14-year-old murderer.

SCHOOL VIOLENCE

School violence is the occurrence of violent crime at school as well as on the way home from school. In the United States, an estimated 55 million students are enrolled in pre-kindergarten through 12th grade (Dinkes, Cataldi, & Lin-Kelly, 2007). Another 15 million students attend colleges and universities across the country (Jamieson, Curry, & Martinez, 1999). Although U.S. schools remain relatively safe, any amount of violence is unacceptable. Parents, teachers, and administrators expect schools to be safe havens of learning. Acts of violence disrupt the learning process and have a negative effect on students, the school itself, and the broader community. School violence is a subset of youth violence, a broader public health problem. Youth violence refers to harmful behaviors that may start early and continue into young adulthood. It includes a variety of behaviors such as bullying, slapping, punching, weapon use, and rape. Victims can suffer serious injury, significant social and emotional damage, or even death. The young person can be a victim, an offender, or a witness to the violence or a combination of these.

The first step in preventing school violence is to understand the extent and nature of the problem. The Centers for Disease Control and Prevention (CDC), the Department of Education, and the Department of Justice gather and analyze data from a variety of sources to gain a more complete understanding of school violence.

School Environment

Approximately 38% of public schools reported at least one incident of violence to police during 2005–2006 (Department of Education, Indicators of School Crime and Safety, 2007). In 2005, 24% of students reported gangs at their schools. Students in urban schools were more likely to report gang activity than suburban and rural students. In 2003–2004, 10% of teachers in city schools reported they were threatened with injury by students, compared with 6% of teachers in suburban schools and 5% in rural schools.

Risk Behaviors

In 2005, a nationwide survey of students in grades 9 to 12 reported the following risk behaviors:

- 6.5% of students carried a weapon on school property in the 30 days preceding the survey. Weapons included a gun, knife, or club.

- 7.9% of students were threatened or injured with a weapon on school property in the 12 months preceding the survey.
- 13.6% of students were involved in a physical fight on school property in the 12 months preceding the survey.
- 8.4% of students attempted suicide one or more times in the 12 months preceding the survey.
- 25.4% of students were offered, sold, or given an illegal drug on school property in the 12 months preceding the survey.

Nonfatal Victimization

In 2005, students ages 12 to 18 were the victims of about 628,200 violent crimes at school (Department of Education Indicators of School Crime and Safety, 2007). The violent crimes included rape, both sexual and aggravated assault, as well as robbery. Approximately 30% of the students in this sample reported moderate ("sometimes") or frequent ("once a week or more") bullying. This included 13% as a bully, 10.6% as a victim, while 6.3% reported both moderate and frequent bullying (Nansel, Overpeck, Ramani, Ruan, Simons-Morton, & Scheidt, 2001). Young people who bully are more likely to smoke, drink alcohol, and get into fights (Olweus, 1993) and (Anderson et al., 2001), these children also vandalize property, skip school, and drop out of school more often. Anderson and colleagues report 60% of boys who were bullies in middle school have had at least one criminal conviction by the age of 24. Among the student perpetrators of school-associated violent deaths, 20% were known to have been victims of bullying (Anderson et al., 2001).

Violent Deaths

Violent deaths at schools accounted for less than 1% of the homicides and suicides among children ages 5 to 18. During the past 7 years, 116 students were killed in 109 separate incidents, and an average of 16.5 student homicides occur each year (CDC, 2008b). Rates of school-associated student homicides decreased between 1992 and 2006. However, they have remained relatively stable in recent years. Violent death rates were significantly higher for males, students in secondary schools, and students in central cities (CDC, 2009). Most school-associated violent deaths occur during transition times before and after school and during lunch (Olweus, 1993). Violent deaths are more likely to occur at the start of each semester (CDC, 2001). Nearly 50% of homicide perpetrators gave some type of warning signal, including making a threat or leaving a note, prior to the event (Anderson et al., 2001).

Short- and Long-Term Health Effects

School-associated violent deaths are only part of the problem. A number of students seek medical care for nonfatal violence-related injuries. Some of these injuries are relatively minor and include cuts, bruises, and broken bones. Other serious injuries include gunshot wounds and head trauma and can lead to permanent disability. It is important to note that not all injuries are visible. Feelings of depression, anxiety, and many other psychological problems, like fear, can result from school violence. In 2005, 6% of high school students participating in a nationwide survey reported not going to school on one or more of the previous 30 days because they feared for their safety. Student fears about safety at school increased between 1993 and 2005 but have not changed significantly since 2005 (CDC, 2008). Another study found that as many as 160,000 students go home early on any given day because they are afraid of being bullied (Pollack, 1998).

Risk Factors for Perpetrating Youth Violence

Research on youth violence has increased our understanding of the factors that make some populations more likely to commit violent acts. These risk factors increase the likelihood that a young person will become violent, but they are not necessarily the direct causes of youth or school violence (U.S. Department of Health and Human Services [DHHS], 2001; CDC, 2008a). Individual risk factors include:

- History of violent victimization
- Attention deficits
- Hyperactivity
- Learning disorders
- A history of early aggressive behavior
- Association with delinquent peers
- Involvement in gangs
- Drugs and alcohol use
- Low IQ or poor academic performance or low commitment to school or failure in school

Individuals engaging in school violence also demonstrate poor behavioral control; deficits in social, cognitive, or information-processing abilities; high emotional distress; antisocial beliefs and attitudes; and social rejection by peers. Exposure to violence and conflict in the family as well as lack of involvement in childhood activities are also risk factors for individuals who engage in school violence.

Relationship risk factors are as follows:

- Harsh, lax, or inconsistent disciplinary practices

- Low parental involvement
- Emotional attachment to parents or caregivers
- Low parental education and income

Parental substance abuse or criminality, poor family functioning (e.g., communication), and poor monitoring and supervision of children are also relationship factors leading to school violence.

Community/societal risk factors are as follows:

- Diminished economic opportunities
- High concentrations of poor residents and transiency
- Family disruption and low levels of community participation

Finally, individuals living in socially disorganized neighborhoods have a high incidence of school violence (CDC, 2008a; DHHS, 2001; Lipsey & Derzon, 1998; Resnick, Ireland, & Borowsky, 2004).

Preventing School Violence

The goal for school violence is simply to stop it from happening in the first place. Prevention efforts should reduce exposure to the risk factors and promote protective factors. In addition, prevention measures should address all levels of school violence risk factors: individual, relationship, community, and society. For example, the Gun Free Schools Act of 1994 requires schools to expel a student for a year if he or she brings a firearm to school. Individual-level strategies or universal school-based prevention programs have been found to reduce rates of aggression and violent behavior among students (CDC, 2007). These programs are delivered to all students in a school or a particular grade and focus on many areas, including emotional self-awareness, emotional control, self-esteem, positive social skills, social problem solving, conflict resolution, and teamwork. Many of these programs help children learn social skills by having them observe and interact with others. Some programs incorporate didactic teaching, modeling, and role playing to enhance social interaction, teach nonviolent methods for resolving conflict, and strengthen nonviolent beliefs among young people. Relationship-level strategies or parent, child, and family-based interventions are designed to improve family relations. There is growing evidence that these interventions, especially those that start early and recognize all risk factors that influence a family, can have substantial long-term effects in reducing violent behavior. Mentoring has also been proven to be an effective intervention to decrease school violence. Matching of a young person with a volunteer who is successful, acts as a supportive, nonjudgmental role model, and comes from a similar background is valuable. This strategy may provide children and adolescents with positive adult influences when they do not otherwise exist (CDC, 2002). Leaders who use mentor programs must take into account that the quality of mentoring programs can vary and success depends, in part, on properly training mentors and equal participation by the mentor and mentee. Research has shown that mentoring, when implemented correctly, can significantly improve school attendance and performance, reduce violent behavior, decrease the likelihood of drug use, and improve relationships with parents and friends (CDC, 2002).

Community-Level Strategies

Strategies at the community level focuses on modifying community characteristics, including school settings that either promote or inhibit violence. Schools have made numerous efforts to improve the overall environment and to reduce negative outcomes on their campuses, such as violence. For example, improved classroom management and teacher/staffing practices, promoting cooperative learning techniques, student monitoring and supervision, and reducing bullying by involving parents/caregivers in the day-to-day operation of the school help to decrease violence in schools (Dahlberg & Butchart, 2005).

GANG VIOLENCE

The idea or organization of gangs is not a new phenomenon. Throughout the world, gangs have been used as a method of survival for centuries. The gangs seen in our communities today are different from the original gangs that were, in some cases, classified as tribes. Groups of people have been classified and distinguished from one another by their dress, rituals, ceremonies, and beliefs since the beginning of time, but those characteristics alone do not necessarily require the use of the word *gang*. Although gangs usually share some of the same historical components as these groups of people, it is the violence associated with groups that warrant the use of the negative word.

Individuals who join gangs do it for various and personal reasons. In 1960, Cloward and Ohlin concluded that young people are likely to join one of three types of gangs—criminal, conflict, or retreatist—because of differential opportunity. Common reasons for joining a gang include, but are not limited to, wanting to belong to a family, protection, economic positioning, and acceptance. In some communities and neighborhoods, joining a gang means unconditional protection from that gang, which can be vital for survival.

The indicators that one is a gang member can be as obvious as the colors he or she wears every day but are often based on who that individual hangs out with. Chances are high that the person is in the gang if they are consistently associated with known gang members. According to Steven R. Wiley, chief of the Violent Crimes and Major Offenders Section of the Federal Bureau of Investigation, in a 1997 report to the Senate Committee on the Judiciary Committee of the U.S. Senate, gangs have certain turfs that they reign over, which can be as small as a single street or neighborhood, or as large as an entire city or coast.

Causes

There are many speculations about why people join gangs, but it is usually because the gang offers something the individual is lacking. People who join gangs believe that members of the gang can provide these missing components—self-image, self-worth, and survival—that are important in their lives. If the needs cannot be met by family members, individuals look elsewhere to have needs met. Not everyone has the same reasons for joining a gang, but some of the common ones are family, economic gain, peer pressure, family affiliation, and protection.

Some young people join gangs because they lack the feeling of belonging to a group or do not feel loved because of their unstable home life. Other individuals who join gangs come from broken homes where a parent, usually the father, is absent. These students often do not receive any positive attention or bond with family members. The lack of positive attention and bonding can be absent for various reasons, such as the parent working long hours to support the family, large families, or parents who are substance abusers. Joining a gang may give certain members the sense of belonging to a family and increase access to multiple father figures.

Joining a gang can also be due to peer pressure and environment. Everyone wants to belong and be accepted by his or her peers, so young people may join gangs because that is what their peers are doing. When acceptance is lacking from a young person's life, that person might do things he or she would not usually do to impress his or her peers. In addition, some young people are in an environment where gangs are prevalent. In neighborhoods like that, gang members are not only looked up to but are idolized as the acceptable way a person from that neighborhood should be (Jankowski, 1991). Some of these young people have family members who are gang members, making membership almost a tradition. Family affiliations can sometimes be generational, and it is expected of the young person. "Many of these individuals have known people who have been in gangs, including family members—often a brother, but even, in a considerable number of cases, a father and grandfather. The fact that their relatives have a history of gang involvement usually influences these individuals to see the gang as part of the tradition of the community" (Jankowski, 1991, p. 46).

Another common factor in young people's joining a gang is money. Poverty causes people to fight just for survival. When impoverished individuals cannot even get necessities that gang members can access, the attraction is even greater. Sharing in illegal activity with a gang can become economically rewarding. The lack of money is often correlated with the lack of education and opportunities because many young people drop out of school and therefore have fewer opportunities when it comes to employment.

Having protection is very important for some youth. In areas with a lot of gangs, someone may feel obliged to join a gang in order to be safe. Joining a gang means that one will be offered protection by the name itself or from its members. Protection from other gangs and perceived general well-being are key factors for joining a gang. Social, economic, and cultural forces also push many adolescents in the direction of gangs (Baccaglini, 1993; Decker & Van Winkle, 1996). There are many threats in some communities that can be lessened by joining or belonging to a gang.

Symptoms

Visible signs and symptoms, such as privacy about activities or time away from home, new or strange friends or acquaintances, or adopting a street nickname are characteristics of being in a gang. Changes in school and dress are other signs that may indicate a young person is in a gang. Changes in social habits such as low school grades, lack of interest in school activities, and change of peer groups also are common signs of gang membership. Clothing is also a good indicator of gang membership because only one color or specific colors are worn by members of a specific gang (www.safeyouth.org/scripts/faq/prevgangs.asp).

The signs or symptoms of gang membership just described are serious; however, they are not as dangerous as possession or use of weapons, involvement in drugs, or negative involvement with law enforcement like drive-by shootings, breaking and entering, and numerous other criminal offenses. Criminal offenses are dangerous and suffer harsh consequences. Sudden increase in the youth's material possessions that the parents did not purchase is a common indicator of gang activity. Another link to gangs are tattoos or ink drawings of gang symbols on skin or walls as graffiti. Tattoos can be of the name of the gang, a street or turf where the gang resides, or even the street name of the gang member. Graffiti can be found on belongings such as notebooks, jackets, and clothing or on bedroom walls and furniture (www.helpinggangyouth.com).

Several prevention techniques are used to make sure that neighborhoods have limited crime. Prevention is paramount to minimize the existence of gangs. Several strategies can be implemented to facilitate the evacuation of gang violence and the influence of gangs on youth. These strategies may include after-school programs for all youth and shortening the amount of time in between classes to decrease mingling or loitering. Requiring students to volunteer for something useful in their communities and neighborhoods is a strategy that could connect the students positively to their neighborhood as an alternative to being in a gang (www.safeyouth.org/scripts/faq/prevgangs.asp).

Treatment

Getting help is the first step for the treatment process. Mothers Against Gangs (MAG) is a support group that helps victims of gang violence. They offer aid for youths leaving gangs. Andrew P. Thomas, a Maricopa County attorney, started MAG, which is made up of volunteer mothers who learn how to listen and communicate with the teens who are usually hanging out on the streets. Offering help to the youths helps the youth and mothers build a foundation of trust, which causes the youths to become involved in MAG. The members of the organization believe they should intervene with positive actions, healing, and helping, which makes a difference in the life of the youths.

Prevention

Gang prevention programs have been rare because there is a general lack of consensus about why gangs emerge and why juveniles join gangs. Therefore, it is more difficult to develop gang prevention programs that assess their impact. Nevertheless, there are three types of prevention efforts. *Primary prevention* focuses on the entire population at risk and the identification of those conditions (personal, social, and environmental) that promote criminal behavior. The purpose of primary prevention is to help discourage at-risk youth from engaging in criminal behavior and becoming involved in a gang. School-based prevention programs provide a common ground for youth in the United States because most growing children participate in the public education system. Schools should conduct leadership training classes to assist students in developing insight and skills that enable them to work harmoniously with diverse individuals and groups. Offering classes and incorporating curricula on life skills, resistance to peer pressure, values clarification, and cultural sensitivity is a great way to prevent gang violence in school. A school-based program called Gang Resistance Education and Training (GREAT) was introduced by the Phoenix Police Department in 1991 to educate youth about the consequences of gang involvement and to reduce gang activity. The curriculum consists of nine lessons, which include a discussion about gangs and their effects on the quality of life and address the topic of resisting peer pressure (www.ncjrs.gov/html/ojjdp/2009_9_2/page3.html).

Secondary prevention provides outreach to individuals identified as at high risk of becoming delinquent or involved in gangs. Organizing crisis intervention teams to counsel students coping with violence in and near school, as well as implementing victim or offender programs requiring juvenile offenders to make restitution to victims for damage or loss incurred, are great ways to reach youth at risk of gang involvement. Programs such as the Boys & Girls Clubs of America, the Montreal Preventive Treatment Program, and Gang Prevention Through Targeted Outreach consists of structured recreational, educational, and life skills programs. These programs target youths who are at risk of becoming involved in gangs and seeks to alter their attitudes, behaviors, and perception and improve conflict resolution skills (www.ncjrs.gov/html/ojjdp/2009_9_2/page3.html).

Tertiary prevention targets individuals who are already involved in criminal activity or who are gang members. There were several gang prevention programs that law enforcement has experimented with as suppression tactics, such as the "Flying Squad" and the Community Resources Against Street Hoodlums (CRASH). Evaluations of suppression efforts are lacking, but the consensus is that suppression programs are effective means of combating gang crime. Law enforcement agencies have responded to gangs and juvenile violence with suppression tactics like anti-loitering laws, curfew laws, and civil conjunctions that limit the ability of certain groups of people (based on age or group affiliation) to congregate in public places. These laws and restrictions are under scrutiny because they have raised constitutional concerns; thus, evaluations of these city ordinances are mixed (www.ncjrs.gov/html/ojjdp/2009_9_2/page3.html).

The purpose of the primary, secondary, and tertiary programs is to prevent and reduce gang membership using positive reinforcement by encouraging extracurricular activities. Programs are typically in the form of training or instruction and may focus on a variety of areas such as building conflict resolution skills, behavioral modification, and/or educating youths about the negative aspects of gang involvement (www.jrsa.org/jjec/programs/gang/index.html).

Programs especially for tertiary prevention use law enforcement to focus on gang activity through the creation of a gang unit specifically tasked with gang suppression activities. Mental health care providers can advise parents to watch for signs of gang involvement and can encourage them to take the following steps:

- Supervise children's activities and know their friends
- Get their children involved in supervised, positive group activities
- Develop good communication with their children
- Spend positive time with their children
- Become involved in their children's education
- Express to their children at an early age their disapproval of gangs and gang-related activity
- Keep their children from attracting the attention of gangs (e.g., gang-style clothing and gang gestures)
- Learn about gang and drug activity in the community (www.safeyouth.org)

Another way to prevent gang violence is to establish ongoing professional development and in-service training programs for all school employees, including training techniques in classroom management and in dealing with disruptive students and parents, campus intruders, and cultural diversity.

It is important for us, as functioning members of society, to recognize and respect the problems associated with the existence of gangs. It is even more critical to work at understanding the complex world that makes gangs what they are. There is no standard of gang activity, membership, or method of operation, so it is difficult, if not impossible, to understand how and why gangs operate unless you are a member of that gang. What is possible is recognizing that every gang is different, and the world of gang violence is always changing. What may be acceptable behavior to one gang may be deplorable to another gang. It is difficult to begin to change the course of gang violence when there are no constants in the gangs themselves or among the individual members.

If members of society can focus on outreach programs to keep youths out of gangs, we can move toward social change. By informing each other about the dangers of gang membership and making positive efforts toward preventing youths from joining a gang, we can put a pulse on decreasing gang violence.

People join gangs for many different reasons, so it is impossible to put all gang members in one category. Prevention and treatment programs need to constantly evolve and be fluid in order to make the smallest difference in the reduction of gang violence. Some, especially younger, individuals may join a gang for protection, whereas others may join a gang because they want to be accepted and have a form of support. These two individuals will have different views on being in a gang, thus they require different approaches on why they should try to leave their respective gangs.

CHAPTER SUMMARY

Community mental health professionals are in key positions to detect community problems that might affect individuals who are mentally ill, and they play a key role in addressing violence across the lifespan. It is important that community mental health professionals, law enforcement personnel, and government officials discover ways to have an impact on domestic violence in our communities. In this chapter we discussed violence to the unborn that takes place during pregnancy to homicide through gang and school violence. In addition to knowing the risk factors leading to violence, community mental health professionals must specialize in assessing, designing, and implementing programs that help people change destructive behaviors and protect others from harm. In addition, the community mental health professional needs to know what programs and resources are available in the local area, what they charge, eligibility, and what degree of success has been reported. Community mental health professionals are also trained to identify gaps in services and develop evidence-based programs targeting violence.

REVIEW

1. Discuss violence across the lifespan.
2. Define the risk factors for perpetrating youth violence.
3. Explain the impact of physical abuse during pregnancy on the emotional and physical well-being of a pregnant woman and her unborn child.
4. Describe primary and secondary prevention actions related to violence that community mental health professionals can take.
5. Discuss the role of the community mental health provider in preventing and treating violence across the lifespan.

ACTIVITIES

1. Drive by a school and identify potential signs of gang or school violence.
2. Design a community-based program addressing school violence or domestic violence.
3. Develop a community-based program targeting abused pregnant women.
4. Explore the resources for domestic violence in your community.

REFERENCES AND FURTHER READINGS

Anderson, M., Kaufman, J., Simon, T. R., Barrios, L., Paulozzi, L., Ryan, G., . . . Potter, L. (2001). School-associated violent deaths in the United States, 1994–1999. *Journal of the American Medical Association*, *286*(21):2695–2702.

Baccaglini, W. F. (1993). *Project Youth Gang-Drug Prevention: A Statewide Research Study*. Rensselaer, NY: New York State Division for Youth.

California Courts Self-Help Center. (n.d.). *Can a Domestic Violence Restraining Order Help Me*? Retrieved from http://www.courtinfo.ca.gov

California Department of Public Safety. (2007). *Information for Victims of Domestic Violence*. Retrieved from http://www.dps.state.ak.us/

Centers for Disease Control and Prevention [CDC]. (2001). Temporal variations in school-associated student homicide and suicide events—United States, 1992–1999. *Morbidity and Mortality Weekly Report*, *50*(31):657–660.

Centers for Disease Control and Prevention [CDC]. (2008a). National youth risk behavior survey 1991–2005: Trends in the prevalence of selected risk behaviors. Retrieved from http://www.cdc.gov/HealthyYouth/yrbs/pdf/trends_YRBS_Risk_Behaviors.pdf

Centers for Disease Control and Prevention [CDC]. (2008b). School-associated student homicides–United States, 1992–2006. *Morbidity and Mortality Weekly Report*, *57*(2):33–36.

Centers for Disease Control and Prevention [CDC]. (2009). *School associated violent deaths*. Retrieved from www.cdc.gov/ncipc

Cloward, R., & Ohlin, L. (1960). *Delinquency and opportunity*. Glencoe, IL: Free Press.

Dahlberg, L. L., & Butchart, A. (2005). State of the science: Violence prevention efforts in developing and developed countries. *International Journal of Injury Control and Safety Promotion*, *12*(2):93–104.

Decker, S. H., & Van Winkle, B. (1996). *Life in the gang: Family, friends, and violence*. New York: Cambridge University Press.

Dinkes, R., Cataldi, E. F., & Lin-Kelly, W. (2007). *Indicators of School Crime and Safety: 2007* (NCES 2008-021/NCJ 219553). National Center for Education Statistics, Institute of Education Sciences, U.S. Department of Education, and Bureau of Justice Statistics, Office of Justice Programs, U.S. Department of Justice. Washington, DC.

Esbensen, F. (2000). Preventing adolescent gang involvement. Retrieved from http://www.ncjrs.gov/

"Expert encourages alternate treatments for men who abuse women." (2005). *Purdue News*. Retrieved from http://www.purdue.edu/newsroom/

Families. (n.d.). The CDC publication. Retrieved from http://www.cdc.gov/mmwr

Gangs and youth violence. (2007). Retrieved from http://safestate.org/UCSF

Gang Prevention/Intervention. (n.d.). Retrieved from http://www.jrsa.org

Helpguide.org. (2007). Domestic violence and abuse: Signs and symptoms of abusive relationships. Retrieved from http://www.helpguide.org

Jamieson, A., Curry, A., & Martinez, G. (1999). School enrollment in the United States: Social and economic characteristics of students (Current Population Reports). Washington, DC: U.S. Census Bureau. Retrieved from www.census.gov/prod/2001/pubs/P20-533.pdf

Jankowski, M. S. (1991). *Islands in the streets: Gangs and American urban society*. Berkeley: University of California Press.

Lee, M., Sebold, J., & Uken, A. (2003). *Solution-focused treatment of domestic violence offenders*. New York: Oxford University Press.

Lipsey, M. W., & Derzon, J. H. (1998). Predictors of violent and serious delinquency in adolescence and early adulthood: A synthesis of longitudinal research. In R. Loeber & D. P. Farrington (Eds.), *Serious and violent juvenile offenders: Risk factors and successful interventions* (pp. 86–105). Thousand Oaks, CA: Sage.

Lohr, J. M., DeMaio, C., & McGlynn, F. D. (2003). Specific and nonspecific treatment factors in the experimental analysis of behavioral treatment efficacy. *Behavior Modification*, *27*, 322–367.

Murphy, C. M., & Eckhardt, C. I. (2005). *Treating the abusive partner: An individualized, cognitive-behavioral approach*. New York: Guilford Press.

Nansel, T. R., Overpeck, M. D., Haynie, D. L., Ruan, W. J., & Scheidt, P. C. (2003). Relationships between bullying and violence among US youth. *Archives of Pediatric Adolescent Medicine*, *157*, 348–353.

Nansel, T. R., Overpeck, M., Ramani, P. S., Ruan, W. J., Simons-Morton, B., & Scheidt, P. (2001). Bullying behaviors among US youth. *Journal of the American Medical Association*, *285*, 2094–2100.

National Center for Victims of Crime: *Child abuse* (1997). Retrieved from http://www.ncvc.org/

National Center on Child Abuse Prevention Research. (1997). Prevent Child Abuse America. Current trends in child abuse reporting and fatalities: The results of the 1997 annual fifty state survey.

National Clearinghouse on Child Abuse & Neglect Information. (2005). Long term consequences of child abuse & neglect. Retrieved from http://nccanch.acf.hhs.gov/pubs/factsheets/long_term_consequences.cfm

National Coalition Against Domestic Violence [NCADV]. (n.d.). Domestic Violence Awareness Month. Retrieved from http://www.ncadv.org/takeaction Domestic Violence AwarenessMonth_134.html

National Eating Disorders Association. (2008). Body image. Retrieved from http://www.nationaleatingdisorders.org/

New Generation. *Health Center*. (2007). Retrieved from www.ucsf.edu

Office of Juvenile and Delinquency Preventions. Prevent gang violence in school. Retrieved from http://www.safeyouth.org

Olweus, D. (1993). *Bullying at school: What we know and what we can do*. Malden, MA: Blackwell.

Pollack, W. (1998). *Real boys: Rescuing our sons form the myths of boyhood*. New York: Henry Holt.

Resnick, M. D., Ireland, M., & Borowsky, I. (2004). Youth violence perpetration: What protects? What predicts? Findings from the National Longitudinal Study of Adolescent Health. *Journal of Adolescent Health*, *35*(424), e1–e10.

Rice, M. (2007, May). *Domestic violence*. National Center for PTSD, United States Department of Veteran Affairs. Retrieved from http://www.ncptsd.va.gov/

Safe Alternatives to Violent Environments [SAVE]. (2007). Retrieved from http://www.save-dv.org

Safe Schools Healthy Students. Retrieved from www.sshs.samhsa.gov/

San Francisco Child Abuse Prevention Center. (2005). *Programs: Overview*. Retrieved from http://www.sfcapc.org/programs.htm

Sarkar, N. N. (2008).The impact of intimate partner violence on women's reproductive health and pregnancy outcome. *Journal of Obstetrics and Gynaecology*, *28*(3), 266–271.

Teen Birth Rates. (n.d.) How does the United States compare? Retrieved from http://www.teenpregnancy.org/

Thomas, A. P. (n.d.). Maricopa County Attorney: Gang violence. Retrieved from http://www.maricopacountyattorney.org/

Understanding and combating elder abuse in minority communities. (1997). Proceedings of a 1997 conference sponsored by the National Center on Elder Abuse (NCEA) and funded by the Archstone Foundation. Single copies are available at no cost from the Archstone Foundation.

U.S. Department of Education and Justice. (2007). Washington, DC: U.S. Government Printing Office. Washington, DC: U.S. Government Printing Office. Retrieved from http://www.acf.dhhs.gov/programs/cb/publications/cmreports.htm

U.S. Department of Health and Human Services. (1999). *Mental health: A report of the Surgeon General*. Rockville, MD: Author.

U.S. Department of Health and Human Services. (2001.) Youth violence: A report of the surgeon general. Retrieved from www.surgeongeneral.gov/library/youthviolence/toc.html

U.S. Department of Health and Human Services. (2001). *Youth violence: A report of the Surgeon General*. Rockville, MD: Author.

U.S. Department of Health and Human Services. (2004, June). *Silence hurts: Alcohol abuse and violence against women*. Retrieved from http://www.pathwayscourses

U.S. Department of Health and Human Services. (2005). *Child Maltreatment 2005, Chapter 3 Figures and Tables*. Retrieved from http://www.acf.hhs.gov/programs/cb/pubs/cm05/threetabfig.htm

U.S. Department of Health and Human Services. (2005). Summary child maltreatment 2005. Retrieved from http://www.acf.dhhs.gov/

U.S. Department of Health and Human Services, Administration for Children & Families. (2003). Child maltreatment: Summary of key findings.

CHAPTER 13

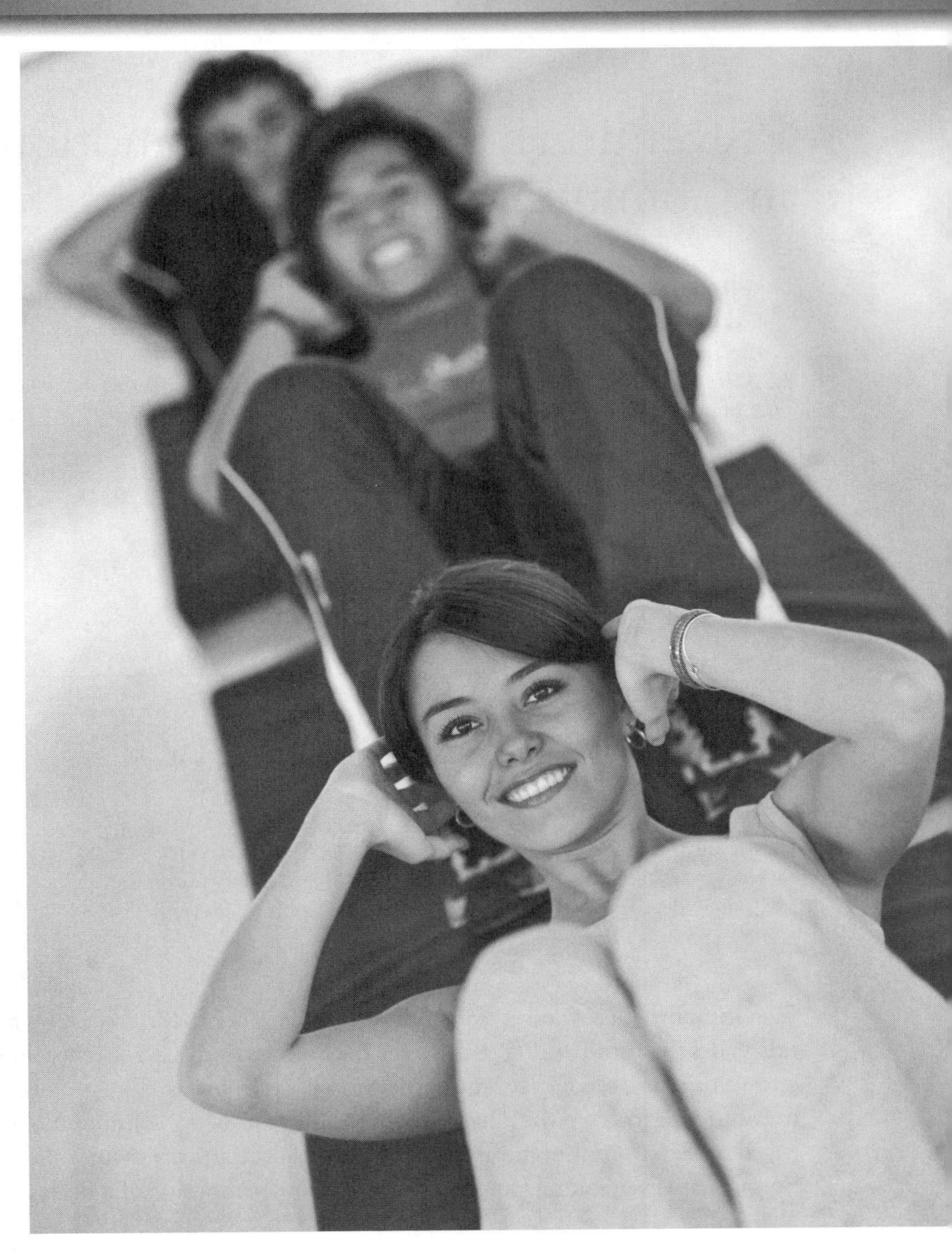

Prevention and Health Promotion in Community Mental Health

CHAPTER OBJECTIVES

1. List data sources for where community health information can be found.
2. List three criteria for conducting a community needs assessment and performing an evaluation.
3. Write an action plan based on the conclusions and recommendations that result from the community needs assessment process.
4. Define the three-tiered prevention classification system.
5. Identify and organize steps in program evaluation practice, as well as concepts that comprise each step.
6. Discuss primary, secondary, and tertiary prevention.
7. Define the components of the health promotion model.
8. List the components of a program evaluation.

KEY TERMS

- Community participatory research
- Cross-tabbing
- Delphi Process
- Focus Group
- Morbidity
- Mortality
- Neurophysiological deficits
- Primary data
- Primary prevention
- Protective factors
- Quality of life
- Random sample
- Risk
- Risk reduction
- Secondary data
- Secondary prevention
- Tertiary prevention

In community health care, prevention is any activity that reduces the burden of **mortality**, death, or **morbidity**, the presence of illness or disease. Prevention of disease occurs at primary, secondary, and tertiary prevention levels. The importance of primary prevention is to avoid the development of a disease. Most community- and population-based health promotion measures are primary preventive activities. Secondary prevention initiatives are aimed at detecting signs and symptoms of a disease early and in so doing increase the opportunity for interventions to prevent progression of the disease and emergence of late-stage signs and symptoms.

Community health professionals play a pivotal role in promoting and providing legitimization of planned community-based programs, participating in program planning, and assessing and evaluating community mental health programs. In this chapter, examples and frameworks related to prevention, health promotion, program evaluation, and community assessment are described. Using the foundations presented in this chapter will give you a foundation to develop programs aimed at improving the mental health status for the entire community.

OVERVIEW OF PREVENTION

Public health and mental health professionals recognize the importance of prevention to keep a major health problem from occurring. The principles of healthcare prevention were first applied to infectious diseases in the establishment of mass vaccination, water safety, and other public hygiene programs. As preventive methodologies proved to be successful, prevention principles were applied to other areas of health, including chronic diseases (Institute of Medicine [IOM], 1994a). In 1994, the IOM published a pivotal report that extended the concept of prevention to mental disorders (IOM, 1994a). In the report *Reducing Risks for Mental Disorders*, the body of research on the prevention of mental disorders was evaluated, offering a new definition of prevention, and provided recommendations on federal policies, programs, and goals.

It is a known fact that preventing a disease or mental illness from occurring is better than treating the disease or mental illness after the onset. In many areas of health, increased knowledge of the etiology and the role of risk and protective factors in the onset of health problems have propelled prevention forward. In the mental health domain, however, progress has been slow because of the two fundamental and interrelated problems described in Chapter 2. First, for major mental disorders, there is insufficient awareness about the etiology of the condition, and second, there is an inability to modify the known etiology of a particular mental disorder. Although these facts have hindered the development of prevention interventions, some successful strategies have emerged in the absence of a full understanding of the etiology of mental illness in the community setting.

Scientific trials have documented successful prevention programs for conditions such as dysthymia and major depressive disorders (Clarke et al., 1995; Muñoz et al., 1995), suicide prevention (Mann et al., 2005), risky behaviors leading to HIV infection (Kalichman, Simbayi, Vermaakk, Jooste, & Cain, 2008), and low birthweight babies (Jablensky, Morgan, Zubrick, Bower, & Yellachich, 2005). Progress also has been made to prevent the incidence of lead poisoning, which, if unchecked, can lead to serious and persistent cognitive deficits in children (Brody et al., 1994; Centers for Disease Control and Prevention [CDC], 1991). Finally, historical landmarks in the prevention of mental illness have led to the successful eradication of neurosyphilis, pellagra, and measles encephalomyelitis (invasion of measles into the brain) in the developed world.

DEFINITIONS OF PREVENTION

Although the term *prevention* is operationalized to mean the prevention of disease, it can have different meanings in different healthcare settings. The classic definition of the term used in the public health settings distinguishes the difference between primary prevention, secondary prevention, and tertiary prevention. The meaning of **primary prevention** in this text is the prevention of a disease or mental illness before the disease or mental illness occurs. For example, prenatal and postnatal visits by nurses and community outreach workers to young mothers have been shown to be successful at preventing poor child care, child abuse, and postpartum depression and improving child-parent attachment as well as fostering good parenting skills.

Secondary prevention focuses on the minimization of recurrences of some of the characteristics of a mental disorder. Prevention strategies in these instances are interventions carried out primarily to help individuals who have displayed signs of mental illness, such as bullying or illicit drug use. Secondary prevention strategies can reduce the severity of the disorder and possibly eliminate behaviors and problems that already exist. **Tertiary prevention** is the reduction and management of disability caused by a disease or mental illness to achieve the highest level of function. Examples include outreach programs that monitor persons with mental disorders who live in the community to ensure that they adhere to their prescribed medication regimens and in inpatient psychiatric hospitals.

The IOM has identified several challenges in applying the principles of prevention to the mental health field (IOM, 1994a). The challenges are primarily due to the difficulty of diagnosing mental disorders and the shifts in the definitions of mental disorders over time. Therefore, the IOM redefined the definition of prevention for the mental health field in terms of three core activities: prevention, treatment, and maintenance (IOM, 1994a). According to the IOM report, prevention resembles the classic concept of primary prevention from the public health arena, which refers to interventions to protect against the initial onset of a mental disorder. Treatment in the proposed framework refers to the identification of individuals with mental disorders and the standard treatment for those disorders, which includes interventions to reduce the likelihood of future co-occurring disorders. Health maintenance refers to interventions that are geared to reduce relapse and recurrence of a disease or mental illness and to provide rehabilitation. (Health maintenance incorporates what the public health field defines as some aspects of secondary prevention and all aspects of tertiary prevention.)

Although the IOM's new definitions of prevention have been very important in conceptualizing the nature of prevention activities for mental health disorders; mental health researchers have not universally adopted the terms. The first onset of a symptom or behavioral change in an individual is the initial point when a mental health problem meets the full criteria for a diagnosis of a mental disorder.

The concepts of **risk** and **protective factors**, **risk reduction**, and enhancement of protective factors are central to most empirically based prevention programs. In the next section, we discuss the risk and protective factors associated with mental health disorders.

RISK FACTORS AND PROTECTIVE FACTORS

Understanding risk factors and protective factors also are important for the community mental health professional. Risk factors are characteristics, variables, or vulnerabilities present that make it more likely that an individual experiencing these characteristics rather than someone selected at random will develop a disorder (Garmezy, 1983; IOM, 1994a; Werner & Smith, 1992). A risk factor is a variable that precedes or leads to the onset of a disorder. Risk factors are not static. A risk factor can change in relation to a developmental phase or a new stressor in an individual's life, and the risk factor can reside within the individual, family, community, or institution. Other risks factors, such as gender and family history, are predetermined, meaning they are not adaptable to change. Risk factors such as lack of social support, inability to read, and exposure to bullying or drugs can be altered by strategic and vigorous interventions (Chaux, Molano, & Podlesky, 2009; Lincoln et al., 2008; Ringwalt et al., 2009). Research has focused on the interplay between biological risk factors and psychosocial risk factors and how they can be modified. Even with a highly inherited condition such as schizophrenia, some studies show that in over half of identical twins, the second twin does not have schizophrenia. This suggests the possibility of modifying the environment to eventually prevent the biological risk factor (i.e., the unidentified genes that contribute to schizophrenia) from being expressed.

Prevention focuses on protective factors as well as the risk factors associated with a particular disease or mental illness. Protective factors improve an individual's response to some environmental hazards resulting in an adaptive outcome (Rutter, 1979). Such risk factors can live in an individual, within the family, or in the community. These risk factors, however, might not promote normal development in the absence of the risk factors. However, the risk factors make a difference on the influence related to the risk factors (IOM, 1994a). There is still a great deal to be learned in the mental health field about the role of protective factors across the lifespan, within families as well as at the community level. The potential for altering these factors in intervention studies will be a major accomplishment.

Researchers who focus on prevention use risk factor status to identify populations for interventions, and then they target risk factors that are thought to be contributory to disease and adaptable to target protective factors that are enhanced through a targeted intervention. If the interventions are successful, the amount of risk decreases, protective factors increase, and the probability of a potential mental problem decreases. The risk factors for an onset of a disorder are more likely to be different from the risks involved in relapse of a previously diagnosed mental problem. This distinction is important because terminology customary to mental illness is customary throughout the mental health intervention continuum. The optimal redesign of at-risk terminology for an individual with a serious mental illness diagnosis aims to reduce the length of time the disorder exists, stop the progress of severity, prevent the recurrence of the original disorder, and increase the length of time between episodes (IOM, 1994a). To accomplish these goals, an assessment of the individual's specific risks for recurrence must take place.

Mental health problems, especially those in childhood, share similar risk factors for the initial onset of a mental illness. Thus, targeting those factors can result in positive outcomes in multiple areas. Risk factors that are common to many mental disorders include individual factors such as **neurophysiological deficits**, difficult temperament, chronic physical illness, and below-average intelligence. Additionally, the mental health professional must consider family factors such as severe marital conflict, social disadvantage, overcrowding or large family size, paternal criminality, maternal mental disorder, and admission into foster care. Other contributing factors include community factors such as living in an area with a high rate of disorganization, crime, poverty, and inadequate schools (IOM, 1994a). In addition, some individual risk factors can lead to a state of vulnerability in which other risk factors may have more effect. For example, low birthweight is a general risk factor for multiple physical and mental outcomes in newborns; however, when it is combined with a high-risk social environment, low birthweight has poorer outcomes (McGauhey, Starfield, Alexander, & Ensminger, 1991). The accumulation of several risk factors also may increase the likelihood of an onset of a disorder;

however, the presence of protective factors can reduce the onset of mental illness in varying degrees.

The accumulation of risk factors in pathways that draw attention to other risks has led prevention researchers to the concept of "breaking the chain at its weakest links" (IOM, 1994a; Robins, 1970). For example, some risks, even though they contribute considerably to the onset of mental illness, may be less flexible than other risk factors to prevention interventions. The goal of the preventive strategy is to change the risks that are amenable to an intervention. For example, it may be easier to prevent a child from being disruptive and isolated from peers by altering his or her classroom environment and increasing academic achievement than it is to change the home environment where there is severe marital conflict, domestic violence, and substance abuse.

Because mental health is fundamentally related to all aspects of health care, it is important to consider the interactions of risk and protective factors, etiologic links across domains, and multiple outcomes. For example, according to Kaplan and his colleagues (1987), chronic illness, unemployment, substance abuse, and being the victim of violence can be risk factors or attributing variables for the onset of mental health problems. Some of the same risk factors also can be related to the detriment of mental health problems (e.g., depression may lead to substance abuse, which in turn may lead to lung or liver cancer).

Gordon (1987a), in the area of disease prevention, and Kumpfer and Baxley (1997), in the area of substance abuse, proposed a three-tiered preventive intervention classification system: universal, selective, and indicated prevention. The three-tiered typology has gained favor among government, national, and community mental health service providers and is used by the IOM, the National Institute of Drug Abuse, and the European Monitoring Center for Drugs and Drug Addiction. The three-tiered system is as follows:

1. *Universal prevention* addresses the population as a whole (nationally, local community, school, and districtwide). Universal prevention aims to prevent or delay the abuse of alcohol, tobacco, and other substance. All individuals are provided with prevention educational information and skills necessary to prevent a condition like substance abuse from occurring.
2. *Selective prevention*, in contrast, focuses on groups whose risk of developing alcohol abuse or dependence on drugs is high. The subgroups are identified by characteristics such as age, gender, family history, or economic status. An example is drug abuse campaigns in recreational, community, or school settings.
3. *Indicated prevention* involves a screening process. The goal of indicated prevention is to identify individuals who exhibit early signs of substance abuse and other

psychosocial behaviors that might lead to substance abuse. Signs may include falling grades among students, known substance abuse or conduct disorders, and/or alienation from parents, school, and positive peer groups.

4. *Environmental prevention* is not included in the three-tiered model. Environmental prevention approaches are usually managed at the regulatory or community level and focus on interventions to discourage drug abuse. Prohibition and bans (e.g., smoking workplace bans, alcohol advertising bans) is viewed as an environmental restriction. However, in practice, environmental prevention programs embrace various initiatives at the macro and micro level, from government control for alcohol sales, through roadside sobriety or drug tests, worker/pupil/student drug or athletic drug testing, increased policing in susceptible settings (near schools, at street festivals), and legislative guidelines aimed at precipitating punishments (warnings, penalties, fines, and imprisonment). The following sections describe the concepts, emerging evidence, practice, and policy associated with the promotion of positive mental health.

The Roots of Health Promotion

As we look at the past to guide the direction for health promotion activities for this text, we are aware of several common threads that have created the pattern for health promotion as it appears today. Here, we briefly examine these roots with a description of the issues of the past that still exist to some extent today. Notable threads of development that converged to produce contemporary policies in health promotion include (1) reliance on long-standing public health programs, implementation of health education efforts to gain the cooperation of the public; (2) development of mass media communication and outreach campaigns and technologies of the 1950s and 1960s that created recruitment of grassroots organizations reflecting the public's heightened interest of public health issues; (3) the self-care, civil rights, and women's rights movements of the 1960s that demanded the transferring of authority and resources to individuals previously held by others; (4) the inflation and cost containment concerns of the 1970s that led to cutbacks in social programs and caps on expenditures for high-tech medical care; (5) the growing recognition of diminishing returns on investments in medical care and communicable disease control and the increasing attributes of chronic disease to lifestyle and behavior; (6) the strengthening of the scientific base of social, behavioral, and educational research applied to health; and (7) the mounting cynicism and impatience of the public with conventional medical approaches to health, replaced by more imaginative concepts encompassing social, mental, and spiritual qualities of life. We present one of the many models of health promotion later in this chapter.

HEALTH PROMOTION IN MENTAL HEALTH

Health promotion in the mental health setting is a cost-effective way to improve public health and quality of life as well as to decrease the economic costs of mental illness. Local, federal, and state government agencies and health departments are aware that health promotion activities focusing on decreasing psychosocial and mental activities are beneficial; however, traditionally, national healthcare budgets are targeted inevitably for care and treatment services and programs. Although health promotion is known to be cost effective, numerous mental and behavioral healthcare programs are in need of new resources to promote health and address mental health problems that are priority concerns based on *Healthy People 2010*. If we are going to fulfill the mental health objectives set forth by *Healthy People 2020*, it is important to secure long-term funding for community mental health promotion programs that are essential and innovative; thus funding sources are urgently needed to address community mental health programs and initiatives.

One solution to increase health promotion activities is to duplicate efforts like the tobacco tax laws in California to fund national health promotion programs addressing the mentally ill. The creation of the International Network of Health Promotion Foundations (INHPF) demonstrates an innovative way of mobilizing resources for promoting health. The INHPF was established in 1999 to enhance the performance of existing health promotion foundations and to assist the development of new foundations. The mission of the INHPF is to strengthen the capacities of countries to promote population health through health promotion foundations at national and subnational levels.

Presently health promotion scholars and policymakers encourage the adoption of participatory approaches to the evaluation process and recommend meaningful opportunities for involvement of community advocates, patients, and family members with interest in a particular health promotion initiative to participate in that initiative and program evaluation. Some public policies require that a minimum of 10% of the total funding for a health promotion initiative be allocated to evaluation and that a combination of process and outcome information be used to evaluate all health promotion initiatives. The INHPF supports the use of multiple methods to evaluate health promotion initiatives. It also supports further research into the development of appropriate approaches to evaluating health promotion initiatives. Creating additional training and education infrastructure to develop expertise in the evaluation of health promotion initiatives is also important to support opportunities for sharing evaluation methodologies used in health promotion through conferences, workshops, networks, and other educational settings.

Implementing program evaluations in an ethical and effective manner requires complex professional skills in conducting recurrent cycles of program planning, implementation, and evaluation leading to enhanced quality and effectiveness of health promotion over time (Davies & Macdonald, 1998; Minkler, 1997). Many health promotion models exist in the literature. For example, Green and Kreuter's (2005) PRECEDE–PROCEED model is widely used for communitywide programs and applications within community settings such as workplaces and schools. A number of other models also are in wide use, such as the Multilevel Approach to Community Health (MATCH), CDCynergy, SMART (Social Marketing Assessment and Response Tool), and A Systematic Approach to Health Promotion (*Healthy People 2010*).

There are a number of common features in all health promotion practice models. First, action is preceded by a considerable period of meticulous study of a community's needs, resources, priorities, history, and structure. The study of the community's needs is conducted in collaboration with the community. This method of assessment represents an underlying philosophy of "doing in collaboration with" rather than "doing to the community." Second, an assessment team agrees to a plan of action, the required resources are gathered, implementation of the assessment begins, and monitoring of action and change processes is carried out. Practice models emphasize the need for flexibility in planning and implementation to meet the demands of new or changing conditions and constant surveillance of and reflection over practice, change processes, and outcomes to inform better quality of practice. Third, the importance of evaluation is stressed, and dissemination of best practices occurs at this stage. It is important to pay attention to maintaining and improving quality as dissemination of the data unfolds.

Healthcare professionals working in mental health promotion can learn from the experiences of public health promotion initiatives. The key lessons for mental health promotion are outlined in **Box 13-1**.

BOX 13-1 Key Lessons from Health Promotion Relevant to Mental Health

Combine individual and structural strategies with advocacy.
Work with an array of public and private sectors, not just the health sector.
Emphasize positive mental health as well as prevention and treatment.
Use professional tools for program planning, implementation, and evaluation.
Strive to increase people's control over their own mental health.
Avoid over-dependence on "expert-driven" approaches.
Adopt a capacity building approach with individuals and communities.

Source: Centers for Disease Control and Prevention. (1999). Framework for program evaluation in public health. *Morbidity and Mortality Weekly Report, 48*(No. RR-11).

Health Promotion Model

The health promotion model (HPM) shown in **Figure 13-1** was intended to be a complementary counterpart to models of health protection. The HPM proposed by Nola J. Pender (1982; revised, 1996) defines health as a positive dynamic state not merely the absence of disease. Health promotion, in contrast, is aimed at increasing a client's level of well-being. The HPM illustrates the multidimensional nature of a person as he or she interacts within the environment to pursue health. Pender's

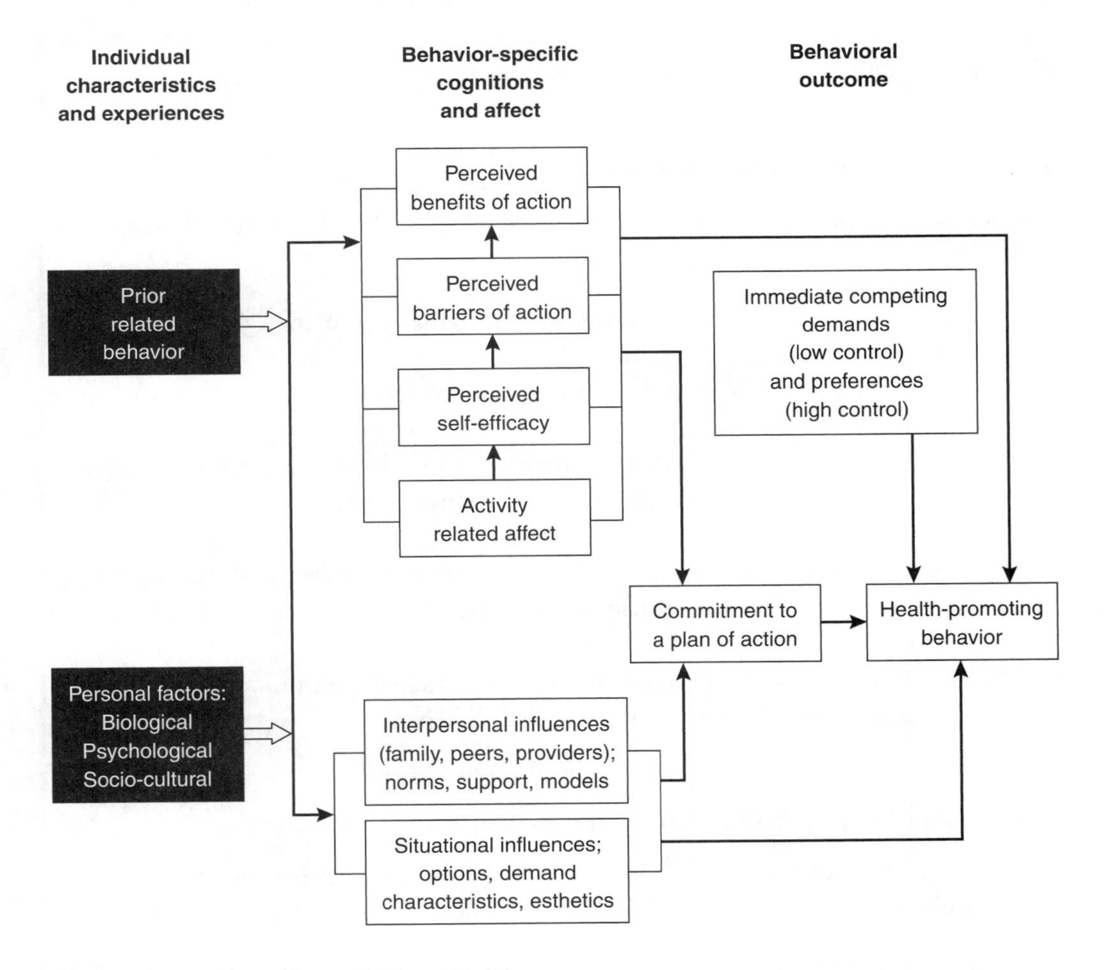

FIGURE 13-1 Health Promotion Model
Source: Pender, N. J., Murdaugh, C., & Parsons, M.A. (2006). *Health Promotion in Nursing Practice* (5th ed.). Upper Saddle River, NJ: Prentice Hall Health.

model focuses on the following three areas: individual characteristics and experiences, behavior-specific cognitions, and affective behavioral outcomes.

The health promotion model explains that each person has distinctive personal characteristics and experiences that influence subsequent actions. The set of variables for behavioral-specific knowledge and affect have important motivational significance. These variables can be modified through nursing and health professional actions. Health-promoting behavior is the desired behavioral outcome and is the end in the HPM. Health-promoting behaviors should bring about improved health, enhanced functional ability, and better quality of life at all stages of development. The final behavioral demand is also subject to the immediate challenging demands and preferences that can disrupt any intended health-promoting actions.

Assumptions of the Health Promotion Model

Reflecting both nursing and behavioral science perspectives, the HPM is based on the following assumptions:

- Persons seek to create circumstances of living where they can express their unique human health potential.
- Persons have the ability for reflective self-awareness, including assessment of their own competencies.
- An individual values growth in positive directions viewed as attempts to achieve a personally acceptable balance between change and stability.
- Individuals seek to regulate actively their own behavior.
- Individuals interact with the environment, progressively transforming the environment and being transformed over time while dealing with all of their biopsychosocial complexities.
- Health professionals are a part of the interpersonal environment, which exerts influence on individuals throughout their lifespan.

Theoretical Propositions of the Health Promotion Model

Theoretical statements significant to the HPM provide a basis for investigative work on health behaviors. The HPM is based on the following theoretical propositions:

- Previous behaviors and inherited and acquired characteristics influence beliefs, affect, and enactment of health-promoting behaviors.

- Individuals commit to connecting behaviors from areas they anticipate draw from personally valued benefits.
- Perceived barriers can restrain a commitment to action, a mediator of behavior as well as actual behavior.
- Perceived competence or self-efficacy to execute a given behavior increases the likelihood of commitment to action and actual performance of the behavior.
- Greater perceived self-efficacy results in fewer perceived barriers to a specific health behavior.

Finally, a positive affect toward a behavior results in greater perceived self-efficacy, which in turn can result in increased positive affect. When positive emotions have an effect on a behavior, the probability of commitment and action is increased. Individuals are more likely to commit to and engage in health-promoting behaviors when significant others model the behavior, anticipate the behavior, and provide assistance and support to enable the behavior.

Families, peers, and healthcare providers are important sources of interpersonal influence who can increase or decrease commitment to an individual engaging in positive health-promoting behavior. Situational influences in the external environment can enhance or diminish commitment or participation in health-promoting behavior. The greater the commitments to a specific plan of action, the more likely the health-promoting behaviors will be maintained over time.

Commitment to a plan of action is less likely to affect the desired behavior when competing demands occur that individuals have little or no control over and require immediate attention. Commitment to a plan of action is less likely to result in the desired behavior when other actions are more appealing and thus preferred over the target behavior. Persons can amend cognitions, affect, and the interpersonal and physical environment to create incentives for health actions.

THE MAJOR CONCEPTS AND DEFINITIONS OF THE HEALTH PROMOTION MODEL

Individual Characteristics and Experience

Prior Related Behavior

Behavioral change depends on the direct and indirect effects or the likelihood of engaging in health-promoting behaviors as well as the frequency of similar behaviors in the past.

Personal Factors

Personal factors are categorized as biological, psychological, and sociocultural. These factors are predictive of a given behavior and formed by the nature of the target behavior being considered.

Personal biological factors include variables such as age, gender, body mass index, pubertal status, aerobic capacity, strength, agility, balance, self-esteem, self-motivation, personal competence, perceived health status, and definition of health.

Personal sociocultural factors comprise variables such as race, ethnicity, acculturation, education, and socioeconomic status.

Behavioral-Specific Cognition and Affect

- Perceived benefits of action: Probable positive outcomes that will occur from health behavior.
- Perceived barriers to action: Imagined, real, or perceived obstructions and personal costs of understanding a given behavior action.
- Perceived self-efficacy: The judgment of personal ability to organize and execute a health-promoting behavior. In addition, perceived self-efficacy influences perceived barriers to action so higher efficacy results in lower perceptions of barriers to the performance of the behavior.
- Activity-related affect: Activity-related affect influences perceived self-efficacy, which means the more positive the subjective feeling, the greater the feeling of efficacy. In turn, increased feelings of efficacy can generate further positive affect. This concept also includes subjective positive or negative feelings that occur before, during, and following behavior based on the stimulus properties of the behavior itself.
- Interpersonal influences: Concerned with cognition concerning behaviors, beliefs, or attitudes of the other. Interpersonal influences include norms (expectations of significant others), social support (instrumental and emotional encouragement), and modeling (vicarious learning through observing others engaged in a particular behavior). Primary sources of interpersonal influences are families, peers, and healthcare providers.
- Situational influences: These influences review personal perceptions and cognitions of any given situation or context that can facilitate or impede behavior. They include perceptions or options available, demand characteristics, and aesthetic features of the environment in which given health-promoting behavior is proposed to take place. Situational influences may have direct or indirect influences on health behavior.

Behavioral Outcome

Commitment to Plan of Action

Commitment to plan of action is the concept of intention and recognition of a planned strategy leading to implementation of health behavior.

Immediate Competing Demands and Preferences

Competing demands are alternative behaviors that individuals have low control over because of environmental emergencies such as work or family care responsibilities. Competing preferences include alternative behaviors over which individuals apply reasonably high control, such as choice of ice cream or carrots for a snack or taking prescribed mental health medications or not.

Health-Promoting Behavior

Health-promoting behaviors are the end point or action outcomes directed toward attaining positive health outcomes such as optimal well-being, personal fulfillment, and productive living and improved quality of life.

PROMOTING QUALITY OF LIFE IN THE MENTAL HEALTH SETTING

In the current environment, it is important to add quality of life to any conceptual framework of mental health. Early attempts to bring "quality of life" and "social well-being" into a discussion about the value of population health were made by health practitioners, rather than by social scientists and philosophers in the 1960s and 1970s (Campbell, Converse, & Rodgers, 1976; Katschnig, 1997). Despite the fact that the World Health Organization's 1948 definition of health was broad and indicated a conceptualization of health going beyond the physiologic, anatomic, or chemical dimensions, measures of health at both population and individual levels were comparatively narrow until a few decades ago. Traditional statistics on births, deaths, life expectancy, and survival periods were the accepted indexes of health and outcome until consumers and human rights advocates raised concerns about their appropriateness. A portion of the advocate's motivation to address these concerns was the need to capture indexes of social and economic well-being and to address the importance that consumers attach to things like autonomy, choice, life satisfaction, and self-actualization.

Given the breadth and depth of the construct of quality of life, a need soon arose to define a more specific range of variables relating directly to health distinct from those that were not perceived as being directly related to health. Thus, in defining health-related quality of life, issues such as housing, income, freedom, and social support have traditionally been excluded from the definition (Patrick & Erickson, 1993). Health-related quality of life concepts in early health promotion discussion were in physical medicine, in areas such as oncology and arthritis. The quality of life concept had a late entry into psychiatry; however, the assessment of nondisease aspects of the mentally ill such as impairments, disabilities, social functioning, and patient satisfaction has had a long tradition in the field (Katschnig, 1997).

For psychiatry and mental health, the concept of quality of life has generated much controversy (Barry, Crosby, & Bogg, 1993; Gill & Feinstein, 1994; Hunt, 1997). A portion of the controversy connects to the common characteristics between a number of the dimensions included in the quality-of-life assessment and the traditional psychopathological domains that are regarded as indicators of mental illness. The redundancy in the measurement raises the question of whether assessing quality of life in people with mental illness adds value to the psychiatric evaluation. Oliver, Huxley, Priebe, and Kaiser (1997) argue that the conceptualization of health-related quality of life excludes issues like as housing, social support, and autonomy. Oliver et al. (1997) further argue that these characteristics are controversial in psychiatry because the issues are of direct relevance to mental health. Additionally, placing emphasis on subjective reports of well-being in quality of life assessments is repetitious in the mental health setting where subjective experiences are a core feature of the exploration of health or illness. Moreover, reliance on subjective reports as a way of evaluating quality of life has other crucial limitations in psychiatry, where patients' reports of the quality of their lives may deviate significantly from what may be predicted by objective or social norms (Atkinson, Zibin, & Chuang, 1997).

Despite these limitations, few health professionals question the relevance of a quality-of-life assessment discussion about health problems today. For example, the primary need for autonomy, human rights, and freedom from the experience of stigma to an informed concept of mental health is considered relevant. The importance of being emotionally involved to evaluating quality of life is displayed in the range and number of assessment tools that have been developed to measure quality of life within the mental health field over the past two decades (Lehman, 1996). Of particular importance is the fact that the current tools focus on the negative factors of quality of life that may weaken quality of life but also the positive factors that may enhance general well-being. The WHO (WHOQOL Group, 1995) defines **quality of life** as "an individual's perception of his/her position in life in the context of the culture and value systems in which he/she lives, and in relation to his/her goals, expectations, standards and concerns." Quality of life is also a broad view of well-being including social indicators, happiness, and health status. For many healthcare professionals in the field of mental health, the definition of quality of life gives voice to the previously voiceless mentally ill and emphasizes the interaction between personal and environmental factors in health. The definition also reflects the utility of the concept of quality of life for describing health, including mental health, in terms that go beyond the presence or absence of signs and symptoms of a mental illness and captures positive aspects of coping, satisfaction, and autonomy.

It is important that health professionals understand the importance of how quality-of-life issues interface with mental illness as well as other health issues that might influence mental health. To that end, the ability to conduct a community needs assessments is becoming an important skill for health professionals. Designing community-based mental health programs without research and community needs assessments is practice based on tradition without validation. Community mental health programs are constantly undergoing tremendous changes and challenges. To meet social challenges and needs, healthcare delivery must be research based (Lanuza, 1999). The next sections define the components for defining a community and the community assessment process.

DEFINING COMMUNITY

There are numerous definitions of community in the literature. Shamanksy and Pesznecker (1991) noted the wide and variable use of the word *community*. The term has existed for several years, has surpassed different eras, cultures, and has been modified over time by interpretation and meaning. Derived from the Latin word *communitas*, community has over 100 variations in the health field. For the healthcare professional, the community can be defined as a setting of practice. Laffrey and Craig (1995), however, report that community as a setting of practice is an important definition but not "sufficient" for community practice (p. 127). Communities are seen as an area in which healthcare professions practice as well as a focus on services. Blum (1975) defines several different types of communities, including face-to-face communities, neighborhood, and community identifiable need, community of ecology, community of concern, community of special interest, community of viability, community of action capability, community of political jurisdiction, resource community, and community of solution. These community definitions are structural and suggest that the community is a neighborhood within a defined region, and functional aspects of community are where special interest groups cross geopolitical boundaries.

Other theorists' definitions describe the specific aspects of the community. For example, Anderson and McFarlane (2008) indicate that a community comprises eight components: physical environment, education, safety and transportation, politics and government, health and social services, communication, economics, and recreation. Moreover, Higgs and Gustafson (1985) list the attributes of a community to include size, population groups, culture, spatial characteristics or boundaries, organizations, laws, socioeconomic status, community history, occupations, schools, and community resources.

Community as a Client

According to Higgs and Gustafson (1985), the concept of community as a client is the strongest conceptualization of a community and is important for the health professional to understand. Within this conceptualization, a community is defined as a group or aggregate of people within a geopolitical boundary and is the unit of practice. The early public health movement's desire to prevent communicable diseases developed the concept community as a client. The concept of community as a client has offered great results in reducing the overall morbidity and mortality rates in the population (Anderson & McFarlane, 2008; Higgs & Gustafson, 1985). In the mid to late 1800s, the primary focus of public health was on the prevention of disease such as cholera and smallpox. Sanitation, clean drinking water, and environmental influences on the incidence of disease came under security. In the next section of this chapter we discuss the purpose and importance of conducting a community needs assessment. The section ends with the community assessment process and the importance of reporting the findings.

COMMUNITY ASSESSMENTS

Purpose

As community-assessment teams begin to view the community as a client, at times they must determine if a community needs assessment is warranted. If they elect to conduct a community needs assessment, they must consider the steps necessary to create program or community changes. Often members of the assessment team realize they do not have sufficient knowledge to make decisions leading to changing the components of a program. At times program changes are made based on selected "stories" or anecdotal information. The implications of anecdotes are frequently contradictory. Between the vision of an agency's future development and implementation of a plan to achieve its goals, community planners may also realize there is more than one way to accomplish their vision. Results from a well-designed community assessment cannot generalize the findings to the entire community. A well-designed community assessment, however, will allow community planners to feel a sense of confidence when they use the assessment findings as a foundation for decision making. The most significant mental health problem within a population is an organization's inability and lack of capacity to address specific health problems with the most promising interventions and best practices related to the identified problem.

What Is a Community Assessment?

Once the community is defined, the next step is an assessment to identify the needs, the problems, and the community to be served. Assessing the needs of the community is a critical step in the planning process because it provides objective data to define key mutual health problems. It also sets priorities for program implementation as well as establishes baseline data for evaluating an intervention. Peterson and Alexander (2001) suggest that a needs assessment should answer the following questions:

- Who is the priority population?
- What are the needs of the priority population?
- Which subgroups within a community have the greatest needs?
- Where are the subgroups located geographically?
- What is currently being done to resolve identified needs?
- How well have the identified needs been addressed in the past?

Several approaches exist to determine the needs and priorities of a community. A community assessment, also known as a needs assessment, is the process of gathering, analyzing, and reporting information about the needs of a community and the strengths currently available in the community to meet those needs. A community assessment starts by convening a team of collaborators, establishing a vision, and prioritizing the issues that require investigation or change. Developing a collaborative effort between the community and mental health care providers establishes a foundation for a community assessment that includes professionals who have expertise on mental health issues and community members, patients, and advocates who are likely to be affected by planned changes (such as children and parents). The vision provides a focus for the community assessment—a clear picture of where the team wants to be in the future. Once the assessment is complete, findings are used to prioritize program changes and to select the appropriate information needed to make decisions that create change.

Characteristics of Successful Community Assessment

A successful community assessment presents comprehensive and accurate information for decision making. Community assessments with reliable results and useful information begin with an assessment of the community's current situation. Depending on the focus of the assessment, an evaluation component also may be included. The current capacities of the community—services and other resources provided by public health agencies, institutions, and associations, and the skills and abilities of individuals and the community—are identified.

During the needs assessment process, information can be collected through data that already exists **(secondary data)** and through newly collected data, also known as **primary data**. Conclusively, the gap between current service resources and needs in the community are identified, and ideas on how to eliminate gaps can be generated. Successful community assessments begin with a vision of the future and allow questions to drive the information-gathering process. With the recent increase and availability of information due to technology changes, the assessment team may find a large amount of information applicable to the issue or issues being studied. Identifying the questions that will be answered by the community assessment allows team members to be more selective in collecting data and judging the usefulness of the data. A preliminary list of questions acts as a framework for collection of new information through surveys, **focus groups**, or public meetings.

Finally, community assessments leading to useful, comprehensive information address issues that stakeholders—people with an interest in the issue such as mental health providers, parents, students, agency personnel, government officials—perceive as important. Moreover, a community assessment leading to the desired change by the planning team communicates the information gathered back to stakeholders and involves them in the planning process.

Steps Involved in Conducting a Community Assessment

The steps required in conducting a community assessment vary, depending on the problems the planning team feels the community is facing. The planning team might prepare for a community assessment by including stakeholders, developing a vision for the future for the community, and creating a list of questions that need to be answered by the community assessment. The questionnaire might include the following:

1. What is currently known: Be prepared to interpret the data collected and explain the rationale of collecting the data.
2. What still needs to be known: Identify all information needed to address the problem. What questions are partially or totally unanswered?

Collecting the Data

Select a methodology to collect the data. The planning team may suggest additional data sets. For example, secondary data sources can be analyzed or assist with understanding data that is gathered. The team might elect to collect new, also known as primary, data through a telephone or mail survey of a random sample of community residents or collect primary data using focus groups, face-to-face interviews, a public forum (such as a town hall meeting or community forum), or through the nominal group process. Using any of these four methods can yield qualitative and quantitative information that can be useful in planning and decision making. The team could consider using a combination of data collection methods. For example, they could follow a mail survey with focus groups or a public forum. Hosting a focus group may provide supporting data and richer information to the results of a mailed survey. **Table 13-1** suggests possible ways data can be collected for a community assessment and ways to find that data. It is also important to remember, however, that the data needed for the assessment might vary from this list. The assessment team should also consider other data sources that are available to assess a community and understand both the problems and solutions that exist using a particular data set, for example cost and accessibility.

Selecting the Sample

Another critical decision the assessment team must make is what extent community members or mental health care organizations will participated in the research assessment. **Community participatory research** has gained popularity in the past 10 years by government funders like the National Institutes of Health. Identifying the characteristics of the people who will provide information for a community assessment can be a lengthy and difficult process. Ideally, if time and resources were available, data would be collected from everyone in the geographic area or community who has the characteristics in which the assessment team is interested (for example, homeless mental health patients). However, collecting information from everyone is not possible.

The preferred method of data collection is a **random sample**. A random sample is a smaller group of the population who are asked to participate in the assessment. Everyone has an equal chance of being selected to participate. Regardless of the sampling procedure, each participant must understand the purpose of the study, be given information about confidentiality, and must sign an informed consent. Additionally, participants need to know how the information they provide will be used, the measures taken to protect their identity, and understand that they can choose not to participate without disruption of any community mental health services they are receiving.

TABLE 13-1 Table of Data Sources for Program Evaluation

Data Domains: What Data Do You Want?	Data Sources: Who Collects This Data?	Data Access Points: Where Can You Find This Data?
Demographic data, such as age, gender, school/level, race/ethnicity, etc.	U.S. Census Local program data Local survey data	Substance Abuse and Mental Health Services Administration's Prevention Platform GIS Mapping Tools
Socioeconomic data, such as income, employment, housing, etc.	U.S. Census U.S. Department of Labor U.S. Housing & Urban Development	Public records Prevention Platform GIS Mapping Tools
Crime and delinquency data, such as arrests, reported crimes, violence and substance-related offenses, etc.	Local law enforcement agencies U.S. Department of Justice Bureau of Justice Statistics Office of Juvenile Justice Delinquency Prevention (OJJDP)	*Sourcebook of Criminal Justice Statistics* *Uniform Crime Reports* Drug Abuse Warning Network Drug Use Forecasting System OJJDP Statistical Briefing Book
Public health data, such as mortality/morbidity, teen pregnancy, immunizations, illnesses, etc.	Department of Public Health Centers for Disease Control	Vital health statistics Hospital records Coroner's office Hospital emergency rooms' discharge data sets
Education data, such as academic achievement, graduation/completion, attendance/enrollment, dropout, suspensions and expulsions	U.S. Department of Education State Departments of Education Local School Districts	Education public records, reports, and data
Traffic/transportation data, such as car crashes, licenses, etc.	U.S. Department of Transportation State Department of Motor Vehicles National Highway Traffic Safety Administration	Traffic and transportation public records, reports, and data
Other public data sources, especially systematically collected survey data	National surveys, such as the Youth Risk Behavior Survey, Behavioral Risk Factor Surveillance System, Monitoring the Future, National Survey on Drug Use and Health, Communities That Care, Assets Survey	State surveys Local community surveys School surveys
Program/grant funding data, such as Block Grant and Discretionary Grant Information Systems, etc.	National Funds Data Systems (e.g., BGAS) State and community management information systems	Federal, state, and community agencies

Source: Adapted from Library of Economics and Liberty: US Data Sources. Retrieved from http://www.econlib.org/library/sourcesUS.html. Accessed August 16, 2010.

What to Ask

Designing the questionnaire, also known as the instrument or protocol for collecting data, is a complex process. The wording of the questions influences the answers given and may influence the likelihood of getting an answer. Consideration must be given to issues such as the order of the questions, response options, the number of questions, and the way the questionnaire is constructed (font size, spacing, highlighting or emphasis, and literacy level). Sample questions include, "Do you feel you have control over the things that affect your health?" as an opened-ended question, and "I take a positive attitude toward myself—strongly disagree, disagree, agree, or strongly agree."

Community Indicators

The assessment team must define what community concerns or indicators they would like to assess. Indicators are measurements that give information about both past and current trends. Indicators assist community mental health professionals, state officials, and community leaders in making decisions that affect future program outcomes. Community indicators provide insight into the overall direction of the mental health status of a community, whether certain conditions, for example, homelessness among the chronically mentally ill, are improving, declining, or stagnating or some mix of the three. Community indicators are important measurements because they reflect the interplay among social, environmental, and economic factors affecting a community's well-being.

Indicators that might be of most concern to a community partnership include the following issues pertaining to age, gender, or economics:

- Adolescent substance abuse
- Child abuse and neglect
- Gang activity
- Juvenile arrest/adjudication
- Youth violence rates
- Homelessness rates
- Elder abuse rates
- Placement of children and youth in foster care facilities
- Juvenile weapons/gun violation arrests
- Suicide rates
- Graduation rates
- Unemployment rate

Places in the community to concentrate assessment efforts include:

- City or town block
- Schools
- Senior centers
- Homeless shelters
- Community-based and faith-based programs
- Neighborhood
- City or town
- County

It is important to determine a specific population to focus on the assessment:

- Youths ages 10 to 19
- Men
- Women
- Children
- Adults ages 19 to 45
- Families from diverse populations
- Low-income families
- Single-parent families
- Families with children
- Families with different education levels
- Families with varying employment statuses

Here is a possible outline for a community assessment report:

Introduction: State the purpose of the assessment and explain the goals of the assessment and your plans to accomplish the goals. Summarize the information you have to share.
Key findings: Present the major findings of the community assessment and the central problems that emerged as well as identify priorities.
Additional factors: Present the associated risks that were identified and talk about the community perceptions that need to be considered in addressing these problems.
Strengths and resources: Map out the available resources in the community to address these issues.
Action plan: Arrange the plan of action to include the strategies you will put into practice to address the needs uncovered during the assessment.
Measures of success: Propose ways to determine the success of the implementation plan.

Challenges: Identify the challenges to be addressed to ensure that the assessment is successful.

Conclusions: Present the conclusions in the community where the assessment took place and invite the community and assessment team to participate.

Data Collection

Volunteers or staff from the planning team or external evaluation team can distribute questionnaires in the community. Volunteers must be trained in the distribution of the questionnaires. Conducting telephone interviews, face-to-face interviews, focus groups, and other methods listed previously requires special training and skills. Community health professionals must be familiar with the data collection process. Mailed surveys may be less time consuming than face-to-face interviews; however, return rates usually do not yield high results.

Compiling the Data

At this point in the assessment, the team must analyze all of the data collected, with the group identifying and prioritizing mental health problems. Data analysis can be formal or informal. The difference between using formal and informal analysis is the use of standard measures. Data analysis can be the most complicated part of the assessment. Thus community mental health professionals should serve in a leadership role for the data analysis for the community assessment. They can assist in developing a database to analyze the information collected using computer-based statistical data-analysis software.

Methods for presenting the data include developing frequencies calculated for responses to questions. In addition, analyses can look at the difference in response between groups of respondents (e.g., are respondents with higher educational levels more likely to answer a question a certain way than those with lower educational levels or mental illness?). This can be conducted by **cross-tabbing** the information. Creating transcriptions of the responses to open-ended questions (from the mailed and telephone surveys) and comments collected during focus groups and face-to-face interviews will have important information to include in the final report.

Reporting the Findings

Once the data is collected, it is essential to have the information summarized in a report and disseminated to community mental health groups, mental health officials, foundations, and public health departments. Report findings also can be disseminated by creating a Web site, a press release, offering workshops and trainings, and by writing an article for an academic journal. Illustrating the results in charts, tables, or graphs that simplify the information for the lay audience is important.

Completing a community assessment that provides information, which has a high level of validity as a basis for decision making, is only the beginning of the assessment process. Unfortunately, some assessment teams see a survey or assessment as the end of their efforts instead of the means of the beginning of a new revelation for healthcare planning. The completion of the assessments also marks the beginning of the next phase of the change effort. The planning process must begin again. The community mental health professional can serve as a facilitator to guide the community and health team through a review of the findings and the group's vision, formulating a statement of the problems that have been identified and generating solutions and a plan of action that uses existing strengths in the community.

Assigning Value to Program Activities

When addressing the value of a program, questions regarding values generally involve three interrelated issues: merit (i.e., quality), worth (i.e., cost effectiveness), and significance (i.e., importance) (Scriven, 1998; Shadish, Cook, & Leviton, 1991). When judging if a program is meritorious, questions regarding the cost and worth of the program might arise. Questions can also arise concerning whether or not valuable programs contribute important differences.

When developing a program evaluation, several questions must be addressed: What will be evaluated? (That is, what is the program offering, and in what context does the program exist in the community?) What viewpoint of the program will be considered when critiquing program performance? What standards, goals, and objectives (i.e., type or level of performance) must be reached for the program to be considered successful? What type of evidence will be used to indicate how the program has performed over time? What conclusions regarding the program's performance are acceptable when comparing the available evidence to the selected standards? How will the lessons learned from the investigation be used to improve public program effectiveness? Addressing these questions among others at the beginning of a program evaluation is important. These questions should be reassessed throughout implementation of the program evaluation. The framework described in the next section provides a systematic approach for answering these questions.

EVALUATING COMMUNITY MENTAL HEALTH PROGRAMS

Community mental health officials often find themselves under pressure to evaluate and validate the need for mental health promotion programs. Demands can stem from administrative requirements, funding sources, or a board of directors. Community health officials often view the evaluation process as daunting, directing funds, time, and energy away from program delivery and having little benefit to the program. For an evaluation to be useful, the results must be considered when decisions are made to model a new direction for the program. Evaluation can be tied to routine business operations when the emphasis is on practical ongoing evaluation that involves all program staff and stakeholders. Public health professionals have routinely used the evaluation processes to answer questions from concerned individuals, the community, and consulting partners (Love, 1991).

These evaluation processes are adequate for ongoing program assessment to guide small changes to improve program functions and objectives. However, when the stakes of potential decisions or program changes increase (e.g., when deciding what services to offer for a national health promotion program), employing evaluation procedures that are explicit, formal, and justifiable becomes important (Sanders, 1993).

Framework for Program Evaluation in Public Health

Effective program evaluation is a systematic approach to improve and account for public health and community mental health actions by involving procedures that yield useful, feasible, ethical, and accurate findings. The recommended framework used in this text was developed to guide public health professionals in using program evaluation. The approach is a practical, nonprescriptive tool, designed to summarize and organize the essential elements of program evaluation (see **Figure 13-2**) (CDC, 1999; Scriven, 1998).

The public health framework for program evaluation is composed of six steps. The steps can be tailored to any evaluation or to a particular public health endeavor. The steps are all interdependent; thus they might be encountered in a nonlinear sequence. Each step builds the foundation for subsequent steps in the framework. Decisions considered on how to execute a step should not be finalized until all previous steps have been thoroughly addressed. The steps are as follows:

Step 1: Engage stakeholders in the evaluation.
Step 2: Provide a program description.
Step 3: Focus the evaluation design.

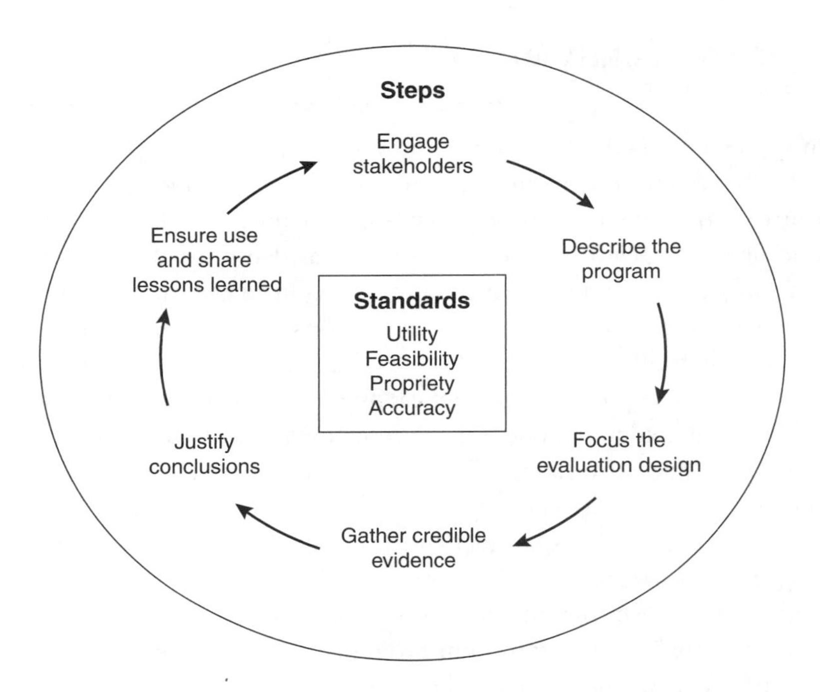

FIGURE 13-2 Recommended Framework for Program Evaluation
Source: Centers for Disease Control and Prevention. (1999). Framework for program evaluation in public health. *Morbidity and Mortality Weekly Report*, *48*(No. RR-11).

Step 4: Collect credible evidence.
Step 5: Validate conclusions.
Step 6: Ensure use and communicate lessons learned.

Following the six steps presented in this framework will facilitate an understanding of a program's context (e.g., the program's history, setting, and organization) and can help improve how most evaluations are conceived and conducted. The second element of the framework includes 30 standards for assessing program evaluation activities and quality. The standards are organized into the following four groups:

Standard 1: Utility
Standard 2: Feasibility
Standard 3: Propriety
Standard 4: Accuracy

These four standards are adopted from the Joint Committee on Standards for Educational Evaluation (1994). They are approved by the American National Standards Institute (ANSI) and endorsed by the American Evaluation Association as well as 14 other professional organizations (ANSI Standard No. JSEE-PR 1994, Approved March 15, 1994).

Steps in Program Evaluation

Step 1: Engaging Stakeholders in the Evaluation Process

To be successful, the evaluation cycle begins by engaging stakeholders. Stakeholders are persons or organizations that have an investment in the outcome of the evaluation. Stakeholders must be engaged in the inquiry to ensure that their perspectives and information needs are understood.

Stakeholders involved in the evaluation process must ensure that the three principal stakeholder groups are represented in the evaluation : (1) individuals involved in program operations (e.g., sponsors, collaborators, coalition partners, funding officials, administrators, managers, and staff); (2) those served or influenced by the program (e.g., clients, family members, neighborhood organizations, academic institutions, elected officials, advocacy groups, professional associations, opponents, and staff of related or competing organizations); and (3) primary users of the evaluation outcomes such as policymakers and healthcare officials.

Primary users of the program evaluation findings are in decision-making roles. In practice, primary users are a subset of all stakeholders identified. To conduct a successful evaluation, primary users should be designated early in the process. In addition, it is important to maintain frequent contact with the stakeholders during the evaluation process to make certain the evaluation addresses their unique informational needs (1997a).

The scope and level of stakeholder involvement in the evaluation process will vary for each program evaluation. Various activities reflect the requirement to engage stakeholders in the evaluation process as demonstrated in **Box 13-2** (CDC, 1997). For example, they should be involved directly in designing and conducting the evaluation and be informed concerning the progress of the evaluation through periodic meetings, reports, and other means of communication. Shared governance and resolving conflicts together helps avoid overemphasis of values held by any specific stakeholder (Mertens, 1999).

BOX 13-2 Engaging Stakeholders

Definition

Fostering input, participation, and power-sharing among those persons who have an investment in the conduct of the evaluation and the findings; it is especially important to engage primary users of the evaluation.

Role

Helps increase chances that the evaluation will be useful; can improve the evaluation's credibility, clarify roles and responsibilities, enhance cultural competence, help protect human subjects, and avoid real or perceived conflicts of interest.

- Consulting insiders (e.g., leaders, staff, clients, and program funding sources) and outsiders (e.g., skeptics);
- Taking special effort to promote the inclusion of less powerful groups or individuals;
- Coordinating stakeholder input throughout the process of evaluation design, operation, and use; and
- Avoiding excessive stakeholder identification, which might prevent progress of the evaluation.

Source: Centers for Disease Control and Prevention. (1999). Framework for program evaluation in public health. *Morbidity and Mortality Weekly Report, 48*(No. RR-11).

Step 2: Describing the Program

Program descriptions express the mission, goals, and objectives of the program being evaluated as shown in **Box 13-3**. The description should be detailed to ensure understanding of program goals and strategies. The description should also address the program's capacity to effect change, its stage of program development, and how the program fits into the organization and community. Program descriptions set the frame of reference for all subsequent decisions in an evaluation. The description allows comparisons with similar programs and facilitates attempts to connect program components to their effects (Joint Committee on Standards for Educational Evaluation, 1994).

Evaluations completed without an agreement of the program definition are less likely to be beneficial. At times, negotiating with stakeholders to formulate a clear and logical program description before data are collected to evaluate program effectiveness will benefit the evaluation results (1997a). Features to include in a program description are need, expected effects, activities, resources, stage of development, context, and logic model. Each component is explained in detail here.

BOX 13-3 Examples of Activities Describing the Program

Definition
Scrutinizing the features of the program being evaluated, including its purpose and place in a larger context. Description includes information regarding the way the program was intended to function and the way that it actually was implemented. Also includes features of the program's context that are likely to influence conclusions regarding the program.

Role
Improves evaluation's fairness and accuracy; permits a balanced assessment of strengths and weaknesses and helps stakeholders understand how program features fit together and relate to a larger context.

- Characterizing the need (or set of needs) addressed by the program;
- Listing specific expectations as goals, objectives, and criteria for success;
- Clarifying why program activities are believed to lead to expected changes;
- Drawing an explicit logic model to illustrate relationships between program elements and expected changes;
- Assessing the program's maturity or stage of development;
- Analyzing the context within which the program operates;
- Considering how the program is linked to other ongoing efforts; and
- Avoiding creation of an overly precise description for a program that is under development.

Source: Centers for Disease Control and Prevention. (1999). Framework for program evaluation in public health. *Morbidity and Mortality Weekly Report, 48*(No. RR-11).

A *statement* of need expresses the problem that the program addresses and implies how the program proposes to respond to a problem. Important features for defining a program's statement of need include (1) the nature and magnitude of the problem, (2) which populations are affected, (3) if the need is changing, and (4) what approach will be taken to change identified needs. In addition to a statement of need, the program should include descriptions of the outcomes that must be accomplished to consider the assessment successful (i.e., program effects). For some programs, the effects develop over time; for that reason, the descriptions of expectations should be organized by time, ranging from specific (i.e., immediate) to broad (i.e., long-term) consequences. The program's mission, goals, and objectives all represent varying levels of specificity regarding the program's outcomes. Describing program activities is also key to program evaluation (i.e., what the program does to effect change). It permits specific steps, strategies, or actions to be displayed in logical sequence. Arranging the program activities in a logical manner demonstrates how each program activity relates to another and clarifies the program's hypothesized mechanism or theory of change (Chen, 1990; Connell & Kubisch, 1998).

Program resources should define the amount and intensity of program services offered in the community and highlight situations where a disparity exists between desired program activities and available resources to execute program activities. Economic evaluations require an awareness of all direct and indirect program inputs, capital, and costs (CDC, 1992; Gold, Russell, Siegel, & Weinstein, 1996; Haddix, Teutsch, Shaffer, & Duñet, 1996).

Most public health programs advance and change over time; as a result, a program's stage of development reflects its growth and development. Programs that have recently received start-up funding will differ from those that have been operating continuously for a long period. The growth of a program should be considered during the evaluation process (Eoyang & Berkas, 1999). At least three stages of development should be recognized: planning, implementation, and effects. During the planning phase, program activities are untested, and the goal of evaluation is to refine the program plans. During the implementation phase, the program activities are field-tested and modified; the goal of the evaluation is to characterize actual, as opposed to ideal, program activities and components as well as to improve program operations, by revising program plans. During the last stage of the evaluation, the program's effects should emerge; the goal of the evaluation is to identify and account for both intended and unintended effects.

Following the program effects, the evaluation should address the program's context. The components assessed should include the setting and environmental influences (e.g., history, geography, politics, social and economic conditions, and efforts of related or competing programs) in the program's geographic area of operation (Worthen, Sanders, & Fitzpatrick, 1996). Understanding these environmental influences is required to design a context-sensitive evaluation and aid users in interpreting findings accurately and assessing the generalizability of the findings.

Logic models are also used in program evaluation as depicted in **Figure 13-3**. A logic model describes the sequence of events for bringing about change in a program by synthesizing the main program elements into a picture of how the program is intended to work (Julian, 1997; Rossing & Geran, 1998; Rush & Ogbourne, 1991; Scriven, 1998; Taylor-Powell & Weiss, 1997). The logic model is displayed in a flow chart, map, or table to portray the sequence of steps leading to program results (Figure 13-3A–C). A quality of a logic model is the ability to summarize the overall program's mechanism of change by linking processes (e.g., laboratory diagnosis of disease and noncompliance with psychotropic medication to anticipated effects [e.g., reduced tuberculosis incidence in a mental health shelter and decreased manic occurrences or depression in a person with bipolar disease]). The logic model also can display the infrastructure needed to support program operations. Elements connected within a logic model vary. Generally, the elements include inputs (e.g., trained staff), activities (e.g., identification of cases), outputs (e.g., persons completing treatment), and results ranging from immediate (e.g., curing affected persons or providing mental health counseling) intermediate (e.g., reduction in tuberculosis rate or depression) to long-term effects (e.g., improvement of population health status).

Creating a logic model allows stakeholders to clarify the program's strategies; therefore, including the evaluation process in the logic model can improve and better focus the program direction. The logic model also reveals assumptions concerning conditions for program effectiveness and provides a frame of reference for evaluating the program in the future. A detailed logic model also can strengthen claims of causality and be a basis for estimating program effects on end points that are not directly measured but are linked in a causal chain supported by prior research (Lipsey, 1993).

A variety of logic models can be created to display a program at different levels of detail, from different perspectives, or for different audiences. Program descriptions vary for each evaluation, and various activities reflect the requirement to describe the program (e.g., using multiple sources of information to construct a well-rounded description) as shown in Box 13-3. The accuracy of a program description can be confirmed by consulting with diverse stakeholders, and reported descriptions of program practice can be validated against direct observation of activities in the field. A narrow program description can be improved by addressing such factors as staff turnover, inadequate resources, political pressures, or strong community participation that might affect program performance.

Step 3: Targeting the Evaluation Design

This step entails making sure that the stakeholder's needs are being met. The evaluation as shown in **Box 13-4** is targeted to assess the areas of greatest concern and should meet the information needs of stakeholders. The items that should be considered when targeting the focus of an evaluation are purpose, users, uses, questions, methods, and agreements.

Verbalizing the purpose (i.e., intent) of an evaluation before it begins prevents premature decision making regarding how the evaluation is conducted. Four purposes of evaluation exist in public health, which are described in the following paragraphs.

The first purpose is to gain insight into the program, for example, assessing the feasibility of an innovative new approach to community mental health practice. Knowledge from the evaluation provides information concerning the practicality of

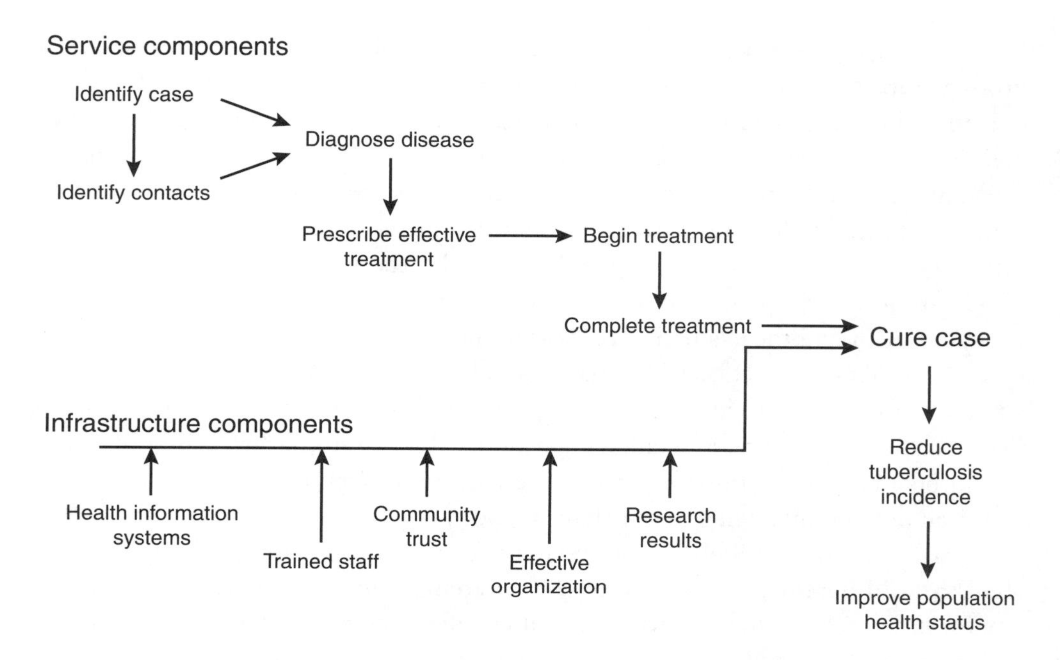

FIGURE 13-3A Logic Model for a Tuberculosis Case
Source: Adapted from Centers for Disease Control and Prevention. (1999). Framework for program evaluation in public health. *Morbidity and Mortality Weekly Report*, *48*(No. RR-11).

a new approach, which can be used to design a program that will be tested for its effectiveness. A developing program, for example, can review prior evaluations to provide insight and clarify how the program activities should be designed to bring about expected changes and desired outcomes.

A second purpose for program evaluation is to change or improve practice. Evaluations assessing practice usually occur in the implementation stage of the program. The evaluation seeks to describe what the program has accomplished and to what extent. The gathered information is used to better describe the program processes, improve how the program operates, and to perfect the overall program strategy. Evaluations carried out for this purpose include efforts to improve the quality, effectiveness, or efficiency of program activities.

A third purpose for program evaluation is to assess program effects. Evaluations completed to assess the effects of a program examine the relationship between program activities and observed outcomes. Outcome evaluations are appropriate for programs that can define what type of interventions were delivered to what proportion

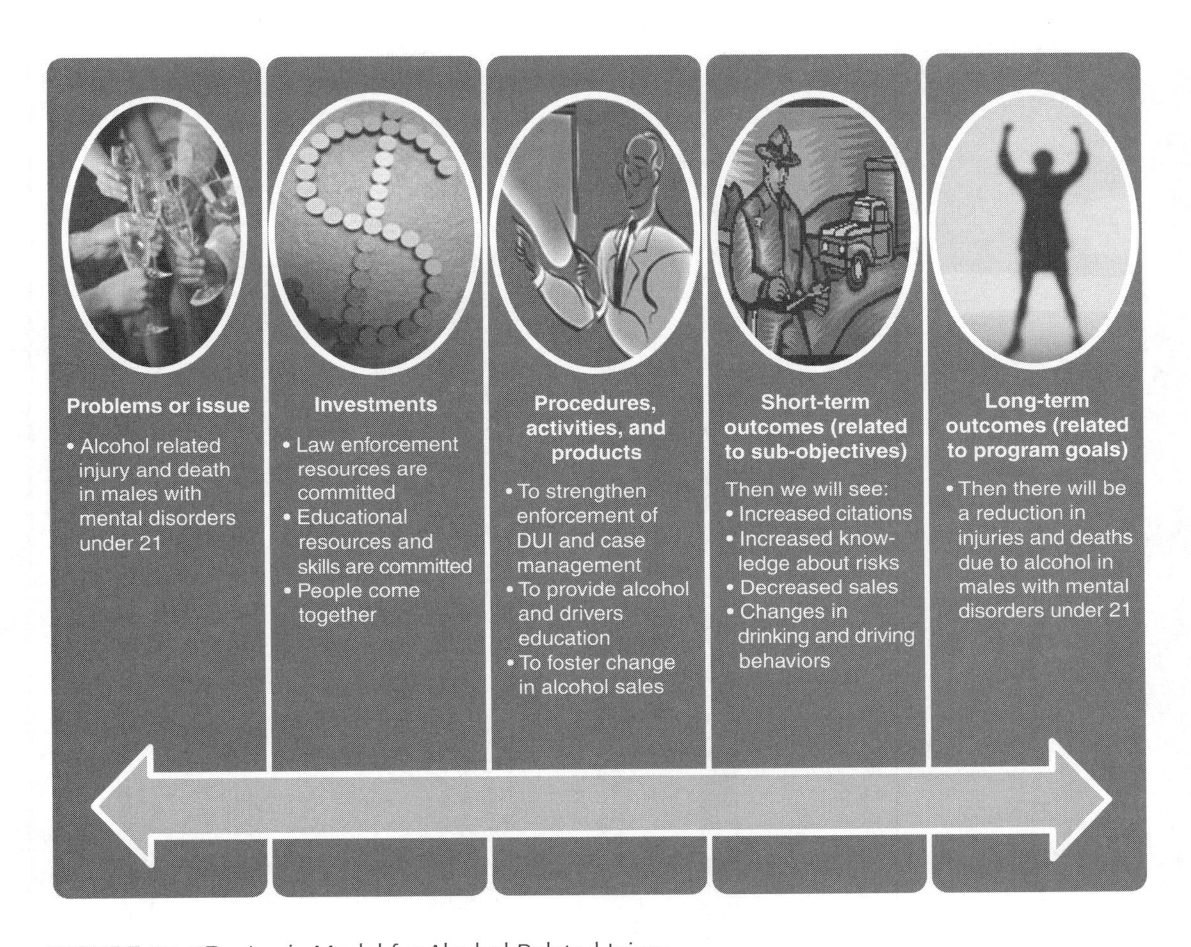

FIGURE 13-3B Logic Model for Alcohol-Related Injury
Source: Adapted from Centers for Disease Control and Prevention. (1999). Framework for program evaluation in public health. *Morbidity and Mortality Weekly Report, 48*(No. RR-11).

of the target population. Knowing where to find potential program effects can ensure that significant effects are not overlooked. Effects might arise from a direct cause-and-effect relationship of the program. Through the evaluation, evidence can be found to attribute the effects exclusively to the program. In addition, effects might arise from a causal process involving issues of contribution as well as attribution. For example, if a mental health case management to increase medication adherence activities is aligned with that of another program operating in the same setting, certain effects (e.g., a drug treatment program) cannot be attributed solely to one program or another. In

The VERB™ Campaign Logic Model: A Tool for Planning and Evaluation

Parental support occurs through verbal recognition and praise and through direct support, such as paying for an activity, transporting a child to and from a physical activity event, and attending that event. It also includes participating with the child in physical activity.

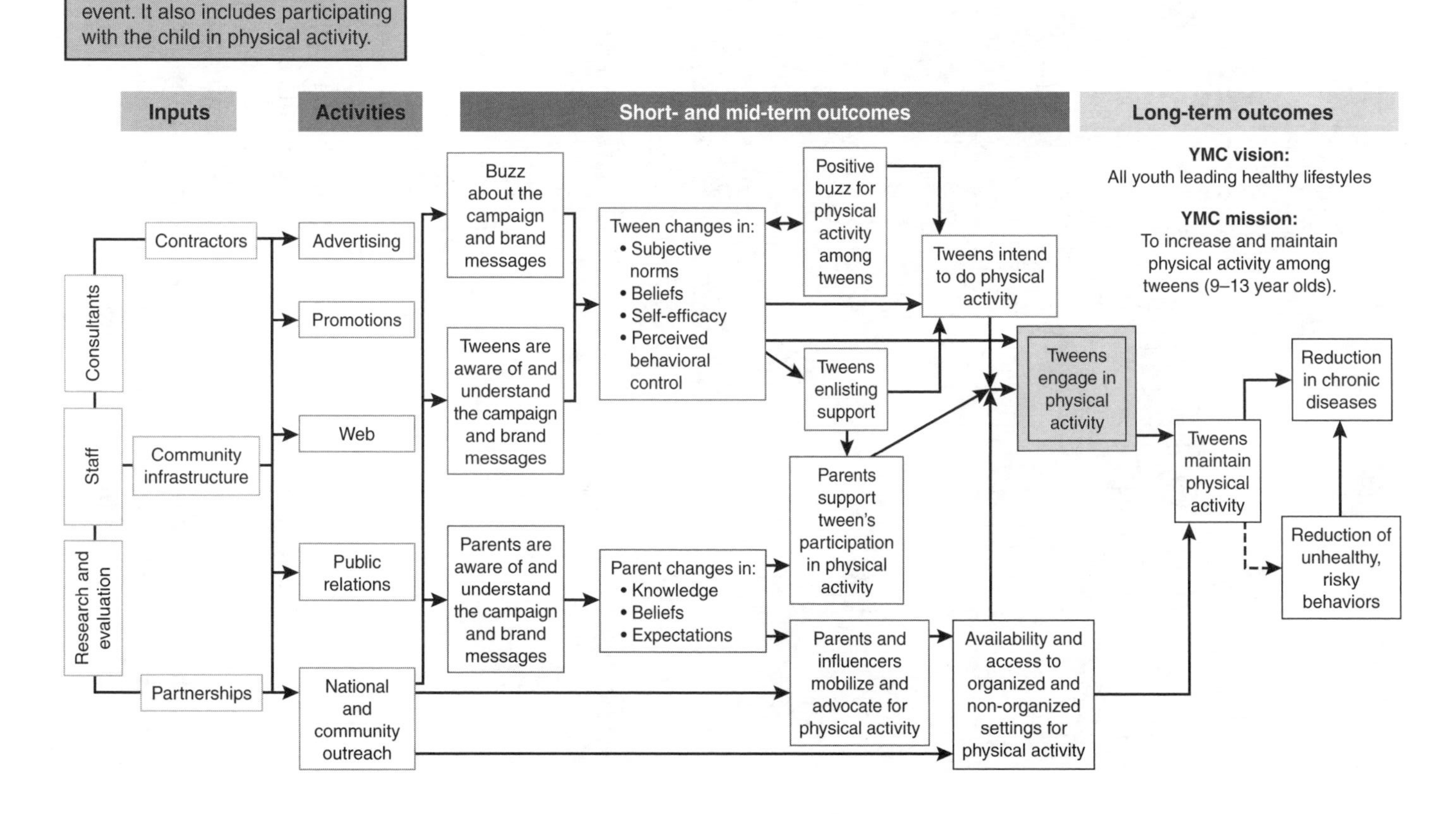

VERB Campaign Vision: All youth leading healthy lifestyles.
VERB Campaign Mission: To increase and maintain physical activity among tweens (children aged nine to 13 years).

The *inputs* of the campaign are:

- Consultants
- Staff
- Research and evaluation
- Contractors
- Community infrastructure
- Partnerships

All *inputs* contribute to campaign *activities*. Campaign activities include:

- Advertising
- Promotions
- Web
- Public relations
- National and community outreach

All *activities* lead to short-term outcomes for both tween and parent audiences. The short-term outcome for the campaign is tween and parent awareness of and buzz about the campaign brand and its messages. Awareness and buzz lead to mid-term outcomes, which include changes in:

- Subjective norms
- Beliefs
- Self-efficacy
- Perceived behavioral control

The logic indicates that if these changes occur, *positive buzz* will be created among tweens about physical activity. Tweens will enlist support from their parents and generate intentions to take part in physical activity.

Awareness and understanding of the campaign and brand messages by parents lead to changes for parents in *knowledge*, *beliefs*, and *expectations*.

The logic indicates that if these changes take place among parents, and if tweens are enlisting their parents' support, parents will support tweens' participation in physical activity, and *parents and influencers will mobilize and advocate for physical activity*.

The mobilization of parents and influencers and advocacy for physical activity as well as national and community outreach lead to the *availability and access to organized and non-organized settings for physical activity*.

Tweens' behavioral intention as well as parent support and available and accessible settings are likely to result in tweens engaging in physical activity.

The *long-term outcomes* include tweens engaging in and maintaining physical activity, thereby reducing chronic diseases. The model also indicates a possible displacement strategy: tweens who participate in physical activity may also have a *reduction of unhealthy, risky behavior*.

PREVENTING CHRONIC DISEASE
PUBLIC HEALTH RESEARCH, PRACTICE, AND POLICY
Volume 1: No. 3, July 2004

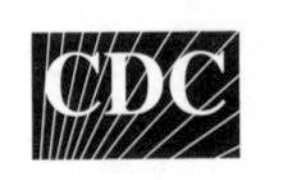

FIGURE 13-3C Logic Model: The VERB Model
Source: Centers for Disease Control and Prevention. (2004). Preventing chronic disease. *Public Health Research, Practice, and Policy, 1*(3).

BOX 13-4 Selected Uses for Evaluation in Public Health Practice by Category of Purpose: Gain Insight

- Assess needs, desires, and assets of community members.
- Identify barriers and facilitators to service use.
- Learn how to describe and measure program activities and effects.
- Change practice.
- Refine plans for introducing a new service.
- Characterize the extent to which intervention plans were implemented.
- Improve the content of educational materials.
- Enhance the program's cultural competence.
- Verify that participants' rights are protected.
- Set priorities for staff training.
- Make midcourse adjustments to improve patient/client flow.
- Improve the clarity of health communication messages.
- Determine if customer satisfaction rates can be improved.
- Mobilize community support for the program.
- Assess effects.
- Assess skills development by program participants.
- Compare changes in provider behavior over time.
- Compare costs with benefits.
- Find out which participants do well in the program.
- Decide where to allocate new resources.
- Document the level of success in accomplishing objectives.
- Demonstrate that accountability requirements are fulfilled.
- Aggregate information from several evaluations to estimate outcome effects for similar kinds of programs.
- Gather success stories.
- Affect participants.
- Reinforce intervention messages.
- Stimulate dialogue and raise awareness regarding health issues.
- Broaden consensus among coalition members regarding program goals.
- Teach evaluation skills to staff and other stakeholders.
- Support organizational change and development.

Source: Centers for Disease Control and Prevention. (1999). Framework for Program Evaluation in Public Health. *Morbidity and Mortality Weekly Report*, *48*(No. RR-11).

such situations, the goal for evaluation is to gather credible evidence that describes each program's contribution in the combined change. Establishing accountability for program results is predicated on the ability to conduct evaluations that assess both of these kinds of effects.

A fourth purpose of program evaluation applies at any stage of program development. It involves using the evaluation process to affect those who participate in the inquiry. An evaluation can be initiated with the intent of generating a positive influence on stakeholders. Such influences might be to supplement the program intervention (e.g., using a follow-up questionnaire to reinforce program messages); empower program participants (e.g., increasing a client's sense of control over the program's direction); promote staff development (e.g., teaching staff how to collect, analyze, and interpret evidence); contribute to organizational growth (e.g., clarifying how the program relates to the organization's mission); or facilitate social transformation (e.g., advancing a community's struggle for self-determination) (Fetterman, Kaftarian, & Wandersman, 1996; Patton, 1997b; Wandersman et al., 1998).

Users of the evaluation are the specific persons who will receive evaluation findings. The intended users directly experience the consequences of unavoidable design exchanges; therefore, they should participate in selecting the evaluation focus (Patton, 1997a). User involvement in the evaluation process is required for clarifying intended uses, information needed, methods used, and preventing the evaluation from becoming misguided or irrelevant.

The methods essential for program evaluation drawn from scientific research options, particularly those developed in the social, behavioral, and health sciences (Bickman & Rog, 1998; Cook & Reichardt, 1979; Patton, 1990, 1997a; Rossi, Freeman, & Lipsey, 1999; Trochim, 1999; Weiss, 1998a; Worthen et al., 1996), are discussed in the following section. A classification of design types includes experimental, quasi-experimental, and observational designs.

Evaluation methods should be selected to provide the appropriate information to address stakeholders' questions. For example, experimental designs use random assignment to compare the effect of an intervention with otherwise equivalent groups (Boruch, 1998). Quasi-experimental methods, in contrast, compare nonequivalent groups (e.g., program participants versus those on a waiting list) or a variety of data to set up a comparison (e.g., interrupted time series) (Cook &Campbell, 1979; Reichardt & Mark, 1998). Observational methods use comparisons within a group to explain unique features of the members (e.g., comparative case studies or cross-sectional surveys) (Patton, 1990; Yin, 1994, 1998). Various activities are required to focus the evaluation design, as shown in **Box 13-5**.

BOX 13-5 Focusing the Evaluation Design

Definition

Planning in advance where the evaluation is headed and what steps will be taken; process is iterative (i.e., it continues until a focused approach is found to answer evaluation questions with methods that stakeholders agree will be useful, feasible, ethical, and accurate); evaluation questions and methods might be adjusted to achieve an optimal match that facilitates use by primary users.

Role

Provides investment in quality; increases the chances that the evaluation will succeed by identifying procedures that are practical, politically viable, and cost effective; failure to plan thoroughly can be self-defeating, leading to an evaluation that might become impractical or useless; when stakeholders agree on a design focus, it is used throughout the evaluation process to keep the project on track.

Examples of Activities

- Meeting with stakeholders to clarify the intent or purpose of the evaluation;
- Learning which persons are in a position to actually use the findings and then orienting the plan to meet their needs;
- Understanding how the evaluation results are to be used;
- Writing explicit evaluation questions to be answered;
- Describing practical methods for sampling, data collection, data analysis, interpretation, and judgment;
- Preparing a written protocol or agreement that summarizes the evaluation procedures, with clear roles and responsibilities for all stakeholders; and
- Revising parts or all of the evaluation plan when critical circumstances change.

Source: Centers for Disease Control and Prevention. (1999). Framework for program evaluation in public health. *Morbidity and Mortality Weekly Report*, *48*(No. RR-11).

All interested parties should be consulted to ensure that the proposed evaluation questions are politically feasible (i.e., responsive to the varied positions of interest groups). A list of options of potential evaluation uses appropriate for the program's stage of development and context could be circulated among stakeholders to determine which is most compelling.

Step 4: Collection of Credible Evidence

The ultimate goal of the evaluation is to collect information that will provide a snapshot of the program so the evaluation's primary users see the information as credible, reasonable, and relevant for answering the evaluation questions. At this point of the evaluation, stakeholders must decide on the measurements, indicators, sources of evidence, quality, and quality of evidence, and method of collecting the data.

Having credible evidence strengthens evaluation results and the recommendations. Even though all types of data have limitations, an evaluation's overall credibility can be improved by using multiple procedures for gathering, analyzing, and interpreting data. Encouraging participation by stakeholders also can enhance perceived credibility.

Step 5: Validating Conclusions

- Conclusions of the evaluation are validated when they are linked to the evidence gathered and concluded against the agreed-upon values and standards set by the stakeholders. Stakeholders must agree that conclusions are validated before they will use the evaluation findings with confidence. Validating conclusions on the basis of evidence includes standards, analysis and synthesis, interpretation, judgment, and recommendations.
- Standards reflect the values held by stakeholders. Values provide the basis for forming judgments concerning the program's performance. In practice, when stakeholders define and negotiate their values, they become the standards for judging whether a given program's performance will be considered successful, adequate, or unsuccessful. A collection of value systems might serve as a source of norm-referenced or criterion-referenced standards (**Box 13-6**).
- Analysis and synthesis of findings of an evaluation might detect patterns in evidence, either by isolating important findings (analysis) or by combining sources of information to reach a larger understanding (synthesis). Mixed method evaluations require the separate analysis of each evidence element and a synthesis of all sources for examining patterns of agreement, convergence (reaching a common point of view), or complexity (co-presence of attributes in society). Interpreting facts from a body of evidence involves making a decision how to organize, classify, interrelate, compare, and display information (Patton, 1997b). Guided by the questions asked, the types of data available and input from stakeholders and primary users direct the final decision.
- Interpretation of the data is the effort of figuring out what the findings mean and is part of the overall effort to understand the evidence gathered in an evaluation (Rogers & Hough, 1995). Uncovering the facts regarding a program's performance is not sufficient to draw evaluative conclusions, because evaluation evidence must first be interpreted to determine the practical significance

BOX 13-6 Selected Sources of Standards for Judging Program Performance

- Needs of participants;
- Community values, expectations, norms;
- Degree of participation;
- Program objectives;
- Program protocols and procedures;
- Expected performance, forecasts, estimates;
- Feasibility;
- Sustainability;
- Absence of harms;
- Targets or fixed criteria of performance;
- Change in performance over time;
- Performance by previous or similar programs;
- Performance by a control or comparison group;
- Resource efficiency;
- Professional standards;
- Mandates, policies, statutes, regulations, laws;
- Judgments by reference groups (e.g., participants, staff, experts, and funding officials);
- Institutional goals;
- Political ideology;
- Social equity;
- Political will; and
- Human rights.

Source: Centers for Disease Control and Prevention (1999). Framework for program evaluation in public health. *Morbidity and Mortality Weekly Report, 48*(No. RR-11).

of what has been learned. Interpretations must draw on information and perspectives that are brought to the evaluation inquiry and can be strengthened through active participation or interaction.

- Judgments made by evaluators based on the data from a needs assessment are accounts concerning the merit, value, or significance of the program. The judgments are formed by comparing the findings and interpretations of the program against standards in community mental health like *Healthy People 2015*, Cultural Competence Standards in Managed Care Mental Health Services: Four Underserved/Underrepresented Racial/Ethnic Groups, and Mental Health America Standards for Affiliates. Standards can be applied to any given program element. For example, program managers using a standard of improved performance over time might judge positively a program that increases its outreach by 10% from the previous year. However, community members might feel that despite improvements, a minimum threshold of access to services has not been reached. Moreover, conflicting claims regarding a program's quality, value, or importance often indicate that stakeholders might be using different standards of judgment. In the context of an evaluation, such disagreement can be a catalyst for clarifying relevant values and for negotiating the appropriate bases on which the program should be judged.

Forming recommendations is a distinct element of program evaluation that requires information beyond what is necessary to form a judgment regarding program performance (Scriven, 1998). Having the knowledge that a program is able to reduce homelessness among the mentally ill does not automatically translate into a recommendation to continue the effort, particularly when competing priorities or other effective program alternatives exist. Recommendations for continuing, expanding, redesigning, or terminating a program are based on a different viewpoint from judgments regarding the program's effectiveness. More important, recommendations that lack sufficient evidence or those that are not aligned with stakeholders' values can undermine an evaluation's credibility. Alternatively, an evaluation can be strengthened by recommendations that anticipate the political sensitivities of intended users and highlight areas that users can control or influence (1997b).

Various activities for validating conclusions in an evaluation are displayed in **Box 13-7**. Conclusions of an assessment can be strengthened by (1) summarizing the plausible mechanisms of change; (2) delineating the temporal sequence between activities and effects; (3) searching for alternative explanations and showing why they are unsupported by the evidence; and (4) showing that the effects can be repeated. When different but equally well-supported conclusions exist, each should be presented with a summary of the strengths and weaknesses.

Finally, creative techniques, for example, the **Delphi process**, allow all stakeholders or members of a community group to communicate to generate ideas, establish consensus for dealing with complex problems, and assign value judgments (Adler & Ziglio, 1996). Techniques for analyzing, synthesizing, and interpreting findings should be agreed on before data collection begins to ensure that all necessary evidence will be available.

Step 6: Ensuring Use and Reporting Lessons Learned

The final stage of the evaluation process focuses on the lessons learned summarized in **Box 13-8**. The final stage of the evaluation is an effort needed to ensure that the evaluation processes and findings are used and disseminated appropriately. Five elements

BOX 13-7 Justifying Conclusions

Definition
Making claims regarding the program that are warranted on the basis of data that have been compared against pertinent and defensible ideas of merit, worth, or significance (i.e., against standards of values); conclusions are justified when they are linked to the evidence gathered and consistent with the agreed on values or standards of stakeholders.

Role
Reinforces conclusions central to the evaluation's utility and accuracy; involves values clarification, qualitative and quantitative data analysis and synthesis, systematic interpretation, and appropriate comparison against relevant standards for judgment.

Examples of Activities

- Using appropriate methods of analysis and synthesis to summarize findings;
- Interpreting the significance of results for deciding what the findings mean;
- Making judgments according to clearly stated values that classify a result (e.g., as positive or negative and high or low);
- Considering alternative ways to compare results (e.g., compared with program objectives, a comparison group, national norms, past performance, or needs);
- Generating alternative explanations for findings and indicating why these explanations should or should not be discounted;
- Recommending actions or decisions that are consistent with the conclusions; and
- Limiting conclusions to situations, time periods, persons, contexts, and purposes for which the findings are applicable.

Source: Centers for Disease Control and Prevention. (1999). Framework for program evaluation in public health. *Morbidity and Mortality Weekly Report, 48*(No. RR-11).

critical to ensure appropriate evaluation findings are used for decision making are as follows: design, preparation, feedback, follow-up, and dissemination.

Designing the evaluation refers to how the evaluation's questions, methods, and overall processes are assembled. As discussed in the third step of this framework, organizing the design of the evaluation should start in the developmental stage in order to achieve the intended outcome. Establishing a clear purposeful design helps to know how to use the findings, who will benefit from participating in the evaluation process, and who will use the results.

Evaluation results are often presented orally to stakeholders and sometimes at conferences. Primary users and other stakeholders could be given a set of hypothetical results and asked to explain what decisions or actions they would make based on the

BOX 13-8 Ensuring Use and Sharing Lessons Learned

Definition
Ensuring that (1) stakeholders are aware of the evaluation procedures and findings; (2) the findings are considered in decisions or actions that affect the program (i.e., findings use); and (3) those who participated in the evaluation have had a beneficial experience (i.e., process use).

Role
Ensures that evaluation achieves its primary purpose—being useful; however, several factors might influence the degree of use, including evaluator credibility, report clarity, report timeliness and dissemination, disclosure of findings, impartial reporting, and changes in the program or organization context.

Examples of Activities

- Designing the evaluation to achieve intended use by intended users;
- Preparing stakeholders for eventual use by rehearsing throughout the project how different kinds of conclusions would affect program operations;
- Providing continuous feedback to stakeholders regarding interim findings, provisional interpretations, and decisions to be made that might affect likelihood of use;
- Scheduling follow-up meetings with intended users to facilitate the transfer of evaluation conclusions into appropriate actions or decisions; and
- Disseminating both the procedures used and the lessons learned from the evaluation to stakeholders, using tailored communications strategies that meet their particular needs.

Source: Centers for Disease Control and Prevention. (1999). Framework for program evaluation in public health. *Morbidity and Mortality Weekly Report, 48*(No. RR-11).

new knowledge. Preparing to use the data and sharing the outcome also gives stakeholders time to explore positive and negative implications of potential results and time to identify options for program improvement.

Follow-up refers to the technical and emotional support that users need during the evaluation process and after receiving the evaluation findings. It is important that follow-up stay active to remind intended users of the planned use of the findings. Follow-up might also be required to prevent lessons learned from becoming lost or ignored in the process of making complex or politically sensitive decisions.

Program evaluation results are always bound by the context in which the evaluation was conducted. Results taken out of context or used for purposes other than those agreed is unethical. For instance, inappropriately generalizing the evaluation findings from a single case study to make decisions that affect programs on a national level would constitute misuse of the case study evaluation. Similarly, a program can be undermined if the results are misused by overemphasizing negative findings without giving regard to the program's positive attributes. Finally, careful consideration should be given for disseminating or communicating polices and procedures or the lessons learned from the evaluation to relevant audiences in a timely, unbiased, and consistent fashion. Like all other elements of the evaluation, the reporting strategy should be discussed in advance with intended users and other stakeholders. Planning effective communication also requires considering the timing, style, tone, message source, vehicle, and format of information products. The goal for dissemination of the report is to achieve full disclosure of the evaluation. A checklist of items to consider when developing evaluation reports includes tailoring the report content for the audience, explaining the focus of the evaluation and its limitations, and listing both the strengths and weaknesses of the evaluation (**Box 13-9**) (Worthen et al., 1996).

BOX 13-9 Checklist for Ensuring Effective Evaluation Reports

- Provide interim and final reports to intended users in time for use.
- Tailor the report content, format, and style for the audience(s) by involving audience members.
- Include a summary.
- Summarize the description of the stakeholders and how they were engaged.
- Describe essential features of the program (e.g., including logic models).
- Explain the focus of the evaluation and its limitations.
- Include an adequate summary of the evaluation plan and procedures.
- Provide all necessary technical information (e.g., in appendices).
- Specify the standards and criteria for evaluative judgments.
- Explain the evaluative judgments and how they are supported by the evidence.
- List both strengths and weaknesses of the evaluation.
- Discuss recommendations for action with their advantages, disadvantages, and resource implications.
- Ensure protections for program clients and other stakeholders.
- Anticipate how people or organizations might be affected by the findings.
- Present minority opinions or rejoinders where necessary.
- Verify that the report is accurate and unbiased.
- Organize the report logically and include appropriate details.
- Remove technical jargon.
- Use examples, illustrations, graphics, and stories.

Source: Centers for Disease Control and Prevention. (1999). Framework for program evaluation in public health. *Morbidity and Mortality Weekly Report*, *48*(No. RR-11).

Engagement in the logic, reasoning, and values of the evaluation can lead to lasting impacts (e.g., basing decisions on systematic judgments instead of on unfounded assumptions) (Patton, 1997a). Additional process uses for evaluation includes defining indicators to discover what matters to decision makers and making outcomes matter by changing the structural reinforcements connected with outcome attainment (e.g., by paying outcome dividends to programs that save money through their prevention efforts) (Fawcett et al., 2001).

Standards for Effective Evaluation

Community mental health professionals will recognize that the basic steps in the framework presented for program evaluation are part of their routine work. In day-to-day public health practice, stakeholders are consulted; program goals are defined; guiding questions are stated; data are collected, analyzed, and interpreted; judgments are formed; and lessons are shared. Even though an informal evaluation occurs through routine clinical practice and healthcare delivery, standards exist to consider whether a set of evaluative activities are well designed and working to their capability. The Joint Committee on Standards for Educational Evaluation (1994) has developed program evaluation standards for this purpose. These standards, designed to assess evaluations of educational programs, are relevant for public health programs as well. The American Evaluation Association, an international professional association of evaluators, also has developed guiding principles for evaluators, as follows:

- Systematic inquiry: Evaluators conduct systematic, data-based inquiries.
- Competence: Evaluators provide competent performance to stakeholders.
- Integrity/Honesty: Evaluators display honesty and integrity in their own behavior, and they attempt to ensure the honesty and integrity of the entire evaluation process.
- Respect for people: Evaluators respect the security, dignity, and self-worth of respondents, program participants, clients, and other evaluation stakeholders.
- Responsibilities for general and public welfare: Evaluators articulate and take into account the diversity of general and public interests and values that may be related to the evaluation.

Evaluation is the only way to separate programs that promote health and prevent injury, disease, mental illness, or disability from those that do not. Evaluation is the driving force for planning effective public health strategies, improving existing programs, and demonstrating the results of resource investments. Because it focuses attention on the common purpose of public health programs, evaluation also asks whether the magnitude of investment matches the tasks to be accomplished (Schorr, 1997). The recommended framework for conducting an evaluation is both a synthesis of existing evaluation practices and a standard for further improvement. It supports a practical approach to evaluation and is based on steps and standards applicable in public health settings. Because the framework is general, it provides a guide for designing and conducting specific evaluation projects across many different program areas.

CHAPTER SUMMARY

In this chapter, we defined operating principles, frameworks, and models to guide you through the understanding of prevention, community assessment, promotion, and program evaluation. Understanding these principles and concepts will help you assess, evaluate, and design community mental health services. The evaluation and health promotion frameworks will also help you determine if a particular program is considered a best practice model and how mental health programs are planned, managed, and evaluated. The concepts presented in this chapter underscore the need for professionals developing programs to create clear plans, inclusive partnerships, and feedback systems that allow learning and ongoing improvement to occur.

The health promotion model (HPM) proposed by Nola J. Pender was presented in the chapter. The model defines health as a positive dynamic state, not merely the absence of disease. Conducting a successful community assessment is also important to understand. The community assessment provides comprehensive, usable, and accurate information for decision making. Thus the community assessments process was incorporated in the chapter.

Finally, information about effective program evaluation was built into the chapter. Program evaluation is a systematic way to improve and account for mental health care programs by developing procedures that are useful, feasible, ethical, and accurate. The evaluation framework will guide you in program evaluations. The framework encourages an approach to evaluation that is integrated with routine program operations. The emphasis is on practical, ongoing evaluation strategies that involve all program stakeholders, not just evaluation experts. Understanding and applying the evaluation framework presented can be a driving force for planning effective mental health strategies, improving existing programs, and demonstrating the results of resource investments.

REVIEW

1. Determine what factors should be considered in delineating evaluation questions.
2. Conduct a community needs assessment of mental health services in your city, county, or state.
3. Develop a community mental health program using Pender's health promotion model.
4. Develop a community mental health program using the concepts of prevention.
5. Evaluate a community mental health program.

ACTIVITIES

1. Discuss a framework to conduct a community mental needs assessment.
2. Explore logic models developed for mental health programs in your community. Discuss the inputs and outputs of the logic model.
3. Discuss primary, secondary and tertiary approaches to mental health.
4. Review the findings of a community needs assessment.
5. Discuss the findings of an evaluation of a community mental health program.

REFERENCES AND FURTHER READINGS

Adler, M., & Ziglio, E. (1996). *Gazing into the oracle: The Delphi method and its application to social policy and public health*. Bristol, PA: Jessica Kingsley.

Ahuja, N. (2002). *A short text book of psychiatry* (5th ed.). New Delhi, India: Jaypee.

Ahuja, R. (2001). *Research methods*. New Delhi, India: Rawat Publications.

American Psychiatric Association. (1994). *Diagnostic and statistical manual of mental disorders* (4th ed.). Washington, DC: Author.

Anderson, E. T., & McFarland, J. (2008). *Community as partner: Theory and practice in nursing* (5th ed.). Philadelphia: Lippincott.

Anderson, K., Kubisch, A. C., & Connell, J. P. (1998). *New approaches to evaluating community initiatives: Theory, measurement, and analysis*. Washington, DC: Aspen Institute.

Atkinson, M., Zibin, S., & Chuang, H. (1997). Characterizing quality of life among patients with chronic mental illness: A critical examination of the self-report methodology. *American Journal of Psychiatry*, *154*(1), 99–105.

Barry, M. M., Crosby, C., & Bogg, J. (1993). Methodological issues in evaluating the quality of life of long-stay psychiatric patients. *Journal of Mental Health*, *2*, 43–56.

Bickman, L., & Rog, D. J. (1998). *Handbook of applied social research methods*. Thousand Oaks, CA: Sage.

Blum, J. L. (1975). *Planning for health*. New York: Behavioral Publications.

Boruch, R. F. (1998). Randomized controlled experiments for evaluation and planning. In L. Bickman & D. J. Rog (Eds.), *Handbook of applied social research methods* (pp. 161–192). Thousand Oaks, CA: Sage.

Brody, D. J., Pirkle, J. L., Kramer, R. A., Flegal, K. M., Matte, T. D., Gunter, E. W., & Paschal, D. C. (1994). Blood lead levels in the US population. Phase 1 of the Third National Health and Nutrition Examination Survey (NHANES III, 1988 to 1991). *Journal of the American Medical Association*, *272*(4), 277–283.

Campbell, A., Converse, P. E., & Rodgers, W. L. (1976). *The quality of American life: Perceptions, evaluations, and satisfactions*. New York: Russell Sage Foundation.

Center for Mental Health Services. (1998). *Cultural competence standards in managed care: Mental health services for four underserved/ underrepresented racial/ethnic groups*. Rockville, MD: Author.

Centers for Disease Control and Prevention [CDC]. (1991). *Strategic plan for the elimination of childhood lead poisoning*. Atlanta, GA: Author.

Centers for Disease Control and Prevention [CDC]. (1992). Framework for assessing the effectiveness of disease and injury prevention. *Morbidity and Mortality Weekly Report*, *41*(No. RR-3), 1–13.

Centers for Disease Control and Prevention [CDC]; Public Health Practice Program Office. (1997). *Principles of community engagement*. Atlanta, GA: Author. Retrieved from http://www.cdc.gov/phppo/pce/

Chaux, E., Molano, A., & Podlesky, P. (2009). Socio-economic, socio-political and socio-emotional variables explaining school bullying: A country-wide multilevel analysis. *Aggressive behavior*, *35*(6), 520–529.

Chen, H. T. (1990). *Theory driven evaluations*. Newbury Park, CA: Sage.

Clarke, G. N., Hawkins, W., Murphy, M., Sheeber, L. B., Lewinsohn, P. M., & Seeley, J. R. (1995). Targeted prevention of unipolar depressive disorder in an at-risk sample of high school adolescents: A randomized trial of a group cognitive intervention. *Journal of the American Academy of Child and Adolescent Psychiatry*, *34*, 312–321.

Connell, J. P., & Kubisch, A. C. (1998). Applying a theory of change approach to the evaluation of comprehensive community initiatives: Progress, prospects, and problems. In K. Fulbright-Anderson, A. C. Kubisch, & J. P. Connell (Eds.), *New approaches to evaluating community initiatives* (pp. 15–44). Washington, DC: Aspen Institute.

Conwell, Y. (1996). *Diagnosis and treatment of depression in late life*. Washington, DC: American Psychiatric Press.

Cook, J. A., & Jonikas, J. A. (1996). Outcomes of psychiatric rehabilitation service delivery. *New Directions in Mental Health Services*, *71*, 33–47.

Cook, K., & Timberlake, E. M. (1989). Cross-cultural counseling with Vietnamese refugees. In D. Koslow & E. Salett (Eds.), *Crossing cultures in mental health* (pp. 84–100). Washington, DC: SIETAR International.

Cook, T. D., & Campbell, D. T. (1979). *Quasi-experimentation: Design and analysis issues for field settings*. Boston: Houghton Mifflin.

Cook, T. D., & Reichardt, C. S. (1979). *Sage Research Progress Series in Evaluation: Vol. 1 Qualitative and quantitative methods in evaluation research*. Beverly Hills, CA: Sage.

Davies, J., & Macdonald, G. (1998). *Quality, evidence, and effectiveness in health promotion: Striving for certainties*. London UK: Routledge.

Denzin, N. K., & Lincoln, Y. S. (1994). Introduction: Entering the field of qualitative research. In N. K. Denzin & Y. S. Lincoln (eds.). *Handbook of qualitative research*. Thousand Oaks, CA: Sage.

Eoyang, G. H., & Berkas, T. (1999). Evaluation in a complex adaptive system. In M. Lissack & H. Gunz (Eds.), *Managing complexity in organizations*. Westport, CT: Quorum.

Erikson, E. (1950). *Childhood and society*. New York: Norton.

Fawcett, S. B., Paine-Andrews, A., Francisco, V. T., Schultz, J., Richter, K. P., Berkley-Patton, J., . . . Evensen, P. (2001). Evaluating community initiatives for health and development. *WHO Regional Publications European Series, 92*, 241–270.

Fetterman, D. M., Kaftarian, S. J., & Wandersman, A. (1996). *Empowerment evaluation: Knowledge and tools for self-assessment and accountability*. Thousand Oaks, CA: Sage.

Fitzpatrick, J. L., & Morris, M. (1999). *New Directions for Program Evaluation: Vol. 82. Current and emerging ethical challenges in evaluation*. San Francisco: Jossey-Bass.

Garmezy, N. (1983). Stressors of childhood. In N. Garmezy & M. Rutter (Eds.), *Stress, coping, and development in children* (pp. 43–84). New York: McGraw-Hill.

General Accounting Office. (1977). *Returning the mentally disabled to the community: Government needs to do more*. Washington, DC: Author.

Gill, T. M., & Feinstein, A. R. (1994). A critical appraisal of the quality of life measurements. *Journal of the American Medical Association, 272*(8), 619–626.

Gold, M. E., Russell, L. B., Siegel, J. E., & Weinstein, M. C. (1996). *Cost-effectiveness in health and medicine*. New York: Oxford University Press.

Gordon, M. F. (1964). *Assimilation in American life*. New York: Oxford University Press.

Gordon, R. (1987). An operational classification of disease prevention. In J. A. Steinberg, & M. M. Silverman (Eds.) *Preventing mental disorders* (pp. 20–26). Rockville, MD: Department of Health and Human Services.

Green, L. W., & Kreuter, M. W. (2005). *Health program planning: An educational and ecological approach* (4th ed.). New York: McGraw-Hill.

Haddix, A. C., Teutsch, S. M., Shaffer, P. A., & Duñet, D. O. (1996). *Prevention effectiveness: A guide to decision analysis and economic evaluation*. New York: Oxford University Press.

Higgs, Z. R., & Gustafson, D. D. (1985). Descriptive approach to community assessment. In *Community as a Client: Assessment and Diagnosis*. Philadelphia: F.A. Davis.

Hunt, S. M. (1997). The problem of quality of life. *Quality of Life Research, 6*, 205–212.

Institute of Medicine [IOM]. (1990). *Broadening the base of treatment for alcohol problems: Report of a study by a committee of the Institute of Medicine, Division of Mental Health and Behavioral Medicine*. Washington, DC: National Academy Press.

Institute of Medicine [IOM]. (1994a). *Adverse events associated with childhood vaccines: Evidence bearing on causality*. Washington, DC: National Academy Press.

Institute of Medicine [IOM]. (1994b). *Reducing risks for mental disorders: Frontiers for preventive intervention research*. Washington, DC: National Academy Press.

Institute of Medicine & Committee for the Study of the Future of Public Health. (1988). *The future of public health*. Washington, DC: National Academy Press.

Interagency Council on the Homeless. (1991). *Reaching out: A guide for service providers*. Rockville, MD: National Resource Center on Homelessness and Mental Health.

Jablensky, A. V., Morgan, V., Zubrick, S. R., Bower, C., & Yellachich, L. A. (2005). Pregnancy, delivery, and neonatal complications in a population cohort of women with schizophrenia and major affective disorders. *American Journal of Psychiatry, 162*, 79–91.

Joint Committee on Standards for Educational Evaluation. (1988). *Personnel evaluation standards: How to assess systems for evaluating educators*. Newbury Park, CA: Sage.

Joint Committee on Standards for Educational Evaluation. (1994). *Program evaluation standards: How to assess evaluations of educational programs* (2nd ed.). Thousand Oaks, CA: Sage.

Julian, D. (1997).Utilization of the logic model as a system level planning and evaluation device. *Evaluation and Program Planning*, *20*(3), 251–257.

Kalichman, S. C., Simbayi, L. C., Vermaakk, R., Jooste, S., & Cain, D. (2008). HIV/AIDS risks among men and women who drink at informal alcohol serving establishments (Shebeens) in Cape Town, South Africa. *Prevention Science*, *9*, 55–62.

Kaplan, G. A., Roberts, R. E., Camacho, T. C., & Coyne, J. C. (1987). Psychosocial predictors of depression. Prospective evidence from the human population laboratory studies. *American Journal of Epidemiology*, *125*, 206–220.

Katschnig, H. (1997). How useful is the concept of quality of life in psychiatry? *Current Opinion in Psychiatry*, 10, 337–345.

Koplan, J. P. (1995). CDC sets millennium priorities. US Medicine 1999; 4–7.

Kumpfer, K. L., & Baxley, G. B. (1997). *Drug abuse prevention: What works?* Rockville, MD: National Institute on Drug Abuse.

Laffrey, S. C., & Craig, D. M. (1995). "Health promotion for communities and aggregates: An integrated model." In M. Stewart (Ed.), *Community nursing: Promoting Canadians' health* (pp. 125–146). Toronto, ON: W. B. Saunders.

Lanuza, D. M. (1999). Research and practice. In M. A. Mathew, & K. T. Kirchoff (Eds.), *Using and Conducting Nursing Research in the Clinical Setting* (2nd ed.) (pp. 2–12). Philadelphia: W. B. Saunders.

Lehman, A. F. (1996). Measures of quality of life among persons with severe and persistent mental disorders. *Social Psychiatry and Psychiatric Epidemiology*, *2*, 78–88.

Lincoln, A., Espejo, D., Johnson, P., Paasche-Orlow, M., Speckman, J., Webber, T., & White, R. F. (2008). Limited literacy and psychiatric disorders among users of an urban safety-net hospital's mental health outpatient clinic. *Journal of Nervous & Mental Disease*, *196*: 687–693. Retrieved from http://search.ebscohost.com

Lipsey, M. W. (1993). Theory as method: Small theories of treatments. *New Directions for Program Evaluation*, *57*, 5–38.

Love, A. (1991). *Applied Social Research: Vol. 24. Internal evaluation: Building organizations from within*. Newbury Park, CA: Sage.

Mann, J. J., Apter, A., Bertolote, J., Beautrais, A., Currier, D., Haas, A., . . . Hendin, H. (2005). Suicide prevention strategies. A systematic review. *Journal of the American Medical Association*, *294*, 2064–2074.

McEwan, K. L., & Bigelow, D. A. (1997). Using a logic model to focus health services on population health goals. *Canadian Journal of Program Evaluation*, *12*(1):167–174.

McGauhey, P., Starfield, B., Alexander, C., & Ensminger, M. E. (1991). Social environment and vulnerability of low birth weight children: A social-epidemiological perspective. *Pediatrics*, *88*, 943–953.

Mertens, D. M. (1999). Inclusive evaluation: Implications of transformative theory for evaluation. *American Journal of Evaluation*, *20*(1), 1–14.

Muñoz, R. F., Ying, Y. W., Bernal, G., Pérez-Stable, E. J., Sorensen, J. L., Hargreaves, W. A., . . . Miller, L. S. (1995). Prevention of depression with primary care patients: A randomized controlled trial. *American Journal of Community Psychology*, *2*, 199–222.

Oliver, J. P., Huxley, P. J., Priebe, S., & Kaiser, W. (1997). Measuring the quality of life of severely mentally ill people using the Lancashire Quality of Life Profile. *Social Psychiatry and Psychiatric Epidemiology*, *32*(2), 76–83.

Patrick, D. L., & Erickson, P. (1993). *Health status and health policy: Quality of life in health care evaluation and resource allocation*. New York: Oxford University Press.

Patton, M. Q. (1990). *Qualitative evaluation and research methods* (2nd ed.). Newbury Park, CA: Sage.

Patton, M. Q. (1997a). Toward distinguishing empowerment evaluation and placing it in a larger context. *Evaluation Practice*, *18*(2), 147–163.

Patton, M. Q. (1997b). *Utilization-focused evaluation: The new century text* (3rd ed.). Thousand Oaks, CA: Sage.

Peterson, D. J., & Alexander G. R. (2001) *Needs assessment in public health: A practical guide for students and professionals*. New York: Kluwer Academic/Plenum Publishers.

Reichardt, C. S., & Mark, M. M. (1998). Quasi-experimentation. In L. Bickman & D. J. Rob (Eds.), *Handbook of applied social research methods* (pp. 193–228). Thousand Oaks, CA: Sage.

Ringwalt, C., Vincus, A., Hanley, S., Ennett, S., Bowling, J., & Rohrbach, L. (2009). The prevalence of evidence-based drug use prevention curricula in U.S. middle schools in 2005. *Prevention Science*, *10*(1), 33–40. Retrieved from http://search.ebscohost.com

Robins, L. N. (1970). Follow-up studies investigating childhood disorders. In E. H. Hare & J. K. Wayne (Eds.), *Psychiatric epidemiology* (pp. 29–68). London: Oxford University Press.

Rogers, P. J., & Hough, G. (1995). Improving the effectiveness of evaluations: Making the link to organizational theory. *Evaluation and Program Planning*, *18*(4), 321–332.

Rossi, P. H., Freeman, H. E., & Lipsey, M. W. (1999). *Evaluation: A systematic approach* (6th ed.). Thousand Oaks, CA: Sage.

Rush, B., & Ogbourne, A. (1991). Program logic models: Expanding their role and structure for program planning and evaluation. *Canadian Journal of Program Evaluation*, *6*(2), 95–106.

Rutter, M. (1979). Protective factors in children's responses to stress and disadvantage. *Annals of the Academy of Medicine, Singapore*, *8*, 324–338.

Sanders, J. R. (1993). Uses of evaluation as a means toward organizational effectiveness. In S. T. Gray (Ed.), *Leadership IS: A vision of evaluation; a report of learnings from Independent Sector's work on evaluation*. Washington, DC: Independent Sector.

Schorr, L. B. (1997). *Common purpose: Strengthening families and neighborhoods to rebuild America*. New York: Doubleday/Anchor.

Scriven, M. (1998). Minimalist theory of evaluation: The least theory that practice requires. *American Journal of Evaluation*, *19*, 57–70.

Shadish, W. R., Cook, T. D., & Leviton, L. C. (1991). *Foundations of program evaluation: Theories of practice*. Thousand Oaks, CA: Sage.

Shamansky, S., & Pesznecker, B. (1981). A community is. . . . *Nursing Outlook*, *29*,182–185.

Smith, M. K. (1996, 2001, 2007). Action research, the encyclopedia of informal education. Retrieved from www.infed.org/research/b-actres.htm

Taylor-Powell, E., Rossing, B., & Geran, J. (1998). *Evaluating collaboratives: Reaching the potential.* Madison: University of Wisconsin-Madison Cooperative Extension.

Torres, R. T., Preskill, H., & Piontek, M. (1997). Public Health Research. Education and Development Program.

Trochim, W. M. K. (1999). *Research methods knowledge base* (2nd ed.). Retrieved from http://trochim.human.cornell.edu

U.S. Department of Health and Human Services. (1998). DHHS Pub No. (SMA) 99-3285 (pp. 82–98). Washington, DC: U.S. Government Printing Office.

U.S. General Accounting Office. (1990). Case study evaluations. U.S. General Accounting Office Pub. No. GAO/PEMD-91-10.1.9. Washington, DC: Author.

U.S. General Accounting Office. (1991). Designing evaluations. Pub. No. GAO/PEMD-10.1.4. Washington, DC: Author.

U.S. General Accounting Office. (1992). Evaluation synthesis. Pub. No. GAO/PEMD-10.1.2. Washington, DC: Author.

U.S. General Accounting Office. (1998). Managing for results: Measuring program results that are under limited federal control. Pub. No. GAO/GGD-99-16. Washington, DC: Author.

United Way of America. (1996). *Measuring program outcomes: A practical approach*. Alexandria, VA: Author.

Wandersman, A., Morrissey, E., Davino, K., Seybolt, D., Crusto, C., Nation, M., Goodman, R., & Imm, P. (1998). Comprehensive quality programming and accountability: Eight essential strategies for implementing successful prevention programs. *Journal of Primary Prevention*, *19*(1): 3–30.

Weiss, C. H. (1995). Nothing as practical as a good theory: Exploring theory-based evaluation for comprehensive community initiatives for families and children. In J. P. Connell, A. C. Kubisch, L. B. Schorr, & C. H. Weiss (Eds.), *New approaches to evaluating community initiatives: Concepts, methods, and contexts*. Washington, DC: Aspen Institute.

Weiss, C. H. (1997). How can theory-based evaluation make greater headway? *Evaluation Review*, *21*, 501–524.

Weiss, C. H. (1998a). *Evaluation: Methods for studying programs and policies* (2nd ed.). Upper Saddle River, NJ: Prentice Hall.

Weiss, C. H. (1998b). Have we learned anything new about the use of evaluation? *American Journal of Evaluation*, *19*(1), 21–33.

Werner, E., & Smith, R. (1992). *Overcoming the odds: High-risk children from birth to adulthood*. New York: Cornell University Press. (ED 344 979)

WHOQOL Group. (1994). Development of the WHOQOL: Rationale and current status. *International Journal of Mental Health*, *23*(3), 24–56.

WHOQOL Group. (1995). The World Health Organization Quality of Life Assessment (WHOQOL): Position paper from the World Health Organization. *Social Science & Medicine*, *41*, 1403–1409.

Worthen, B. R., Sanders, J. R., & Fitzpatrick, J. L. (1996). *Program evaluation: Alternative approaches and practical guidelines* (2nd ed.). New York: Longman.

Yin, R. K. (1994). *Applied Social Research Methods Series: Vol. 5. Case study research: Design and methods* (2nd ed.). Thousand Oaks, CA: Sage.

Yin, R. K. (1998). Abridged version of case study research: Design and method. In L. Bickman & D. J. Rob (Eds.), *Handbook of applied social research methods* (pp. 229–260). Thousand Oaks, CA: Sage.

UNIT V Looking into the Future

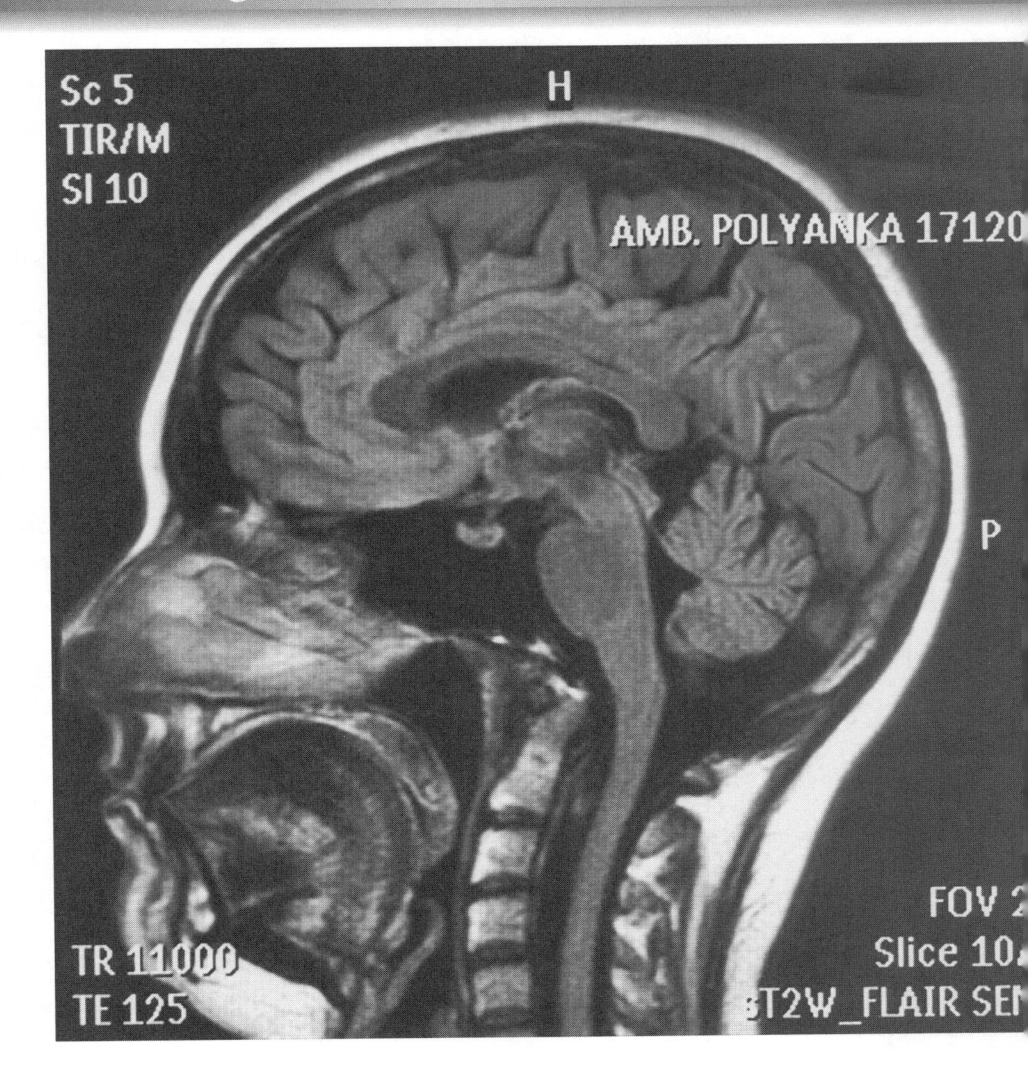

CHAPTER 14

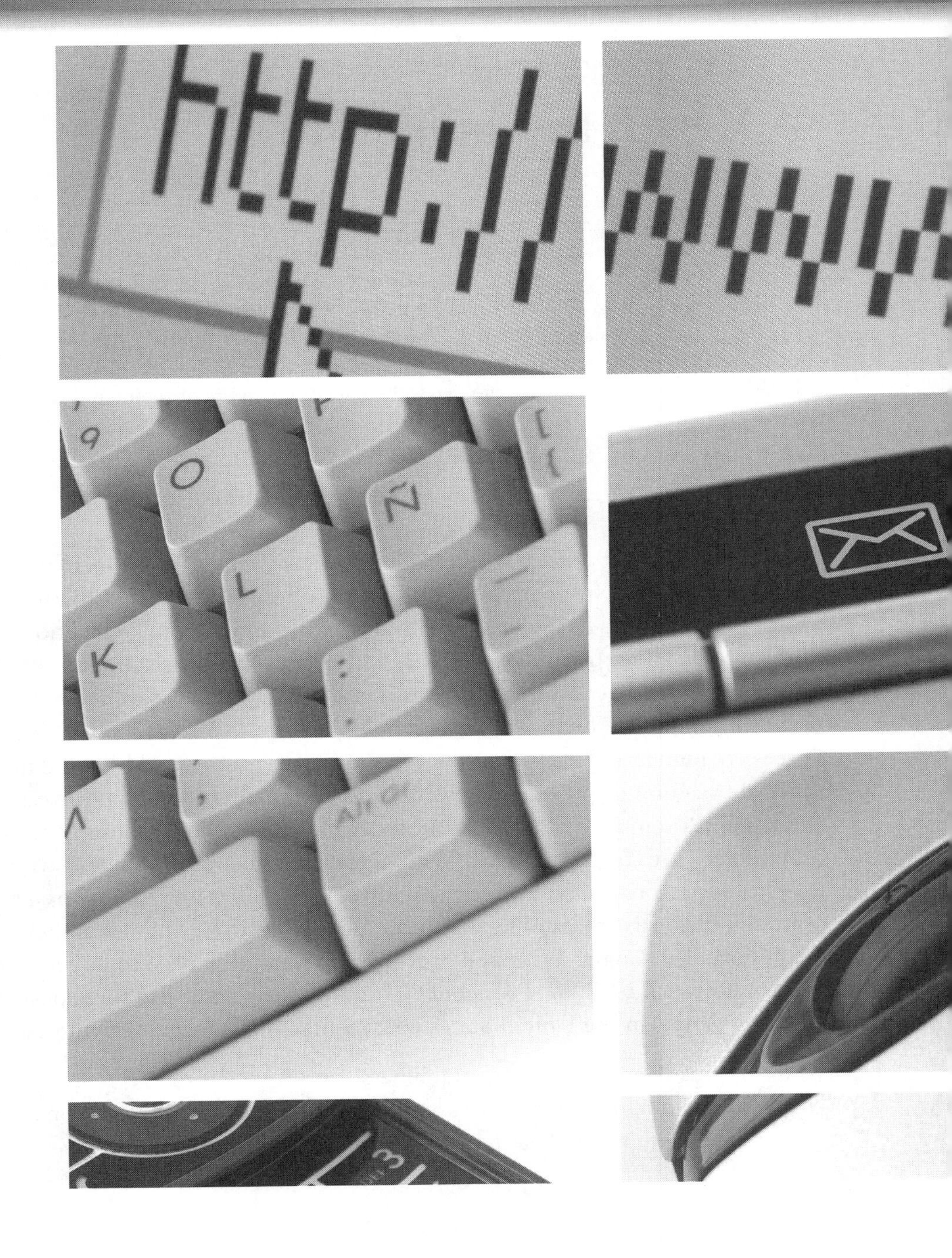

A Vision for the Future

CHAPTER OBJECTIVES

1. Identify the three obstacles to preventing mentally ill people from receiving excellent care outlined in the *President's New Freedom Commission on Mental Health Report.*
2. Identify the eight goals outlined in *Mental Health: A Report of the Surgeon General.*
3. Identify the six goals outlined in the *President's New Freedom Commission on Mental Health Report.*
4. Explain the recommendations to achieve those goals.
5. Explain how genetics and technology will influence the future of community mental health.

KEY TERMS

- Best practice
- Evidence-based practice

Mental health is a core and foundational component to the functioning of human beings, which is why there needs to be more research directed toward discovering ways to prevent and treat mental illness. Information about prevention lags behind information about treatment; there should be more emphasis on prevention. Prevention is essential because mental illness has a negative impact on individuals, families, and communities. There are high economic costs tied to mental illness along with excessive human suffering. Everyone in our nation is impacted by it. All mental illness probably cannot be prevented, which is why treatment methods and access to care are essential. Prompt and effective treatment can manage the symptoms and prevent further deterioration and disability. With proper treatment, most people with mental illness can have productive and engaging lives. Treatment must be tailored to the needs of the individuals and families and be culturally sensitive. Stigmas and others barriers (e.g., financial, language, limited providers) to treatment need to be reduced or eliminated. On April 29, 2002, President George W. Bush identified three obstacles to preventing people in the United States with mental illness from receiving excellent care:

1. Stigma that surrounds mental illness,
2. Unfair treatment limitations and financial requirements placed on mental health benefits in private health insurance, and

3. The fragmented mental health service delivery system. (*President's New Freedom Commission on Mental Health Report*, p. 1)

Reducing and eliminating these barriers along with accelerating progress toward identifying effective prevention and treatment methods and improving services and access is needed to achieve our vision. This is the vision statement contained in the *President's New Freedom Commission on Mental Health Report* (2002, p. 1):

> We envision a future when everyone with a mental illness will recover, a future when mental illness can be prevented and cured, a future when mental illnesses are detected early, and a future when everyone with a mental illness at any stage of life has access to effective treatment and supports—essentials for living, working, learning, and participating fully in the community.

This chapter describes the steps needed to achieve this vision. The goals outlined in two federal publications are included in this chapter: *Mental Health: A Report of the Surgeon General* and *President's New Freedom Commission on Mental Health Report*. The latter report focuses on changes that need to be made to the delivery of mental health services; the former report is broader in scope. We also discuss how genetics and technology will impact community mental health in the future.

MENTAL HEALTH: A REPORT OF THE SURGEON GENERAL

In September 1997, the Substance Abuse and Mental Health Services Administration (SAMHSA) was authorized by the Office of the Surgeon General to take the lead on writing the surgeon general's report on mental health. SAMHSA and the National Institute of Mental Health (NIMH) partnered to develop the report under the guidance of Surgeon General David Satcher. SAMHSA and NIMH created a planning board composed of mental health experts from academics as well as mental health professionals, researchers in neuroscience and service delivery, and self-identified consumers of mental health services and family members of consumers of mental health services. Individuals representing federal operating divisions, offices, centers, and institutes, and private nonprofit foundations with interests in mental health also participated in the planning board.

The planning board wrote *Mental Health: A Report of the Surgeon General*. In the report the board outlined eight goals:

1. Continue to build the science base.
2. Overcome stigma.

3. Improve public awareness of effective treatment.
4. Ensure the supply of mental health services and providers.
5. Ensure delivery of state-of-the-art treatments.
6. Tailor treatment to age, gender, race, and culture.
7. Facilitate entry into treatment.
8. Reduce financial barriers to treatment (U.S. Department of Health and Human Services, 1999).

What follows is a description of these eight goals.

Goal 1: Continue to Build the Science Base

Our knowledge base has increased because of research about mental health and illness during the past several decades. This includes knowledge of new technology and genetics. Genetic research holds promise to provide new and accurate targets for additional medications and psychosocial interventions. This research has the potential to reduce stigma, which can eliminate misconceptions and stereotypes about mental illness and the burdens experienced by persons who have these disorders.

Future research needs to make a concerted effort to fill in the knowledge gaps base, particularly those related to mental health promotion and illness prevention. Other gaps include information about culturally sensitive research on mental health and illness and effective ways to reduce stigmas and health disparities.

Goal 2: Overcome Stigma

Stigma that surrounds mental illness deters people from seeking treatment. The stigma manifests itself through prejudice and discrimination, fear, distrust, and stereotyping. It prompts many people to avoid working, socializing, and living with people who have a mental disorder and contributes to myths such as the mentally ill being more violent than those who do not suffer from such illness. Stigma is a deterrent for people seeking help for fear that the confidentiality of their diagnosis or treatment will be breached. Stigma prevents people from acknowledging their own mental health problems and discussing them with others. For our country to reduce the burden of mental illness, improve access to care, improve preventive services, and advance research on the topic, stigma must be reduced and ultimately eliminated.

Goal 3: Improve Public Awareness of Effective Treatment

Americans are often unaware of the vast array of choices for effective mental health treatments. Public awareness is needed so that people can make informed decisions about the treatment method that they select in order to choose one that they feel comfortable and confident with and that meets their personal preferences and styles. If the path of help-seeking leads to only limited improvement, an array of options still exists: The intensity of treatment may be changed, new treatments may be introduced, or another provider may be sought. Social support systems such as clergy, family members, and friends often can help by encouraging a distressed person to seek help.

All human services professionals, not just health professionals, have an obligation to be better informed about mental health treatment resources in their communities. Insurance companies need to publish clear information about their mental health benefits. People may not know that they have coverage for mental health issues and/or where to get help for such problems.

Goal 4: Ensure the Supply of Mental Health Services and Providers

The fundamental components of effective service delivery include integrated community-based services, continuity of providers and treatments, family support services, and services that are culturally sensitive. For people with severe mental health problems, effective service delivery also requires housing and employment assistance. For adults and children with less severe conditions, primary health care, schools, and other human services must be prepared to assess and, at times, to treat individuals who come seeking help. All services for those with a mental disorder should be consumer oriented and focused on promoting recovery. In addition, efforts need to be made to reduce or eliminate the short supply of mental health care professionals and treatment centers, particularly in certain geographic regions such as rural communities.

Goal 5: Ensure Delivery of State-of-the-Art Treatments

State-of-the-art treatments and community-based services that have been shown to be effective are not being utilized. A gap exists in the introduction and application of these advances in services in local communities, and many people with mental illness are being denied the most up-to-date and advanced forms of treatment. One reason for this is the time lag between reporting the research results and getting it into practice. Other reasons include providers' lack of knowledge of research results and the cost of introducing innovations in health systems.

Goal 6: Tailor Treatment to Age, Gender, Race, and Culture

To be effective, the diagnosis and treatment of mental illness must be tailored to individual circumstances while taking into account age, gender, race, culture, and other characteristics that shape a person's image and identity. Services that take these demographic factors into consideration have the greatest chance of engaging people in treatment, keeping them in treatment, and helping them to recover. The successful experiences of individual patients will positively influence attitudes toward mental health services and service providers, thus encouraging others who may share similar concerns or interests to seek help.

Although women and men experience mental disorders at almost equal rates, some mental disorders such as depression, panic disorder, and eating disorders affect women disproportionately. The mental health service system should be tailored to focus on unique needs of both genders. In addition, members of racial and ethnic minority groups account for an increasing proportion of the nation's population so providers of mental health services need to be informed and responsive to cultural context. Culturally competent services are needed to enhance the appropriate use of services and effectiveness of treatments for consumers. Also, members of ethnic and racial minority groups may prefer to be treated by mental health professionals of similar background. There is an insufficient number of mental health professionals from racial and ethnic minority groups, which is a problem that needs to be corrected.

Goal 7: Facilitate Entry into Treatment

The mental health service system is highly fragmented, leaving many who seek treatment confused and frustrated by the complexity. Progress has been made in coordinating services for those with severe mental illness, but more can be accomplished. Public and private agencies have an obligation to facilitate entry into treatment. There are multiple portals of entry to mental health care and treatment, including a range of community and faith-based organizations. Primary health care could be an important portal of entry for children and adults of all ages with mental disorders. The schools and child welfare system are the initial points of contact for most children and adolescents, and they can be useful sources of first-line assessment and referral, provided that expertise is available. The juvenile justice and correctional systems represent another pathway, although many overburdened facilities tend to lack the staff required to deal with the magnitude of the mental health problems encountered.

It is essential for first-line contacts in the community to recognize mental illness and mental health problems, to respond sensitively, to know what resources exist, and to make proper referrals and/or to address problems effectively themselves. For the general public, primary care represents a prime opportunity to obtain mental health treatment or an appropriate referral. Yet primary healthcare providers vary in their capacity to recognize and manage mental health problems, and they may not be aware of referral sources or do not have the time to help their patients find services.

Goal 8: Reduce Financial Barriers to Treatment

Economic barriers can prevent or discourage people from seeking treatment and from staying in treatment. Recent legislative efforts to mandate equitable insurance coverage for mental health services is a step in the right direction toward eliminating barriers to care. Still, for the millions of Americans who have no health insurance, equity of mental health and other health benefits is irrelevant.

THE *PRESIDENT'S NEW FREEDOM COMMISSION ON MENTAL HEALTH REPORT*

As mentioned previously, President Bush created the New Freedom Commission on Mental Health. That commission established six goals to improve the mental health care delivery system. Those six goals in a transformed mental health system contained in the *President's New Freedom Commission on Mental Health Report* (2003) are explained in this section.

Goal 1: Americans Understand That Mental Health Is Essential to Overall Health

Americans will seek mental health care when they need it. The barrier of stigma will be reduced or eliminated. This can occur through national educational efforts to dispel misconceptions about mental illness. With the understanding about mental illness people will be more likely to seek treatment. The commission identified two recommendations to aid in the transformation of the mental health system for this goal:

1. Advance and implement a national campaign to reduce the stigma of seeking care and a national strategy for suicide prevention.
2. Address mental health with the same urgency as physical health. (*President's New Freedom Commission on Mental Health Report*, 2002, p. 7)

BOX 14-1 Model Program: Suicide Prevention and Changing Attitudes About Mental Health Care

Program	Air Force Initiative to Prevent Suicide
Goal	To reduce the alarming rate of suicide. Between 1990 and 1994, one in every four deaths among active duty U.S. Air Force personnel was from suicide. After unintentional injuries, suicide was the second leading cause of death in the Air Force.
Features	In 1996, the Air Force Chief of Staff initiated a community-wide approach to prevent suicide through hard-hitting messages to all active duty personnel. The messages recognized the courage of those confronting life's stresses and encouraged them to seek help from mental health clinics—actions that were once regarded as career hindering, but were now deemed "career-enhancing." Other features of the program: education and training, improved surveillance, critical incident stress management, and integrated delivery systems of care.
Outcomes	From 1994 to 1998, the suicide rate dropped from 16.4 to 9.4 suicides per 100,000. By 2002, the overall decline from 1994 was about 50%. Researchers also found significant declines in violent crime, family violence, and deaths that resulted from unintentional injuries. Air Force leaders have emphasized community-wide involvement in every aspect of the project.
Biggest challenge	Sustaining the enthusiasm by service providers as the program has become more established.
How other organizations can adopt	The program can be transferred to any community that has identified leaders and organization, especially other military services, large corporations, police forces, firefighters, schools, and universities.
Sites	All U.S. Air Force locations throughout the world.

Source: *President's New Freedom Commission on Mental Health Report*, 2002, p. 25.

Goal 2: Mental Health Care Is Consumer and Family Driven

The diagnosis of mental illness will initiate a well-planned and coordinated array of services and treatment, which will be defined in a single care plan. A personalized road map will be tailored to the needs of the individual and guide the way for appropriate treatment and supports that are needed for recovery. Service providers and consumers will actively participate in designing the plan. The commission made five recommendations specific to this goal:

1. Develop an individualized plan of care for every adult with a serious mental illness and child with a serious emotional disturbance.
2. Involve consumers and families fully in orienting the mental health system toward recovery.
3. Align relevant federal programs to improve access and accountability for mental health services.
4. Create a comprehensive state mental health plan.
5. Protect and enhance the rights of people with mental illnesses. (*President's New Freedom Commission on Mental Health Report*, 2002, p. 9)

BOX 14-2 Model Program: Integrated System of Care for Children with Serious Emotional Disturbances and Their Families

Program	Wraparound Milwaukee
Goal	To offer cost-effective, comprehensive, and individualized care to children with serious emotional disturbances and their families. The children and adolescents that the program serves are under court order in the child welfare or juvenile justice system; 64% are African American.
Features	Provides coordinated system of care through a single public agency (Wraparound Milwaukee) that coordinates a crisis team, provider network, family advocacy, and access to 80 different services. The program's $30 million budget is funded by pooling child welfare and juvenile justice funds (previously spent on institutional care) and by a set monthly fee for each Medicaid-eligible child. (The fee is derived from historical Medicaid costs for psychiatric hospitalization or related services.)
Outcomes	Reduced juvenile delinquency, higher school attendance, better clinical outcomes, lower use of hospitalization, and reduced costs of care. Program costs $4,350 instead of $7,000 per month per child for residential treatment or juvenile detention.
Biggest challenge	To expand the program to children with somewhat less severe needs who are at risk for worse problems if they are unrecognized and untreated.
How other organizations can adopt	Encourage integrated care and more individualized services by ensuring that funding streams can support a single family-centered treatment plan for children whose care is financed from multiple sources.
Sites	Milwaukee and Madison, Wisconsin; Indianapolis, Indiana; and the State of New Jersey.

Source: *President's New Freedom Commission on Mental Health Report*, 2002, p. 36.

Goal 3: Disparities in Mental Health Services Are Eliminated

This goal focuses on giving all Americans an equal share in the best available services and outcomes regardless of demographic variables such as race and geographic location. The mental health workforce will include people of diverse backgrounds and live in rural and remote geographic areas. Research and training related to proving appropriate interventions tailored to consumer needs will be conducted. This includes recognizing factors such as age, gender, race, ethnicity, culture, and locale. The two specific recommendations are:

1. Improve access to quality care that is culturally competent.
2. Improve access to quality care in rural and geographically remote areas. (*President's New Freedom Commission on Mental Health Report*, 2002, p. 10)

BOX 14-3 Model Program: A Culturally Competent School-Based Mental Health Program

Program	Dallas School Based Youth and Family Centers
Goal	To establish the first comprehensive, culturally competent, school-based program in mental health care in the 12th largest school system in the nation. The program overcomes stigma and inadequate access to care for underserved minority populations.
Features	Annually serves the physical and mental health care needs of 3,000 low-income children and their families. The mental health component features partnerships with parents and families, treatment (typically 6 sessions), and follow-up with teachers. The well-qualified staff, who reflect the racial and ethnic composition of the population they serve (more than 70% Latino and African American), train school nurses, counselors, and principals to identify problems and create solutions tailored to meet each child's needs.
Outcomes	Improvements in attendance, discipline referrals, and teacher evaluation of child performance. Preliminary findings reveal improvement in children's standardized test scores in relation to national and local norms.
Biggest challenge	To sustain financial and organizational support of collaborative partners despite resistance to change or jurisdictional barriers. Program's $3.5 million funding comes from the school district and an additional $1.5 million from Parkland Hospital.
How other organizations can adopt	Recognize the importance of mental health for the school success of all children, regardless of race or ethnicity. Rethink how school systems can more efficiently partner with and use State and Federal funds to deliver culturally competent school-based mental health services.
Sites	Dallas and Fort Worth, Texas.

Source: *President's New Freedom Commission on Mental Health Report*, 2002, p. 53.

Goal 4: Early Mental Health Screening, Assessment, and Referral to Services Are Common Practice

In the transformed mental health care system, routine and comprehensive testing and screening for mental health problems in children and adults will be expected and typically occur. Preventive interventions will occur when signs of difficulties first appear to keep problems from escalating. These are the specific recommendations:

1. Promote the mental health of young children.
2. Improve and expand school mental health programs.
3. Screen for co-occurring mental and substance use disorders and link with integrated treatment strategies.
4. Screen for mental disorders in primary health care, across the lifespan, and connect to treatment and supports. (*President's New Freedom Commission on Mental Health Report*, 2002, p. 11)

BOX 14-4 Model Program: Collaborative Care for Treating Late-Life Depression in Primary Care Settings

Program	IMPACT—Improving Mood: Providing Access to Collaborative Treatment for Late Life Depression
Goal	To recognize, treat, and prevent future relapses in older patients with major depression in primary care. About 5%–10% of older patients have major depression, yet most are not properly recognized and treated. Untreated depression causes distress, disability, and, most tragically, suicide.
Features	Uses a team approach to deliver depression care to elderly adults in primary care setting. Older adults are given a choice of medication from a primary care physician or psychotherapy with a mental health provider. If they do not improve, their level of care is increased by adding supervision by a mental health specialist.
Outcomes	The intervention, compared to usual care, leads to higher satisfaction with depression treatment, reduced prevalence and severity of symptoms, or complete remission.
Biggest challenge	To ensure that the intervention is readily adapted from the research setting into the practice setting.
How other organizations can adopt	Be receptive to organizational changes in primary care and devise new methods of reimbursement.
Sites	Study sites in California, Texas, Washington, North Carolina, Indiana.

Source: *President's New Freedom Commission on Mental Health Report*, 2002, p. 66.

Goal 5: Excellent Mental Health Care Is Delivered and Research Is Accelerated

The emphasis of this goal is to have the mental health system use evidence-based state-of-the art treatments and for them to be standard practice used throughout the system. Research discoveries will be routinely available. Knowledge about **evidence-based practices** (treatments and services that have well-documented effectiveness) and **best practices** (treatments and services that are promising but have less evidence) should be widely circulated and utilized. These are the recommendations made by the commission:

1. Accelerate research to promote recovery and resilience, and ultimately to cure and prevent mental illnesses.
2. Advance evidence-based practices using dissemination and demonstration projects and create a public-private partnership to guide their implementation.
3. Improve and expand the workforce providing evidence-based mental health services and supports.
4. Develop the knowledge base in four understudied areas: mental health disparities, long-term effects of medications, trauma, and acute care. (*President's New Freedom Commission on Mental Health Report*, 2002, p. 13)

Goal 6: Technology Is Used to Access Mental Health Care and Information

The intent of this goal is to empower consumers and give providers a tool to deliver the best possible care through the use of advanced communication and information technology. The technology will enable consumers and families to communicate regularly with the agencies and personnel that deliver treatment and support services and that are accountable for achieving the goals outlined in the individual plan of care. The technology will enable providers to access information about recent medical advances and studies of optimal outcomes to facilitate the best care options and information about illnesses, effective treatments, and the services in their community. The two commission recommendations are:

1. Use health technology and telehealth to improve access and coordination of mental health care, especially for Americans in remote areas or in underserved populations.
2. Develop and implement integrated electronic health record and personal health information systems. (*President's New Freedom Commission on Mental Health Report*, 2002, p. 15)

BOX 14-5 Model Program: Critical Time Intervention with Homeless Families

Program	Family Critical Time Intervention model (FCTI). The program was jointly funded by NIMH and the Center for Mental Health Services/Center for Substance Abuse Treatment Homeless Families Program.
Goal	To apply effective, time-limited, and intensive intervention strategies to provide mental health and substance abuse treatment, trauma recovery, housing, support and family preservation services to homeless mothers with mental illnesses and substance use disorders who are caring for their dependent children.
Features	The Critical Time Intervention model (CTI) was developed in New York City as a program to increase housing stability for persons with severe mental illnesses and long-term histories of homelessness. Its principal components are rapid placement in transitional housing, fidelity to a CTI model for families (i.e., provision of an intensive, 9-month case management intervention, with mental health and substance use treatments), a focused team approach to service delivery, with the aim of reducing homelessness, and brokering and monitoring the appropriate support arrangements to ensure continuity of care.
Outcomes	Data indicate that mothers in this group tend to be poorly educated; have meager work histories; and face multiple medical, mental health, and substance use problems. Their children's lives have lacked stability in terms of housing, education, and periods of separation from their mothers. African American and Latina women were over-represented in study sites in proportions greater than the national average for homeless populations.
Biggest challenge	The CTI model for families challenges the assumption that homeless mothers with children who have mental health or substance use disorders require confinement and extended stays in congregate shelter living before they can independently manage their own households. This can be addressed by acquiring buy-in from collaborators and involved agencies, acquiring needed housing resources, evaluating the project with respect to model fidelity, and attaining ongoing involvement of practice innovators to establish thoughtful compromises within local contexts.
How other organizations can adopt	The program is transferable to any community that can align resources needed for housing and conduct relevant training for providers in a CTI model for families.
Sites	Westchester County, NY

Source: *President's New Freedom Commission on Mental Health Report*, 2002, p. 73.

BOX 14-6 Model Program: Veterans Administration Health Information and Communication Technology System

Program	U.S. Department of Veterans Affairs (VA), Veterans Health Administration (VHA): Use of Health Information and Communication Technology.
Goal	Improve the quality, access, equity and efficiency of care by using a fully integrated electronic health record system, personal health information systems, and telemedicine.
Features	VHA is the largest integrated health care system in the U.S., with approximately 1,300 sites providing a full continuum of health care services. VA provided mental health services to more than 750,000 veterans in 2002. All VHA medical facilities (clinics, hospitals, and nursing homes) use a fully integrated electronic medical record that is capable of supporting a paperless health record system. The VA system incorporates clinical problem lists, clinic notes, hospital summaries, laboratory, images and reports from diagnostic tests and radiological procedures, pharmacy, computerized order entry, a bar-code medication administration system, clinical practice guidelines, reminders and alerts, and a specialized package of mental health tools. In addition, VA uses innovative information technology and communication systems to give beneficiaries information on benefits and services, allow web-based enrollment, support a national electronic provider credentialing system, provide veterans and their families access to health information, and support health care provider education. Telemedicine is used to increase access to primary and specialty care for rural and underserved populations. VA provided approximately 350,000 telemedicine visits and consultations last year. Telemedicine mental health consultations and follow-up visits provide access to these services at locations where they would otherwise be unavailable.
Outcomes	In 2002, the Institute of Medicine reported, "VA's integrated health care information system, including its framework of performance measures, is considered to be one of the best in the nation." Utilizing an electronic health record with a clinical reminder system, VA screens 89% of primary care patients for depression and 81% for substance abuse. In VA, 80% of patients hospitalized for mental illnesses receive follow-up outpatient appointments within 30 days; the next best reported performance by National Committee for Quality Assurance is 73%, and the Medicaid average is only 55%.
Biggest challenge	The public's lack of confidence in the privacy and security of the electronic health record and the lack of national standards for data and communications represent the biggest challenges to implementing such a system.
How other organizations can adopt	High-performance, reliable electronic health record and information systems are currently available for use by any provider, clinic, hospital, or health system. Incentives for adopting electronic health records would speed wider use.
Sites	All VHA clinics, hospitals, and nursing home facilities nationwide.

Source: *President's New Freedom Commission on Mental Health Report*, 2002, p. 82.

GENETICS AND COMMUNITY MENTAL HEALTH

We know that some mental health disorders tend to run in families, indicating genetic links, but if other factors did not play a role, then 100% of all monozygotic twins would have the same mental health disorders. This is not the case. For example, Carey (2003) noted that the risk for schizophrenia for the general population is 1%, and it is 48% for monozygotic (genetically identical) twins. If genes were the only factor, then we would expect a 100% risk for monozygotic twins. Therefore, environmental factors play a role, and this is where community health and genetics are integrated.

Genetic variation interacts with environmental factors and sociocultural influences, such as infections, stress, and exposure to toxins, which modify the risk of various disorders and behavioral problems. New genetic information and technologies are being integrated into community health, and it may provide additional insight and understanding into the linkages between genes and mental health, including antisocial behavior, alcohol and other substance abuse, and violence. This information may assist community mental health professionals with developing and implementing more effective primary and secondary prevention programs.

In the future, community mental health professionals will increasingly use genetic technologies and information in risk assessments and genetic testing, research, policy, and program development. This same process is expected to occur in all subspecialties in health care. This may lead to a better understanding of the interaction between the environment and expression of genetically linked mental health disorders as well as identify more effective prevention measures and methods of treatment.

TECHNOLOGY AND COMMUNITY MENTAL HEALTH

The use of technology is expanding rapidly. It is increasingly being used for education, research, the delivery of healthcare services, and behavior modification. For example, the Internet is being used to educate people about mental health problems. Telemedicine, as discussed in Chapter 5, is used to provide mental health services, particularly to remote and medically underserved regions. Text messaging can be used to remind patients to take their medications or not to miss their appointments.

Another technology that is playing an increasing role in mental health is 3D virtual platforms. Second Life, the largest virtual platform, is being used by organizations, schools, colleges, hospitals, governments, and nonprofits because it provides a powerful platform for training and education, research, meetings, conferences, and collaborative work. It also has become a positive force in the lives of people with certain disabilities. In particular, a person who has difficulty dealing in social situations (such as an individual with autism or Asperger's syndrome) or who has a physical disfigurement finds himself or herself suddenly in a world where the person is on the same playing field as everyone else. Second Life becomes, literally, a second chance.

Users of Second Life, called residents, create their own virtual selves, called avatars, and interact within a simulated 3D environment. Users can search for places to visit, people to meet, and groups to join, and they can even create buildings, change their appearance, and walk, fly, swim, and teleport from one location to another. Avatars can communicate just like in real life. They can change their voice volume and facial expressions, for example. Avatars can publicly or privately communicate with each other either through voice or text tools, such as instant messaging. There are museums, libraries, bars, and even a deaf café to visit.

An example of how Second Life is being used in the mental health field is Virtual Hallucinations. The Virtual Hallucinations site, created by the University of California, Davis, aims to educate people about the perceptual abnormalities experienced by schizophrenics by simulating common auditory and visual hallucination experiences. In the Virtual Hallucinations pilot project, the researcher found that users reported a greater understanding of hallucinations and schizophrenia as a result of the simulation (see **Box 14-7**).

BOX 14-7 Virtual Hallucinations

Schizophrenia is a severe mental illness causing experiences of auditory hallucinations ("hearing voices") and visual hallucinations. Schizophrenic patients often feel alienated, isolated, and unable to express the severity and depth of their experiences, feelings, and symptoms (Yellowlees & Cook, 2006). In an attempt to facilitate greater understanding and sympathy in caregivers, the Internet-accessible, three-dimensional simulation of the hallucinations of psychosis was created using Second Life (SL) (Yellowlees & Cook, 2006).

The researchers created an inpatient hospital ward in SL and constructed simulations such as a poster in which the text would change to obscenities; multiple voices could be heard, which would sometimes overlap, criticizing the user; and a person's reflection in a mirror would appear to die, becoming gaunt, with bleeding eyes.

Method

This pilot project used SL to facilitate a virtual environment that simulates patient accounts of schizophrenic auditory and visual hallucinations.

- Eight hundred and sixty-three SL users took a self-guided tour that activated psychosis symptoms when the user "moved" through the hospital ward.
- At the end of the tour, users were asked to complete a survey about the experience. Survey responses were considered valid if seven of the nine questions were answered (Yellowlees & Cook, 2006).

- A 5-point Likert scale was used to evaluate subjective questions.
- A small incentive was offered to SL users who completed the survey after the tour (Yellowlees & Cook, 2006).

Results

The virtual psychosis environment on SL was toured 836 times over a two-month period. It is reported by Yellowlees and Cook that 579 (69%) of valid surveys were completed at the end of the self-guided tour.

- Of the survey responders, 440 (76%) thought the environment improved their understanding of auditory hallucinations;
- 69% (N = 400) of survey responders felt the SL simulated visual hallucinations facilitated a better understanding of these symptoms;
- 82% (N = 476) of survey responders agreed that they would recommend the SL environment to a friend;
- The majority of responders were male (N = 366, 63%); and
- The common age ranges were 25 to 35 (N = 186, 32%) and 18 to 25 (N = 182, 31%)

The Yellowlees and Cook pilot project demonstrated that using SL is an accessible and effective way to create simulations of hallucinations for educational purposes. The pilot also was successful in integrating evaluation tools into a virtual reality environment. Self-referred users of the program who completed the survey reported that the SL hallucination simulation improved their understanding of the experience of hallucinations (Yellowlees & Cook, 2006).

Source: Yellowlees, P. M., & Cook, J. N. (2006). Using technology to teach clinical care. Education about hallucinations using an Internet virtual reality system: A qualitative survey. *Academic Psychiatry*, *30*(6), 534–538. Retrieved from http://ap.psychiatryonline.org. Accessed August 16, 2010.

Geographic information system (GIS) is a mapping system that is increasingly being used in community health, including mental health. GIS captures, analyzes, manages, and presents data. The manner is which the data is presented allows people to visualize the information and enables the viewer to easily identify relationships, patterns, and trends in the form of maps, globes, reports, and charts (see **Figure 14-1**).

An example of how GIS is being used in community mental health includes using maps to identify where sex offenders reside. As a result of Megan's law (a law in California that mandates that the public with Internet access has detailed information on registered sex offenders), a Web site has been created that allows people to view GIS maps that illustrate where sex offenders reside. Users can enter a zip code, city, and/or county. Specific home addresses are displayed of offenders in the communities. Other examples of how GIS is being used include the illustration of demographic data and crime maps, including prostitution arrests.

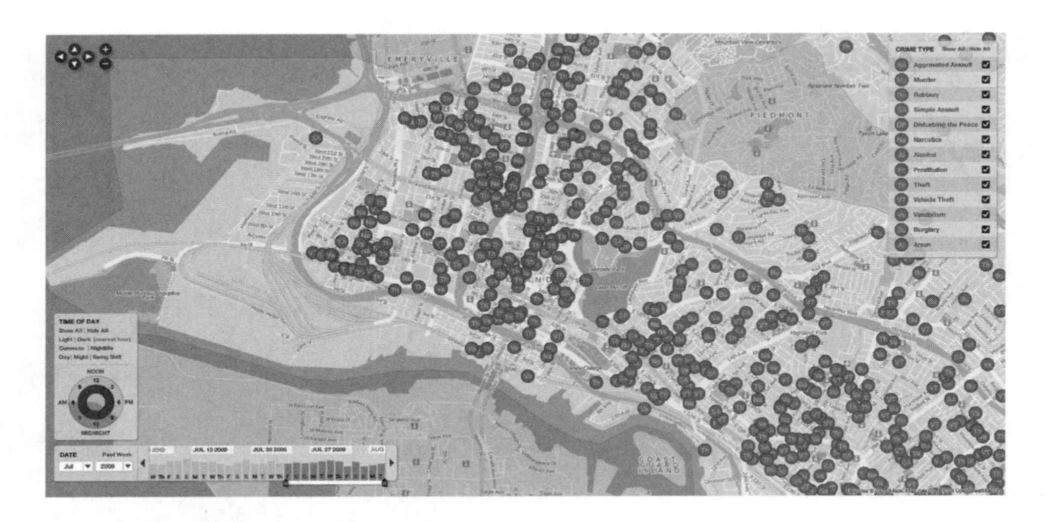

FIGURE 14-1 GIS Mapping System

CHAPTER SUMMARY

This chapter identified eight goals for our nation to improve the mental health of all who live here. Also explained were the six goals for reforming the mental health care system. These two sets of goals overlap, and both federal documents support the need for changes to improve the mental health of people living in the United States. Genetics and technology also are expected to continue to influence the field of community mental health.

Although this is the final chapter of this book, it is not an end point but a point of departure. The journey ahead must firmly establish mental health as a cornerstone of health; place mental illness treatment in the mainstream of healthcare services; and ensure consumers of mental health services access to respectful, evidence-based, and reimbursable care.

REVIEW

1. List the three obstacles to preventing mentally ill people from receiving excellent care outlined in the *President's New Freedom Commission on Mental Health Report*.
2. List and explain the eight goals to improve mental health outlined in the surgeon general's report.

3. List and explain the six goals laid out in the *President's New Freedom Commission on Mental Health Report* for improving the mental health care system.
4. Identify the recommendations for achieving these goals.
5. Explain how genetics and technology are being used in community mental health.

ACTIVITIES

1. Select one of the goals outlined in the two reports in this chapter. How do you envision fitting into that goal? What organization(s) would you like to work with, what role would you like to have, and what activities would you like to be involved with? Are there evidence-based practices that you would use? If so, which one(s) and why?
2. Visit a site in Second Life that is related to mental health. Describe how it is being used and ways that it can be used to prevent mental health problems, treat mental illness, and/or reduce stigmas.

REFERENCES AND FURTHER READINGS

Carey, G. (2003). *Human genetics for the social sciences*. Thousand Oaks, CA: Sage.

President's New Freedom Commission on Mental Health Report. (2002). Rockville: MD. Retrieved from http://www.mentalhealthcommission.gov/reports/reports.htm

U.S. Department of Health and Human Services. (1999). *Mental Health: A Report of the Surgeon General—Executive Summary*. Rockville, MD: U.S. Department of Health and Human Services, Substance Abuse and Mental Health Services Administration, Center for Mental Health Services, National Institutes of Health, National Institute of Mental Health.

GLOSSARY OF KEY TERMS

CHAPTER 1

Assertive community training (ACT) A way of delivering comprehensive and effective services to people with severe mental illness that includes support services.

Asylum An institution for the care of the mentally ill.

Community A group of people who share common characteristics.

Community mental health The development and delivery of programs for a defined group of people to promote, protect, and treat mental health and mental health problems.

Culture The set of learned behaviors, beliefs, attitudes, values, and ideals that are characteristic of a particular society or population.

Diagnostic and Statistical Manual of Mental Disorders (DSM) The standard manual used for diagnosis of mental disorders in the United States.

Disability-adjusted life year (DALY) A measure that expresses years of life lost to premature death and years lived with a disability of specified severity and duration.

Electroconvulsive therapy Electroshock treatment in which seizures are electrically induced in anesthetized patients for therapeutic effect; usually used to treat severe major depression that has not responded to other treatment.

Lobotomy A surgical technique that involves making an incision in the brain's frontal lobe, severing several nerve tracts.

Mental disorders Health conditions characterized by alterations in thinking, mood, or behavior (or some combination thereof) associated with distress and/or impaired functioning.

Mental health The successful performance of mental function, resulting in productive activities, fulfilling relationships with other people, and the ability to adapt to change and to cope with adversity; from early childhood until late life, mental health is the springboard of thinking and communication skills, learning, emotional growth, resilience, and self-esteem (U.S. Department of Health and Human Services, 1999).

Mental health problems The signs and symptoms are of insufficient intensity or duration to meet the criteria for any mental disorder.

Mental illness Refers collectively to all mental disorders, which are health conditions that are characterized by alterations in thinking, mood, or behavior (or some combination thereof) associated with distress and/or impaired functioning (U.S. Department of Health and Human Services, 1999).

Psychopathology The study of the origin, development, and manifestations of mental or behavioral disorders.

Public health The prevention of disease and the promotion of health by government agencies that is concerned with the health of the community as a whole.

Seasonal affective disorder Also known as winter depression or winter blues, it is a mood disorder in which people who have normal mental health throughout most of the year experience depressive symptoms during certain times of the year, usually in the winter.

Somatic A medical term that derives from the Greek word *soma* for the body; somatic conditions are those in which alterations in non-mental functions predominate.

CHAPTER 2

Behavior therapy Psychotherapy that seeks to extinguish or inhibit abnormal or maladaptive behavior by reinforcing desired behavior and extinguishing undesired behavior.

Biopsychosocial model of disease A model that posits that biological, psychological, or social factors all play a role in health and illness.

Cognitive therapy Psychological therapy in which cognition (thinking) is seen as the most significant factor in psychological problems and their treatment.

Crisis hotline A phone number people can call to get immediate over-the-phone emergency counseling, which is usually provided by trained volunteers.

Curanderismo A traditional folk healer or shaman in the Hispanic culture.

Delusion A false belief or opinion.

Disease Conditions with known pathology (detectable physical change).

Disorder Clusters of symptoms and signs associated with distress and disability (i.e., impairment of functioning), yet the pathology and etiology are unknown.

Naturopathy A drugless system of therapy based on the use of physical forces such as heat, water, light, air, and massage.

Pediatric autoimmune neuropsychiatric disorders (PANDAS) A psychiatric disorder that entails a sudden onset of symptoms like those of obsessive-compulsive disorder following infection with streptococcus bacteria, caused by an autoimmune reaction that affects the basal ganglia in the brain.

Psychosis A symptom or feature of mental illness typically characterized by radical changes in personality, impaired functioning, and a distorted or nonexistent sense of objective reality.

Tourette syndrome A neurologic condition that causes the affected person to make sounds or words (vocal tics) and body movements (motor tics) that are beyond his or her control.

CHAPTER 3

Acculturation The process of adapting to another culture by acquiring the majority group's culture.

Cultural competence An ability to interact effectively with people of different cultures.

Culture A system of shared meanings.

Culture-bound syndromes The particular symptoms, course, and social response influenced by local cultural factors that frame coherent meanings for certain repetitive, patterned, and troubling sets of experiences and observations.

Dominant culture The predominant way of organizing the society, including values, norms, institutions, and symbols.

Ethnicity Relating to large groups of people classed according to common racial, national, tribal, religious, linguistic, or cultural origin or background.

Ethnocentricity When a person believes that his or her culture is superior to another one or when a person views the world only through the perspective of his or her own cultural values.

Ethnopsychiatry (also known as cultural psychiatry) The examination of how the social, cultural, and biological contexts interact to shape illnesses and reactions to them.

Ethnopsychopharmacology Investigates cultural variations and differences that influence the effectiveness of pharmacotherapies used in the mental health field.

Ghost sickness A culture-bound syndrome that some Native American tribes believe to be caused by association with the dead or dying and is sometimes associated with witchcraft.

Idioms of distress Cultural idioms through which emotional distress is experienced and communicated.

***Mal de ojo* (evil eye)** In the Hispanic culture it is an illness thought to be caused by jealousy. Translated into Spanish it means "bad eye."

Minority Used to signify a group's limited political power and social resources, as well as their unequal access to opportunities, social rewards, and social status.

Naturalistic system Illness is explained in terms of a disturbed equilibrium of the physical body.

Personalistic system Illness is seen as being caused by the intentional intervention of an agent who may be a supernatural being (a deity or ancestral spirits) or a human being with special powers (a witch or sorcerer).

Race The concept of dividing people into populations or groups on the basis of visible traits and beliefs about common ancestry.

Somatization The expression of mental distress in terms of physical suffering.

Susto In the Hispanic culture, an illness caused by fright.

CHAPTER 4

Accountability Being answerable legally, morally, ethically, or socially to someone for something one has done.

Advanced directives A written or oral statement by which a competent person makes known treatment preferences and/or designates a surrogate decision maker.

Advocacy The act of an individual or by an advocacy group normally aims to influence public policy and resource allocation decisions within political, economic, and social systems and institutions; it may be motivated from moral, ethical, or faith principles or simply to protect an asset of interest.

Aggregate The sum.

Autonomy Independence or freedom, as of the will or one's actions: the autonomy of the individual.

Belief The psychological state in which an individual holds a proposition or premise to be true.

Beneficence The doing of good; active goodness or kindness; charity.

Block grant Formula funds that are not allocated to a specific category and are more flexibly distributed. The grant seeker applies directly to the state for these funds, and the state sets up procedures for their disbursement.

Caring A form of involving self with others that is directly related to concern about how other individuals experience their world.

Client's rights Services, programs, goods, and health provider behaviors that consumers are entitled to in order to maintain or achieve health or to exist.

Code of Ethics Set of statements encompassing rules that apply to people in professional roles.

Confidentiality An ethical principle associated with several professions (e.g., medicine, law, religion, professional psychology, and journalism). In ethics and health care, the dialogue between patient and healthcare professionals as well as the diagnosis and treatment of a patient is "privileged" and may not be discussed or divulged to third parties. In those jurisdictions in which the law makes provision for such confidentiality, there are usually penalties for its violation.

Duty of disclosure In the United States, it is mandatory to report cases of child abuse, neglect, and elder abuse. Additionally, it is mandatory for healthcare professionals to warn potential victims that a client has made a credible threat to kill themselves or others.

Ethical decision making Using a systematic model to make ethical decisions in difficult clinical, community, and individual situations.

Ethics The science or study of moral values; a code of principles and ideals that guide action.

Grant to consent to carry out for a person: allow fulfillment of grant a request or to permit as a right, privilege, or favor luggage allowances granted to passenger.

Informed consent A client's rights to receive enough information to make a decision about treatment and to communicate the decision to others.

Justice The quality of being just; righteousness, equitableness, or moral rightness; to uphold the justice of a cause.

Mental Health Services Act (aka Prop 63) Expands mental health services to persons who have serious mental illness or who are seriously emotionally disturbed and whose service needs are not being met through other funding sources. MHSA is funded through an additional 1% income tax on Californians.

Nonmaleficence The act of doing no evil or harm.

Right to Health Care Right to goods, resources, and to maintain and improve one's state of health (a positive right).

Rule of Utility Rule derived from the principle of beneficence. Includes the moral duty to weigh and balance benefits and reduce the occurrence of harm.

Ryan White Care Act The legislation called the Ryan White HIV/AIDS Treatment Extension Act of 2009 (Public Law 111-87, October 30, 2009) was first enacted in 1990 as the Ryan White CARE (Comprehensive AIDS Resources Emergency) Act. It has been amended and reauthorized four times—in 1996, 2000, 2006, and 2009. The Ryan White legislation has been adjusted with each reauthorization to accommodate new and emerging needs, such as an increased emphasis on funding of core medical services and changes in funding formulas.

Value Ideas of life, customs, and ways of behaving that members of a society or a culture regard as desirable.

Veracity A duty to tell the truth and not lie or deceive others.

CHAPTER 5

Catchment area Providing comprehensive mental health services in a specific area. A catchment area consists of 75,000 to 200,000 people.

Child protective services The Adoption Assistance and Child Welfare Act of 1980 (P.L. 96-272) that focuses on state economic incentives to substantially decrease the length and number of foster care placements.

De facto mental health system Mental disorders and mental health problems are treated by a variety of caregivers who work in diverse, relatively independent, and coordinated facilities and services both public and private.

Housing plan A delineated set of strategies to address the housing needs of persons with mental illness.

Individualized Treatment Plan A person-centered treatment plan that meets the unique needs of an individual.

National Institute of Mental Health (NIMH) Part of the federal government of the United States and the largest research organization in the world specializing in mental illness.

Recovery Orientation All of the 45 reporting SMHAs have adopted a mission statement or policy about the potential of consumers to recover from their illnesses and are seeking to reorient the mental health system to be more recovery oriented. SMHA recovery initiatives include drafting recovery mission statements, changing the array of services funded by the SMHA, working with consumers and families to promote recovery concepts, and moving toward evidence-based practices.

Specialty mental health The sector that consists of mental health professionals such as psychiatrists, psychologists, psychiatric nurses, community mental health outreach workers, and psychiatric social workers who are trained specifically to treat people with mental disorders.

CHAPTER 6

Anxiety disorders Includes several different forms of abnormal, pathologic anxieties, fears, and phobias.

Attachment theory A theory that posits that the human infant has a need for a secure relationship with adult caregivers that fosters social, emotional, and cognitive skills.

Attention deficit hyperactivity disorder (ADHD) A mental health disorder characterized by two distinct sets of symptoms: inattention and hyperactivity-impulsivity.

Autism A developmental disorder characterized by impaired social interaction; problems with verbal and nonverbal communication; and unusual, repetitive, or severely limited activities and interests.

Bipolar disorder A mood disorder in which episodes of mania alternate with episodes of depression.

Disruptive disorders A group of mental disorders of children and adolescents consisting of behavior that violates social norms and is disruptive.

Dysthymic disorder A mood disorder that is considered chronic depression.

Eating disorder An often long-term illness that involves extreme emotions, attitudes, and behaviors involving weight and food.

Pervasive developmental disorder A group of developmental conditions that affect children and involve delays or impairments in communication and social skills (e.g., autism).

Posttraumatic stress disorder (PTSD) An anxiety disorder associated with serious traumatic events.

Reactive attachment disorder (RAD) An attachment disorder in which individuals have difficulty forming lasting relationships.

Temperament The inherent, relatively consistent traits or dispositions that underlie behavior and determine how people react to the world around them.

Tourette syndrome A neurologic condition that causes the affected person to make sounds or words (vocal tics) and body movements (motor tics) that are beyond his or her control.

CHAPTER 7

Agoraphobia Severe and pervasive anxiety about being in situations from which escape might be difficult or avoidance of situations such as being alone outside of the home; traveling in a car, bus, or airplane; or being in a crowded area.

Anhedonia The inability to experience pleasure.

Cyclothymia Alternating manic and depressive states that, although protracted, do not meet criteria for bipolar disorder.

Delirious mania A relatively rare and serious psychiatric disorder that is characterized by the sudden onset of complete disorientation to time and place.

Dysphoria A negative or aversive mood state.

Dysthymia A chronic form of depression.

Generalized anxiety disorder Defined by a protracted period (6 months or longer) of anxiety and worry, accompanied by multiple associated symptoms.

Jaques's theory Elliott Jaques emphasized the importance of the midlife crisis in individual development and coined the term "midlife crisis."

Midlife crisis The phrase used to describe a period of self-doubt felt by some individuals during the midpoint of their lives.

Neuroticism An enduring tendency to experience negative emotional states.

Schizophrenia A psychiatric disorder in which two or more of the following symptoms occur for a significant time during a 1-month period: delusions, hallucinations, disorganized speech, grossly disorganized or catatonic behavior, or negative symptoms.

Social phobia (also known as social anxiety disorder) Describes people with marked and persistent anxiety in social situations, including performances and public speaking.

Sociopath A person with antisocial personality disorder who does not usually care about other people, has a complete disregard for rules, and lies constantly.

Trichotillomania Compulsive hair pulling.

Type A personality Temperament characterized by excessive ambitiousness, competitiveness, aggressiveness, impatience, and the need for control.

CHAPTER 8

Alzheimer's disease One of the most feared mental disorders because of its gradual, yet relentless, attack on memory. Symptoms extend to other cognitive deficits in language, object recognition, and executive functioning.

Crystallized intelligence Accumulated information and vocabulary acquired from school and everyday life. Also encompasses the application of skills and knowledge to solving problems.

Delirium An acute change in mental functioning and/or acute confusion.

Dementia An acquired loss of intellectual functioning that occurs over a long period of time.

Fluid intelligence The ability to think and reason. Includes the speed with which information can be analyzed and attention and memory capacity.

Normal aging Changes attributed to aging itself and the common complex of diseases and impairments that occur in many elderly people.

Polypharmacy The use of multiple medications by a patient.

CHAPTER 9

Chronically homeless An unaccompanied homeless individual with a disabling condition (e.g., substance abuse, serious mental illness, developmental disability, or chronic physical illness) who has been continuously homeless either for a year or more or has had at least four episodes of homelessness in the past 3 years.

Discrimination The beliefs, attitudes, and practices that defame individuals or groups because of the color of their skin, gender, age, ethnic, religious group affiliation, or other characteristic.

Poverty The state of having little or no money and few or no material possessions.

Racism The belief that race accounts for differences in human character or ability and that a particular race is superior to others.

CHAPTER 10

Abstinence The act or practice of refraining from indulging an appetite or desire, especially for alcoholic drink or sexual intercourse.

Addiction A chronic, often relapsing brain disease that causes compulsive drug-seeking behavior and use despite harmful consequences to the individual who is addicted to drugs and to those in his or her presence.

Alcohol abuse Excessive use of alcohol and alcoholic drinks.

Alcohol dependence Also known as "alcoholism," a psychiatric diagnosis in which an individual uses alcohol despite significant areas of dysfunction, evidence of physical dependence, and/or related hardship.

Anabolic Refers to the synthetic phase of metabolism; some athletes take anabolic steroids to increase muscle size temporarily.

Androgenic Refers to increased male sexual characteristics.

Blood alcohol concentration The concentration of alcohol in the blood, expressed as the weight of alcohol in a fixed volume of blood and used as a measure of the degree of intoxication in an individual. The concentration depends on body weight, the quantity and rate of alcohol ingestion, and the rates of alcohol absorption and metabolism. Also called *blood alcohol level*.

Detoxification The process of cleaning toxins from the body and withdrawing from the drugs safely.

Drug addiction Drug addiction is considered a brain disease because overuse of drugs leads to structural and functional changes of the brain. For most people the initial decision to take drugs is voluntary; over time, however, changes in the brain caused by repeated drug abuse can affect a person's self-control and ability to make sound decisions. Additionally the brain will send intense impulses to the individual to take drugs.

Drug dependence Drug dependence occurs when there is a psychological change in the central nervous system caused by frequent abuse of drugs that prevents withdrawal symptoms.

Glutamate A neurotransmitter that influences the reward circuit and the ability to learn.

Inhalant Diverse group of volatile substances whose chemical vapors can be inhaled to produce psychoactive (mind-altering) effects.

Late-onset alcoholism Addiction to alcohol that begins after age 60.

Steroids A class of drugs that can be legally prescribed to treat conditions resulting from steroid hormone deficiency, such as delayed puberty, but also body wasting in patients with AIDS and other diseases that result in loss of lean muscle mass.

Substance abuse The use of any substance that impairs a person's social or economic well-being and jeopardizes a person's health.

Tolerance The need for an abuser of drugs to require larger amounts of the drug to achieve a dopamine high.

Withdrawal Symptoms of withdrawal include irritability, craving, cognitive and attention defects, and sleep disturbances.

CHAPTER 11

Affective violence The verbal expression of intense anger and emotions such as bullying, taunts, disrespect, alienation, and physical threats.

Assault A crime of violence against another person. An assault is often defined to include not only violence but any physical contact with another person without their consent.

Child abuse Cruelty to children (younger than age 18).

Child neglect Failure to provide the basic needs of a child.

Emotional abuse or psychological abuse Form of abuse characterized by a person subjecting or exposing another to behavior that is psychologically harmful.

Homicide The killing of one human being by the act or omission of another.

Incest Sexual abuse committed by a family member.

Munchausen syndrome by proxy (MSBP) A mental health problem in which a caregiver makes up or causes an illness or injury in a child under his or her care. The caregiver is usually a mother, and the victim is her child. Because children are the victims, MSBP is a form of child abuse.

Neglect A passive form of abuse in which the perpetrator is responsible to provide care for a victim who is unable to care for oneself but fails to provide adequate care to meet the victim's needs, thereby resulting in the victim's demise.

Physical abuse Abuse involving contact intended to cause pain, injury, or other physical suffering or harm.

Rape The unlawful compelling of someone through physical force or duress to have sexual intercourse.

Suicide bomber A suicide attack (also known as suicide bombing, homicide bombing, or *kamikaze*) that is an attack intended to kill others and inflict widespread damage, in which the attacker expects or intends to die in the process.

CHAPTER 12

Infanticide The practice of intentionally killing an infant.

CHAPTER 13

Community participatory research Research that is conducted as an equal partnership between traditionally trained "experts" and members of a community or patients of a particular health issue like mental health.

Cross-tabbing The process of creating a contingency table from the multivariate frequency distribution of statistical variables. Cross-tabbing is common in survey research.

Delhi process A process that allows all stakeholders or members of a community group to communicate to generate ideas and establish consensus for dealing with complex problems and assigning value judgments.

Focus group A form of qualitative research in which a group of people or sample of selected people are asked about their perceptions, beliefs, knowledge, and attitudes toward a service, concept, or health issue.

Morbidity The presence of illness or disease.

Mortality Death from an illness or disease.

Neurophysiological deficits Altered perceptions and behavior, including derealization; depersonalization; distortions of perception of time, space, and body.

Primary data Newly collected data.

Primary prevention Prevention of a disease or mental illness before symptoms arise.

Protective factors Factors that improve an individual's response to some environmental hazards, resulting in an adaptive outcome.

Quality of life The WHO (WHOQOL Group, 1995) defines quality of life as "an individual's perception of his/her position in life in the context of the culture and value systems in which he/she lives, and in relation to his/her goals, expectations, standards and concerns." Quality of life is also a broad view of well-being including social indicators, happiness, and health status.

Random sample Randomly selecting a group of people to participate in a research study, for example selecting every fourth person to participate in a study; a random sample is a smaller group of the population who are asked to participate in a study.

Risk factor Characteristics, variables, or vulnerabilities present that make it more likely that an individual experiencing these characteristics rather than someone selected at random will develop a disorder.

Risk reduction The decrease in risk of a given activity or unhealthy behavior.

Secondary data Data that already exists.

Secondary prevention Prevention interventions carried out primarily to help individuals who have displayed signs of mental illness, such as bullying or illicit drug use. Secondary prevention strategies can reduce the severity of the disorder and possibly eliminate behaviors and problems that already exist.

Tertiary prevention The reduction and management of disability caused by a disease or mental illness to achieve the highest level of function. Examples include outreach programs that monitor persons with mental disorders who live in the community to ensure that they adhere to their prescribed medication regimens and in inpatient psychiatric hospitals.

CHAPTER 14

Best practices Treatments and services that are promising but have limited evidence of effectiveness.

Evidence-based practices Treatments and services that have well-documented effectiveness.

PHOTO CREDITS

Unit Opener I © Ghislain & Marie Davi/age fotostock

Chapter 1
Opener, page 9, page 10 © National Library of Medicine

Chapter 2
Opener © Andy Z./ShutterStock, Inc.

Chapter 3
Opener © Serdar Tibet/Dreamstime.com; **page 72** Courtesy of the U.S. Census Bureau

Unit Opener II © Henryk Sadura/ShutterStock, Inc.

Chapter 4
Opener © Creativ Studio Heinem/age fotostock; **4-2** © Comstock Images/Alamy Images; **inset** © jean schweitzer/ShutterStock, Inc.; **4-3 (left)** © PhotoCreate/ShutterStock, Inc.; **(right)** © Franz Pfluegl/Dreamstime.com

Chapter 5
Opener Courtesy of James Gathany/CDC

Unit Opener III © Big Cheese Photo/Jupiterimages

Chapter 6
Opener © corepics/ShutterStock, Inc.

Chapter 7
Opener © Edward Bock/Dreamstime.com

Chapter 8
Opener © Ariel Skelley/age fotostock

Unit Opener IV © Andrew Kazmierski/Dreamstime.com

Chapter 9

Opener © Xavier Marchant/Dreamstime.com; **9-2 (airplane)** © Kamil Macniak/Dreamstime.com; **(guitar and amp)** © Cgidesigner/Dreamstime.com; **(lawn mower)** © R. Gino Santa Maria/ShutterStock, Inc.; **(blender)** © ZTS/ShutterStock, Inc.; **(city)** © Zina Seletskaya/ShutterStock, Inc.; **(people talking)** © Barbara Oleksa/Dreamstime.com; **(car)** © Mike C.t. Tan/ Dreamstime.com; **(living room)** © Phaedra Wilkinson/Dreamstime.com; **(moon)** © Cammeraydave/Dreamstime.com; **(people whispering)** © David Davis/ShutterStock, Inc.; **(tree)** © Pavelk/ShutterStock, Inc.

Chapter 10

Opener © Ray Grover/Alamy Images

Chapter 11

Opener © Digital Vision/age fotostock

Chapter 12

Opener © Design Pics/age fotostock

Chapter 13

Opener © Andres Rodriguez/Dreamstime.com

Unit Opener V © Basov Mikhail/ShutterStock, Inc.

Chapter 14

Opener © Luis Francisco Cordero/ShutterStock, Inc.; **14-1** Courtesy of Stamen Design

INDEX

Note: Page numbers followed by *f* indicate figures; numbers followed by *t* indicate tables.

V

W

Y

Z